# USERS' GUIDES TO THE MEDICAL LITERATURE

## A Manual for Evidence-Based Clinical Practice

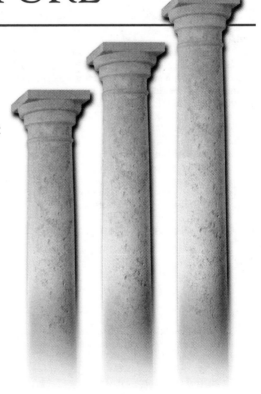

The Evidence-Based Medicine Working Group

*Edited by*
Gordon Guyatt, MD
Drummond Rennie, MD

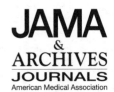

JAMA
&
ARCHIVES
JOURNALS
American Medical Association

## AMA Press

**Vice President, Business Products:** Anthony J. Frankos
**Editorial Director:** Mary Lou White
**Director, Production and Manufacturing:** Jean Roberts
**Senior Acquisitions Editor:** Barry Bowlus
**Developmental Editor:** Susan Moss
**Director, Marketing:** JD Kinney
**Marketing Manager:** Amy Roberts
**Senior Production Coordinator:** Rosalyn Carlton
**Senior Print Coordinator:** Ronnie Summers
**Project Manager:** Katharine Dvorak

**McMaster University and University of Alberta Staff:**
Christina Lacchetti and Tanya Voth

*JAMA* **Book Liaison:** Annette Flanagin

Additional copies of this book may be ordered by calling 800 621-8335 or visiting the Web site at www.ama-assn.org.
Mention product number OP427700.

ISBN 1-57947-174-9
BP92:0129-00:07/01

*To my professional mentors, David Sackett, Jack Hirsh, and William Goldberg; my personal mentors, Sam Auron and Maureen Meade; and my friends and colleagues, Roman Jaeschke, Deborah Cook, and Alba DiCenso.*

**GG**

*To Deb, who has watched over and tended me while I have watched over and tended this wonderful group of authors, with gratitude for her love and her good humor.*

**DR**

# CONTENTS

## Part 1
## The Basics: Using the Medical Literature

## Part 2
## Beyond the Basics: Using and Teaching the Principles of Evidence-Based Medicine

# FOREWORD

When I was attending school in wartime Britain, staples of the curriculum, along with cold baths, mathematics, boiled cabbage, and long cross-country runs, were Latin and French. It was obvious that Latin was a theoretical exercise—the Romans were dead, after all. However, while France was clearly visible just across the Channel, for years it was either occupied or inaccessible, so learning the French language seemed just as impractical and theoretical an exercise. It was unthinkable to me and my teachers that I would ever put it to practical use—that French was a language to be spoken.

This is the relationship too many practitioners have with the medical literature—clearly visible but utterly inaccessible. We recognize that practice should be based on discoveries announced in the medical journals. But we also recognize that every few years the literature doubles in size, and every year we seem to have less time to weigh it,[1] so every day the task of taming the literature becomes more hopeless. The translation of those hundreds of thousands of articles into everyday practice appears to be an obscure task left to others. And as the literature becomes more inaccessible, so does the idea that the literature has any utility for a particular patient become more fanciful.

This book is designed to change all that. It's designed to make the clinician fluent in the language of the medical literature in all its forms. To free the clinician from practicing medicine by rote, by guesswork, and by their variably integrated experience. To put a stop to clinicians being ambushed by drug company representatives, or by their patients, telling them of new therapies the clinicians are unable to evaluate. To end their dependence on out-of-date authority. To enable the practitioner to work with the patient and use the literature as a tool to solve the patient's problems. To provide the clinician access to what is relevant and the ability to assess its validity and whether it applies to a specific patient. In other words, to put the clinician in charge of the single most powerful resource in medicine.

## The Users' Guides Series in *JAMA*

I have left it to Gordon Guyatt, the moving force, principal editor, and most prolific co-author of the "Users' Guides to the Medical Literature" series in *JAMA*, to describe the history of this series and of this book in the accompanying Preface. But where did *JAMA* come into this story?

In the late 1980s, at the invitation of my friend David Sackett, I visited his department at McMaster University to discuss another Sackett/*JAMA* venture— a series examining the evidence behind the clinical history and examination. Following these discussions, a series of articles and systematic reviews was developed and, with the enthusiastic support of then *JAMA* editor-in-chief, George Lundberg, *JAMA* began publishing the "Rational Clinical Examination" series in 1992.[1] By that time, I had formed an excellent working relationship with the brilliant group at McMaster. Like Sackett, their leader, they tended to be iconoclastic, expert at working together and forming alliances with new and talented workers, and intellectually exacting. Like their leader, they delivered on their promises.

So, when I heard that they were thinking of updating the wonderful series of "Readers' Guides" published in 1981 in the *Canadian Medical Association Journal*, I took advantage of this working relationship to urge that they update and expand the series for *JAMA*. Together with Sackett, and first with Andy Oxman, and then with Gordon Guyatt taking the lead (when Oxman left to take his present position in Oslo), the Users' Guides Series was born. We began publishing articles in the series in *JAMA* in 1993.[2,3]

At the start, we thought we might have eight or 10 articles, but the response from readers was so enthusiastic, and the variety of types of article in the literature so great, that 7 years later I still found myself receiving, sending for review, and editing new articles for the series. In the end, Gordon Guyatt and I closed this series at 25, appearing as 33 separate journal articles.

The passage of 8 years during the preparation of the series had a particularly useful result. Some subjects that in 1992-1993 were scarcely discussed in the major medical journals, but that have burgeoned recently, could receive the attention that had become their due. For instance, in 2000, *JAMA* published two Users' Guides on how readers should approach reports of qualitative research in health care.[4,5] To take another example, systematic reviews and meta-analyses, given a huge boost by the activities of the Cochrane Collaboration, have become prominent features of the literature. An article in the series discusses how to use such studies.[6] Another example would be the guide on electronic health information resources.[7]

## The Book

From the start, readers kept urging us to put the series together as a book. That had been our intention right from the start, but each new article delayed its implementation. How fortunate! When the original "Readers' Guides" appeared in the *CMAJ* in 1981, Gordon Guyatt's phrase "evidence-based medicine" had never been coined, and only a tiny proportion of health care workers possessed computers. The Internet did not exist and electronic publication was only a dream. In 1992, the Web—for practical purposes—had scarcely been invented, the dot.com bubble hadn't appeared, let alone burst, and the health professions were only beginning to become computer-literate. But at the end of the 1990s, when Guyatt and I approached AMA Press with the idea of publishing not merely the standard printed book, but also Web-based and CD-ROM formats of the book, they were immediately receptive. Putting the latter part into practice has been the notable achievement of Dr Rob Hayward, of the University of Alberta.

In addition, the science and art of evidence-based medicine, which this series does so much to reinforce, has developed remarkably during the past 8 years, and this is reflected in every page of the book.

The requirements for individual articles in a journal series are different from those of separate chapters in a book. To make it possible to understand each article by itself, a good deal of redundancy had to be built in, and one of Guyatt's tasks when editing the book was to remove this extra material. In addition, the

Evidence-Based Medicine Working Group has updated the articles in the series so that they all reflect the latest practice.

First, I must thank Gordon Guyatt, who has become a good friend over the years, for making my own task, first as editor of the *JAMA* series and then as co-editor of the book, extraordinarily easy and pleasant, as well as educational. I know personally and greatly admire a good number of his colleagues, but it would be invidious to name them, given the huge collective effort this 9-year effort has entailed. On the *JAMA* side, I must thank Annette Flanagin, a wonderfully efficient, creative, and diplomatic colleague at *JAMA*. The book would not exist without the vision of Tony Frankos and the hard work, enthusiasm, and dedication of Barry Bowlus, both of AMA Press. Susan Moss has been an exemplary book editor, meticulous, thoughtful, and long-suffering. Between her and Gordon, I was left little to do. I also wish to thank Jean Roberts, Katharine Dvorak, and Amy Roberts of AMA Press. Finally, I thank my wonderful new boss, Cathy DeAngelis, Editor-in-Chief of *JAMA*, for her strong backing of me, my colleagues, and this project; for her tolerance; and for keeping up everyone's spirits with her dreadful jokes.

**Drummond Rennie, MD**
*University of California, San Francisco*
*Deputy Editor, JAMA*

## References

1. Durack DT. The weight of medical knowledge. *N Engl J Med*. 1978;298:773-775.

2. Sackett DL, Rennie D. The science of the art of the clinical examination. *JAMA*. 1992;267:2650-2652.

3. Guyatt GH, Rennie D. Users' guides to the medical literature. *JAMA*. 1993;270:2096-2097.

4. Giacomini MK, Cook DJ. Users' guides to the medical literature, XXIII: qualitative research in health care. A. Are the results of the study valid? Evidence-Based Medicine Working Group. *JAMA*. 2000;284:357-362.

5. Giacomini MK, Cook DJ. Users' guides to the medical literature, XXIII: qualitative research in health care. B. What are the results and how do they help me care for my patients? Evidence-Based Medicine Working Group. *JAMA*. 2000;284:478-482.

6. Oxman AD, Cook DJ, Guyatt GH. Users' guides to the medical literature, VI: how to use an overview. Evidence-Based Medicine Working Group. *JAMA*. 1994;272:1367-1371.

7. Hunt DL, Jaeschke R, McKibbon KA. Users' guides to the medical literature, XXI: using electronic health information resources in evidence-based practice. Evidence-Based Medicine Working Group. *JAMA*. 2000;283:1875-1879.

## Users' Guides to Medical Literature Series in *JAMA*

I. Oxman AD, Sackett DL, Guyatt GH. How to get started. The Evidence-Based Medicine Working Group. *JAMA*. 1993;270:2093-2095.

II. Guyatt GH, Sackett DL, Cook DJ. How to use an article about therapy or prevention. A. Are the results of the study valid? Evidence-Based Medicine Working Group. *JAMA*. 1993;270:2598-2601.

II. Guyatt GH, Sackett DL, Cook DJ. How to use an article about therapy or prevention. B. What are the results and will they help me in caring for my patients? Evidence-Based Medicine Working Group. *JAMA*. 1994;271:59-63.

III. Jaeschke R, Guyatt G, Sackett DL. How to use an article about a diagnostic test. A. Are the results of the study valid? Evidence-Based Medicine Working Group. *JAMA*. 1994;271:389-391.

III. Jaeschke R, Guyatt GH, Sackett DL. How to use an article about a diagnostic test. B. What are the results and will they help me in caring for my patients? Evidence-Based Medicine Working Group. *JAMA*. 1994;271:59-63.

IV. Levine M, Walter S, Lee H, Haines T, Holbrook A, Moyer V. How to use an article about harm. Evidence-Based Medicine Working Group. *JAMA*. 1994;271:1615-1619.

V. Laupacis A, Wells G, Richardson WS, Tugwell P. How to use an article about prognosis. Evidence-Based Medicine Working Group. *JAMA*. 1994;272:234-237.

VI. Oxman AD, Cook DJ, Guyatt GH. How to use an overview. Evidence-Based Medicine Working Group. *JAMA*. 1994;272:1367-1371.

VII. Richardson WS, Detsky AS. How to use a clinical decision analysis. A. Are the results of the study valid? Evidence-Based Medicine Working Group. *JAMA*. 1995;273:1292-1295.

VII. Richardson WS, Detsky AS. How to use a clinical decision analysis. B. What are the results and will they help me in caring for my patients? Evidence Based Medicine Working Group. *JAMA*. 1995;273:1610-1613.

VIII. Hayward RS, Wilson MC, Tunis SR, Bass EB, Guyatt G. How to use clinical practice guidelines. A. Are the recommendations valid? The Evidence-Based Medicine Working Group. *JAMA*. 1995;274:570-574.

VIII. Wilson MC, Hayward RS, Tunis SR, Bass EB, Guyatt G. How to use clinical practice guidelines. B. What are the recommendations and will they help you in caring for your patients? The Evidence-Based Medicine Working Group. *JAMA*. 1995;274:1630-1632.

IX. Guyatt GH, Sackett DL, Sinclair JC, Hayward R, Cook DJ, Cook RJ. A method for grading health care recommendations. Evidence-Based Medicine Working Group. *JAMA*. 1995;274:1800-1804.

X. Naylor GH, Guyatt GH. How to use an article reporting variations in the outcomes of health services. The Evidence-Based Medicine Working Group. *JAMA*. 1996;275:554-558.

# PREFACE

This book grew out of a series of 25 articles published in *JAMA* between 1993 and 2000, the original Users' Guides to the Medical Literature. Clinicians and medical educators have found this series, which includes contributions by approximately 50 clinicians expert in evidence-based medicine, to be invaluable.

*Users' Guides to the Medical Literature: A Manual for Evidence-Based Clinical Practice* goes beyond the Users' Guides in a number of ways. First, it incorporates the advances in clinical research that have taken place during the past 7 years relevant to understanding sources of bias in research studies, quantifying the magnitude of benefits and risks, and incorporating patient values. Second, it incorporates what we have learned about how to better teach evidence-based medicine (EBM) concepts and approaches to clinicians. Third, it clearly distinguishes what we believe every clinician should know about EBM (Part 1 of this book) from what those who wish to role-model and teach EBM should know (Part 2). Fourth, we have eliminated redundancies, linked different sections, and ensured consistency of style and conceptual presentation. Fifth, the focus on clinical decision making, already prominent in the Users' Guides, has been further strengthened through the addition of clinical examples* and through highlighting of the role of patient values in choosing optimal therapy. Sixth, Part 2 provides a much more comprehensive and in-depth exploration of key concepts in understanding and applying clinical research to patient problems.

Finally, this book is available in both paper and electronic formats. Robert Hayward has taken primary responsibility for translation of the material into both CD-ROM and Web-based formats, the latter of which includes a large number of additional aids for the practice of EBM. Rob has done a magnificent job as coeditor of the electronic versions, and his contribution, representing an enormous expenditure of both time and energy, has been vital.

## How It All Began

During the late 1970s, a group of clinical epidemiologists at McMaster University, led by David Sackett and including Brian Haynes, Peter Tugwell, and Victor Neufeld, were planning a series of articles advising clinicians on how to read clinical journals. The series appeared in the *Canadian Medical Association Journal* beginning in 1981. The group proposed the term *critical appraisal* to describe the application of the basic rules of evidence presented in that series. After teaching critical appraisal for a number of years, members of the group became increasingly aware of both the necessity and the challenges of motivating clinicians to go beyond merely browsing the literature and, rather, to actually use the information in solving patient problems. David Sackett suggested the term *bringing critical appraisal to the bedside* to describe the process of the practical application of

---

* Most clinical scenarios and their resolutions were finalized at the end of August 2000; they do not include evidence that has appeared since that time.

evidence from the medical literature to patient care.

In 1990, I assumed the position of Residency Director of the internal medicine program at McMaster. Through Dave Sackett's leadership, the concept of bringing critical appraisal to the bedside had evolved into a philosophy of medical practice based on knowledge and understanding of the medical literature supporting each clinical decision. We believed this represented a fundamentally different style of practice warranting a formal term that would capture this difference.

In the spring of 1990, with the mission to train physicians who would practice this new brand of medicine, I presented our plans for changing the program to the members of the Department of Medicine, many of whom were not sympathetic. The term I suggested to describe the new approach was *scientific medicine*. Those already hostile to the challenge to the traditional sources of medical authority were incensed by the term; specifically, they were disturbed at the implication that they had previously been unscientific. My second try at a name for our philosophy of medical practice, *evidence-based medicine*, proved felicitous.

The term *evidence-based medicine* first appeared in the autumn of 1990 in an informational document intended for residents entering or considering application to our residency program. An excerpt follows:

> Residents are taught to develop an attitude of "enlightened scepticism" toward the application of diagnostic, therapeutic, and prognostic technologies in their day-to-day management of patients. This approach, which has been called "evidence-based medicine," is based on principles outlined in the text "Clinical Epidemiology." The goal is to be aware of the evidence on which one's practice is based, the soundness of the evidence, and the strength of inference the evidence permits. The strategy employed requires a clear delineation of the relevant question(s); a thorough search of the literature relating to the questions; a critical appraisal of the evidence, and its applicability to the clinical situation; and a balanced application of the conclusions to the clinical problem.

The term subsequently appeared in print in the *ACP Journal Club* in 1991.[1] Meanwhile, our group of enthusiastic evidence-based medical educators at McMaster, led by Deborah Cook, Roman Jaeschke, Jim Nishikawa, Pat Brill-Edwards, and Akbar Panju, in addition to the four original innovators, were refining our practice and teaching of EBM. Because the process proved exciting and productive, we concluded that the concept of a new approach to medical practice would prove useful for the larger community of medical educators.

Consequently, we linked up with a larger group of academic physicians, primarily from the United States, to form the first international Evidence-based Medicine Working Group, and we published an article that expanded greatly on the existing description of evidence-based medicine, labeling it a paradigm shift.[2]

The Evidence-based Medicine Working Group then addressed the task of producing a new set of articles, the successor to the *Canadian Medical Association Journal* "Readers' Guides" series, to present a much more practical approach to applying the medical literature to clinical practice. Although many people made important contributions, the non-McMaster faculty who provided the greatest input to the intensive development of educational strategies included Scott Richardson, Mark Wilson, Robert Hayward, and Virginia Moyer. With the unflagging support and wise counsel of *JAMA* editor Drummond Rennie, the Evidence-based Medicine Working Group created a 25-part series called "The Users' Guides to the Medical Literature." This series was published in *JAMA* between 1993 and 2000,[3] and the book you are now reading is the direct descendent of those Users' Guides.

It did not take long for health care practitioners to realize that the principles of EBM were equally applicable to such allied health care workers as nurses, dentists, orthodontists, physical therapists, occupational therapists, chiropractors, podiatrists, and others. Thus, terms such as *evidence-based health care* or *evidence-based practice* are appropriate to cover the full range of clinical applications of the evidence-based approach to patient care. However, since this book is directed primarily to physicians, we have stayed with the term *evidence-based medicine* (EBM).

## Who Should Read This Book?

Any clinician who wishes to understand the medical literature, and to use it more effectively in solving patient problems, will benefit from this book. Those who wish to develop a core knowledge of basic concepts will read Part 1 of the book thoroughly and delve into Part 2 only for issues that catch their particular interest. Most medical students, residents, and community practitioners will likely be satisfied with this level of understanding. They will find Part 1 filled with case scenarios and clinical examples that facilitate their understanding, and they will also uncover tips for finding the best information and applying it to their practice.

Those who wish to reach a higher level of proficiency in using the medical literature in their patient care—in particular, those who wish to teach others the practice of evidence-based medicine—will find the in-depth discussions of Part 2 useful. Many physicians involved in continuing medical education, along with faculty members of medical schools, will wish to master the concepts we present in Part 2. They will appreciate the extensive use of teaching tips and strategies for making difficult concepts comprehensible.

## A Note About Authorship

Among the innovative aspects of this book is the way we have dealt with authorship, which is shared by all 50 members of the EBM Working Group. For most sections of the book, we began with the relevant Users' Guides as they appeared in *JAMA*; in most cases, the authors of those guides participated in their revision and retain authorship. In addition to the input of the primary authors, other members of the EBM Working Group have reviewed each section in detail. In certain instances, the magnitude of their input has warranted a coauthorship role. In other cases, we have acknowledged their valuable suggestions by means of prominent placement of their names immediately below the author byline. On page xvii we acknowledge the members of the EBM Working Group who participated in the creation of this book.

Producing this book has proved to be an enormously stimulating collaborative adventure. We hope the results provide a sense of how exciting it is to practice evidence-based medicine.

**Gordon Guyatt, MD**
*McMaster University*

## References

1. Guyatt GH. Evidence-based medicine. *ACP Journal Club*. 1991;114:A-16.

2. Evidence-Based Medicine Working Group. Evidence-based medicine: a new approach to the teaching of medicine. *JAMA*. 1992;268:2420-2425.

3. Guyatt GH, Rennie D. Users' Guides to the Medical Literature [editorial]. *JAMA*. 1993;270:2096-2097.

# Contributors

John Attia, MD, MSc, PhD
Centre for Clinical Epidemiology and
 Biostatistics
Royal Newcastle Hospital
Newcastle, NSW, Australia

Alexandra Barratt, MBBS, MPH, PhD
Public Health and Community
 Medicine
University of Sydney
Sydney, NSW, Australia

Eric Bass, MD, MPH
Division of Internal Medicine
Johns Hopkins University School of
 Medicine
Baltimore, Maryland, USA

Patrick Bossuyt, PhD
Clinical Epidemiology and
 Biostatistics
University of Amsterdam
Amsterdam, the Netherlands

Heiner Bucher, MD
Department of Internal Medicine
University Hospital Basel
Basel, Switzerland

Deborah Cook, MD, MSc
Department of Medicine
Faculty of Health Sciences
McMaster University
Hamilton, Ontario, Canada

Jonathan Craig, FRACP, PhD
Department of Public Health and
 Community Medicine
Faculty of Medicine
University of Sydney
Sydney, NSW, Australia

Robert Cumming, MB BS, MPH, PhD,
 FAFPHM
Department of Public Health and
 Community Medicine
University of Sydney
Sydney, NSW, Australia

Antonio Dans, MD
Clinical Epidemiological Unit
University of the Philippines
Manila, Philippines

Leonila Dans, MD
Clinical Epidemiological Unit
University of the Philippines
Manila, Philippines

Alan Detsky, MD, PhD
Department of Clinical Epidemiology
 and Biostatistics
McMaster University
Hamilton, Ontario, Canada

P J Devereaux, BSc, MD
Department of Medicine
McMaster University
Hamilton, Ontario, Canada

Michael Drummond, BSc, MCom,
 DPhil
Centre for Health Economics
University of York
York, England, UK

Mita Giacomini, PhD
Centre for Health Economics and
 Policy Analysis
McMaster University
Hamilton, Ontario, Canada

**Paul Glasziou, MBBS, PhD**
Department of Social and Preventative
  Medicine
University of Queensland Medical
  School
Herston, QLD, Australia

**Lee Green, MD, MPH**
Department of Family Medicine
University of Michigan Medical Centre
Ann Arbor, Michigan, USA

**Trisha Greenhalgh, MA, MD, FRCP,
FRCGP**
Unit for Evidence-Based Practice
  and Policy
Royal Free and University College
  Medical School
London, England, UK

**Gordon Guyatt, MD, MSc**
Chair, Evidence-Based Medicine
  Working Group
Clinical Epidemiology and
  Biostatistics and Medicine
McMaster University
Hamilton, Ontario, Canada

**Ted Haines, MD, MSc**
Departments of Clinical Epidemiology
  and Biostatistics, and Occupational
  Health Program
McMaster University
Hamilton, Ontario, Canada

**David Haslam, MD, FRCPC**
North Bay Psychiatric Hospital
North Bay, Ontario, Canada

**Rose Hatala, MD, MSc, FRCPC**
Department of Medicine
McMaster University
Hamilton, Ontario, Canada

**Brian Haynes, MD, MSc, PhD**
Department of Clinical Epidemiology
  and Biostatistics
McMaster University
Hamilton, Ontario, Canada

**Robert Hayward, MD, MPH, FRCPC**
Centres for Health Evidence
University of Alberta
Edmonton, Alberta, Canada

**Daren Heyland, MD, FRCPC, MSc**
Medicine and Community Health and
  Epidemiology
Queen's University
Kingston, Ontario, Canada

**Anne Holbrook, MD, PharmD, MSc**
Centre for Evaluation of Medicines
Faculty of Sciences
McMaster University
Hamilton, Ontario, Canada

**Dereck Hunt, MD**
Health Information Research Unit
Faculty of Health Sciences
McMaster University
Hamilton, Ontario, Canada

**Les Irwig, MBBCh, PhD, FFPHM**
Department of Public Health and
  Community Medicine
University of Sydney
Sydney, NSW, Australia

**Roman Jaeschke, MD, MSc**
Department of Medicine
McMaster University
Hamilton, Ontario, Canada

**Elizabeth Juniper, MCSP, MSc**
Department of Clinical Epidemiology
  and Biostatistics
McMaster University
Hamilton, Ontario, Canada

**Regina Kunz, MD, MSc**
Department of Nephrology
Charite Humboldt-University
Berlin, Germany

**Christina Lacchetti, MHSc**
Departments of Clinical Epidemiology
and Biostatistics and Medicine
McMaster University
Hamilton, Ontario, Canada

**Andreas Laupacis, MD, MSc**
Departments of Medicine and
Epidemiology and Community
Medicine
University of Ottawa
Ottawa, Ontario, Canada

**Hui Lee, MD, MSc, FRCPC**
Department of Medicine
McMaster University
Hamilton, Ontario, Canada

**Luz Letelier, MD**
General Internal Medicine
Servicio de Medicina
Hospital Dr. Sotero del Rio
U.D.A. Universidad Catolica de Chile
Santiago, Chile

**Raymond Leung, MDCM**
Centres for Health Evidence
Department of Cardiology
University of Alberta
Edmonton, Alberta, Canada

**Mitchell Levine, MD, MSc**
Centre for Evaluation of Medicines
St. Joseph's Hospital
Hamilton, Ontario, Canada

**Jeroen Lijmer, MD**
Clinical Epidemiology and
Biostatistics
University of Amsterdam
Amsterdam, the Netherlands

**Finlay McAlister, MD, MSc, FRCPC**
Department of Medicine
University of Alberta
Edmonton, Alberta, Canada

**Thomas McGinn, MD**
Primary Care Medicine
Mount Sinai Medical Center
New York, New York, USA

**Ann McKibbon, MLS**
Department of Clinical Epidemiology
and Biostatistics
Health Information Research Unit
McMaster University
Hamilton, Ontario, Canada

**Maureen Meade, MD, FRCPC, MSc**
Department of Medicine
McMaster University
Hamilton, Ontario, Canada

**Victor Montori, MD**
Department of Medicine
Mayo Clinic and Foundation
Rochester, Minnesota, USA

**Virginia Moyer, MD, MPH**
Department of Pediatrics
University of Texas
Houston, Texas, USA

**David Naylor, MD DPhil**
Faculty of Medicine
University of Toronto
Toronto, Ontario, Canada

**Thomas Newman, MD, MPH**
Departments of Epidemiology and
Biostatistics, Pediatrics and
Laboratory Medicine
University of California, San Francisco
San Francisco, California, USA

**Jim Nishikawa, MD, FRCPC**
Departments of Clinical Epidemiology
  and Biostatistics and Medicine
McMaster University
Hamilton, Ontario, Canada

**Bernie O'Brien, PhD**
Centre for Evaluation of Medicines
St. Joseph's Hospital
Hamilton, Ontario, Canada

**Andrew Oxman, MD, MSc**
Health Services Research Unit
National Institute of Public Health
Oslo, Norway

**Peter Pronovost, MD, PhD**
Anesthesiology and Critical Care
  Medicine
Johns Hopkins University
Baltimore, Maryland, USA

**Adrienne Randolph, MD, MSc**
The Children's Hospital
Boston, Massachusetts, USA

**Drummond Rennie, MD**
Institute for Health Policy Studies
University of California, San Francisco
San Francisco, California, USA

**Scott Richardson, MD**
Audie L. Murphy Memorial Veterans
  Hospital
San Antonio, Texas, USA

**Holger Schünemann, MD**
Departments of Medicine and Social
  and Preventative Medicine
University at Buffalo
Buffalo, New York, USA

**Jack Sinclair, MD**
Departments of Clinical Epidemiology
  and Biostatistics and Pediatrics
McMaster University
Hamilton, Ontario, Canada

**Martin Stockler, MBBS, MSc, FRACP**
Department of Medicine
University of Sydney
Sydney, NSW, Australia

**Sharon Straus, MD**
Department of Medicine
  University of Toronto
and Mount Sinai Hospital
Toronto, Ontario, Canada

**Peter Tugwell, MD, MSc**
Clinical Epidemiology Unit and
  Departments of Medicine and
  Epidemiology
University of Ottawa
Ottawa, Ontario, Canada

**Stephen Walter, PhD**
Department of Clinical Epidemiology
  and Biostatistics
McMaster University
Hamilton, Ontario, Canada

**George Wells, MSc, PhD**
Clinical Epidemiology Unit and
  Departments of Medicine and
  Epidemiology
University of Ottawa
Ottawa, Ontario, Canada

**Mark Wilson, MD, MPH**
Department of Medicine
Wake Forest University School of
  Medicine
Winston-Salem, North Carolina, USA

**Jeremy Wyatt, MD**
Knowledge Management Centre
University College London
London, England, UK

**Peter Wyer, MD**
Department of Medicine
Columbia University College of
  Physicians and Surgeons
Pelham, New York, USA

# HOW TO USE
# THIS BOOK

Gordon Guyatt

The following EBM Working Group members also made substantive contributions to this section: John Attia, Roman Jaeschke, Maureen Meade, Andrew Oxman, Trisha Greenhalgh, Jack Sinclair, Anne McKibbon, Deborah Cook, and Eric Bass

Like evidence-based medicine (EBM), this book is about clinical decision making. In particular, our objective is to make efficient use of the published literature to help with patient care. What does the published literature comprise? Our definition is broad. Evidence may be published in a wide variety of sources, including original journal articles, reviews and synopses of primary studies, practice guidelines, and traditional and innovative medical textbooks. Increasingly, clinicians can most easily access many of these sources through the World Wide Web. In the future, the Internet may be the only route of access for some resources.

## PART 1: THE BASICS: USING THE MEDICAL LITERATURE

Part 1 of our clinicians' guide covers the basics: what every medical student, every intern and resident, and every practicing physician should know about reading the medical literature. We have kept this section as simple and succinct as possible. From an instructor's point of view, Part 1 constitutes a curriculum for a short course in using the literature for medical students or house staff; it is also appropriate for a continuing education program for practicing physicians.

Part 1 of this book teaches a systematic approach that involves three steps to using an article from the medical literature. The clinician should ask whether new information is likely to be true, what the information says about patient care, and how the information can be used. In the first step, the clinician considers the validity or likelihood of bias. In the second and third steps, the clinician comes to understand the results and to apply those results to the care of individual patients. These three steps provided the inspiration for the three pillars that you see on the cover of this book. To help demonstrate the clinical relevance of this approach, we begin each section with a clinical scenario, demonstrate a search for relevant literature, and present a table that summarizes criteria for using the three steps.

Although Part 1 of this book is concise, after you have mastered its concepts you will be able to ensure that your practice is evidence-based. You will have learned:

- To distinguish stronger evidence from weaker evidence;

- To become familiar with the full process of detailed critical appraisal, summarization of evidence, and balancing of benefits and risks that should precede management decisions;

- To identify, locate, and understand preappraised evidence summaries and evidence-based recommendations; and

- To understand the issues involved in applying evidence from the literature to your clinical practice and, in particular, to individualizing the application to each unique patient.

A wide array of preappraised evidence-based resources already exist and most are easily accessed by computer. The number and quality of these resources are certain to increase dramatically during the next few years. Part 1A1, "Finding the Evidence," will teach you how to identify the right databases—ones providing evidence that is both valid and applicable to your practice—and to find the information you want within them. Sections B through F of Part 1 will teach you how to make optimal use of what you find to address patient management problems.

In fact, you need not read all of Part 1. The book is designed so that each section is largely self-contained. If all you need is guidance on formulating and carrying out searches, read only Part 1A1. If the only original articles you are interested in are primary studies concerning therapy and systematic reviews of those studies, read only the Therapy and Harm section of Parts 1B, 1B1, and 1B2 and the systematic reviews section in Part 1E. We have avoided excessive redundancy, so there are times when we do not repeat a concept common to two sections. You will find such instances clearly denoted.

# PART 2: BEYOND THE BASICS: USING AND TEACHING THE PRINCIPLES OF EVIDENCE-BASED MEDICINE

Part 2 of this book is directed to clinicians who want to practice EBM at a more sophisticated level. Reading Part 2 will deepen your understanding of study methodology, of statistical issues, and of how to use the numbers that emerge from medical research in helping each patient make the best health care choices.

We wrote Part 2 mindful of an additional audience: those who teach evidence-based practice. You will find that many entries in Part 2 read like a guideline for an interactive discussion with a group of learners in tutorial, or on the ward. That is natural enough, as the material originated in just such small-group settings.

You need not read Part 2 from beginning to end in the order presented. Our intent is for you to take a flexible, nonlinear approach: You will read sections of Part 2 as the need arises, when considering issues that emerge in the critical appraisal and application of articles that may guide your clinical practice.

How should you use Part 2? Note first that the organization of Part 2 roughly parallels that of Part 1. Each major section includes more detailed discussion of concepts introduced in the corresponding section of Part 1. For instance, in the Therapy and Harm section of Part 2 you will find discussions concerning standards for appraising studies that address cost issues, studies evaluating screening programs, and studies evaluating computer decision support systems. We judged each of these as being outside the core knowledge needed for a basic application of EBM in your practice.

Each expansion in Part 2 has a corresponding cross-reference in Part 1. For instance, you will find an expanded version of our introductory discussion of the philosophy of EBM in Part 2A. In most cases, the expansion in Part 2 will be directly linked to core knowledge presented in Part 1. For instance, Part 1 tells you that when using an article about therapy, you need to ask whether the investigators have measured all important outcomes of treatment, both good and bad. It mentions that health-related quality of life is often an important outcome, and it includes some brief remarks about how it should be measured. Part 2, by contrast, includes a major expansion of this topic, with a full discussion of quality-of-life measurement.

What else have we included in Part 2? We believe our discussion of criticisms of EBM may amuse you and our historical note may interest you; these are sections we could not justify classifying as "core knowledge." You will find these discussions in Part 2A, "Expanded Philosophy of Evidence-Based Medicine."

Thus, we anticipate that clinicians may be selective in their reading of Part 1 and will certainly be selective in reading Part 2. On the first read, you may choose only a few sections in Part 2 that interest you. If, as you use the medical literature, you find the need to expand your understanding of quality-of-life measurement, for instance, or of the use of surrogate endpoints, you can return to Part 2 to familiarize or reacquaint yourself with the issues.

Some may find the CD-ROM version, in which a mouse-click moves you from Part 1 to the relevant section of Part 2, easier to use than the written text. Either way, many will find the glossary of terms a useful reminder of formal definition of terms used in the book. We hope that this organization is well suited to the needs of any clinician who is eager to achieve an evidence-based practice.

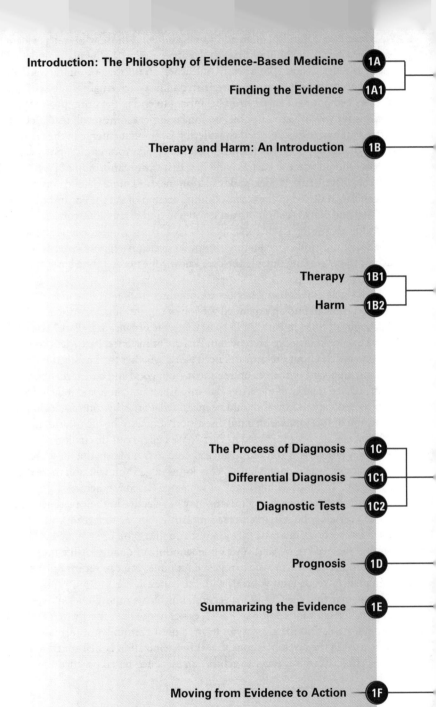

# The Basics: Using The Medical Literature

C linicians are primarily interested in making accurate diagnoses and selecting optimal treatments for patients in their practice. They must also avoid harmful exposures and offer patients prognostic information. Part 1 of this book provides clinicians with the essential skills they need to use the medical literature for these four aspects of patient care.

Before clinicians can incorporate the best evidence, they must find it. Part 1 begins with an approach to formulating clinical questions and locating the best studies that address those questions. Opportunities for efficient searching have grown enormously during in recent years, and our section concerning "Finding the Evidence" (see Section 1A1) incorporates the latest developments.

## Primary Studies

One can distinguish between individual studies presenting original data—which we shall call primary studies—and reports that summarize a number of primary studies. After we have offered instruction on how to find the best evidence, we provide an approach to critically appraising primary studies and applying the results to patient care. The principles of assessing articles on therapy and harm are closely linked, as are the principles of assessing diagnostic and prognostic studies. Throughout, our discussion highlights these links.

## Systematic Reviews

When someone has gone to the trouble of systematically summarizing primary studies addressing a specific clinical question, clinicians should take advantage of that summary. Indeed, efficient evidence-based practice dictates bypassing the critical assessment of primary studies and moving straight to the evaluation of rigorous systematic literature reviews. Thus, clinicians must be aware of how to recognize a systematic review, appraise its methodologic quality, and apply its results to patients in their practice. After discussing primary studies, Part 1 provides clinicians with the skills needed to use a systematic review.

## Treatment Recommendations

Even more efficient than using a systematic review is moving directly to a treatment recommendation. Ideally, treatment recommendations—which are summarized in practice guidelines or decision analyses—will rigorously incorporate the best evidence and make explicit the value judgments used in moving from evidence to recommendations for action. Once again, there are methodologically weak practice guidelines and decision analyses that clinicians should ignore—and methodologically rigorous recommendations to which they should attend. Our section on "Moving From Evidence to Action" (see Section 1F) provides instruction in how to differentiate weak practice guidelines and decision analyses from strong ones, to understand their limitations, and to judiciously use these recommendations in clinical practice.

# INTRODUCTION: THE PHILOSOPHY OF EVIDENCE-BASED MEDICINE

Gordon Guyatt, Brian Haynes, Roman Jaeschke,
Deborah Cook, Trisha Greenhalgh, Maureen Meade,
Lee Green, C. David Naylor, Mark Wilson, Finlay McAlister,
and W. Scott Richardson

The following EBM Working Group members also made substantive
contributions to this section: Victor Montori and Heiner Bucher

## IN THIS SECTION

## CLINICAL SCENARIO

### Who's Right?

**A** senior resident, a junior attending physician, a senior attending physician, and an emeritus professor were discussing evidence-based medicine over lunch in a hospital cafeteria. "EBM," announced the resident with some passion, "is a revolutionary development in medical practice." She went on to describe EBM's fundamental innovations in solving patient problems. "A compelling exposition," remarked the emeritus professor. "Wait a minute," the junior attending exclaimed with some heat, and then proceeded to present an alternative position: that EBM has merely provided a set of additional tools for traditional approaches to patient care. "You make a strong and convincing case," the emeritus professor commented. "Something's wrong here," the senior attending exclaimed to her older colleague, "their positions are diametrically opposed. They can't both be right." The emeritus professor looked thoughtfully at the puzzled doctor and, with the barest hint of a smile, replied, "Come to think of it, you're right too."

Evidence-based medicine (EBM) is about solving clinical problems.[1] In 1992, we described EBM as a shift in medical paradigms.[2] In contrast to the traditional paradigm of medical practice, EBM acknowledges that intuition, unsystematic clinical experience, and pathophysiologic rationale are insufficient grounds for clinical decision making; and it stresses the examination of evidence from clinical research. In addition, EBM suggests that a formal set of rules must complement medical training and common sense for clinicians to interpret the results of clinical research effectively. Finally, EBM places a lower value on authority than the traditional medical paradigm does.

We continue to find this paradigm shift a valid way of conceptualizing EBM. As our opening vignette about the lunchtime conversation suggests, the world is often complex enough to invite more than one useful way of thinking about an idea or a phenomenon. In this section, we describe the way of thinking about EBM that currently appeals to us most. We explain two key principles of EBM relating to the value-laden nature of clinical decisions, along with a hierarchy of evidence. We note the additional skills necessary for optimal clinical practice, and we conclude with a discussion of the challenges facing EBM in the new millennium.

# Two Fundamental Principles of EBM

As a distinctive approach to patient care, EBM involves two fundamental principles. First, evidence alone is never sufficient to make a clinical decision. Decision makers must always trade the benefits and risks, inconvenience, and costs associated with alternative management strategies, and in doing so consider the patient's values.[1] Second, EBM posits a hierarchy of evidence to guide clinical decision making.

## 1. Clinical Decision Making: Evidence Is Never Enough

Picture a patient with chronic pain resulting from terminal cancer. She has come to terms with her condition, has resolved her affairs and said her goodbyes, and she wishes to receive only palliative therapy. The patient develops pneumococcal pneumonia. Now, evidence that antibiotic therapy reduces morbidity and mortality from pneumococcal pneumonia is strong. Almost all clinicians would agree, however, that even evidence this convincing does not dictate that this particular patient should receive antibiotics. Despite the fact that antibiotics might reduce symptoms and prolong the patient's life, her values are such that she would prefer a rapid and natural death.

Now envision a second patient—an 85-year-old man with severe dementia, who is incontinent, contracted, and mute, without family or friends, who spends his days in apparent discomfort. This man develops pneumococcal pneumonia. Although many clinicians would argue that those responsible for this patient's care should not administer antibiotic therapy because of his circumstances, others, by contrast, would suggest that they should do so. Again, evidence of treatment effectiveness does not automatically imply that treatment should be administered. The management decision requires a judgment about the tradeoff between risks and benefits; and because values or preferences differ, the best course of action will vary from patient to patient and among clinicians.

Finally, picture a third patient—a healthy, 30-year-old mother of two children who develops pneumococcal pneumonia. No clinician would doubt the wisdom of administering antibiotic therapy to this patient. However, this does not mean that an underlying value judgment has been unnecessary. Rather, our values are sufficiently concordant, and the benefits so overwhelm the risks, that the underlying value judgment is unapparent.

In current health care practice, judgments often reflect clinical or societal values concerning whether intervention benefits are worth the cost.[2] Consider the decisions regarding administration of tissue plasminogen activator (tPA) versus streptokinase to patients with acute myocardial infarction, or administration of clopidogrel versus aspirin to patients with transient ischemic attack. In both cases, evidence from large randomized trials suggests that the more expensive agents are more effective. In both cases, many authorities recommend first-line treatment with the less expensive, less effective drug, presumably because they believe society's resources would be better used in other ways. Implicitly, they are making a value or preference judgment about the tradeoff between deaths and strokes prevented, and resources spent.

By *values* and preferences, we mean the underlying processes we bring to bear in weighing what our patients and our society will gain—or lose—when we make a management decision. The explicit enumeration and balancing of benefits and risks that is central to EBM brings the underlying value judgments involved in making management decisions into bold relief.

Acknowledging that values play a role in every important patient care decision highlights our limited understanding of eliciting and incorporating societal and individual values. Health economists have played a major role in developing a science of measuring patient preferences.[3,4] Some decision aids incorporate patient values indirectly: If patients truly understand the potential risks and benefits, their decisions will likely reflect their preferences.[5] These developments constitute a promising start. Nevertheless, many unanswered questions remain concerning how to elicit preferences and how to incorporate them in clinical encounters already subject to crushing time pressures. Addressing these issues constitutes an enormously challenging frontier for EBM. We discuss these issues in more detail in Part 2F, "Moving From Evidence to Action, Incorporating Patient Values."

## 2. A Hierarchy of Evidence

What is the nature of the "evidence" in EBM? We suggest a broad definition: any empirical observation about the apparent relation between events constitutes potential evidence. Thus, the unsystematic observations of the individual clinician constitute one source of evidence, and physiologic experiments constitute another source. Unsystematic observations can lead to profound insight, and experienced clinicians develop a healthy respect for the insights of their senior colleagues in issues of clinical observation, diagnosis, and relations with patients and colleagues. Some of these insights can be taught, yet rarely appear in the medical literature.

At the same time, unsystematic clinical observations are limited by small sample size and, more importantly, by deficiencies in human processes of making inferences.[6] Predictions about intervention effects on clinically important outcomes based on physiologic experiments usually are right, but occasionally are disastrously wrong. We provide a number of examples of just how wrong predictions based on physiologic rationale can be in Part 2B1, "Therapy and Validity, Surprising Results of Randomized Controlled Trials."

Given the limitations of unsystematic clinical observations and physiologic rationale, EBM suggests a hierarchy of evidence. Table 1A-1 presents a hierarchy of study designs for treatment issues; very different hierarchies are necessary for issues of diagnosis or prognosis. Clinical research goes beyond unsystematic clinical observation in providing strategies that avoid or attenuate spurious results. Because few—if any—interventions are effective in all patients, we would ideally test a treatment in a patient to whom we would like to apply that treatment. Numerous factors can lead clinicians astray as they try to interpret the results of conventional open trials of therapy. These include natural history, placebo effects, patient and health worker expectations, and the patient's desire to please.

**TABLE 1A–1**

## A Hierarchy of Strength of Evidence for Treatment Decisions

- N of 1 randomized controlled trial
- Systematic reviews of randomized trials
- Single randomized trial
- Systematic review of observational studies addressing patient-important outcomes
- Single observational study addressing patient-important outcomes
- Physiologic studies (studies of blood pressure, cardiac output, exercise capacity, bone density, and so forth)
- Unsystematic clinical observations

The same strategies that minimize bias in conventional therapeutic trials involving multiple patients can guard against misleading results in studies involving single patients.[7] In the N of 1 randomized controlled trial (RCT), patients undertake pairs of treatment periods in which they receive a target treatment during one period of each pair, and a placebo or alternative during the other. Patients and clinicians are blind to allocation, the order of the target and control is randomized, and patients make quantitative ratings of their symptoms during each period. The N of 1 RCT continues until both the patient and clinician conclude that the patient is, or is not, obtaining benefit from the target intervention. N of 1 RCTs are often feasible,[8,9] can provide definitive evidence of treatment effectiveness in individual patients, and may lead to long-term differences in treatment administration (see Part 2B1, "Therapy and Validity, N of 1 Randomized Controlled Trials").[10]

When considering any other source of evidence about treatment, clinicians are generalizing from results in other people to their patients, inevitably weakening inferences about treatment impact and introducing complex issues of how trial results apply to individual patients. Inferences may nevertheless be very strong if results come from a systematic review of methodologically strong RCTs with consistent results. However, inferences generally will be somewhat weaker if only a single RCT is being considered, unless it is very large and investigators have enrolled a diverse patient population (see Table 1A-1). Because observational studies may under-estimate treatment effects in an unpredictable fashion,[11,12] their results are far less trustworthy than those of randomized trials. Physiologic studies and unsystematic clinical observations provide the weakest inferences about treatment effects.

This hierarchy is not absolute. If treatment effects are sufficiently large and consistent, for instance, observational studies may provide more compelling evidence than most RCTs. By way of example, observational studies have allowed extremely strong inferences about the efficacy of insulin in diabetic ketoacidosis or that of hip replacement in patients with debilitating hip osteoarthritis. At the same time, instances in which RCT results contradict consistent results from observational studies reinforce the need for caution. Defining the extent to which clinicians should temper the strength of their inferences when only observational studies are available remains one of the important challenges for EBM. The challenge is particularly important given that much of the evidence regarding the harmful effects of therapies comes from observational studies.

The hierarchy implies a clear course of action for physicians addressing patient problems: they should look for the highest available evidence from the hierarchy. The hierarchy makes clear that any statement to the effect that there is no evidence addressing the effect of a particular treatment is a non sequitur. The evidence may be extremely weak—it may be the unsystematic observation of a single clinician or a generalization from physiologic studies that are related only indirectly—but there is always evidence.

Next we will briefly comment on additional skills that clinicians must master for optimal patient care and the relation of those skills to EBM.

# CLINICAL SKILLS, HUMANISM, SOCIAL RESPONSIBILITY, AND EBM

The evidence-based process of resolving a clinical question will be fruitful only if the problem is formulated appropriately. One of us, a secondary care internist, developed a lesion on his lip shortly before an important presentation. He was quite concerned and, wondering if he should take acyclovir, proceeded to spend the next 2 hours searching for the highest quality evidence and reviewing the available RCTs. When he began to discuss his remaining uncertainty with his partner, an experienced dentist, she quickly cut short the discussion by exclaiming, "But, my dear, that isn't herpes!"

This story illustrates the necessity of obtaining the correct diagnosis before seeking and applying research evidence in practice, the value of extensive clinical experience, and the fallibility of clinical judgment. The essential skills of obtaining a history and conducting a physical examination and the astute formulation of the clinical problem come only with thorough background training and extensive clinical experience. The clinician makes use of evidence-based reasoning—applying the likelihood ratios associated with positive or negative physical findings, for instance—to interpret the results of the history and physical examination. Clinical expertise is further required to define the relevant treatment options before examining the evidence regarding the expected benefits and risks of those options.

Finally, clinicians rely on their expertise to define features that have an impact on the generalizability of the results to the individual patient. We have noted that, except when clinicians have conducted N of 1 RCTs, they are attempting to generalize (or, one might say, particularize) results obtained in other patients to the individual patient before them. The clinician must judge the extent to which differences in treatment (local surgical expertise or the possibility of patient noncompliance, for instance), the availability of monitoring, or patient characteristics (such as age, comorbidity, or concomitant treatment) may impact estimates of benefit and risk that come from the published literature.

Thus, knowing the tools of evidence-based practice is necessary but not sufficient for delivering the highest quality of patient care. In addition to clinical expertise, the clinician requires compassion, sensitive listening skills, and broad perspectives from the humanities and social sciences. These attributes allow understanding of patients' illnesses in the context of their experience, personalities, and cultures. The sensitive understanding of the patient links to evidence-based practice in a number of ways. For some patients, incorporation of patient values for major decisions will mean a full enumeration of the possible benefits, risks, and inconvenience associated with alternative management strategies that are relevant to the particular patient. For some of these patients and problems, this discussion should involve the patients' family. For other problems—the discussion of screening with prostate-specific antigen with older male patients, for instance—attempts to involve other family members might violate strong cultural norms.

Many patients are uncomfortable with an explicit discussion of benefits and risks, and they object to having what they perceive as excessive responsibility for decision making being placed on their shoulders.[13] In such patients, who would tell us they want the physician to make the decision on their behalf, the physician's responsibility is to develop insight to ensure that choices will be consistent with patients' values and preferences. Understanding and implementing the sort of decision-making process patients desire and effectively communicating the information they need requires skills in understanding the patient's narrative and the person behind that narrative.[14, 15] A continuing challenge for EBM—and for medicine in general—will be to better integrate the new science of clinical medicine with the time-honored craft of caring for the sick.

Ideally, evidence-based technical skills and humane perspective will lead physicians to become effective advocates for their patients both in the direct context of the health system in which they work and in broader health policy issues. Most physicians see their role as focusing on health care interventions for their patients. Even when they consider preventive therapy, they focus on individual patient behavior. However, we consider this focus to be too narrow.

Observational studies have documented the strong and consistent association between socioeconomic status and health. Societal health is associated more strongly with income gradients than with the total wealth of the society. In other words, the overall health of the populace tends to be higher in poorer countries with a relatively equitable distribution of wealth than in richer countries with larger disparities between rich and poor. These considerations suggest that physicians concerned about the health of their patients as a group, or about the health of the community, should consider how they might contribute to reducing poverty.

Observational studies have shown a strong and consistent association between pollution levels and respiratory and cardiovascular health. Physicians seeing patients with chronic obstructive pulmonary disease will suggest that they stop smoking. But should physicians also be concerned with the polluted air that patients are breathing? We believe they should.

# ADDITIONAL CHALLENGES FOR EBM

In 1992, we identified skills necessary for evidence-based practice. These included the ability to precisely define a patient problem and to ascertain what information is required to resolve the problem, conduct an efficient search of the literature, select the best of the relevant studies, apply rules of evidence to determine their validity, extract the clinical message, and apply it to the patient problem as the skills necessary for evidence-based practice.[1] To these skills we would now add an understanding of how the patient's values impact the balance between advantages and disadvantages of the available management options and the ability to appropriately involve the patient in the decision.

A further decade of experience with EBM has not changed the biggest challenge to evidence-based practice: time limitation. Fortunately, new resources to assist clinicians are available and the pace of innovation is rapid. One can consider a classification of information sources that comes with a mnemonic device, 4S: the individual study or studies, the systematic review of all the available studies on a given problem, a synopsis of individual studies or systematic reviews or both, and systems of information. By systems we mean summaries that link a number of synopses related to the care of a particular patient problem (for example, acute upper gastrointestinal bleeding) or type of patient (for example, an outpatient with diabetes) (Table 1A-2). Evidence-based selection and summarization is becoming increasingly available at each level (see Part 1A1, "Finding the Evidence").

**TABLE 1A–2**

## A Hierarchy of Preprocessed Evidence

| | |
|---|---|
| **Studies** | Preprocessing involves selecting only those studies that are both highly relevant and characterized by study designs that minimize bias and thus permit a high strength of inference. |
| **Systematic Reviews** | Systematic reviews provide clinicians with an overview of all of the evidence addressing a focused clinical question. |
| **Synopses** | Synopses of individual studies or of systematic reviews encapsulate the key methodologic details and results required to apply the evidence to individual patient care. |
| **Systems** | Practice guidelines, clinical pathways, or evidence-based textbook summaries of a clinical area provide the clinician with much of the information needed to guide the care of individual patients. |

This book deals primarily with decision making at the level of the individual patient. Evidence-based approaches can also inform health policy making,[16] day-to-day decisions in public health, and systems-level decisions such as those facing hospital managers. In each of these arenas, EBM can support the appropriate goal of gaining the greatest health benefit from limited resources. On the other hand, evidence—as an ideology, rather than a focus for reasoned debate—has been used as a justification for many agendas in health care, ranging from crude cost cutting to the promotion of extremely expensive technologies with minimal marginal returns.

In the policy arena, dealing with differing values poses even more challenges than in the arena of individual patient care. Should we restrict ourselves to alternative resource allocation within a fixed pool of health care resources, or should we be trading off health care services against, for instance, lower tax rates for individuals or lower health care costs for corporations? How should we deal with the large body of observational studies suggesting that social and economic factors may have a larger impact on the health of populations than health care delivery? How should we deal with the tension between what may be best for a person and what may be optimal for the society of which that person is a member? The debate about such issues is at the heart of evidence-based health policy making, but, inevitably, it has implications for decision making at the individual patient level.

# References

1. Haynes RB, Sackett RB, Gray JMA, Cook DC, Guyatt GH. Transferring evidence from research into practice, 1: the role of clinical care research evidence in clinical decisions. *ACP Journal Club*. Nov-Dec 1996 ;125:A-14-15.

2. Napodano RJ. *Values in Medical Practice*. New York, NY: Human Sciences Press; 1986.

3. Drummond MF, Richardson WS, O'Brien B, Levine M, Heyland DK, for the Evidence-Based Medicine Working Group. Users' Guides to the Medical Literature XIII. How to use an article on economic analysis of clinical practice. A. Are the results of the study valid? *JAMA*. 1997;277:1552-1557.

4. Feeny DH, Furlong W, Boyle M, Torrance GW. Multi-attribute health status classification systems: health utilities index. *Pharmacoeconomics*. 1995;7:490-502.

5. O'Connor AM, Rostom A, Fiset V, et al. Decision aids for patients facing health treatment or screening decisions: systematic review. *BMJ*. 1999;319:731-734.

6. Nisbett R, Ross L. *Human Inference*. Englewood Cliffs, NJ: Prentice-Hall; 1980.

7. Guyatt GH, Sackett DL, Taylor DW, et al. Determining optimal therapy: randomized trials in individual patients. *N Engl J Med*. 1986;314:889-892.

8. Guyatt GH, Keller JL, Jaeschke R, Rosenbloom D, Adachi JD, Newhouse MT. The n-of-1 randomized controlled trial: clinical usefulness. Our three-year experience. *Ann Intern Med*. 1990;112:293-299.

9. Larson EB, Ellsworth AJ, Oas J. Randomized clinical trials in single patients during a 2-year period. *JAMA*. 1993;270:2708-2712.

10. Mahon J, Laupacis A, Donner A, Wood T. Randomised study of n of 1 trials versus standard practice. *BMJ.* 1996;312:1069-1074.

11. Guyatt GH, DiCenso A, Farewell V, Willan A, Griffith L. Randomized trials versus observational studies in adolescent pregnancy prevention. *J Clin Epidemiol*. 2000;53:167-174.

12. Kunz R, Oxman AD. The unpredictability paradox: review of empirical comparisons of randomised and non-randomised clinical trials. *BMJ.* 1998;317: 1185-1190.

13. Sutherland HJ, Llewellyn-Thomas HA, Lockwood GA, Tritchler DL, Till JE. Cancer patients: their desire for information and participation in treatment decisions. *J R Soc Med*. 1989;82:260-263.

14. Greenhalgh T. Narrative based medicine: narrative based medicine in an evidence based world. *BMJ*. 1999;318:323-325.

15. Greenhalgh T, Hurwitz B. Narrative based medicine: why study narrative? *BMJ*. 1999;318:48-50.

16. Muir Gray FA, Haynes RB, Sackett DL, Cook DJ, Guyatt GH. Transferring evidence from research into practice, III: developing evidence-based clinical policy. *ACP Journal Club*. 1997;A14.

# 1A1 FINDING THE EVIDENCE

Ann McKibbon, Dereck Hunt, W. Scott Richardson,
Robert Hayward, Mark Wilson, Roman Jaeschke,
Brian Haynes, Peter Wyer, Jonathan Craig,
and Gordon Guyatt

The following EBM Working Group members also made substantive
contributions to this section: Patrick Bossuyt, Trisha Greenhalgh,
Sharon Straus, and Deborah Cook

## IN THIS SECTION

# WAYS OF USING THE MEDICAL LITERATURE

This book is about using the medical literature. But not, as we describe in the following section, in the ways medical students most typically use it.

## Background and Foreground Questions

There are several reasons that medical students, early in their training, seldom consult the original medical literature. First, they are not usually responsible for managing patients and solving specific patient problems. Even if they attend a school that uses problem-oriented learning as an educational strategy, their interest is primarily in understanding normal human physiology and the pathophysiology associated with a patient's condition or problem. Once they have grasped these basic concepts, they will turn to the prognosis, available diagnostic tests, and possible management options. Finally, when students are presented with a patient-related problem, their questions are likely to include, for example, what is diabetes, why did this patient present with polyuria, and how might we manage the problem.

By contrast, experienced clinicians responsible for managing a patient's problem ask very different sorts of questions. They are interested less in the diagnostic approach to a presenting problem and are more interested in how to interpret a specific diagnostic test; less in the general prognosis of a chronic disease and more in a particular patient's prognosis; less in the management strategies that might be applied to a patient's problems and more in the risks and benefits of a particular treatment in relation to an alternative management strategy.

Think of the first set of questions, those of the medical student, as background questions; think of the second set as foreground questions. In most situations, you need to understand the background thoroughly before it makes sense to address issues in the foreground.

On her first day on the ward, a medical student will still have a great deal of background knowledge to acquire. However, in deciding how to manage the first patient she sees, she may well need to address a foreground issue. A senior clinician, while well versed in all issues that represent the background of her clinical practice, may nevertheless also occasionally require background information. This is most likely when a new condition or medical syndrome appears (consider the fact that as recently as 20 years ago, experienced clinicians were asking, "What is the acquired immunodeficiency syndrome?") or when a new diagnostic test ("How does PCR work?") or treatment modality ("What are COX-2 inhibitors?") is introduced into the clinical arena. At every stage of training and experience, clinicians' grasp of the relevant background issues of disease inform their ability to identify and formulate the most pertinent foreground questions for an individual patient.

Figure 1A-1 represents the evolution of the questions we ask as we progress from being novices (who pose almost exclusively background questions) to being experts (who pose almost exclusively foreground questions). This book is devoted to how clinicians can use the medical literature to solve their foreground questions.

**FIGURE 1A-1**

## Asking Questions

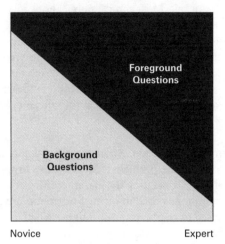

Foreground
Questions

Background
Questions

Novice                    Expert

## Browsing and Problem Solving

Traditionally, clinicians subscribed to a number—sometimes a large number—
of target medical journals in which articles relevant to their practice were likely to
appear. They would keep up to date by skimming the table of contents and reading
articles relevant to their practice. One might label this the browsing mode of using
the medical literature.

Traditional approaches to browsing have major limitations of inefficiency and
resulting frustration. Picture a clinician with a number of subscriptions placing
journals in a pile on her desk awaiting browsing review. She may even be aware
that less than 10% of articles that are published in the core medical journals are
both high quality and clinically useful. Unable to spend sufficient time to browse,
she finds the pile growing until it becomes intimidating. At this point, she tosses
the whole pile and starts the process again.

Although it is somewhat of a parody, most experienced clinicians can relate
easily to this scenario. Physicians at every stage of training often feel overwhelmed
by the magnitude of the medical literature. Evidence-based medicine offers some
solutions to this problem.

Browse Secondary Journals. Perhaps the most efficient strategy is to restrict
your browsing to secondary journals. For internal and general medicine, *ACP
Journal Club* (www.acponline.org/journals/acpjc/jcmenu.htm) publishes synopses
of articles that meet criteria of both clinical relevance and methodologic quality.
We describe such secondary journals in more detail later in this section.

Many specialties and subspecialties do not yet have devoted secondary journals. This is likely to be a temporary phenomenon, at least for the major specialties. In the meantime, you can apply your own relevance and methodologic screen to articles in your target journals. Most clinical publications serve a dual purpose: as a forum for both investigator-to-investigator communication and investigator-to-clinician communication.[1] However, only the latter articles will be directly relevant to your practice. Part 1 of this book is devoted to providing the tools that will allow you to screen journals for high-quality, relevant evidence. When you have learned the skills, you will be surprised both at the small proportion of studies to which you need to attend—and at the efficiency with which you can identify them.

**Operate in a Problem-Solving Mode.** Another part of the solution to the overwhelming-amount-of-literature problem is for clinicians to spend more of the time they have available for consulting the literature in what we call a problem-solving mode. Here, questions raised in caring for patients are defined and then the literature is consulted to resolve these questions. Whether you are operating in the browsing mode or problem-solving mode, this book can help you to judge the validity of the information in the articles you are examining, gain a clear understanding of their results, and apply them to patients.

The remainder of this section focuses on skills you will need to use the literature effectively when you are in the problem-solving mode.

# FRAMING THE QUESTION

Clinical questions often spring to practitioners' minds in a form that makes finding answers in the medical literature a challenge. Dissecting the question into its component parts to facilitate finding the best evidence is a fundamental EBM skill.[2,3] Most questions can be divided into three parts.

1. **The population**. Who are the relevant patients?

2. **The interventions or exposures** (diagnostic tests, foods, drugs, surgical procedures, etc). What are the management strategies we are interested in comparing, or the potentially harmful exposure about which we are concerned? For issues of therapy or harm, there will always be two or more parts to this: the intervention or exposure and a control or alternative intervention(s) or exposure(s).

3. **The outcome**. What are the patient-relevant consequences of the exposure in which we are interested?

We will now provide examples of the transformation of unstructured clinical questions into the structured questions that facilitate use of the medical literature.

## Example 1: Diabetes and Target Blood Pressure

A 55-year-old white woman presents with type 2 diabetes mellitus and hypertension. Her glycemic control is excellent on metformin and she has no history of complications. To manage her hypertension, she takes a small daily dose of a thiazide diuretic. Over a 6-month period, her blood pressure hovers around a value of 155/88 mm Hg.

**Initial Question:** When treating hypertension, at what target blood pressure should we aim?

**Digging Deeper:** One limitation of this formulation of the question is that it fails to specify the population in adequate detail. The benefits of tight control of blood pressure may differ in diabetic patients vs nondiabetic patients, in type 1 vs type 2 diabetes mellitus, as well as in those with and without diabetic complications. We may wish to specify that we are interested in the addition of a specific antihypertensive agent. Alternatively, the intervention of interest may be any antihypertensive treatment. Furthermore, a key part of the intervention will be the target for blood pressure control. For instance, we might be interested in knowing whether it makes any difference if our target diastolic blood pressure is < 80 mm Hg vs < 90 mm Hg. The major limitation of the initial question formulation is that it fails to specify the criteria by which we will judge the appropriate target for our hypertensive treatment. The target outcomes of interest would include stroke, myocardial infarction, cardiovascular death, and total mortality.

**Improved (Searchable) Question:** A searchable question would specify the relevant patient population, the management strategy and exposure, and the patient-relevant consequences of that exposure as follows:

- *Patients:* Hypertensive type 2 diabetic patients without diabetic complications

- *Intervention:* Any antihypertensive agent aiming at a target diastolic blood pressure of 90 mm Hg vs a target of 80 mm Hg

- *Outcomes:* Stroke, myocardial infarction, cardiovascular death, total mortality

## Example 2: Suspected Unstable Angina

A 39-year-old man without previous chest discomfort presented to the emergency department at the end of his working day. Early that day he had felt unwell and nauseated; he had had a vague sensation of chest discomfort and had begun to sweat profusely. The unpleasant experience lasted for about 2 hours, after which the patient felt tired but otherwise normal. At the end of his work day, feeling rather nervous about the episode, he came to the emergency department. The patient has no family history of coronary artery disease. He has had hypertension for 5 years that is controlled with a thiazide, has a 15-pack-year smoking history, and has a normal lipid profile. His physical examination, electrocardiogram (ECG), creatine kinase level, and troponin I level are all normal.

**Initial Question:** Can I send this man home or should I admit him to a monitored hospital bed?

**Digging Deeper:** The initial question gives us little idea of where to look in the literature for an answer. We can break down the issue by noting that the patient has suspected unstable angina. However, a number of distinguishing features differentiate him from other patients with possible unstable angina. He is relatively young, he has some risk factors for coronary artery disease, his presentation is atypical, he is now pain free, there is no sign of heart failure, and his ECG and cardiac enzymes are unremarkable.

The management strategies we are considering include admitting him to a hospital for overnight monitoring or sending him home with the appropriate follow-up, including an exercise test. Another way of thinking about the issue, however, is that we need to know the consequences of sending him home. Would discharge be a safe course of action, with an acceptably low likelihood of adverse events? Thinking of our question that way, the exposure of interest is time. Time is usually the exposure of interest in studies about patients' prognosis.

What would be our objective in admitting the patient to a coronary care unit? By doing this, we will not be able to prevent more distant events (such as a myocardial infarction a month later). We are interested primarily in events that might occur during the next 72 hours, the maximum time the patient is likely to be monitored in the absence of complications. What adverse events might we prevent if the patient is in a hospital bed with cardiac monitoring? Should he develop severe chest pain, cardiac failure, or myocardial infarction, we would be able to treat him immediately. Most important, should he develop ventricular fibrillation or another life-threatening arrhythmia we would be able to administer cardioversion and save his life.

**Improved (Searchable) Question:** A searchable question would specify the relevant patient population, the management strategy and exposure, and the patient-relevant consequences of that exposure as follows:

- *Patients:* Young men with atypical symptoms and normal ECG and cardiac enzymes presenting with possible unstable angina

- *Intervention/Exposure:* Either admission to a monitored bed vs discharge home, or time

- *Outcomes:* Severe angina, myocardial infarction, heart failure, or arrhythmia, all within the next 72 hours

## Example 3: Squamous Cell Carcinoma

A 60-year-old, 40-pack-year smoker presents with hemoptysis. A chest radiograph shows a parenchymal mass with a normal mediastinum, and a fine needle aspiration of the mass shows squamous cell carcinoma. Aside from the hemoptysis, the patient is asymptomatic and physical examination is entirely normal.

Initial Question: What investigations should we undertake before deciding whether to offer this patient surgery?

Digging Deeper: The key defining features of this patient are his non-small-cell carcinoma and the fact that his history, physical examination, and chest radiograph show no evidence of intrathoracic or extrathoracic metastatic disease. Alternative investigational strategies address two separate issues: Does the patient have occult mediastinal disease, and does he have occult extrathoracic metastatic disease? For this discussion, we will focus on the former issue. Investigational strategies for addressing the possibility of occult mediastinal disease include undertaking a mediastinoscopy or performing a computed tomographic (CT) scan of the chest and proceeding according to the results of this investigation.

What outcomes are we trying to influence in our choice of investigational approach? We would like to prolong the patient's life, but the extent of his underlying tumor is likely to be the major determinant of survival and our investigations cannot change that. The reason we wish to detect occult mediastinal metastases if they are present is that if the cancer has spread to the mediastinum, resectional surgery is very unlikely to benefit the patient. Thus, in the presence of mediastinal disease, patients will usually receive palliative approaches and avoid an unnecessary thoracotomy. Thus, the primary outcome of interest is an unnecessary thoracotomy.

Improved (Searchable) Question: A searchable question would specify the relevant patient population, the management strategy and exposure, and the patient-relevant consequences of that exposure as follows:

- *Patients:* Newly diagnosed non-small-cell lung cancer with no evidence of extrapulmonary metastases

- *Intervention*: Mediastinoscopy for all or chest CT-directed management

- *Outcome:* Unnecessary thoracotomy

Another way of structuring this question is as an examination of the test properties of the chest CT scan. Looking at the problem this way, the patient population is the same, but the exposure is the CT scan and the outcome is the presence or absence of the target condition, mediastinal metastatic disease. As we will subsequently discuss (see Part 1C2, "Diagnostic Tests"), this latter way of structuring the question is less likely to provide strong guidance about optimal management.

These examples illustrate that constructing a searchable question that allows you to use the medical literature to generate an answer is often no simple matter.

It requires an in-depth understanding of the clinical issues involved in patient management. The three examples above illustrate that each patient may trigger a large number of clinical questions, and that clinicians must give careful thought to what they really want to know. Bearing the structure of the question in mind—patient, intervention or exposure, and outcome—is extremely helpful in arriving at an answerable question.

Once the question is posed, the next step in the process is translating the question into an effective search strategy. By first looking at the components of the question, putting the search strategy together is easier.

## SEARCHING FOR THE ANSWER

In this section, we will introduce you to the electronic resources available for quickly finding the answers to your clinical questions. We will demonstrate how the careful definition of the question, including specification of the population, the intervention, and the outcome, can help you develop a workable search strategy. However, you must also consider a fourth component. What sort of study do you hope to find? By sort of study, we mean the way the study is organized or constructed—the study design.

### Determining Question Type

To fully understand issues of study design, we suggest that you read the entire Part 1 of this book. Following is a brief introduction.

There are four fundamental types of clinical questions. They involve:

- **Therapy:** determining the effect of different treatments on improving patient function or avoiding adverse events

- **Harm:** ascertaining the effects of potentially harmful agents (including the very therapies we would be interested in examining in the first type of question) on patient function, morbidity, and mortality

- **Diagnosis:** establishing the power of an intervention to differentiate between those with and without a target condition or disease

- **Prognosis:** estimating the future course of a patient's disease

To answer questions about a therapeutic issue, we identify studies in which a process analogous to flipping a coin determines participants' receipt of an experimental treatment or a control or standard treatment, the so-called *randomized controlled trial* or *RCT* (see Part 1B1, "Therapy"). Once the investigator allocates participants to treatment or control groups, he or she follows them forward in time looking for whether they have, for instance, a stroke or heart attack—what we call the *outcome* of interest (Figure 1A-2).

**FIGURE 1A–2**

**Randomized Controlled Trial**

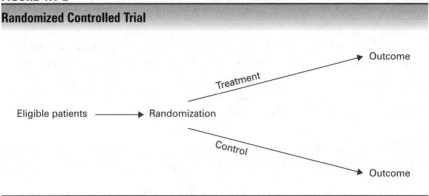

Ideally, we would also look to randomized trials to address issues of harm. However, for many potentially harmful exposures, randomly allocating patients is neither practical nor ethical. For instance, one could not suggest to potential study participants that an investigator will decide by the flip of a coin whether or not they smoke during the next 20 years or whether they will be exposed to potentially harmful ionizing radiation. For exposures like smoking and radiation, the best one can do is identify studies in which personal choice, or happenstance, determines whether people are exposed or not exposed. These observational studies provide weaker evidence than randomized trials.

Figure 1A-3 depicts a common observational study design in which patients with and without the exposure of interest are followed forward in time to determine whether they experience the outcome of interest. For smoking or radiation exposure, one important outcome would likely be the development of cancer.

**FIGURE 1A–3**

**Observational Study: Assessing Exposure**

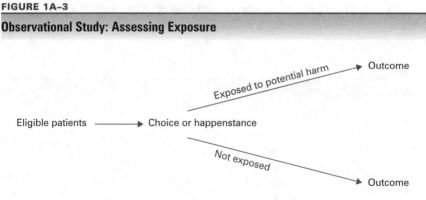

For establishing how well a diagnostic test works (what we call its properties or operating characteristics) we need yet another study design. In diagnostic test studies, investigators identify a group of patients who may or may not have the disease or condition of interest (such as tuberculosis, lung cancer, or iron-deficiency anemia), which we will call the *target condition*. Investigators begin by collecting a group of patients whom they suspect may have the target condition. These patients undergo both the new diagnostic test and a *gold standard* (that is, the test considered to be the diagnostic standard for a particular disease of condition; synonyms include *criterion standard, diagnostic standard*, or *reference standard*). Investigators evaluate the diagnostic test by comparing its classification of patients with that of the gold standard (Figure 1A-4).

**FIGURE 1A–4**

## Study Design to Assess a Diagnostic Test

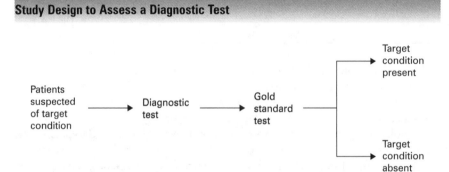

A final type of study examines patients' prognosis and may identify factors that modify that prognosis. Here, investigators identify patients who belong to a particular group (such as pregnant women, patients undergoing surgery, or patients with cancer) with or without factors that may modify their prognosis (such as age or comorbidity). The exposure here is time, and investigators follow patients to determine if they experience the target outcome, such as a problem birth at the end of a pregnancy, a myocardial infarction after surgery, or survival in cancer (Figure 1A-5).

**FIGURE 1A–5**

## Observational Study Assessing Prognosis

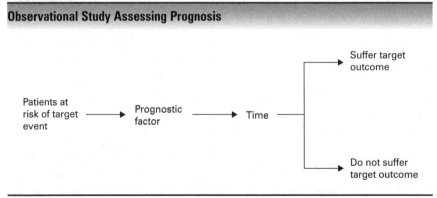

One of the clinician's tasks in searching the medical literature is to correctly identify the category of study that will address her question. For example, if you look for a randomized trial to inform you of the properties of a diagnostic test (as opposed to whether patients benefit from its application), you are unlikely to find the answer you seek.

Think back to the questions we identified in the previous section. Determining the best strategy for managing hypertension is clearly a treatment issue. However, we may also be interested in rare and delayed adverse effects of the medications we use to lower blood pressure, which is an issue of harm.

Considering the second scenario we presented, we can formulate the question in two ways. If we ask, How likely is myocardial infarction or death among young men with symptoms suggestive but atypical of unstable angina? the issue is one of prognosis. If we ask, What is the impact of alternative management strategies, such as admission to a coronary care unit or discharge? we are interested in treatment and would look for a randomized trial that allocated patients to the alternative approaches.

We can also formulate the question from the third scenario in two ways. If we ask, How well does CT scanning of the chest distinguish between non-small-cell lung cancer patients with and without mediastinal metastases? we would look for a study design that can gauge the power of a diagnostic test (see Figure 1A-4). We might also ask, "What is the rate of unnecessary thoracotomy in non-small-cell lung cancer patients who go straight to mediastinoscopy vs those who have CT scan-directed management?" For this treatment issue, we will seek a randomized trial (see Figure 1A-2).

## Is Searching the Medical Literature Worthwhile?

Because our time for searching is limited, we would like to ensure that there is a good chance that our search will be productive. Consider the following clinical questions:

**Example:** In patients with pulmonary embolism, to what extent do those with pulmonary infarction have a poorer outcome than those without pulmonary infarction?

Before formulating our search strategy and beginning our literature search to answer this question, we should think about how investigators would differentiate between those with and without infarction. Since there is no reliable way, short of autopsy, of making this differentiation, our literature search is doomed before we even begin.

**Example:** Consider also a 50-year-old woman who has suffered an uncomplicated myocardial infarction 4 days previously and who asks, before discharge home, when she can resume sexual intercourse.

Were we to formulate a question that would allow us to address her inquiry, its components would look something like this:

- *Patients:* Women after uncomplicated myocardial infarction

- *Intervention:* Advice to resume intercourse as soon as so inclined vs waiting, say, 8 weeks

- *Outcomes:* Recurrent infarction, unstable angina, cardiovascular and total mortality, health-related quality of life

- *Type of question:* Therapy, therefore we would look for a randomized trial.

How likely is it that investigators have conducted a randomized trial of this question? Highly improbable. It is slightly less implausible that investigators have conducted an observational study of timing of return to sexual intercourse (here, patients would report when they had returned to sexual intercourse and investigators would compare outcomes in those who had started early vs those who had waited until later).

These two examples illustrate situations in which you will not want to use the medical literature to solve your patient management problems. The medical literature will not help you when there is no feasible study design that investigators could use to resolve the issue. Your search will also be fruitless if there is a feasible design, but it is very unlikely that anyone has taken the time and effort to carry out the necessary study. Before embarking on a search, carefully consider whether the yield is likely to be worth the time expenditure.

# SOURCES OF EVIDENCE

You can look to local specialists, subspecialists, and more experienced clinical colleagues not only for opinion, but also for evidence to address your clinical problem (see Part 1A, "The Philosophy of Evidence-Based Medicine"). Their experience and advice are particularly crucial when the medical literature is unlikely to be helpful. Furthermore, experts who stay current on the latest evidence in their field may be able to quickly provide you with the most relevant citations.

Clinicians will not need this book to advise them to consult respected colleagues—they do not neglect this source of data. Where clinicians might need help is in the use of online resources. We focus on online rather than print products because they are generally easier to search and more current than print products (Table 1A-3).[4] With the relatively recent appearance of many of the resources we recommend, however, little research specifically addresses their relative merits. The approaches we describe reflect our own experiences and those of our colleagues working individually or with medical trainees.

**TABLE 1A-3**

## Online Medical Information Resource Contact Information

| Resource | Internet Address | Annual Cost* |
|---|---|---|
| *ACP Journal Club* | www.acponline.org/journals/acpjc/jcmenu.htm | $65 |
| Best Evidence | www.acponline.org/catalog/electronic/best_evidence.htm | $85 |
| Cochrane Library | www.update-software.com/cochrane/cochrane-frame.html | $225 |
| UpToDate | www.uptodate.com | $495 |
| MEDLINE<br>  PubMed | www.ncbi.nlm.nih.gov/PubMed | Free |
|   Internet<br>  Grateful Med | igm.nlm.nih.gov | Free |
|   Other sources | www.medmatrix.org/info/medlinetable.asp | Free |
| *Scientific American Medicine* | www.samed.com | $245<br>($159 for online access alone) |
| Clinical Evidence | www.evidence.org | $115 |
| Harrison's Online | www.harrisonsonline.com | $89 |
| *emedicine* | www.emedicine.com | Free |
| Medscape | www.medscape.com/Home/Topics/homepages.html | Free |
| Medical Matrix | www.medmatrix.org/index.asp | Free |
| ScHARR Netting the Evidence | www.shef.ac.uk/~scharr/ir/netting/ | Free |
| Medical World Search | www.mwsearch.com | Free |
| Journal listings | www.nthames-health.tpmde.ac.uk/connect/journals.htm<br>www.pslgroup.com/dg/medjournals.htm | Free |
| Clinical practice guidelines | www.guidelines.gov<br>www.cma.ca/cpgs | Free |
| MD Consult | www.mdconsult.com | $200 |
| Evidence-based Medicine Reviews (OVID) | www.ovid.com/products/clinical/ebmr.cfm<br>(available through many medical libraries) | $1995 |

* Costs as of 2000

## Selecting the Best Medical Information Resource

What is the optimal medical information resource? To a large extent, it depends on the type of question that you have and the time you have available.[5] During the late 1980s, observational studies suggested that clinicians could identify one to two unanswered questions per patient in an outpatient setting[6] and up to five per patient in a hospital setting.[7] More recent studies in family practice in the United Kingdom[8] and the United States[9] have found the rate of questions arising in patient care to be 0.32 question per patient.

Be sure to match your question to the source of information that could likely provide the most appropriate answer. To take extreme examples, MEDLINE is not the best source of information on gross anatomy, and the hospital information system is the best place to provide laboratory data for a specific patient. Table 1A-4 summarizes the types of questions that clinicians ask, along with the optimal study designs, online sources of data, and MEDLINE searching terms to match the methodologic type.

**TABLE 1A-4**

## Asking Focused and Answerable Clinical Questions

| Question Type | Population | Intervention/ Exposure | Outcome | Best Feasible Study Designs | Suitable Databases | Best Single MEDLINE Search Term for Appropriate Study Type |
|---|---|---|---|---|---|---|
| Diagnosis | In patients with lung cancer | What is the test performance of CT scan | For detecting mediastinal metastatic disease | Cross-sectional analytic study | Best Evidence, UpToDate, MEDLINE | Sensitivity.tw |
| Harm | In men | Does vasectomy | Cause testicular cancer | Cohort study, population-based case-control study | Best Evidence, UpToDate, MEDLINE | Risk.tw |
| Prognosis | In young men with atypical chest pain | Sent home from the emergency department, in the next 72 hours | Suffer appreciable rates of unstable angina, heart failure, arrhythmia, myocardial infarction, or sudden death | Cohort study | Best Evidence, UpToDate, MEDLINE | Explode cohort studies |
| Treatment | In patients with hypertension and type 2 diabetes mellitus | Does a target DBP of 80 compared with DBP of 90 mm Hg | Lower risk of stroke, MI, cardiovascular death, and all-cause mortality | RCT or systematic review of RCTs | Cochrane Library, Best Evidence, UpToDate, MEDLINE | Meta-analysis.pt (for systematic reviews) or Clinical trial.pt (for RCTs) |

CT indicates computed tomographic; DBP, diastric blood pressure; MI, myocardial infarction; RCT, randomized controlled trial

To answer focused foreground clinical questions, the most efficient approach is to begin with a prefiltered evidence-based medicine resource such as Best Evidence, the Cochrane Library, or Clinical Evidence (see Table 1A-3). By pre-filtered, we mean that someone has reviewed the literature and chosen only the methodologically strongest studies. The authors of these products have designed them in such a way as to make searching easy. The sources are updated regularly—from months to a couple of years—with methodologically sound and clinically important studies.

**Textbooks.** To find answers to general background medical questions, prefiltered evidence-based medicine resources are unlikely to be helpful. Referring to a textbook that is well referenced and updated frequently is likely to be faster and more rewarding. UpToDate and *Scientific American Medicine* are updated regularly—from months to years, depending on the rapidity with which important new evidence is accumulating; they are heavily referenced so that you can assess how current the material is and you can even read the original articles. Other textbooks available in electronic formats, such as *Harrison's Principles of Internal Medicine*, can also provide valuable general background information. Additionally, new textbooks that are entirely Internet based, such as *emedicine*, are now available. As texts become more evidence based and routinely are updated as new evidence is published, they will provide an increasingly important source of answers to foreground as well as background questions. Our own experience suggests that UpToDate and Clinical Evidence are already well along the path to becoming evidence-based sources to answer foreground questions.

**MEDLINE.** MEDLINE, the bibliographic database maintained by the US National Library of Medicine, is useful primarily to answer focused foreground questions. The size and complexity of this database, however, make searching somewhat more difficult and time consuming. As a result, we recommend using MEDLINE only when searching prefiltered sources has proved fruitless (or when prior knowledge suggests, before beginning the search, that prefiltered sources will prove barren).

We will now review the databases suitable for answering a specific clinical question, illustrating their use with the example of the optimal blood pressure target level in patients with diabetes.

## Using Prefiltered Medical Information Resources

A good starting point in the evidence-seeking process is to look for a systematic review article on your topic. A systematic review addresses a targeted clinical question using strategies that decrease the likelihood of bias. The authors of a rigorous systematic review will have already done the work of accumulating and summarizing the best of the published (and ideally unpublished) evidence. You will find both Best Evidence and the Cochrane Library useful for finding high-quality systematic reviews quickly and effectively. Both are also good sources to consult for original studies.

**Best Evidence**

Best Evidence is one of the quickest available routes to systematic reviews and original studies that address focused clinical questions. Available in CD-ROM format or on the Internet through OVID Technology's Evidence-Based Medicine Reviews, Best Evidence is the cumulative electronic version of two paper-based secondary journals: *ACP Journal Club* and *Evidence-Based Medicine.* (These journals were combined into one journal, *ACP Journal Club,* in North, South, and Central America in January 2000. *Evidence-Based Medicine* is available only outside the United States.) The editorial team for these journals systematically searches 170 medical journals on a regular basis to identify original studies and systematic reviews that are both methodologically sound and clinically relevant, especially for the more common diseases and conditions. By methodologically sound, we mean that they meet validity criteria (see Part 1B1, "Therapy"; Part 1B2, "Harm"; Part 1C, "The Process of Diagnosis"; Part 1C1, "Differential Diagnosis"; Part 1C2, "Diagnostic Tests"; and Part 1D, "Prognosis"). For example, the treatment section includes only randomized trials with 80% follow-up, and the diagnosis section includes only studies that make an independent, blind comparison of a test with a gold standard.

*ACP Journal Club* and *Evidence-Based Medicine* present structured abstracts of studies that meet these criteria, along with an accompanying commentary by an expert who offers a clinical perspective on the study results. In a section of Best Evidence entitled "Other Articles Noted," clinicians can find other studies that meet methodologic criteria but have been judged less relevant. Best Evidence is updated annually and now includes over 2000 abstracted articles that relate to general internal medicine, dating back to 1991. The editors review each article every 5 years to make sure that it has not become dated in view of more recent evidence. In addition to general internal medicine, Best Evidence includes a broader range of articles since 1995 that encompass obstetrics and gynecology, family medicine, pediatrics, psychiatry, and surgery.

Because Best Evidence includes only articles that reviewers have decided meet basic standards of methodologic quality, it is substantially smaller than many other medical literature databases, and thus is easier to search. The downside of this small size is that it is not comprehensive; a search restricted to Best Evidence will not be complete and will put you at risk for receiving a biased selection of articles. However, we believe that the uniformly relatively high methodologic quality of the articles, and the very quick searches that Best Evidence allows, compensate for this limitation.

**Example of Best Evidence Search.** To locate information on blood pressure control in people with type 2 diabetes mellitus, we used the "Search" option in Best Evidence 4 (Figure 1A-6). We entered the phrase representing the question aspects,

*"hypertension AND diabetes AND mortality"*

resulting in a list of 109 articles. Many of these citations, however, dealt with the prognosis of patients with diabetes and were not directly relevant to our question.

Therefore, we returned to the search option, entered the same terms but changed the search strategy from "All topics" to "Selected topics," and clicked on the "Therapeutics" option before completing the search. This yielded a shorter list of 27 articles, all pertaining to therapy (Figure 1A-7). Five were review articles but none of these addressed our topic. Of the 22 original studies, the first was entitled "Tight Blood Pressure Control Reduced Diabetes Mellitus-Related Death and Complications and Was Cost-effective in Diabetes" (Figure 1A-8). Double-clicking on this title produced a structured abstract[10] describing a randomized trial that enrolled persons with type 2 diabetes mellitus and hypertension and evaluated the effect of aiming for either a blood pressure of less than 150/85 mm Hg or a blood pressure of less than 180/105 mm Hg (Figure 1A-9). After an average of 9 years of follow-up, the tight blood pressure control arm had a 32% reduction in the risk of death related to diabetes (95% confidence interval, 8%-50%; $P=.019$) (Figure 1A-10).

**FIGURE 1A–6**

## Best Evidence—Title Page (CD-ROM version)

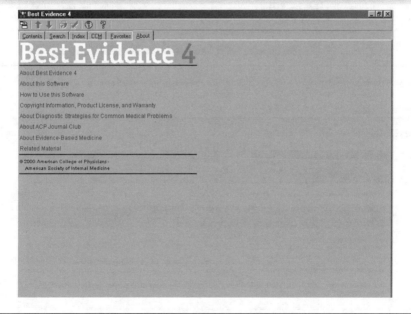

**FIGURE 1A–7**

## Best Evidence—Selected Topic Search

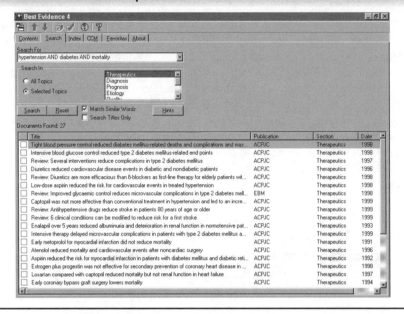

Reproduced with permission from the American College of Physicians-Society of Internal Medicine.

**FIGURE 1A–8**

## Best Evidence—Search Result

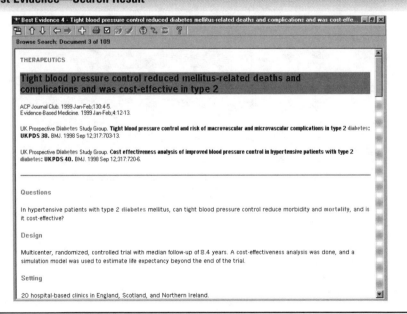

Reproduced with permission from the American College of Physicians-Society of Internal Medicine.

**FIGURE 1A-9**

## Best Evidence—Abstract

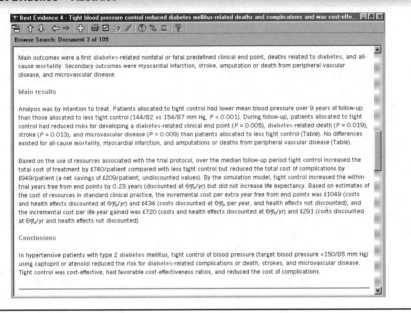

Reproduced with permission from the American College of Physicians-Society of Internal Medicine.

**FIGURE 1A-10**

## Best Evidence—Results Table

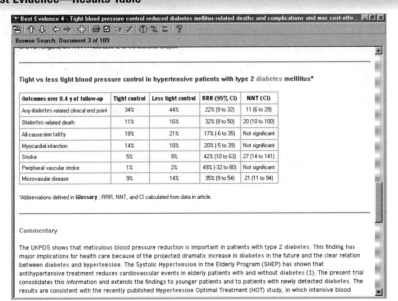

Reproduced with permission from the American College of Physicians-Society of Internal Medicine.

Searching Best Evidence will not always provide an article that answers your question. High-quality evidence is not available or may not have been published in one of the 170 Best Evidence target journals. A relevant trial may have been published after the most recent edition of Best Evidence was released, or before 1991. Rigorous studies published since 1991 will not appear in Best Evidence if the editors believe that they pertain more to subspecialty care than to general internal medicine. Despite these limitations, searching Best Evidence will often be rewarding, especially if you are searching for one of the more common diseases and conditions. And if your search is not rewarding, Best Evidence searches occur so quickly that you will have plenty of time to look elsewhere.

## Cochrane Library

The Cochrane Collaboration, an international organization that prepares, maintains, and disseminates systematic reviews of health care interventions, offers another electronic resource for locating high-quality information quickly. They publish the Cochrane Library, which focuses primarily on systematic reviews of controlled trials of therapeutic interventions. It provides little help in addressing other aspects of medical care, such as the value of a new diagnostic test or a patient's prognosis.

Updated quarterly, the Cochrane Library is available in CD-ROM format or over the Internet. It contains three main sections. The first of these, the Cochrane Database of Systematic Reviews (CDSR), includes the complete reports for all of the systematic reviews that have been prepared by members of the Cochrane Collaboration (716 were in the first issue for 2000) and the protocols for Cochrane systematic reviews that are under way. A second part of the Cochrane Library, the Database of Reviews of Effectiveness (DARE), includes systematic reviews that have been published outside of the collaboration; the first issue for 2000 included 2565 such reviews. Database of Reviews of Effectiveness is searchable outside the Cochrane Library (at http://nhscrd.york.ac.uk); this site also includes access to a database of economic evaluations and health technology assessments.

The third section of the Library, the Cochrane Controlled Trials Registry (CCTR), contains a growing list of over 268,000 references to clinical trials that Cochrane investigators have found by searching a wide range of sources. The sources include the MEDLINE and EMBASE (Excerpta Medica) bibliographic databases, hand searches, and the reference lists of potentially relevant original studies and reviews. Although most citations refer to randomized trials, the database also includes a small number of observational studies. Studies of diagnostic tests will likely be included soon. In addition to the three main sections, the Cochrane Library also includes information about the Cochrane Collaboration and information on how to conduct a systematic review and related methodologic issues.

To search the Cochrane Library, you can enter terms in the first screen that appears after selecting "Search" (Figure 1A-11). If you have access to the CD-ROM version, using the Advanced Search option you can create more complex search strategies that include Medical Subject Headings and logical operators (see the section on MEDLINE for an introduction to Medical Subject Headings and logical operators).

Example of Cochrane Library Search. To find information about blood pressure control in people with diabetes, we entered the search terms

"diabetes AND hypertension AND mortality"

using the 2000 version of the Cochrane Library (Issue 1) (Figure 1A-12). This yielded 36 reports in the CDSR, six citations in the DARE, and 130 citations in the CCTR (Figure 1A-13). A Cochrane review entitled "Antihypertensive therapy in diabetes mellitus"[11] appeared promising (Figure 1A-14). Double-clicking on this item, we found an entire Cochrane Collaboration systematic review, including information on the methodology for the review, the inclusion and exclusion criteria, the results, and a discussion (Figure 1A-15). The results presented the findings in both textual and graphical forms. As was the case with the review article found in Best Evidence, however, this review did not help to resolve the issue of the optimal blood pressure goal for people with diabetes mellitus.

**FIGURE 1A–11**

## The Cochrane Database of Systematic Reviews

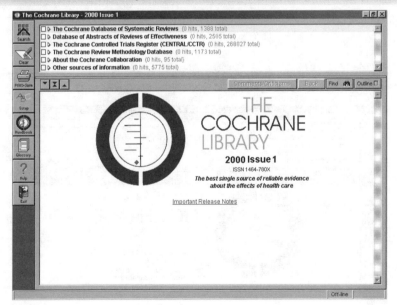

**FIGURE 1A–12**

## The Cochrane Database of Systematic Reviews—Search Strategy

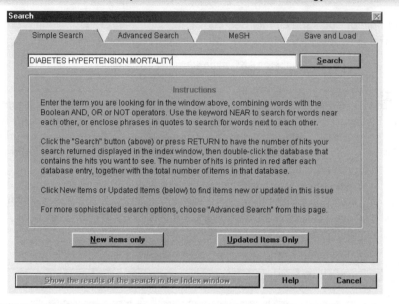

Reproduced with permission from Update Software.

**FIGURE 1A–13**

## The Cochrane Database of Systematic Reviews—Search Results

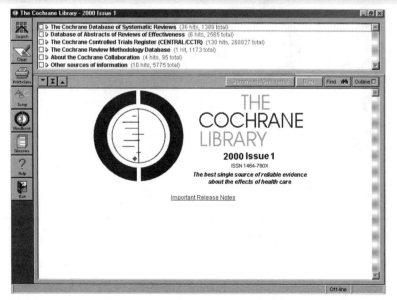

Reproduced with permission from Update Software.

**FIGURE 1A–14**

## The Cochrane Database of Systematic Reviews—Article

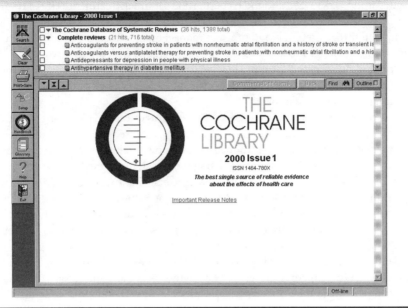

Reproduced with permission from Update Software.

**FIGURE 1A–15**

## The Cochrane Database of Systematic Reviews—Review Article

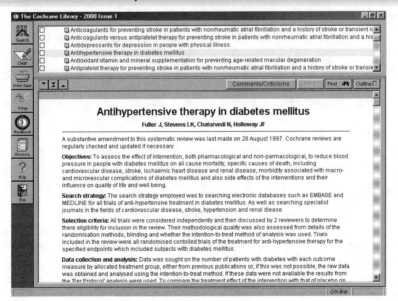

Reproduced with permission from Update Software.

Turning to the CCTR (we double-clicked on the CCTR option to make the citation titles appear), we found both the United Kingdom Prospective Diabetes Study Group (UKPDS)[10] and the Hypertension Optimal Treatment (HOT) trial[12] within the first 26 citations. The HOT trial was a randomized trial that compared three different blood pressure management strategies in persons with hypertension. Subgroup analyses showed that patients with diabetes who reduced their blood pressure to 81.1 mm Hg vs 85.2 mm Hg because of being in the groups randomized to lower target blood pressures had lower rates of cardiovascular events and cardiovascular death.

A second search further illustrates the usefulness of the CCTR database. Recall the patient with non-small-cell lung cancer for whom we were considering alternative investigational strategies of mediastinoscopy for all, or a selective approach based on the results of CT scanning. Using the search term "mediastinoscopy," we found that the clinical trials database yielded 20 citations, of which the fourth and fifth were MEDLINE and EMBASE records of a study a randomized trial in 685 patients with apparently operable non-small-cell carcinoma of the lung. The investigators randomized patients to an arm in which all patients underwent mediastinoscopy or an arm in which all patients underwent CT scanning, with patients with small nodes going straight to thoracotomy and those with larger nodes undergoing mediastinoscopy. The relative risk of an unnecessary thoracotomy in patients in the CT scanning arm was 0.88 (95% confidence interval, 0.71-1.10). The mediastinoscopy strategy cost $708 more per patient (95% confidence interval, $723-$2140). The authors concluded that "the computed tomography strategy is likely to produce the same number of or fewer unnecessary thoracotomies in comparison with doing mediastinoscopy on all patients and is also likely to be as or less expensive."[13]

## UpToDate

UpToDate is a well-referenced online textbook that is carefully updated every 4 months. It exists in digital format because it is too large to print. Although UpToDate, unlike Best Evidence and the Cochrane Database of Systematic Reviews, does not have a set of explicit methodologic quality criteria that included articles must meet, it does reference many high-quality studies chosen by its section authors.

*Example of UpToDate Search.* To locate information on blood pressure control in people with type 2 diabetes mellitus, we entered the term "diabetes" in the search window for version 8.3 (Figure 1A-16). This resulted in a list of 21 key word options and we selected "diabetes mellitus, type 2." This yielded 64 articles, including one entitled "Treatment of Hypertension in Diabetes" that reviewed pathogenesis and included a section on the goal of blood pressure reduction (Figures 1A-17 and 1A-18). This section provided a detailed description of the two large randomized trials, the HOT[12] and UKPDS,[10] trials, that specifically addressed the clinical outcomes associated with more aggressive compared with less aggressive blood pressure management strategies. The text summarized the design and findings, and we were able to retrieve the study abstracts by clicking on the references.

**FIGURE 1A–16**

## UpToDate

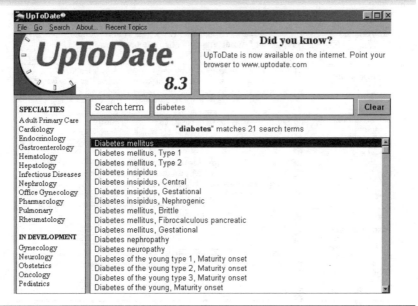

Reproduced with permission from UpToDate.

**FIGURE 1A–17**

## UpToDate—Search Results

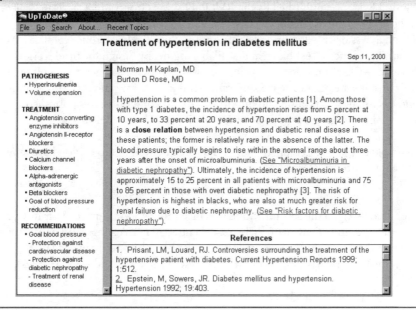

Reproduced with permission from UpToDate.

**FIGURE 1A–18**

**UpToDate—Search Results (continued)**

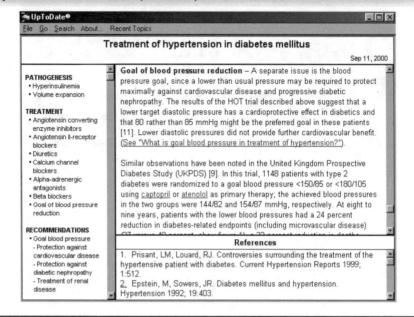

Reproduced with permission from UpToDate.

## Clinical Evidence

Clinical Evidence, published by the *BMJ* Publishing Group and American College of Physicians/American Society of Internal Medicine, is similar to UpToDate, although less oriented to provide bottom-line clinical advice from experts. Clinical Evidence is text based and available online. By design the producers have not written a textbook; instead, they aim to provide a concise account of the current state of knowledge, ignorance, and uncertainty about the prevention and treatment of common and important clinical conditions. It is published biannually and online products are now available (www.evidence.org).

**Example of Clinical Evidence Search.** For the question of target blood pressure in people with diabetes, a search using the terms

"target blood pressure AND diabetes"

took us directly to the section entitled "Which interventions improve cardiovascular outcomes in patients with diabetes?" (Figure 1A-19). A subsection on treatment of hypertension includes a discussion of target levels backed up by evidence from the trials we have found in the other resources (HOT and UKPDS trials).

**FIGURE 1A–19**

## Clinical Evidence—Search Results

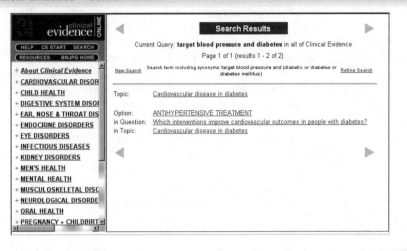

Reproduced with permission from the BMJ Publishing Group.

## Using Unfiltered Medical Information Sources

### MEDLINE

If a search of Best Evidence, the Cochrane Library, UpToDate, and Clinical Evidence does not provide a satisfactory answer to a focused clinical question, it is time to turn to MEDLINE. The US National Library of Medicine maintains this impressive bibliographic database, which includes over 11,000,000 citations of both clinical and preclinical studies. A complementary database known as PreMEDLINE includes citations and abstracts for studies that have been published recently but not yet indexed. MEDLINE is an attractive database for finding medical information because of its relatively comprehensive coverage of medical journals and because it is readily accessible. Anyone with Internet access can search MEDLINE free of charge using PubMed or Internet Grateful Med. In addition, most health sciences or hospital libraries provide access to MEDLINE through a commercial vendor such as OVID, Knowledge Finder, or Silver Platter.

These positive features are balanced with a disadvantage that relates to MEDLINE's size and to the range of publications that it encompasses. Searching MEDLINE effectively often requires careful thought, along with a thorough knowledge of how the database is structured and how publications are indexed. Understanding how to use Medical Subject Headings is essential, as is text word searching and exploding and use of the logical operators AND and OR to combine different search results.

If you are unfamiliar with MEDLINE searching techniques, an article by Greenhalgh[14] presents a good introduction. If you suspect that you may have gaps in your searching skills, strongly consider spending some time with an experienced medical librarian or taking a course on MEDLINE searching. Another potential source for information on searching techniques is to visit an Internet Web site designed to introduce the topic. A listing of tutorials designed to assist users of different MEDLINE systems and at different experience levels is available (www.docnet.org.uk/drfelix/medtut.html). More detailed information on searching MEDLINE and a number of other large bibliographic databases, including EMBASE (Excerpta Medica), is also available in a reference book.[15] In this section, we present only the most crucial and basic MEDLINE searching advice.

The MEDLINE indexers choose Medical Subject Headings (MeSH) for each article. These headings provide one strategy for searching. Note, however, that indexers reference articles under the most specific subject heading available (for example, "ventricular dysfunction, left" rather than the more general term "ventricular dysfunction"). As a result, if you choose the more general heading ("ventricular dysfunction") you risk missing out on many articles of interest. To deal with this problem, use a command known as *explode*. This command identifies all articles that have been indexed using a given MeSH term, as well as articles indexed using more specific terms. For example, in the PubMed MEDLINE system for the 1966 to 2000 file, the MeSH heading "sports" contains 10,806 indexed articles, whereas "explode sports," which picks up more than 20 specific sports from baseball and basketball through weight lifting and wrestling, contains 37,043 indexed articles.

Another fundamental search strategy substitutes reliance on the decisions made by MEDLINE indexers with the choices of study authors regarding terminology. Using "text word" searching makes it possible to identify all articles in which either the study title or abstract includes a certain term. Experience with MEDLINE allows a clinician to develop preferred search strategies. Comprehensive searches will usually utilize both MeSH headings and text words.

**Example of MEDLINE Search.** To search for information pertaining to blood pressure control targets in people with type 2 diabetes mellitus, we used the National Library of Medicine's PubMed MEDLINE searching system. We began by entering the term "diabetes mellitus" and clicking the "Go" button. This yielded a total of 143,691 citations dating back to 1966 (Figure 1A-20). Notice that before searching MEDLINE and PreMEDLINE, the PubMed system processed our request. Rather than simply completing a text word search, PubMed developed a more comprehensive strategy that also included the most appropriate MeSH term. To further increase the yield of citations, PubMed also automatically exploded the MeSH term. PubMed searched MEDLINE and PreMEDLINE using the strategy:

diabetes mellitus (text word) OR explode diabetes mellitus (MeSH term).

The "OR" in the strategy is called a logical operator. It asks MEDLINE to combine the publications found using either the first search term or the second search term to make a more comprehensive list of publications in which diabetes is a topic of discussion.

**FIGURE 1A-20**

## PubMed—Diabetes Mellitus Search

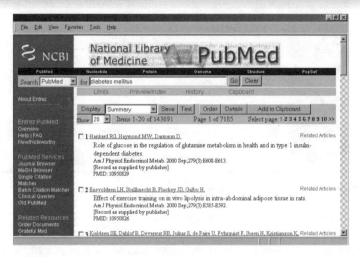

Reproduced with permission from the National Library of Medicine.

We then searched using the term "hypertension" (180,333 references) and the term "mortality" (320,133 references). To combine these three searches, we initially clicked on the "History" button, which showed us a summary. By entering the phrase

"#1 AND #2 AND #3"

into the search window, we were able to ask PubMed to locate only those citations that addressed all of diabetes mellitus, hypertension, and mortality (Figure 1A-21).

**FIGURE 1A-21**

## PubMed—Combining Search Terms

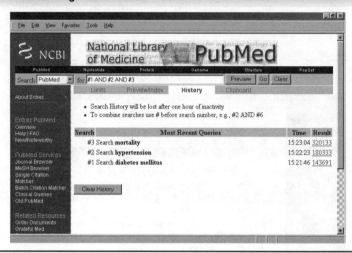

Reproduced with permission from the National Library of Medicine.

Unfortunately, the list of publications that concern all of diabetes, hypertension, and mortality still included 1965 references (Figure 1A-22), prompting us to take advantage of another searching technique designed to help identify particular types of clinical studies. Search hedges or search filters are systematically tested search strategies that help identify methodologically sound studies pertaining to questions of therapy, diagnosis, prognosis, or harm (Figure 1A-23). For example, to retrieve studies related to prognosis, the sensitive search strategy is

> incidence (MeSH) OR explode mortality (MeSH) OR follow-up studies
> (MeSH) OR mortality (subheading) OR prognos: (text word) OR
> predict: (text word) OR course (text word)

and the specific search strategy is

> prognosis (MeSH) OR survival analysis (MeSH).

Sensitive search strategies have comprehensive retrieval with some irrelevant citations, whereas a specific search strategy is not as comprehensive but is less likely to retrieve irrelevant citations. A complete listing of the strategies is available, along with the sensitivities and specificities for each of the different approaches.[16-18] Although the strategies tend to be complex, many MEDLINE searching systems now have them automatically available for use. The PubMed system has a special section with these strategies entitled "Clinical Queries." Access to this option is on the left side of the main searching screen.

## FIGURE 1A-22

# PubMed—Combining Search Terms (Results)

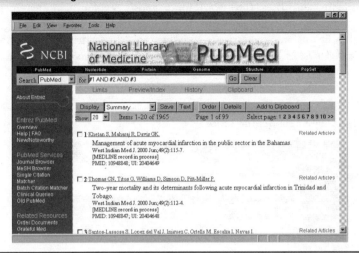

## FIGURE 1A-23

# PubMed—Clinical Queries Search

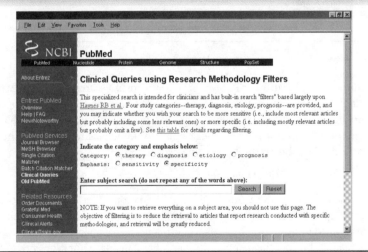

As an alternative to the hedges, clinicians can use "single best terms" for finding higher-quality studies. These terms include "clinical trial" (publication type) for treatment; "sensitivity" (text word) for diagnosis; "explode cohort studies" (MeSH) for prognosis; and "risk" (text word) for harm (see Table 1A-4).

Combining our previous strategy with the term "clinical trial" (publication type) yielded a list of 117 publications (Figure 1A-24). Once again, we found references to the UKPDS trial and the HOT trial in the citation list.

**FIGURE 1A-24**

## PubMed—Single Best Search Term

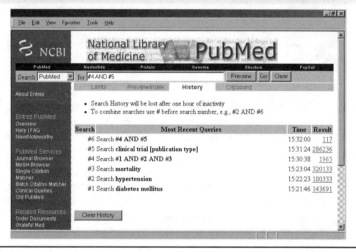

One other useful feature of PubMed is its easy-to-use searching system, which makes knowledge of how to use the various subject heading features and logical operators described above less crucial. The searcher can enter a set of words or phrases into the first window. For example, thinking back to our young man with atypical—possible unstable—angina, we could type

"unstable angina monitor* discharg*"

in the first searching window, and would find 26 citations. The "*" indicates truncation to pick up similar words with varying endings: monitor* picks up "monitor," monitoring, and monitored. The 11th article is a narrative review.[19] By clicking on the "See related" button, the searcher finds another 238 related citations presented in order from the most to least relevant (according to the computer algorithm).

### The World Wide Web

The World Wide Web is rapidly becoming an important source of medical information. A vast number of resources can now be accessed using the Internet—some for a fee, others free of charge. To make these resources more accessible, certain Web sites have been designed specifically to provide links to medical information locations or to facilitate searching for medical information on the Internet. Examples of such Web sites include Medical Matrix, Medscape, ScHARR, and Medical World Search. Clinicians can also use the Internet to access medical journals and clinical practice guidelines.

We must, however, issue a user beware caveat: some of these guidelines may fail to meet *Users' Guides* criteria for evidence-based guidelines (see Part 1F, "Moving From Evidence to Action"). An example of a site that provides access to many resources, including journals, textbooks, and guidelines, albeit for a fee, is MD Consult.

Finally, Web sites produced and maintained by reputable organizations such as the American Cancer Society (www.cancer.org) or the American Diabetes Association (www.diabetes.org) provide another approach for finding information.

# CLINICAL APPLICATION

The health sciences literature is enormous and continues to expand rapidly. To the extent that this reflects ongoing research and the identification of potential improvements for patient care, this is very promising. At the same time, however, it makes the task of locating the best and most current therapy or diagnostic test more challenging. The emergence of new information products specifically designed to provide ready access to high-quality, clinically relevant, and current information is timely and encouraging.

Finding the articles that address your clinical question requires 5 to 30 minutes, depending on the resource you use or your experience with systematic searching.[3] A full assessment of the validity and applicability requires an additional half-hour. The UKPDS study[10] and the HOT study[12] are the closest matches to your patient and the clinical situation. The studies show a clear reduction of diabetes-related mortality with tight blood pressure control in persons with type 2 diabetes mellitus and hypertension. You decide to set target systolic blood pressure at < 150 mm Hg and target diastolic blood pressure at < 80 mm Hg.

# References

1. Haynes RB. Loose connections between peer reviewed clinical journals and clinical practice. *Ann Intern Med.* 1990;113:724-728.

2. Oxman AD, Sackett DL, Guyatt GH, for the Evidence-based Medicine Working Group. Users' guides to the medical literature, I: How to get started. *JAMA.* 1993;270:2093-2095.

3. Richardson WS, Wilson MC, Nishikawa J, Hayward RSA. The well-built clinical question: a key to evidence-based decisions. *ACP Journal Club.* Nov-Dec 1995;123:A-12.

4. McKibbon KA, Richardson WS, Walker Dilks C. Finding answers to well built clinical questions. *Evidence-Based Medicine.* 1999;6:164-167.

5. Sackett DL, Straus SE. Finding and applying evidence during clinical rounds: the "evidence cart." *JAMA.* 1998;280:1336-1338.

6. Covell DG, Uman GC, Manning PR. Information needs in office practice: are they being met? *Ann Intern Med.* 1985;103:596-599.

7. Osheroff JA, Forsythe DE, Buchanan BG, Bankowitz RA, Blumenfeld BH, Miller RA. Physicians' information needs: analysis of questions posed during clinical teaching. *Ann Intern Med.* 1991;114:576-581.

8. Barrie AR, Ward AM. Questioning behaviour in general practice: a pragmatic study. *BMJ.* 1997;315:1515.

9. Ely JW, Osheroff JA, Ebell MH, et al. Analysis of questions asked by family doctors regarding patient care. *BMJ.* 1999;319:358-361.

10. Tight blood pressure control and risk of macrovascular and microvascular complications in Type 2 diabetes mellitus: UKPDS 38. *BMJ.* 1998;317:703-713.

11. Fuller J, Stevens LK, Chaturvedi N, Holloway JF. Antihypertensive therapy in diabetes mellitus (Cochrane Review). In: The Cochrane Library, Issue 4, 1999. Oxford: Update Software.

12. Hansson L, Zanchetti A, Carruthers SG, et al, for the HOT Study Group. Effects of intensive blood-pressure lowering and low-dose aspirin in patients with hypertension: principal results of the Hypertension Optimal Treatment (HOT) randomized trial. *Lancet.* 1998;351:1755-1762.

13. The Canadian Lung Oncology Group. Investigation for mediastinal disease in patients with apparently operable lung cancer. *Ann Thorac Surg.* 1995;60:1382-1389.

14. Greenhalgh T. How to read a paper: the Medline database. *BMJ.* 1997;315:180-183.

15. McKibbon A. *Evidence-based Principles and Practice.* Hamilton: Decker; 1999.

16. Haynes RB, Wilczynski N, McKibbon KA, et al. Developing optimal search strategies for detecting clinically sound studies in MEDLINE. *J Am Med Informatics Assoc*. 1994;1:447-458.

17. Wilczynski NL, Walker CJ, McKibbon KA, Haynes RB. Assessment of methodologic search filters in MEDLINE. *Proc Annu Symp Comp Appl Med Care*. 1994;17:601-605.

18. Devillé WL, Bezemer PD, Bouter LM. Publications on diagnostic test evaluation in family medicine journals: an optimal search strategy. *J Clin Epidemiol*. 2000;53:65-69.

19. Bankwala Z, Swenson LJ. Unstable angina pectoris: what is the likelihood of further cardiac events? *Postgrad Med*. 1995;98:155-158,161-162,164-165.

# THERAPY AND HARM: AN INTRODUCTION

Gordon Guyatt

Peter Wyer also made substantive contributions to this section

## IN THIS SECTION

Clinicians' most compelling questions involve choosing the optimal management strategy for their patients. For example, what are the benefits of prescribing pharmacologic treatment or mandating dietary change to lower blood pressure, cholesterol level, or a patient's weight. What are the benefits of screening women for breast cancer or screening men for prostate cancer, or of instituting a smoking cessation program? What symptomatic benefit or increased longevity might patients anticipate from treatment of their chronic heart failure, asthma, or diabetes? Equally important, what short-term or long-term adverse effects might they expect as a result of their intervention?

These questions address two related issues. First, what risks, if any, will result for patients if they smoke or are overweight, if their blood pressure, cholesterol level, or glucose level is elevated, or if their heart function is abnormal? These are issues of harm. Second, if we intervene to modify their behavior or their bodies' physiology, what benefits will ensue, and will these benefits outweigh any deleterious consequences? These are issues of therapy.

When we address questions of both therapy and harm, we are confronting issues of causation. There are myriad examples. In a particular group of people (healthy men or women, patients with diabetes, or patients with heart failure, for example) is there a causal relationship between an exposure (smoking, obesity, or high blood pressure) or intervention (an antismoking or weight loss program, or a drug that lowers blood pressure) and a particular anticipated outcome (lung cancer, myocardial infarction, or stroke) or unanticipated outcome (eg, the profound visual loss resulting from one antihypertensive medication[1]).

For each of these questions, there is an underlying true answer. If our inferences about the underlying truth are wrong, the consequences may be disastrous. Consider how many lives must have been lost over the course of several hundred years when physicians were convinced that blood-letting was an effective treatment for an extraordinarily wide variety of illnesses. It is impossible to estimate the numbers. By contrast, records of the number of prescriptions and an evaluation of the magnitude of harm from a randomized trial make it possible to estimate the thousands of lives lost resulting from the much more recent administration of class I antiarrhythmia drugs—agents that physicians believed would prevent lethal arrhythmias when, in fact, they were causing them.[2]

Why has the medical community made such disastrous blunders, and what can we do to prevent their repetition? The answer lies in clinicians learning rules of evidence that allow them to differentiate false claims from valid ones. If you are content with a practical approach to determining when you can believe study results and when you cannot, read on. If, however, you would like a deeper conceptual understanding of the foundation of our *Users' Guides to the Medical Literature,* turn now to Part 2B, "Therapy and Harm, Why Study Results Mislead: Bias and Random Error."

# THREE STEPS IN USING AN ARTICLE FROM THE MEDICAL LITERATURE

When using the medical literature to answer a clinical question, approach the study using three discrete steps.

In the first step, ask, *"Are the results of the study valid?"* This question has to do with the believability or credibility of the results. In answering this question, you consider whether the estimate of the treatment effect reported in the article faithfully represents the direction and magnitude of the underlying true effect. Another way to state this question is: "Do these results represent an unbiased estimate of the treatment effect, or have they been influenced in some systematic fashion to lead to a false conclusion?" If the results are valid and the study likely yields an unbiased assessment of the treatment effect, then the results are worth examining further.

In the second step, ask, *"What are the results?"* to consider the size and precision of the treatment's effect. The best estimate of that effect will be the study findings themselves; the precision of the estimate may be superior in larger studies.

Once you understand the results, ask yourself the third question, *"How can I apply these results to patient care?"* This question has two parts. First, can you generalize (or, to put it another way, particularize) the results to your patient? For instance, you should hesitate to institute a treatment if your patient is too dissimilar from those who participated in the trial. Second, if the results are generalizable to your patient, what is the net impact of the treatment? Have the investigators measured all outcomes of importance to patients? The impact depends on both benefits and risks (side effects and toxicity) of treatment and the consequences of withholding treatment. Thus, even therapy that is effective might be withheld when a patient's prognosis is already good without treatment, especially when the treatment is accompanied by important side effects and toxicity.

# THERAPY AND HARM: STUDY DESIGNS

## Randomized Controlled Trials to Assess Treatment

When investigating an issue of treatment, researchers have much more control than when exploring a question of harm. For instance, they can determine who receives the experimental intervention and who receives the control (eg, no treatment or placebo). Ideally, they will allocate patients to groups according to a process analogous to a coin flip, called *randomization,* and they will conduct a randomized controlled trial. In addition, they can design their study so that neither patients nor caregivers are aware of which patients receive the experimental treatment.

## Observational Studies to Assess Harm

By contrast, researchers looking at issues of harm generally do not have this sort of control. They cannot dictate to people whether they should live in high- or low-pollution environments; neither can they allocate them to groups living in spacious or overcrowded settings. Investigators cannot conceal from study participants their living environment—or whether or not they smoke. As a result, investigators use observational study designs. They may follow patients who, as a result of preference or circumstances, have been exposed to a harmful stimulus. They follow them forward in time to determine if they suffer the outcome about which they are concerned, the target outcome (a *cohort* study). Alternatively, researchers may select individuals who have already suffered the target outcome. In addition, they select another group that has not yet suffered the target outcome, and compare the extent to which the two groups had been exposed to the putative harmful agent (a *case-control study*) (see Part 1B2, "Harm").

## Applying Appropriate Criteria

Inferences from studies investigating harm are generally much weaker than those from studies of therapy. As a user of the medical literature, you must apply different criteria to a study of a therapeutic question than to one investigating a harmful exposure. We therefore provide separate *Users' Guides* for coverage of issues of therapy and harm (see Part 1B1, "Therapy," and Part 1B2, "Harm").

There are exceptions to this general rule. Sometimes, the harmful exposure may be a medical intervention, such as a drug, and researchers will perceive the putative harmful effect as occurring quickly and frequently. Under these circumstances, investigators may be able to use the study design usually associated with therapy to determine if there is a causal relation between the drug and the toxic effect.

Similarly, there may be no randomized trials available—or even feasible—addressing a particular therapeutic issue. Investigations of rare conditions, community interventions, the care delivered in different hospitals (see Part 2B, "Therapy and Harm, Outcomes of Health Services"), or the quality of care within a hospital (see Part 2F, "Moving From Evidence to Action, Clinical Utilization Review") do not easily lend themselves to randomized trials. Randomizing health care systems to rely more on primary care physicians or specialists, or to base reimbursement on fee-for-service or capitation, or to public funding vs user-pay, seems, for the foreseeable future at least, improbable.

In all situations when clinicians addressing issues of therapy find that randomized trials are unavailable, they need to rely on cohort and case-control studies—the strongest evidence available. In doing so, they must apply the appropriate criteria for the evaluation of these studies, criteria that ordinarily would be associated with investigations of potentially harmful exposures. When relying on cohort or case-control studies to address issues of therapeutic benefit, however, clinicians must bear in mind that the strength of any inferences about the causal relation between the intervention and the outcome become much weaker than they would if evidence came from a randomized trial.

# References

1. Wright P. Untoward effects associated with practolol administration: oculomucocutaneous syndrome. *BMJ.* 1975;1:595-598.

2. Moore TJ. *Deadly Medicine*. New York, NY: Simon & Schuster; 1995.

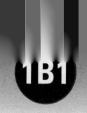

# THERAPY

Gordon Guyatt, Deborah Cook, PJ Devereaux,
Maureen Meade, and Sharon Straus

The following EBM Working Group members also made substantive
contributions to this section: Peter Wyer, Roman Jaeschke,
Daren Heyland, Anne Holbrook, and Luz Maria Letelier

## IN THIS SECTION

# CLINICAL SCENARIO

## The Internet Tells Me Spironolactone Will Prolong My Life: Doctor, Should I Take It?

You are a general internist reviewing a 66-year-old man with idiopathic dilated cardiomyopathy whom you have been following for 3 years. The patient, who has been very involved in decision making with regard to his care, presents you with an Internet summary of a new study stating, "Spironolactone saves lives in heart failure." He is very encouraged by the summary and believes that spironolactone will prolong his life.

For the preceding 18 months, the patient has been stable with mild symptoms that you classify as New York Heart Association (NYHA) class II. His echocardiogram 3 months ago demonstrated unchanged global left-sided ventricular dysfunction with an ejection fraction of 30%. His current medications include enalapril 10 mg twice a day, metoprolol 50 mg twice a day, and furosemide 20 mg once a day. His blood pressure is 110/70 mm Hg and his heart rate is 60 bpm. His blood work from the previous week reveals a creatinine level of 100 mmol/L and potassium level of 4.1 mmol/L. Since enalapril suppresses aldosterone, you wonder how spironolactone, an aldosterone antagonist, could provide additional benefit. You check the *Physician's Desk Reference* (PDR) and read that simultaneous use of enalapril and spironolactone is relatively contraindicated because of the risk of hyperkalemia.[1] You share with the patient your concerns about spironolactone as well as your determination not to overlook its potential benefits, you inform him that you will review the evidence and offer a recommendation when he returns to see you in 1 week.

# FINDING THE EVIDENCE

You begin by formulating your question:

> In patients with NYHA class II heart failure and a decreased
> ejection fraction, what is the impact of spironolactone therapy
> on mortality and quality of life?

Since the study you are seeking was published during the past couple of months, you know that it will not yet be included in Best Evidence, the database you would normally use to begin such a search. You therefore begin with a MEDLINE search using OVID and the following search strategy: "heart failure, congestive" (MH)—which stands for "MeSH heading"—and "spironolactone" (MH) limited to "clinical trials" and the year "1999." This search yields only four articles, one of which is evidently your target.[2]

The article you retrieve reports a trial in which investigators randomized 1663 patients with NYHA class III and class IV heart failure to receive spironolactone 25 mg once daily. In this trial, patients were followed for an average of 2 years. You immediately discern that the patient you are seeing with class II heart failure would not have been eligible for the study. However, you still suspect the trial might be relevant to this patient's care and you decide to review the report carefully before the patient returns to see you.

Although this book discusses evaluation of articles about therapy, we caution that our definition of therapy is a broad one. The principles apply to therapies designed to ameliorate symptoms or reduce morbidity and mortality in those who are acutely or chronically ill (eg, the therapeutic use of spironolactone for patients with heart failure); to interventions designed to prevent chronologically distant morbid or mortal events in patients with known underlying pathology (eg, beta blockade after myocardial infarction); to interventions designed to prevent morbidity and mortality in those at risk but without current evident illness (eg, treatment of high blood pressure); to interventions designed to improve patient outcome by improving the process of care (see Part 2B1, "Therapy and Validity, Computer Decision Support Systems"); to diagnostic tests designed to reduce morbidity or mortality (eg, gastroscopy in those with acute gastrointestinal bleeding); and to the combination of diagnostic testing and subsequent therapy that make up screening programs (eg, screening for fecal occult blood) (see Part 2F, "Moving From Evidence to Action, Recommendations About Screening"). In each of these situations, you risk doing more harm than good when you intervene. Before acting, therefore, ascertain the benefits and risks of the therapy and seek assurance that the societal resources (usually valued in dollars) consumed in the intervention will not be exorbitant.

# ARE THE RESULTS VALID?

As described in "How to Use This Book," we suggest a three-step approach to using an article from the medical literature to guide patient care. We recommend that you first determine whether the study provides valid results, that you next review the results, and, finally, that you consider how the results can be applied to the patients in your practice (Table 1B-1).

Whether the study will provide valid results depends on whether it was designed and conducted in a way that justifies claims about the benefits or risks of a therapeutic regimen. Tests of study methods break down into two sets of four questions. The first set helps you decide whether persons exposed to the experimental therapy had a similar prognosis to patients exposed to a control intervention at the beginning of the study. The second set helps you confirm that the two groups were still similar with respect to prognostic factors throughout the study.

**TABLE 1B–1**

## Users' Guides for an Article About Therapy

**Are the results valid?**

Did experimental and control groups begin the study with a similar prognosis?

- Were patients randomized?
- Was randomization concealed (blinded or masked)?
- Were patients analyzed in the groups to which they were randomized?
- Were patients in the treatment and control groups similar with respect to known prognostic factors?

Did experimental and control groups retain a similar prognosis after the study started?

- Were patients aware of group allocation?
- Were clinicians aware of group allocation?
- Were outcome assessors aware of group allocation?
- Was follow-up complete?

**What are the results?**

- How large was the treatment effect?
- How precise was the estimate of the treatment effect?

**How can I apply the results to patient care?**

- Were the study patients similar to my patient?
- Were all clinically important outcomes considered?
- Are the likely treatment benefits worth the potential harm and costs?

## Were Patients Randomized?

Consider the question of whether, in very sick people, hospital care prolongs life. A study finds that more sick people die in the hospital than in the community. We would easily reject the naive conclusion that hospital care kills because, intuitively, we understand that hospitalized patients are generally much sicker than patients in the community. This difference would lead to a biased assessment, a massive underestimation of the beneficial effect of hospital care. An unbiased comparison would require a comparison of those in the hospital with equally sick patients in the community, a study that an institutional review board is unlikely to approve.

During the 1970s and early 1980s, surgeons frequently performed extracranial-intracranial bypass (ie, anastomosis of a branch of the external carotid artery—the superficial temporal—to a branch of the internal carotid artery—the middle cerebral). They believed it prevented strokes in patients whose symptomatic cerebrovascular disease was otherwise surgically inaccessible. Comparisons of outcomes among nonrandomized cohorts of patients who, for various reasons, did or did not undergo this operation fueled their conviction. These studies suggested that patients who underwent surgery appeared to fare much better than those who did not undergo surgery. However, to the surgeons' surprise, a large multicenter randomized controlled trial (RCT) in which patients were allocated to surgical or medical treatment using a process analogous to flipping a coin demonstrated that the only effect of surgery was to increase adverse outcomes in the immediate postsurgical period.[3]

Other surprises generated by randomized trials that contradicted the results of less rigorous trials include the demonstration that steroid injections do not ameliorate facet-joint back pain,[4] that plasmapheresis does not benefit patients with polymyositis,[5] and that a variety of initially promising drugs increase mortality in patients with heart failure.[6-10] Such surprises occur frequently (see Part 2B1, "Therapy, Surprising Results of Randomized Trials") when treatments are assigned by random allocation, rather than by the conscious decisions of clinicians and patients.

The reason that studies in which patient or physician preference determines whether a patient receives treatment or control (*observational studies*) often yield biased outcomes is that morbidity and mortality result from many causes, of which treatment is only one. Treatment studies attempt to determine the impact of an intervention on such events as stroke, myocardial infarction, or death—occurrences that we call the trial's *target outcomes* or *target events*. A patient's age, the underlying severity of illness, the presence of comorbid conditions, and a host of other factors typically determine the frequency with which a trial's target outcome occurs (*prognostic factors* or determinants of outcome). If prognostic factors—either those we know about or those we don't know about—prove unbalanced between a trial's treatment and control groups, the study's outcome will be biased, either under- or overestimating the treatment's effect. Because known prognostic factors often influence clinicians' recommendations and patients' decisions about taking treatment, observational studies often yield misleading results. Typically, observational studies tend to show larger treatment effects than do randomized trials,[11-14] although systematic underestimation of treatment effects also may occur.[15] Observational studies can theoretically match patients, either in selecting patients for study or in the subsequent statistical analysis, for known prognostic factors (see Part 1B2, "Harm"; and see Part 2B, "Therapy and Harm, Why Study

Results Mislead: Bias and Random Error"). The power of randomization is that treatment and control groups are far more likely to be balanced with respect to both the known and the unknown determinants of outcome.

Randomization does not always succeed in its goal of achieving groups with similar prognosis. Investigators may make mistakes that compromise randomization—if those who determine eligibility are aware of the arm of the study to which the patient will be allocated, or if patients are not analyzed in the group to which they were allocated—or they may encounter bad luck.

## Was Randomization Concealed?

Some years ago, a group of Australian investigators undertook a randomized trial of open vs laparoscopic appendectomy.[16] The trial ran smoothly during the day. At night, however, the attending surgeon's presence was required for the laparoscopic procedure but not the open one; and the limited operating room availability made the longer laparoscopic procedure an annoyance. Reluctant to call in a consultant, and particularly reluctant with specific senior colleagues, the residents sometimes adopted a practical solution. When an eligible patient appeared, the residents checked the attending staff and the lineup for the operating room and, depending on the personality of the attending surgeon and the length of the lineup, held the translucent envelopes containing orders up to the light. As soon as they found one that dictated an open procedure, they opened that envelope. The first eligible patient in the morning would then be allocated to a laparoscopic appendectomy group according to the passed-over envelope (D. Wall, written communication, June 9, 2000). If patients who presented at night were sicker than those who presented during the day, the residents' behavior would bias the results against the open procedure.

This story demonstrates that if those making the decision about patient eligibility are aware of the arm of the study to which the patient will be allocated—if randomization is unconcealed (unblinded or unmasked)—they may systematically enroll sicker—or less sick—patients to either treatment or control groups. This behavior will defeat the purpose of randomization and the study will yield a biased result.[17, 18] Careful investigators will ensure that randomization is concealed, for example, through (a) preparation of blinded medication in a pharmacy, (b) remote randomization, in which the individual recruiting the patient makes a call to a methods center to discover the arm of the study to which the patient is allocated, or (c) (in our view a much less secure approach) ensuring that the envelope containing the code is sealed.

## Were Patients Analyzed in the Groups to Which They Were Randomized?

Investigators can also corrupt randomization by systematically omitting from the results patients who do not take their assigned treatment. Readers might initially agree that such patients who never actually received their assigned treatment should be excluded from the results. Their exclusion, however, will bias the results.

The reasons people do not take their medication are often related to prognosis. In a number of randomized trials, patients who did not adhere to their treatment regimens have fared worse than those who took their medication as instructed, even after taking into account all known prognostic factors and even when their medications were placebos.[19-24] Excluding noncompliant patients from the analysis leaves behind those who may be destined to have a better outcome and destroys the unbiased comparison provided by randomization.

The situation is similar with surgical therapies. Some patients randomized to surgery never have the operation because they are too sick or because they suffer the outcome of interest (eg, stroke or myocardial infarction) before they get to the operating room. If investigators include such poorly destined patients in the control arm but not in the surgical arm of a trial, even a useless surgical therapy will appear to be effective. However, the apparent effectiveness of surgery will come not from a benefit to those who have surgery, but from the systematic exclusion from the surgical group of those with the poorest prognosis.

This principle of attributing all patients to the group to which they were randomized results in an *intention-to-treat analysis,* which is analysis of outcomes based on the treatment arm to which patients were randomized, rather than which treatment they actually received. This strategy preserves the value of randomization: prognostic factors that we know about—and those we do not know about—will be, on average, equally distributed in the two groups; and the effect we see will result simply from the treatment assigned.

In conclusion, when reviewing a report of a randomized trial, look for evidence that the investigators analyzed all patients in the groups to which they were randomized (see Part 2B1, "Therapy and Validity, The Principle of Intention-to-Treat").

## Were Patients in the Treatment and Control Groups Similar With Respect to Known Prognostic Factors?

The purpose of randomization is to create groups whose prognosis, with respect to the target outcome, is similar. Sometimes, through bad luck, randomization will fail to achieve this goal. The smaller the sample size, the more likely the trial will suffer from prognostic imbalance.

Picture a trial testing a new treatment for heart failure enrolling patients in New York Heart Association functional class III and class IV. Patients in class IV have a much worse prognosis than those in class III. The trial is small, with only eight patients. One would not be terribly surprised if all four class III patients were allocated to the treatment group and all four class IV patients were allocated to the control group. Such a result of the allocation process would seriously bias the study in favor of the treatment. Were the trial to enroll 800 patients, one would be startled if randomization placed all 400 class III patients in the treatment arm. The larger the sample size, the more likely randomization will achieve its goal of prognostic balance.

Investigators can check how well randomization has done its job by examining the distribution of all prognostic factors in treatment and control groups.

Clinicians should look for a display of prognostic features of the treatment and control patients at the study's commencement—the baseline or entry prognostic features. Although we never will know whether similarity exists for the unknown prognostic factors, we are reassured when the known prognostic factors are well balanced.

The issue here is not whether there are statistically significant differences in known prognostic factors between treatment groups (eg, in a randomized trial, one knows in advance that any differences that did occur happened by chance, making the frequently cited *P* values unhelpful), but, rather, the magnitude of these differences. If the differences are large, the validity of the study may be compromised. The stronger the relationship between the prognostic factors and outcome, and the greater the differences in distribution between groups, the more the differences will weaken the strength of any inference about treatment impact (ie, you will have less confidence in the study results).

All is not lost if the treatment groups are not similar at baseline. Statistical techniques permit adjustment of the study result for baseline differences. Accordingly, clinicians should look for documentation of similarity for relevant baseline characteristics; if substantial differences exist, they should note whether the investigators conducted an analysis that adjusted for those differences. When both unadjusted and adjusted analyses generate the same conclusion, readers justifiably gain confidence in the validity of the study result.

## Were Patients Aware of Group Allocation?

Patients who take a treatment that they believe is efficacious may feel and perform better than those who do not, even if the treatment has no biologic action. Although we know relatively little about the magnitude and consistency of this *placebo effect*,[25] its possible presence can mislead clinicians interested in determining the biologic impact of a pharmacologic treatment. Even in the absence of placebo effects, patients might answer questions or perform functional tests differently, depending on whether they believe they are taking active medication.

The best way to avoid these problems is to ensure that patients are unaware of whether they are receiving the experimental treatment. For instance, in a trial of a new drug, control group patients can receive an inert tablet or capsule that is identical in color, taste, and consistency to the active medication administered to the treatment group patients. These placebos can ensure that control group patients benefit from placebo effects to the same extent as actively treated patients.

## Were Clinicians Aware of Group Allocation?

If randomization succeeds, treatment and control groups in a study begin with a very similar prognosis. However, randomization provides no guarantees that the two groups will remain prognostically balanced. Differences in patient care other than the intervention under study can bias the results. For example, returning to the spironolactone trial described earlier in this section, if treatment group patients received more intensive treatment with angiotensin-converting enzyme inhibitors or beta blockers than control group patients did, the results would yield an overestimate of the treatment effect. The reason is that both of these classes of cointervention drugs prolong life in heart failure patients.

Clinicians gain greatest confidence in study results when investigators document that all cointerventions that may plausibly impact on the outcome are administered more or less equally in treatment and control groups. The absence of such documentation is a much less serious problem if clinicians are blind to whether patients are receiving active treatment or are part of a control group. Effective blinding eliminates the possibility of either conscious or unconscious differential administration of effective interventions to treatment and control groups.

## Were Outcome Assessors Aware of Group Allocation?

If either the treatment or the control group receives closer follow-up, target outcome events may be reported more frequently. In addition, unblinded study personnel who are measuring or recording outcomes such as physiologic tests, clinical status, or quality of life may provide different interpretations of marginal findings or may offer differential encouragement during performance tests, either one of which can distort results.[26] The study personnel assessing outcome can almost always be kept blind to group allocation, even if (as is the case for surgical therapies or health services interventions) patients and treating clinicians cannot. Investigators can take additional precautions by constructing a blinded adjudication committee to review clinical data and decide issues such as whether a patient has had a stroke or myocardial infarction, or whether a death can be attributed to cancer or cardiovascular disease. The more judgment is involved in determining whether a patient has suffered a target outcome (blinding is less crucial in studies in which the outcome is all-cause mortality, for instance) the more important blinding becomes.

## Was Follow-up Complete?

Ideally, at the conclusion of a trial investigators will know the status of each patient with respect to the target outcome. We often refer to patients whose status is unknown as lost to follow-up. The greater the number of patients who are *lost to follow-up*, the more a study's validity is potentially compromised. The reason is that patients who are lost often have different prognoses from those who are retained; these patients may disappear because they suffer adverse outcomes (even death) or because they are doing well (and so did not return to be assessed). The situation is completely analogous to the reason for the necessity for an intention-to-treat analysis: patients who discontinue their medication may be less or (usually) more likely to suffer the target adverse event of interest.

When does loss to follow-up seriously threaten validity? Rules of thumb (you may run across thresholds such as 20%) are misleading. Consider two hypothetical randomized trials, each of which enters 1000 patients into both treatment and control groups, of whom 30 (3%) are lost to follow-up (Table 1B-2). In trial A, treated patients die at half the rate of the control group (200 vs 400), a reduction in relative risk of 50%. To what extent does the loss to follow-up potentially threaten our inference that treatment reduces the death rate by half? If we assume the worst, ie, that all treated patients lost to follow-up died, the number of deaths in the experimental group would be 230 (23%). If there were no deaths among the control patients who were lost to follow-up, our best estimate of the effect of treatment in reducing the risk of death drops from 200/400, or 50%, to (400 − 230) or 170/400, or 43%. Thus, even assuming the worst makes little difference in the best estimate of the magnitude of the treatment effect. Our inference is therefore secure.

**TABLE 1B–2**

## When Does Loss to Follow-up Seriously Threaten Validity?

| | Trial A | | Trial B | |
|---|---|---|---|---|
| | Treatment | Control | Treatment | Control |
| Number of patients randomized | 1000 | 1000 | 1000 | 1000 |
| Number (%) lost to follow-up | 30 (3%) | 30 (3%) | 30 (3%) | 30 (3%) |
| Number (%) of deaths | 200 (20%) | 400 (40%) | 30 (3%) | 60 (6%) |
| RRR not counting patients lost to follow-up | 0.2/0.4 = 0.50 | | 0.03/0.06 = 0.50 | |
| RRR for worst-case scenario* | 0.17/0.4 = 0.43 | | 0.00/0.06 = 0 | |

* The worst-case scenario assumes that all patients allocated to the treatment group and lost to follow-up died and all patients allocated to the control group and lost to follow-up survived.

RRR indicates relative risk reduction.

Contrast this with trial B. Here, the reduction in the relative risk of death is also 50%. In this case, however, the total number of deaths is much lower; of the treated patients, 30 die—and the number of deaths in control patients is 60. In trial B, if we make the same worst-case assumption about the fate of the patients lost to follow-up, the results would change markedly. If we assume that all patients initially allocated to treatment—but subsequently lost to follow-up—die, the number of deaths among treated patients rises from 30 to 60, which is exactly equal to the number of control group deaths. Let us assume that this assumption is accurate. Since we would have 60 deaths in both treatment and control groups, the effect of treatment drops to 0. Because of this dramatic change in the treatment effect (50% relative risk reduction if we ignore those lost to follow-up; 0% relative risk reduction if we assume all patients in the treatment group who were lost to follow-up died), the 3% loss to follow-up in trial B threatens our inference about the magnitude of the relative risk reduction.

Of course, this worst-case scenario is unlikely. When a worst-case scenario, were it true, substantially alters the results, you must judge the plausibility of a markedly different outcome event rate in the treatment and control group patients

## USING THE GUIDE

**R**eturning to our opening clinical scenario, how well did the study of spironolactone achieve the goal of creating groups with similar prognostic factors? The investigators tell us the study was randomized, but they do not explicitly address the issue of concealment. Of the 822 treated patients, 214 discontinued treatment because of a lack of response, adverse events, or administrative reasons, as did 200 of 841 patients in the control group. The investigators appear to have included all these patients in the analysis, which they state followed intention-to-treat principles. They document the two groups' similarity with respect to age, sex, race, blood pressure, heart rate, ejection fraction, cause of heart failure, and medication use. The one variable for which there was some imbalance is the severity of underlying heart failure: 31% of control patients, vs 27% of treated patients, had NYHA class IV symptoms. This could potentially bias the results in favor of the treatment group. However, the effect is likely to be small, and we are reassured by the investigators' report of an analysis that adjusted for baseline differences in known prognostic factors.

As in many reports of randomized trials, the authors describe their study as "double-blind." Unfortunately, neither clinical epidemiologists nor readers are certain what this term signifies in terms of who is blind to allocation.[27] We will therefore avoid its use and instead, we will specify which groups were unaware of treatment allocation. The spironolactone report implies that patients, caregivers, and those adjudicating outcome were all blinded to allocation, and the editors of Best Evidence have conferred with the authors and reassure us that this is the case.[28]

The authors make no explicit statement about loss to follow-up and their presentation of the data suggests they did not lose any patients. While this is possible for other outcomes, for the outcome of mortality, it seems unlikely.

The final assessment of validity is never a "yes" or "no" decision. Rather, think of validity as a continuum ranging from strong studies that are very likely to yield an accurate estimate of the treatment effect to weak studies that are very likely to yield a biased estimate of effect. Inevitably, the judgment as to where a study lies in this continuum involves some subjectivity. In this case, despite uncertainty about loss to follow-up, we judge that overall, the methods were strong. The study is thus high on the continuum between very low and very high validity, likely provides a minimally biased assessment of spironolactone's impact on heart failure patients, and can help us decide whether to recommend spironolactone to the patient under consideration.

who have not been followed. Investigators' demonstration that patients lost to follow-up are similar with respect to important prognostic variables such as age and disease severity decreases—but does not eliminate—the possibility of a different rate of target events.

In conclusion, loss to follow-up potentially threatens a study's validity. If assuming a worst-case scenario does not change the inferences arising from study results, then loss to follow-up is not a problem. If such an assumption would significantly alter the results, validity is compromised. The extent of that compromise remains a matter of judgment and will depend on how likely it is that treatment patients lost to follow-up did poorly, while control patients lost to follow-up did well.

# WHAT ARE THE RESULTS?

### How Large Was the Treatment Effect?

Most frequently, randomized clinical trials carefully monitor how often patients experience some adverse event or outcome. Examples of these *dichotomous outcomes* ("yes" or "no" outcomes—ones that either happen or do not happen) include cancer recurrence, myocardial infarction, and death. Patients either do or do not suffer an event, and the article reports the proportion of patients who develop such events. Consider, for example, a study in which 20% of a control group died, but only 15% of those receiving a new treatment died. How might these results be expressed?

One way would be as the absolute difference (known as the *absolute risk reduction,* or risk difference), between the proportion who died in the control group ($x$) and the proportion who died in the treatment group ($y$), or $x - y = 0.20 - 0.15 = 0.05$. Another way to express the impact of treatment would be as a *relative risk*: the risk of events among patients on the new treatment, relative to that risk among patients in the control group, or $y/x = 0.15 / 0.20 = 0.75$.

The most commonly reported measure of dichotomous treatment effects is the complement of this relative risk, and is called the *relative risk reduction* (RRR). It is expressed as a percent: $(1 - y/x) \times 100 = (1 - 0.75) \times 100 = 25\%$. An RRR of 25% means that the new treatment reduced the risk of death by 25% relative to that occurring among control patients; and the greater the relative risk reduction, the more effective the therapy. Investigators may compute the relative risk over a period of time, as in a *survival analysis,* and call it a *hazard ratio* (see Part 2B2, "Therapy and Understanding the Results, Measures of Association"). When people do not specify whether they are talking about relative or absolute risk reduction—for instance, "Drug X was 30% effective in reducing the risk of death," or "The efficacy of the vaccine was 92%," they are almost invariably talking about relative risk reduction. Pharmaceutical advertisements, whether they make it explicit or not, almost invariably cite relative risk. See Part 2B2," Therapy and Understanding the Results, Measures of Association," for more detail about how the relative risk reduction results in a subjective impression of a larger treatment effect than do other ways of expressing treatment effects.

## How Precise Was the Estimate of the Treatment Effect?

Realistically, the true risk reduction can never be known. The best we have is the estimate provided by rigorous controlled trials, and the best estimate of the true treatment effect is that observed in the trial. This estimate is called a point estimate, a single value calcuated from observations of the sample that is used to estimate a population value or parameter. The *point estimate* reminds us that, although the true value lies somewhere in its neighborhood, it is unlikely to be precisely correct. Investigators often tell us the neighborhood within which the true effect likely lies by the statistical strategy of calculating *confidence intervals*, a range of values within which one can be confident that that a population parameter is estimated to lie.[29]

We usually (though arbitrarily) use the 95% confidence interval (see Part 2B2, "Therapy, Confidence Intervals"). You can consider the 95% confidence interval as defining the range that includes the true relative risk reduction 95% of the time. You will seldom find the true RRR toward the extremes of this interval, and you will find the true RRR beyond these extremes only 5% of the time, a property of the confidence interval that relates closely to the conventional level of "statistical significance" of $P < .05$ (see Part 2B2, "Therapy and Understanding the Results, Hypothesis Testing"). We illustrate the use of confidence intervals in the following examples.

Example 1. If a trial randomized 100 patients each to treatment and control groups, and there were 20 deaths in the control group and 15 deaths in the treatment group, the authors would calculate a point estimate for the RRR of 25% ($x = 20/100$ or 0.20, $y = 15/100$ or 0.15, and $1 - y/x = [1 - 0.75]$ x 100 = 25%). You might guess, however, that the true RRR might be much smaller or much greater than this 25%, based on a difference of only five deaths. In fact, you might surmise that the treatment might provide no benefit (an RRR of 0%) or might even do harm (a negative RRR). And you would be right—in fact, these results are consistent with both an RRR of −38% (that is, patients given the new treatment might be 38% more likely to die than control patients) and an RRR of nearly 59% (that is, patients subsequently receiving the new treatment might have a risk of dying almost 60% less than that of those who are not treated). In other words, the 95% confidence interval on this RRR is −38% to 59%, and the trial really has not helped us decide whether or not to offer the new treatment.

Example 2. What if the trial enrolled 1000 patients per group rather than 100 patients per group, and the same event rates were observed as before, so that there were 200 deaths in the control group ($x = 200/1000 = 0.20$) and 150 deaths in the treatment group ($y = 150/1000 = 0.15$)? Again, the point estimate of the RRR is 25% ($1 - y/x = 1 - [0.15/0.20]$ x 100 = 25%). In this larger trial, you might think that the true reduction in risk is much closer to 25% and, again, you would be right. The 95% confidence interval on the RRR for this set of results is all on the positive side of zero and runs from 9% to 41%.

What these examples show is that the larger the sample size of a trial, the larger the number of outcome events, and the greater our confidence that the true relative risk reduction (or any other measure of efficacy) is close to what we have observed. In the second example above, the lowest plausible value for the RRR was 9% and the highest value was 41%. The point estimate—in this case, 25%—is the one value most likely to represent the true RRR. As one considers values farther and farther from the point estimate, they become less and less consistent with the observed RRR. By the time one crosses the upper or lower boundaries of the 95% confidence interval, the values are extremely unlikely to represent the true RRR, given the point estimate (that is, the observed RRR).

Figure 1B-1 represents the confidence intervals around the point estimate of a RRR of 25% in these two examples, with a risk reduction of 0 representing no treatment effect. In both scenarios, the point estimate of the RRR is 25%, but the confidence interval is far narrower in the second scenario.

**FIGURE 1B-1**

## Confidence Intervals Around Relative Risk Reduction

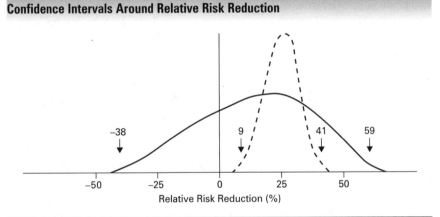

Two studies with the same point estimate, a 25% relative risk reduction, but different sample sizes and correspondingly different confidence intervals. The solid line represents the confidence interval around the first example, in which there were 100 patients per group and the numbers of events in active and control were 15 and 20, respectively. The broken line represents the confidence interval around the first example in which there were 1000 patients per group, and the numbers of events in active and control were 150 and 200, respectively.

It is evident that the larger the sample size, the narrower the confidence interval. When is the sample size big enough[30] (see Part 2B2, "Therapy and Understanding the Results, Confidence Intervals")? In a *positive study*—a study in which the authors conclude that the treatment is effective—one can look at the lower boundary of the confidence interval. In the second example, this lower boundary was +9%. If this RRR (the lowest RRR that is consistent with the study results) is still important (that is, it is large enough for you to recommend the treatment to the patient), then the investigators have enrolled sufficient patients. If, on the other hand, you do not consider an RRR of 9% important, then the study cannot be considered definitive, even if its results are statistically significant (that is, they exclude a risk reduction of 0). Keep in mind that the probability of the true value being less than the lower boundary of the confidence interval is only 2.5%, and that a different criterion for the confidence interval (a 90% confidence interval, for instance) might be as or more appropriate.

The confidence interval also helps us interpret *negative studies* in which the authors have concluded that the experimental treatment is no better than control therapy. All we need do is look at the upper boundary of the confidence interval. If the RRR at this upper boundary would, if true, be clinically important, the study has failed to exclude an important treatment effect. For example, consider the first example we presented in this section—the study with 100 patients in each group. This study does not exclude the possibility of harm (indeed, it is consistent with a 38% increase in relative risk), the associated $P$ value would be greater than .05, and the study would be considered negative in that it failed to show a convincing treatment effect (see Figure 1B-1). Recall, however, that the upper boundary of the confidence interval was an RRR of 59%. Clearly, if this large relative risk reduction represented the truth, the benefit of the treatment would be substantial. We can conclude that, although the investigators have failed to prove that experimental treatment was better than placebo, they have also failed to prove that it is not; they have not excluded a large, positive treatment effect. Once again, you must bear in mind the proviso that the choice of a 95% confidence interval is arbitrary. A reasonable alternative, a 90% confidence interval, would be somewhat narrower.

## When Authors Do Not Report the Confidence Interval

What can you do if the confidence interval around the RRR is not reported in the article? The easiest approach is to examine the $P$ value. If it is exactly .05, then the lower bound of the 95% confidence limit for the RRR has to lie exactly at zero (a relative risk of 1), and you cannot exclude the possibility that the treatment has no effect. As the $P$ value decreases below .05, the lower bound of the 95% confidence limit for the RRR rises above zero.

A second approach involves calculating the confidence intervals yourself[31] or asking the help of someone else (a statistician, for instance) to do so. Once you obtain the confidence intervals, you know how high and low the RRR might be (that is, you know the precision of the estimate of the treatment effect) and can interpret the results as described above.

Not all randomized trials have dichotomous outcomes, nor should they. For example, the authors of the spironolactone study might have reported changes in exercise capacity or quality of life with the drug. In a study of respiratory muscle training for patients with chronic airflow limitation, one primary outcome measured how far patients could walk in 6 minutes in an enclosed corridor.[32] This 6-minute walk improved from an average of 406 to 416 m (up 10 m) in the experimental group receiving respiratory muscle training, and from 409 to 429 m (up 20 m) in the control group. The point estimate for improvement in the 6-minute walk due to respiratory muscle training therefore was negative, at −10 m (or a 10-m difference in favor of the control group).

Here, too, you should look for the 95% confidence intervals around this difference in changes in exercise capacity and consider their implications. The investigators tell us that the lower boundary of the 95% confidence interval was −26 (that is, the results are consistent with a difference of 26 m in favor of the control treatment) and the upper boundary was +5 m. Even in the best of circumstances, adding 5 m to the 400 m recorded at the start of the trial would not be important to the patient, and this result effectively excludes an important benefit of respiratory muscle training as applied in this study.

Having determined the magnitude and precision of the treatment effect, clinicians can turn to the final question of how to apply the article's results to patients in their clinical practice.

## USING THE GUIDE

Of the 822 treated patients, 284 died during the mean 2-year follow-up (35%), as did 386 of 841 control patients (46%). The investigators conducted a survival analysis that takes into account not only the number of people who died by the end of the trial, but the timing of their deaths along the way. Using only the raw death rate, we would compute a relative risk of 76% and a relative risk reduction of 24%. Because patients in the control group not only died more often but at an earlier point than those in the treatment group, the survival analysis yields a relative risk reduction (or hazard ratio) of 35% (95% confidence interval, 18%-48%). The survival curves started to diverge after 6 months of follow-up and showed increasing separation thereafter.

The numbers of patients hospitalized for cardiac causes in the treatment and control groups were, respectively, 336 and 260 (relative risk [RR] 0.70, 95% confidence interval [CI] 0.59-0.82). In the placebo group, about 33% of the patients improved by one or more NYHA functional classes, about 18% were unchanged, and about 48% deteriorated. In the spironolactone group, the comparable percentages were 41%, 21%, and 38%. Chance is a very unlikely explanation for the difference in changes in NYHA functional class ($P < .001$).

In terms of adverse events, nine (1%) of the patients in the control group and 61 (10%) of the treated men developed gynecomastia or breast pain ($P < .001$), and serious hyperkalemia occurred in 10 (1%) and 14 (2%) of the control and treated patients, respectively. The difference in the frequency of serious hyperkalemia was not significant.

# HOW CAN I APPLY THE RESULTS TO PATIENT CARE?

## Were the Study Patients Similar to the Patient in My Practice?

Often, the patient before you has different attributes or characteristics from those enrolled in the trial. She may be older, sicker or less sick, or may suffer from comorbid disease that would have excluded her from participation in the research study. If the patient had qualified for enrollment in the study—that is, if she had met all inclusion criteria and had violated none of the exclusion criteria—you can apply the results with considerable confidence.

Even here, however, there is a limitation. Treatments are not uniformly effective in every individual. Typically, some patients respond extremely well, whereas others achieve no benefit whatsoever. Conventional randomized trials estimate average treatment effects. Applying these average effects means that the clinician will likely be exposing some patients to the cost and toxicity of the treatment without benefit.

Randomized trials in individual patients offer a solution to this dilemma. In these trials, clinicians use the same strategies that minimize bias in conventional trials of therapy involving multiple patients to guard against misleading results in studies involving single patients.[33] In the N of 1 randomized controlled trial, a single patient undertakes a pair of treatment periods in which the patient receives a target treatment in one period of each pair and a placebo or alternative in the other (see Part 2B1, "Therapy and Validity, N of 1 Randomized Controlled Trials"). The patient and clinician are blinded to allocation, the order of the target treatment and control are randomized, and the patient makes quantitative ratings of his or her symptoms during each period. The N of 1 RCT continues until both the patient and clinician conclude that the patient is, or is not, obtaining benefit from the target intervention. When the conditions are right, N of 1 RCTs (a) are feasible,[34,35] (b) can provide definitive evidence of treatment effectiveness in individual patients, and (c) may lead to long-term differences in treatment administration.[36]

On the other hand, N of 1 RCTs are unsuitable for short-term problems, for therapies that cure, or for ascertaining effects on long-term outcomes or those that occur infrequently. Furthermore, they are possible only when patients and clinicians have the interest and time required. In most instances, clinicians must content themselves with applying results of conventional trials of other patients to the individual before them.

What if that individual does not meet a study's eligibility criteria? The study result probably applies even if, for example, she was 2 years too old for the study, had more severe disease, had previously been treated with a competing therapy, or had a comorbid condition. A better approach than rigidly applying the study's inclusion and exclusion criteria is to ask whether there is some compelling reason why the results should not be applied to the patient. A compelling reason usually will not be found, and most often you can generalize the results to the patient with confidence (see Part 2B3, "Therapy and Applying the Results, Applying Results to Individual Patients").

A related issue has to do with the extent to which we can generalize findings from a study using a particular drug to another closely (or not so closely) related agent. This is the issue of drug class effects. The issue of how conservative one should be in assuming class effects is controversial (see Part 2B3, "Therapy and Applying the Results, Drug Class Effects").

A final issue arises when a patient fits the features of a subgroup of patients in the trial report. In articles reporting the results of a trial (especially when the treatment does not appear to be efficacious for the average patient), the authors may have examined a large number of subgroups of patients at different stages of their illness, with different comorbid conditions, with different ages at entry, and the like. Quite often these subgroup analyses were not planned ahead of time, and the data are simply dredged to see what might turn up. Investigators may sometimes overinterpret these data-dependent analyses as demonstrating that the treatment really has a different effect in a subgroup of patients. For example, those who are older or sicker may be held up as benefiting substantially more or less than other subgroups of patients in the trial.

We encourage you to be skeptical of subgroup analyses[37] (see Part 2E, "Summarizing the Evidence, When to Believe a Subgroup Analysis"). The treatment is really likely to benefit the subgroup more or less than the other patients only if the difference in the effects of treatment in the subgroups is large and very unlikely to occur by chance. Even when these conditions apply, the results may be misleading if investigators did not specify their hypotheses before the study began, if they had a very large number of hypotheses, or if other studies fail to replicate the finding.

## Were All Clinically Important Outcomes Considered?

Treatments are indicated when they provide important benefits. Demonstrating that a bronchodilator produces small increments in forced expired volume in patients with chronic airflow limitation, that a vasodilator improves cardiac output in heart failure patients, or that a lipid-lowering agent improves lipid profiles does not necessarily provide a sufficient reason for administering these drugs. What is required is evidence that the treatments improve outcomes that are important to patients, such as reducing shortness of breath during the activities required for daily living, avoiding hospitalization for heart failure, or decreasing the risk of myocardial infarction. We can consider forced expired volume in 1 second, cardiac output, and the lipid profile as substitute or *surrogate endpoints* or outcomes (see Part 2B3, "Therapy and Applying the Results, Surrogate Outcomes"). That is, investigators have chosen to substitute these variables for those that patients would consider important, usually because to confirm benefit on the latter, they would have had to enroll many more patients and follow them for far longer periods of time.

Trials of the impact of antiarrhythmic drugs following myocardial infarction provide a dramatic example of the danger of using substitute endpoints. Because such drugs have been shown to reduce abnormal ventricular depolarizations (the substitute endpoints) in the short run, it made sense that they should reduce the occurrence of life-threatening arrhythmias in the long run. A group of investigators performed randomized trials on three agents (encainide, flecainide, and moricizine) previously shown to be effective in suppressing the substitute end-point of abnormal ventricular depolarizations to determine whether they reduced mortality in patients with asymptomatic or mildly symptomatic arrhythmias following myocardial infarction. The investigators had to stop the trials when they discovered that mortality was substantially higher in patients receiving antiarrhythmic treatment than in those receiving placebo.[38, 39] Clinicians relying on the substitute endpoint of arrhythmia suppression would have continued to administer the three drugs to the considerable detriment of their patients.

Even when investigators report favorable effects of treatment on one clinically important outcome, you must consider whether there may be deleterious effects on other outcomes. For instance, it is likely that a class of lipid-lowering agents, while reducing cardiovascular mortality, increases mortality from other causes.[40] Cancer chemotherapy may lengthen life but decreases its quality (see Part 2B2, "Therapy and Understanding the Results, Quality of Life"). Surgical trials often document prolonged life for those who survive the operation (yielding a higher 3-year survival rate in those receiving surgery), but an immediate risk of dying during or shortly after surgery. Accordingly, users of the reports of surgical trials should look for information on immediate and early mortality (typically higher in the surgical group) in addition to longer-term results. The most common limitation of randomized trials with regard to reporting important outcomes is the omission of documentation of drug toxicity or adverse effects.

Another long-neglected outcome is the resource implications of alternative management strategies. Few randomized trials measure either direct costs, such as drug or program expenses and health care worker salaries, or indirect costs, such as patients' loss of income due to illness. Nevertheless, the increasing resource constraints that health care systems face mandate careful attention to economic analysis, particularly of resource-intense interventions (see Part 2F, "Moving From Evidence to Action, Economic Analysis").

## Are the Likely Treatment Benefits Worth the Potential Harm and Costs?

If you can apply the study's results to a patient, and its outcomes are important, the next question concerns whether the probable treatment benefits are worth the effort that you and the patient must put into the enterprise. A 25% reduction in the relative risk of death may sound quite impressive, but its impact on the patient and your practice may nevertheless be minimal. This notion is illustrated using a concept called *number needed to treat* (NNT), the number of patients who must receive an intervention of therapy during a specific period of time to prevent one adverse outcome or produce one positive outcome.[41]

The impact of a treatment is related not only to its relative risk reduction, but also to the risk of the adverse outcome it is designed to prevent. One large trial suggests that tissue plasminogen activator (tPA) administration reduces the relative risk of death following myocardial infarction by approximately 12% in comparison to streptokinase in the setting of acute myocardial infarction.[42] Table 1B-3 considers two patients presenting with acute myocardial infarction associated with elevation of ST segments on their electrocardiograms.

**TABLE 1B-3**

## Considerations in the Decision to Treat Two Patients With Myocardial Infarction With Tissue Plasminogen Activator or Streptokinase

| | Risk of Death Year After Myocardial Infarction (MI) With Streptokinase | Risk With tPA (Absolute Risk Reduction) | Number Needed to Treat |
|---|---|---|---|
| 40-year-old man with small MI | 2% | 1.76% (0.24% or 0.0024) | 417 |
| 70-year-old man, large MI and heart failure | 40% | 35.2% (4.8% or 0.048) | 21 |

MI indicates myocardial infarction; tPA, tissue plasminogen activator

In the first case, a 40-year-old man presents with electrocardiographic findings suggesting an inferior myocardial infarction. You find no signs of heart failure, and the patient is in normal sinus rhythm with a rate of 90 beats per minute. This individual's risk of death in the first year after infarction may be as low as 2%. In comparison to streptokinase, tPA would reduce this risk by 12% to 1.76%, an absolute risk reduction of 0.24% (0.0024). The inverse of this absolute risk reduction (ARR) (that is, 1 divided by the ARR) is equal to the number of such patients we would have to treat to prevent one event (in this case, to prevent one death following a mild heart attack in a low-risk patient)—the number needed to treat (NNT). In this case, we would have to treat approximately 417 such patients to save a single life (1 / 0.0024 = 417). Given the small increased risk of intracerebral hemorrhage associated with tPA, and its additional cost, many clinicians might prefer streptokinase in this patient.

In the second case, a 70-year-old man presents with electrocardiographic signs of anterior myocardial infarction with pulmonary edema. His risk of dying in the next year is approximately 40%. A 12% RRR of death in such a high-risk patient generates an ARR of 4.8% (0.048), and we would have to treat only 21 such individuals to avert a premature death (1 / 0.048 = 20.8). Many clinicians would consider tPA the preferable agent in this man.

A key element of the decision to start therapy, therefore, is to consider the patient's risk of the adverse event if left untreated. For any given RRR, the higher the probability that a patient will experience an adverse outcome if we do not treat, the more likely the patient will benefit from treatment and the fewer such patients we need to treat to prevent one adverse outcome (see Part 2B2, "Therapy and Understanding the Results, Measures of Association"). Knowing the NNT helps clinicians in the process of weighing the benefits and downsides associated with the management options (see Part 2B3, "Therapy and Applying the Results, Applying Results to Individual Patients"). Part 2B3, "Therapy and Applying the Results, Example Numbers Needed to Treat," presents NNTs associated with clearly defined risk groups in a number of common therapeutic situations.

Trading off benefit and risk requires an accurate assessment of medication adverse effects. Randomized trials, with relatively small sample sizes, are unsuitable for detecting rare but catastrophic adverse effects of therapy. Although RCTs are the correct vehicle for reporting commonly occurring side effects, reports regularly neglect to include these outcomes. Clinicians must often look to other sources of information—often characterized by weaker methodology—to obtain an estimate of the adverse effects of therapy.

The preferences or values that determine the correct choice when weighing benefit and risk are those of the individual patient. Clinicians should attend to the growing literature concerning patients' response to illness (see Part 2B3, "Therapy and Applying the Results, Qualitative Research"). Great uncertainty about how best to communicate information to patients, and how to incorporate their values into clinical decision making, remains. Vigorous investigation of this frontier of evidence-based decision making is, however, under way (see Part 2F, "Moving From Evidence to Action, Incorporating Patient Values").

# CLINICAL RESOLUTION

The spironolactone study addressed a wide variety of relevant endpoints, including mortality, hospitalization rate, and day-to-day function. In addition, the study documents substantial increases in gynecomastia and breast pain in treated men, and a small and nonsignificant increase in episodes of serious hyperkalemia is reported.

For the group as a whole, the ARR of dying from 46% to 35% corresponds to an NNT of 1 / 0.11, or approximately 9. However, not all patients with heart failure have the same prognosis. Class IV patients may have a mortality rate over 2 years of as high as 60%, whereas approximately 40% of class III patients may die during this time period. We would anticipate the mortality rate in class II patients to be approximately 20% during the same period.

Table 1B-4 presents some of the benefits and risks that patients with heart failure might anticipate with spironolactone. Using the point estimate of the RRR, the NNT for those with class IV failure and a higher mortality would be 6; class III and class II, with a lower baseline risk, have higher NNTs of 9 and 17, respectively. This table also highlights the smallest RRR consistent with the data (RRR, 18%), the extreme boundary of the 95% confidence interval and, hence, the largest plausible NNT. For the NYHA class IV, III, and II patients, these NNTs prove to be 9, 14, and 27, respectively. Since breast pain and gynecomastia are likely independent of NYHA functional class, given an incidence of 9%, the number needed to harm (NNH) would be 11 in all three groups (we calculate the NNH in the same way as the NNT: 1 divided by the risk difference; in this case, 1 divided by 0.09). Finally, the drug is inexpensive; the cost of a year's treatment is approximately $25.

**TABLE 1B-4**

## Trading Off Benefits and Risks of Spironolactone Treatment in Three Different Patients With Heart Failure

| NYHA Classification for Heart Failure | Risk of Dying During 2 Years if Untreated | Likely Absolute Risk Reduction and NNT During 2 Years if Treated (30% RRR) | Smallest Plausible Absolute Risk Reduction (18% RRR)* | Risk of Breast Pain or Gynecomastia in Men and NNH |
|---|---|---|---|---|
| Class IV | 60% | 18% NNT 6 | 11% NNT 9 | 9% NNH 11 |
| Class III | 40% | 12% NNT 9 | 7% NNT 14 | 9% NNH 11 |
| Class II | 20% | 6% NNT 17 | 3.6% NNT 27 | 9% NNH 11 |

NNT indicates number needed to treat; RRR, relative risk reduction; NNH, number needed to harm.

* Calculated using lower boundary of 95% confidence interval around the RRR of 18%.

We anticipate that, given these risks and benefits, most patients would choose spironolactone treatment. This is particularly so since, if breast pain or gyneco-mastia develops, men can always stop the medication. However, there were virtu-ally no class II patients who participated in this trial. Can we assume that we would see the same reduction in relative risk in these class II patients as in those with worse heart failure?

There are a number of reasons to think we might. The biology of heart failure remains similar throughout its course. The authors of the study postulate that spironolactone prevented progressive heart failure by reducing sodium retention and myocardial fibrosis, and that it prevented sudden death by averting potassium loss and increasing the myocardial uptake of norepinephrine. Spironolactone may prevent myocardial fibrosis by blocking the effects of aldosterone on the formation of collagen. There is little reason to think these mechanisms, if they indeed explain the results, would not be important in patients with NYHA class II heart failure.

Further reassurance comes from the fact that the RRR appeared similar in participating subgroups of patients with ischemic and nonischemic etiology of their heart failure and those receiving and not receiving beta blockers. Finally, other drugs that lower mortality in heart failure—angiotensin-converting enzyme inhibitors and beta blockers—appear to have similar reductions in relative risk across subgroups of patients with NYHA class II, III, and IV heart failure.[43]

The patient before you is very interested in actively participating in decisions regarding his care. Salient points you must communicate to him include his risk of breast pain or gynecomastia of 9% during a 2-year period and his likely reduction in mortality from 20% to 14%. You must also convey the uncertainty associated with this estimate that arises both from the confidence interval around the estimate of RRR in mortality with spironolactone (which suggests his mortality may drop from 20% to 16%, rather than 14%) and from the exclusion of NYHA class II patients from the trial. When you are satisfied that the patient understands these key concepts, you will be in a position to help him arrive at a final decision about whether he wishes to take the medication.

# References

1. Vasotec tablets: enalapril maleate. In: *Physician's Desk Reference.* 52nd ed. Montvale, NJ: Medical Economics; 1998:1771-1774.

2. Pitt B, Zannad F, Remme WJ, et al. The effect of spironolactone on morbidity and mortality in patients with severe heart failure. *N Engl J Med.* 1999;341: 709-717.

3. Haynes RB, Mukherjee J, Sackett DL, et al. Functional status changes following medical or surgical treatment for cerebral ischemia: results in the EC/IC Bypass Study. *JAMA.* 1987;257:2043-2046.

4. Carette S, Marcoux S, Truchon R, et al. A controlled trial of corticosteroid injections into facet joints for chronic low back pain. *N Engl J Med.* 1991;325:1002-1007.

5. Miller FW, Leitman SF, Cronin ME, et al. Controlled trial of plasma exchange and leukapheresis in polymyositis and dermatomyositis. *N Engl J Med.* 1992;326:1380-1384.

6. The Xamoterol in Severe Heart Failure Group. Xamoterol in severe heart failure. *Lancet.* 1990;336:1-6.

7. Packer M, Carver JR, Rodeheffer RJ, et al, for the PROMISE Study Research Group. Effects of oral milrinone on mortality in severe chronic heart failure. *N Engl J Med.* 1991;325:1468-1475.

8. Packer M, Rouleau JL, Svedberg K, Pitt B, Fisher L, and the Profile investigators. Effect of flosequinan on survival in chronic heart failure: preliminary results of the PROFILE study [abstract]. *Circulation.* 1993;88(suppl I):I-301.

9. Hampton JR, van Veldhuisen DJ, Kleber FX, et al, for the Second Prospective Randomized Study of Ibopamine on Mortality and Efficacy (PRIME II) Investigators. Randomised study of effect of Ibopamine on survival in patients with advanced severe heart failure. *Lancet.* 1997;349:971-977.

10. Califf RM, Adams KF, McKenna WJ, et al. A randomized controlled trial of epoprostenol therapy for severe congestive heart fialure: the FIolan International Randomized Survival Trial (FIRST). *Am Heart J.* 1997;134:44-54.

11. Sacks HS, Chalmers TC, Smith H Jr. Sensitivity and specificity of clinical trials: randomized v historical controls. *Arch Intern Med.* 1983;143:753-755.

12. Chalmers TC, Celano P, Sacks HS, Smith H Jr. Bias in treatment assignment in controlled clinical trials. *N Engl J Med.* 1983;309:1358-1361.

13. Colditz GA, Miller JN, Mosteller F. How study design affects outcomes in comparisons of therapy, I: medical. *Stat Med.* 1989;8:441-454.

14. Emerson JD, Burdick E, Hoaglin DC, et al. An empirical study of the possible relation of treatment differences to quality scores in controlled randomized clinical trials. *Controlled Clin Trials.* 1990;11:339-352.

15. Kunz R, Oxman AD. The unpredictability paradox: review of empirical comparisons of randomised and non-randomised clinical trials. *BMJ*. 1998;317:1185-1190.

16. Hansen JB, Smithers BM, Schache D, Wall DR, Miller BJ, Menzies BL. Laparoscopic versus open appendectomy: prospective randomized trial. *World J Surg*. 1996;20:17-20.

17. Schulz KF, Chalmers I, Hayes RJ, Altman DG. Empirical evidence of bias: dimensions of methodological quality associated with estimates of treatment effects in controlled trials. *JAMA*. 1995;273:408-412.

18. Moher D, Jones A, Cook DJ, et al. Does quality of reports of randomised trials affect estimates of intervention efficacy reported in meta-analyses? *Lancet*. 1998;352:609-613.

19. Coronary Drug Project Research Group. Influence of adherence treatment and response of cholesterol on mortality in the Coronary Drug Project. *N Engl J Med*. 1980;303:1038-1041.

20. Asher WL Harper HW. Effect of human chorionic gonadotropin on weight loss, hunger, and feeling of well-being. *Am J Clin Nutr*. 1973;26:211-218.

21. Hogarty GE, Goldberg SC. Drug and sociotherapy in the aftercare of schizophrenic patients. *Arch Gen Psychiatry*. 1973;28:54-64.

22. Fuller R, Roth H, Long S. Compliance with disulfiram treatment of alcoholism. *J Chronic Dis*. 1983;36:161-170.

23. Pizzo PA, Robichaud KJ, Edwards BK, Schumaker C, Kramer BS, Johnson A. Oral antibiotic prophylaxis in patients with cancer: a double-blind randomized placebo-controlled trial. *J Pediatr*. 1983;102:125-133.

24. Horwitz RI, Viscoli CM, Berkman L, et al. Treatment adherence and risk of death after myocardial infarction. *Lancet*. 1990;336:542-545.

25. Kaptchuk TJ. Powerful placebo: the dark side of the randomised controlled trial. *Lancet*. 1998;351:1722-1725.

26. Guyatt GH, Pugsley SO, Sullivan MJ, et al. Effect of encouragement on walking test performance. *Thorax*. 1984;39:818-822.

27. Devereaux PJ, Manns BJ, Ghali WA, et al. In the dark: physician interpretation of blinding terminology in randomized controlled trials. *JAMA*. In press.

28. Henderson M, Mulrow CD. Commentary on "The effect of spironolactone on morbidity and mortality in patients with severe heart failure." ACP J Club. 2000 Jan-Feb; 132(1):2.

29. Altman DG, Gore SM, Gardner MJ, Pocock SJ. Statistical guidelines for contributors to medical journals. In: Gardner MJ, Altman DG, eds. *Statistics With Confidence: Confidence Intervals and Statistical Guidelines.* London: British Medical Journal; 1989:83-100.

30. Detsky AS, Sackett DL. When was a "negative" trial big enough? How many patients you needed depends on what you found. *Arch Intern Med.* 1985;145:709-715.

31. Sackett DL, Haynes RB, Guyatt GH, Tugwell P. *Clinical Epidemiolog: A Basic Science for Clinical Medicine.* 2nd ed. Boston: Little Brown & Co Inc; 1991:218.

32. Guyatt GH, Keller J, Singer J, Halcrow S, Newhouse M. Controlled trial of respiratory muscle training in chronic airflow limitation. *Thorax.* 1992;47:598-602.

33. Guyatt GH, Sackett DL, Taylor DW, et al. Determining optimal therapy: randomized trials in individual patients. *N Engl J Med.* 1986;314:889-892.

34. Guyatt GH, Keller JL, Jaeschke R, et al. The n-of-1 randomized control trial: clinical usefulness. Our three year experience. *Ann Intern Med.* 1990; 112:293-299.

35. Larson EB, Ellsworth AJ, Oas J. Randomized clinical trials in single patients during a 2-year period. *JAMA.* 1993;270:2708-2712.

36. Mahon J, Laupacis A, Donner A, Wood T. Randomised study of n of 1 trials versus standard practice. *BMJ.* 1996;312:1069-1074.

37. Oxman AD, Guyatt GH. A consumer's guide to subgroup analysis. *Ann Intern Med.* 1992;116:78-84.

38. Echt DS, Liebson PR, Mitchell LB, et al. Mortality and morbidity in patients receiving encainide, flecainide, or placebo: the Cardiac Arrhythmia Suppression Trial. *N Engl J Med.* 1991;324:781-788.

39. The Cardiac Arrhythmia Suppression Trial II Investigators. Effect of the antiarrhythmic agent moricizine on survival after myocardial infarction. *N Engl J Med.* 1992;327:227-233.

40. Muldoon MF, Manuck SB, Matthews KA. Lowering cholesterol concentrations and mortality: a quantitative review of primary prevention trials. *BMJ.* 1990;301:309-314.

41. Laupacis A, Sackett DL, Roberts RS. An assessment of clinically useful measures of the consequences of treatment. *N Engl J Med.* 1988;318:1728-1733.

42. The GUSTO Investigators. An international randomized trial comparing four thrombolytic strategies for acute myocardial infarction. *N Engl J Med.* 1993;329:673-682.

43. Garg R, Yusuf S. Overview of randomized trials of angiotensin-converting enzyme inhibitors on mortality and morbidity in patients with heart failure. *JAMA.* 1995;273:1450-1456.

# HARM

Mitchell Levine, David Haslam, Stephen Walter, Robert Cumming, Hui Lee, Ted Haines, Anne Holbrook, Virginia Moyer, and Gordon Guyatt

The following EBM Working Group members also made substantive contributions to this section: Peter Pronovost and Sharon Straus

## IN THIS SECTION

## CLINICAL SCENARIO

### Do SSRIs Cause Gastrointenstinal Bleeding?

You are a general practitioner considering the optimal choice of antidepressant medication. Your patient is a 55-year-old previously cheerful and well-adjusted individual who, during the past 2 months, has become sad and distressed for the first time in his life. He has developed difficulty concentrating and experiences early morning wakening, but lacks thoughts of self-harm. The patient has attended your practice for the past 20 years and you know him well. You believe he is suffering from a major depressive episode and that he might benefit from antidepressant medication.

During recent years, you have been administering a selective serotonin reuptake inhibitor (SSRI), paroxetine, as your first-line antidepressant agent. However, recent reviews suggesting that the SSRIs are no more effective[1-3] and do not have lower discontinuation rates[1-4] than tricyclic antidepressants (TCAs) have led you to revert to your previous first choice, nortriptyline, in some patients. Patients in your practice usually consider the adverse effects in some depth before agreeing to any treatment decisions and many choose SSRIs on the basis of a preferable side-effect profile.

However, for the past 5 years the patient you are seeing today has been taking ketoprofen (a nonsteroidal anti-inflammatory drug, or NSAID), 50 mg three times per day, which has controlled the pain from his hip osteoarthritis. Your mind jumps to a review article suggesting that SSRIs may be associated with an increased risk of bleeding, and you become concerned about the risk of gastrointestinal bleeding when you consider that the patient is also receiving an NSAID. Unfortunately, an abstract from *Evidence Based Mental Health,*[5] which you have used to obtain a summary of side effects of antidepressant medications, provides no information regarding this issue.

You remember the review article[6] and locate a copy in your files, but at a glance you realize that it will not help answer your question for three reasons: It did not use explicit inclusion and exclusion criteria, it failed to conduct a systematic and comprehensive search, and it did not evaluate the methodologic quality of the original research it summarized (see Part 1E, "Summarizing the Evidence"). In addition, it did not cite any original studies specific to an association between SSRI treatment and gastrointestinal bleeding.

You consider that it is worth following up this issue before you make a final recommendation to the patient. You inform him that he will need antidepressant medication, but you explain your concern about the possible bleeding risk and your need to acquire more definitive information before making a final recommendation. You schedule a follow-up visit 2 days later and you commit to presenting a strategy at that time.

# FINDING THE EVIDENCE

You formulate the following focused question:

> Do adults suffering from depression and taking SSRI medications, compared to patients not taking antidepressants, suffer an increased risk of serious upper gastrointestinal bleeding?

Later that day, you begin your search using prefiltered evidence-based medicine resources—the journal *Evidence Based Mental Health*, Best Evidence4, Clinical Evidence, and the Cochrane Library. For each database, you enter the term "serotonin reuptake inhibitor." Search of *Evidence Based Mental Health* yields eight reviews in volumes 1 (1998) and 2 (1999). Four of these deal with adverse effects associated with SSRI use, but none addresses gastrointestinal bleeding. Searching Best Evidence4 yields 17 equally unhelpful articles. A Clinical Evidence search identifies only a review on treatment of depressive disorders in adults. The Cochrane Library search locates four complete reviews and two abstracts of systematic reviews, but none addresses the issue of gastrointestinal bleeding in SSRI users.

You now turn to the PubMed version of MEDLINE and PreMEDLINE searching system (www.ncbi.nlm.nih.gov/entrez/query.fcgi). For optimum search efficiency, you click on "Clinical queries" under "PubMed Services" to access systematically tested search strategies, or you go to "Search hedges," which will help you identify methodologically sound studies pertaining to your question on harm (see Part 1A1, "Finding the Evidence"). You enter the following: "selective serotonin reuptake inhibitor" AND "bleeding" for the subject search term; and you click on "Etiology" for study category and "Specificity" for emphasis. Your MEDLINE search (from 1966 through 2000) identifies one citation, an epidemiologic study assessing the association between SSRIs and upper gastrointestinal bleeding.[7] This study describes a threefold increased risk of upper gastrointestinal bleeding associated with the use of SSRIs. Thinking that this article may answer your question, you download the full text free of charge from the *British Medical Journal* (*BMJ*) Web site (www.bmj.com) as a portable document format (PDF) file, an electronic version of a printed page or pages.

# ARE THE RESULTS VALID?

Clinicians often encounter patients who are facing potentially harmful exposures, either to medical interventions or environmental agents, and important questions arise. Are pregnant women at increased risk of miscarriage if they work in front of video display terminals? Do vasectomies increase the risk of prostate cancer? Do hypertension management programs at work lead to increased absenteeism? When examining these questions, physicians must evaluate the validity of the data, the strength of the association between the assumed cause and the adverse outcome, and the relevance to patients in their practice.

As when answering any clinical question, our first goal should be to identify a systematic review of the topic that can provide an objective summary of all the available evidence (see Part 1E, "Summarizing the Evidence"). However, interpreting a systematic review requires an understanding of the rules of evidence for observational (nonrandomized) studies. The tests for judging the validity of observational study results, like the validity tests for randomized controlled trials, help you decide whether experimental and control groups began the study with a similar prognosis and whether similarity with respect to prognostic factors persisted after the study was started (see Table 1B-5).

**TABLE 1B–5**

## Users' Guides for an Article About Harm

**Are the results valid?**

Did experimental and control groups begin the study with a similar prognosis?

- Did the investigators demonstrate similarity in all known determinants of outcome; did they adjust for differences in the analysis?

- Were exposed patients equally likely to be identified in the two groups?

Did experimental and control groups retain a similar prognosis after the study started?

- Were the outcomes measured in the same way in the groups being compared?

- Was follow-up sufficiently complete?

**What are the results?**

- How strong is the association between exposure and outcome?

- How precise is the estimate of the risk?

**How can I apply the results to patient care?**

- Were the study patients similar to the patient under consideration in my practice?

- Was the duration of follow-up adequate?

- What was the magnitude of the risk?

- Should I attempt to stop the exposure?

## Did the Investigators Demonstrate Similarity in All Known Determinants of Outcome? Did They Adjust for Differences in the Analysis?

Studies of potentially harmful exposures will yield biased results if the group exposed to the putative harmful agent and the unexposed group begin with a different prognosis. Let us say we are interested in the impact of hospitalization on mortality rate. To investigate this question, we compare mortality in hospitalized individuals to that in people of similar age and sex in the community. Although an examination of the results would lead us to stay clear of hospitals, few would take these results seriously. The reason for skepticism is that people are admitted to hospitals because they are sick and, therefore, are at greater risk of dying. This higher risk results in a spurious (that is, noncausal) association between exposure (hospitalization) and outcome (death). In general, people who seek health care or who take medicine are sicker than people who do not. If clinicians fail to take this into account, they are at high risk of making inaccurate inferences about causal relations between medications and adverse effects.

How can investigators ensure that their comparison groups start a study with a similar likelihood of suffering the target outcome? Randomized controlled trials provide less biased estimates of potentially harmful effects than other study designs because randomization is the best way to ensure that groups are balanced with respect to both known and unknown determinants of outcome (see Part 1B1, "Therapy"). Although investigators conduct RCTs to determine whether therapeutic agents are beneficial, RCTs can also demonstrate harm. The unexpected results of some randomized trials (for example, drugs that investigators expected to show benefit sometimes are associated with increased mortality) have demonstrated the potential of this study design for demonstrating harm (see Part 2B1, "Therapy and Validity, Surprising Results of Randomized Trials").

There are two reasons that we cannot usually find RCTs to help us determine if a putative harmful agent truly has deleterious effects. First, we consider it unethical to randomize patients to exposures that may be harmful (not beneficial). Even if we did not hold these scruples, informed patients would not consent to such an experiment.

Second, we are often concerned about rare and serious adverse effects that occur over prolonged periods of time—ones that become evident only after tens of thousands of patients have consumed the medication. For instance, even a very large randomized trial[8] failed to detect an association between clopidogrel and thrombotic thrombocytopenic purpura, which was detected by a subsequent observational study.[9] Randomized trials specifically addressing side effects may be feasible for adverse event rates as low as 1%[10,11] and meta-analyses may be very helpful when event rates are low.[12] The randomized trials we would need to explore harmful events that occur in less than one in 100 exposed patients—trials characterized by huge sample size and lengthy follow-up—are logistically difficult and prohibitively expensive.

Given that clinicians will not find RCTs to answer most questions about harm, they must understand alternative strategies for ensuring a balanced prognosis in the groups being compared. This understanding requires a familiarity with observational study designs, which we will now describe (Table 1B-6).

**TABLE 1B-6**

## Directions of Inquiry and Key Methodologic Strengths and Weaknesses for Different Study Designs

| Design | Starting Point | Assessment | Strengths | Weaknesses |
|--------|----------------|------------|-----------|------------|
| Cohort | Exposure status | Outcome event status | Feasible when randomization of exposure not possible | Susceptible to bias, limited validity |
| Case-Control | Outcome event status | Exposure status | Overcomes temporal delays, may only require small sample size | Susceptible to bias, limited validity |
| RCT | Exposure status | Adverse event status | Low susceptibility to bias | Feasibility, generalizability |

## Cohort Studies

In a *cohort study*, the investigator identifies exposed and nonexposed groups of patients, each a cohort, and then follows them forward in time, monitoring the occurrence of the predicted outcome. In one such study, for example, investigators assessed perinatal outcomes among infants of men exposed to lead and organic solvents in the printing industry by means of a cohort of all males who had been members of printers' unions in Oslo.[13] The investigators used job classification to categorize fathers as being either exposed to lead and solvents or not exposed to those substances. In this study, exposure was associated with an eightfold increase in preterm births, but it was not linked with birth defects.

Investigators may rely on cohort designs when harmful outcomes occur infrequently. For example, clinically apparent upper gastrointestinal hemorrhage in patients using NSAIDs occurs approximately 1.5 times per 1000 person-years of exposure, in comparison with 1.0 per 1000 person-years in those not taking NSAIDs.[14] Because the event rate in unexposed patients is so low (0.1%), a randomized trial to study an increase in risk of 50% would require huge numbers of patients (sample size calculations suggest about 75,000 patients per group) for adequate power to test the hypothesis that NSAIDs cause the additional bleeding.[15] Such a randomized trial would not be feasible, but a cohort study, in which the information comes from a large administrative database, would be possible.

The danger in using observational studies to assess a possible harmful exposure is that exposed and unexposed patients may begin with a different risk of the target outcome. For instance, in the association between NSAIDs and the increased risk of upper gastrointestinal bleeding, age may be associated both with exposure to NSAIDs and with gastrointestinal bleeding. In other words, since patients taking NSAIDs will be older and older patients are more likely to bleed, this *confounding variable* makes attribution of an increased risk of bleeding to NSAID exposure problematic.

There is no reason patients who self-select (or who are selected by their physician) for exposure to a potentially harmful agent should be similar, with respect to other important determinants of outcome, to the nonexposed patients. Indeed, there are many reasons to expect they will not be similar. Physicians are reluctant to prescribe medications they perceive will put their patients at risk and will selectively prescribe low-risk medications. In one study, for instance, 24.1% of patients who were given a then-new NSAID, ketoprofen, had received peptic ulcer therapy during the previous 2 years in comparison to 15.7% of the control population.[16] The likely reason is that the ketoprofen manufacturer succeeded in persuading clinicians that ketoprofen was less likely to cause gastrointestinal bleeding than other agents. A subsequent comparison of ketoprofen to other agents would be subject to the risk of finding a spurious increase in bleeding with the new agent because higher-risk patients would have been receiving the drug.

The prescription of benzodiazepines to elderly patients provides another example of the way that selective physician prescribing practices can lead to a different distribution of risk in patients receiving particular medications. This is referred to as the *channeling effect*.[17,18] Ray and colleagues[19] found an association between long-acting benzodiazepines and risk of falls (relative risk [RR], 2.0; 95% CI, 1.6-2.5) in data from 1977 to 1979, but not in data from 1984 to 1985 (RR, 1.3; 95% CI, 0.9-1.8). The most plausible explanation for the change is that patients at high risk for falls (those with dementia and anxiety or agitation) selectively received benzodiazepines during the earlier time period. Reports of associations between benzodiazepine use and falls led to greater caution, and the apparent association disappeared when physicians began to avoid benzodiazepine use in those at high risk of falling.

Therefore, investigators must document the characteristics of the exposed and nonexposed participants and either demonstrate their comparability or use statistical techniques to adjust for differences. Since investigators cannot recruit groups that are age-balanced, they must use statistical techniques that correct or adjust for the imbalances.

Effective adjustment for prognostic factors requires the accurate measurement of those prognostic factors. Large administrative databases, while providing a sample size that allows ascertainment of rare events, sometimes have limited quality of data concerning relevant patient characteristics. For example, Jollis and colleagues[20] wondered about the accuracy of information about patient characteristics in an insurance claims database. To investigate this issue, they compared the insurance claims data with prospective data collection by a cardiology fellow. They found that a high degree of chance corrected agreement between the fellow and the administrative database for the presence of diabetes: kappa, a measure of chance-corrected agreement, was 0.83 (see Part 2C, "Diagnosis, Measuring Agreement Beyond Chance"). They also found a high degree of agreement for myocardial infarction (kappa, 0.76), and moderate agreement for hypertension (kappa, 0.56). However, agreement was poor for heart failure (kappa, 0.39) and very poor for tobacco use (kappa, 0.19). We expand on the limitations of administrative databases in another section of this book (see Part 2B, "Therapy and Harm, Outcomes of Health Services").

Even if investigators document the comparability of potentially confounding variables in exposed and nonexposed cohorts and even if they use statistical techniques to adjust for differences, important prognostic factors that the investigators do not know about or have not measured may be unbalanced between the groups and, thus, may be responsible for differences in outcome. Returning to our earlier example, for instance, it may be that the illnesses that require NSAIDs, rather than the NSAIDs themselves, are responsible for the increased risk of bleeding. Thus, the strength of inference from a cohort study will always be less than that of a rigorously conducted RCT.

### Case-Control Studies

Rare outcomes, or those that take a long time to develop, threaten cohort studies' feasibility. An alternative design relies on the initial identification of *cases*—that is, patients who have already developed the target outcome. The investigators then choose *controls*—persons who, as a group, are reasonably similar to the cases with respect to important determinants of outcome such as age, sex, and concurrent medical conditions, but who have not suffered the target outcome. Using this *case-control* design, investigators then assess the relative frequency of exposure to the putative harmful agent in the cases and controls, adjusting for differences in the known and measured prognostic variables. This design permits the simultaneous exploration of multiple exposures that have a possible association with the target outcome.

For example, investigators used a case-control design to demonstrate the association between diethylstilbestrol (DES) ingestion by pregnant women and the development of vaginal adenocarcinomas in their daughters many years later.[21] An RCT or prospective cohort study designed to test this cause-and-effect relationship would have required at least 20 years from the time when the association was first suspected until the completion of the study. Further, given the infrequency of the disease, either an RCT or a cohort study would have required hundreds of thousands of participants. By contrast, using the case-control strategy, the investigators delineated two groups of young women. Those who had suffered the outcome of interest (vaginal adenocarcinoma) were designated as the cases (n = 8) and those who did not experience the outcome were designated as the controls (n = 32). Then, working backward in time, they determined exposure rates to DES for the two groups. The investigators found a strong association between in utero DES exposure and vaginal adenocarcinoma, which was extremely unlikely to be attributable to the play of chance ($P < .00001$). They found their answer without a delay of 20 years and by studying outcomes in only 40 women.

In another example, investigators used a case-control design relying on computer record linkages between health insurance data and a drug plan to investigate the possible relationship between use of beta-adrenergic agonists and mortality rates in patients with asthma.[22] The database for the study included 95% of the population of the province of Saskatchewan in western Canada. The investigators matched 129 cases of fatal or near-fatal asthma with 655 controls who also suffered from asthma but who had not had a fatal or near-fatal asthma attack.

The tendency of patients with more severe asthma to use more beta-adrenergic medications could create a spurious association between drug use and mortality rate. The investigators attempted to control for the confounding effect of disease severity by measuring the number of hospitalizations in the 24 months prior to death (cases) or the index date of entry in to the study (control group) and by using an index of the aggregate use of medications. They found an association between the routine use of large doses of beta-adrenergic agonist metered-dose inhalers and death from asthma (odds ratio [OR], 2.6 per canister per month; 95% CI, 1.7-3.9), even after correcting for their measures of disease severity.

As with cohort studies, case-control studies are susceptible to unmeasured confounding variables, particularly when exposure varies over time. For instance, previous hospitalization and medication use may not adequately capture all the variability in underlying disease severity in asthma. In addition, adverse lifestyle behaviors of asthmatic patients who use large amounts of beta agonists could contribute to the association. Furthermore, choice of controls may inadvertently create spurious associations. For instance, in a study that examined the association between coffee and pancreatic cancer, the investigators chose control patients from the practices of the physicians looking after the patients with pancreatic cancer.[23] These control patients had a variety of gastrointestinal problems, some of which were exacerbated by coffee ingestion. The control patients had learned to avoid coffee; as a result, the investigators found an association between coffee (which the pancreatic cancer patients consumed at general population levels) and cancer. Subsequent investigations, using more appropriate controls, refuted the association.[24,25] These problems illustrate why clinicians can draw inferences of only limited strength from the results of observational studies, even after adjustment for known determinants of outcome.

## Case Series and Case Reports

*Case series* (descriptions of a series of patients) and *case reports* (descriptions of individual patients) do not provide any comparison group, and are therefore unable to satisfy the requirement that treatment and control groups share a similar prognosis. Although descriptive studies occasionally demonstrate dramatic findings mandating an immediate change in physician behavior (eg, recall the consequences when a link was associated between thalidomide and birth defects[26]), there are potentially undesirable consequences when actions are taken in response to weak evidence. Consider the case of the drug Bendectin (a combination of doxylamine, pyridoxine, and dicyclomine used as an antiemetic in pregnancy), whose manufacturer withdrew it from the market as a result of case reports suggesting it was teratogenic.[27] Later, even though a number of comparative studies demonstrated the drug's relative safety,[28] they could not eradicate the prevailing litigious atmosphere—which prevented the manufacturer from reintroducing Bendectin. Thus, many pregnant women who potentially could have benefited from the drug's availability were denied the symptomatic relief it could have offered.

In general, clinicians should not draw conclusions about cause-and-effect relationships from case series but, rather, should recognize that the results may generate questions for regulatory agencies and clinical investigators to address.

## Design Issues—Summary

Just as is true for the resolution of questions of therapeutic effectiveness, clinicians should look first for randomized trials to resolve issues of harm. They will often be disappointed in this search and must make use of studies of weaker design. Regardless of the design, however, they should look for an appropriate control population before making a strong inference about a putative harmful agent. For RCTs and cohort studies, the control group should have a similar baseline risk of outcome, or investigators should use statistical techniques to adjust or correct for differences. Similarly, in case-control studies the derived exposed and nonexposed groups should be similar with respect to determinants of outcome other than the exposure under study. Alternatively, investigators should use statistical techniques to adjust for differences. Even when investigators have taken all the appropriate steps to minimize bias, clinicians should bear in mind that residual differences between groups may always bias the results of observational studies.[29] Since prescribing in the real world is carried out on the basis of evidence, clinician values, and patient values, exposure opportunities in nonrandomized medication studies are likely to differ among patients (channeling bias or effect).

## Were Exposed Patients Equally Likely to Be Identified in the Two Groups?

In case-control studies, ascertainment of the exposure is a key issue. For example, when patients with leukemia are asked about prior exposure to solvents, they may be more likely to recall exposure than would control group members, either because of increased patient motivation (*recall bias*) or because of greater probing by an interviewer (*interviewer bias*). Clinicians should note whether investigators used bias-minimizing strategies such as blinding participants and interviewers to the hypothesis of the study. For example, a case-control study found a twofold increase in risk of hip fracture associated with psychotropic drug use. In this study, investigators established drug exposure by examining computerized claims files of the Michigan Medicaid program, a strategy that avoided both recall and interviewer bias.[30] The study of beta-adrenergic agonist use in patients with asthma suggesting an association with mortality also relied on an administrative database to ascertain exposure.[9] In both cases, the assurance of unbiased exposure status increases our confidence in the studies' findings.

## Were the Outcomes Measured in the Same Way in the Groups Being Compared?

In RCTs and cohort studies, ascertainment of outcome is a key issue. For example, investigators have reported a threefold increase in the risk of malignant melanoma in individuals working with radioactive materials. One possible explanation for some of the increased risk might be that physicians, aware of a possible risk, search more diligently and, therefore, detect disease that might otherwise go unnoticed (or they may detect disease at an earlier point in time). This could result in the exposed cohort having an apparent, but spurious, increase in risk—a situation we refer to as *surveillance bias*.[31]

## Was Follow-up Sufficiently Complete?

As we pointed out in Part 1B1, "Therapy," loss to follow-up can introduce bias because the patients who are lost may have very different outcomes from those still available for assessment. The longer the required follow-up period, the greater the possibility that the follow-up will be incomplete.

For example, in a well-executed study, investigators determined the vital status of 1235 of 1261 white males (98%) employed in a chrysotile asbestos textile operation between 1940 and 1975.[32] The relative risk for lung cancer death over time increased from 1.4 to 18.2 in direct proportion to the cumulative exposure among asbestos workers with at least 15 years since first exposure. Because the 2% missing data were unlikely to affect the results, the loss to follow-up does not threaten the validity of the inference that asbestos exposure causes lung cancer deaths.

## USING THE GUIDE

**R**eturning to our earlier discussion, the study that we retrieved investigating the association between SSRIs and risk of upper gastrointestinal bleeding used a case-control design.[6] Data came from a general practitioner electronic medical record database in the United Kingdom, which included data from more than 3 million people, most of whom had been entered prospectively during a 5-year period.[33-35] The investigators identified cases of upper gastrointestinal bleeding (*n*=1651) and ulcer perforation (*n*=248) among patients aged 40 to 79 years between 1993 and 1997. They then randomly selected 10,000 controls from the at-risk source population that gave rise to cases, choosing their sample so that age, sex, and the year patients were identified were similar among the cases and control groups.

The analysis controlled for a number of possible prognostic factors: previous dyspepsia, gastritis, peptic ulcer and upper gastrointestinal bleeding or perforation, smoking status, and current use of NSAIDs, anticoagulants, corticosteroids, and aspirin. The database included prescription drugs only. The investigators examined the relative frequency of SSRI prescription use in the 30 days before the *index date* (that is, the date of the reported bleeding or perforation) in patients with and without bleeding and perforation after controlling for the prognostic variables. Control patients received a random date as their index date.

Although the investigators controlled for a number of prognostic factors, there are other potential important determinants of bleeding for which they did not control. For example, more patients being treated for depression or anxiety suffer from painful medical conditions than those without depression and anxiety. Patients may have been using over-the-counter NSAIDs for these problems. The database the investigators used does not capture the use of self-medication with over-the-counter analgesics.

Alcohol use is another potential confounder. Although the investigators excluded patients with known alcoholism, many persons afflicted with alcoholism remain unrevealed to their primary care physician, and alcoholism is associated with an increased prevalence of depression and anxiety that could lead to the prescription of SSRIs. Since alcoholism is associated with increased bleeding risk, this prognostic variable fulfills all the criteria for a confounding variable that could bias the results of the study. Finally, it is possible that patients returning for prescription of SSRIs would be more likely to have their bleeding diagnosed in comparison to patients under less intense surveillance (a state of affairs known as *detection bias*).

These biases should apply to all three classes of antidepressants (ie, SSRIs, nonselective serotonin reuptake inhibitors, and a miscellaneous group of other drugs) that the investigators considered. The results of the study, which we will discuss later in this section, showed an association only between gastrointestinal bleeding and SSRIs, rather than between gastrointestinal bleeding and other antidepressant medications. One would expect all these biases to influence the association between any antidepressant agent and bleeding. Thus, the fact that the investigators found the association only with SSRIs decreases our concern about the threats to validity from possible differences in prognostic factors in those receiving—and not receiving—SSRIs.

At the same time, most physicians make decisions regarding the prescription of SSRIs or tricyclic antidepressant agents based on particular patient characteristics. Thus, it remains possible that these characteristics include some that are associated with the incidence of gastrointestinal bleeding. This would be true, for instance, if clinicians differentially used SSRI rather than other antidepressant medications in patients in whom they suspected alcohol abuse.

The major strength of the use of a large database for this study is that it eliminates the possibility of biased assessment of exposure (or recall bias) to SSRIs in the patients who suffered the outcomes as well as in those who did not. The outcomes and exposures were probably measured in the same way in both groups, as most clinicians are unaware that UGI bleeding may be associated with SSRI use. We have no idea, however, about the number of patients lost to follow-up. Although the investigators included only those patients who stayed in the practices of the participating primary care physicians from the beginning to the end of the study, we do not know, for instance, how many people in the database began to receive SSRIs but subsequently left those practices.

In summary, the study suffers from the limitation inherent in any observational study: that exposed and unexposed patients may differ in prognosis at baseline. In this case, at least two unmeasured variables, over-the-counter NSAID use and alcohol consumption, might create a spurious association between SSRIs and gastrointestinal bleeding. The other major limitation of the study is the lack of information regarding completeness of follow-up. That said, although these limitations weaken any inferences we might make, we are likely to conclude that the study is strong enough to warrant a review of the results.

# WHAT ARE THE RESULTS?

## How Strong Is the Association Between Exposure and Outcome?

We have described the alternatives for expressing the association between the exposure and the outcome, the relative risk and the odds ratio, in other sections of this book (see Part 1B1, "Therapy"; see also Part 2B2, "Therapy and Understanding the Results, Measures of Association"). In a cohort study assessing in-hospital mortality after noncardiac surgery in male veterans, 23 of 289 patients with a history of hypertension died, compared with three of 185 patients without the condition. The relative risk for hypertension and mortality, (23/289)/(3/185), was 4.9.[36] The relative risk tells us that death after noncardiac surgery occurs almost five times more often in patients with hypertension than in normotensive patients.

The estimate of relative risk depends on the availability of samples of exposed and unexposed patients, where the proportion of the patients with the outcome of interest can be determined. The relative risk is therefore not applicable to case-control studies in which the number of cases and controls—and, therefore, the proportion of individuals with the outcome—is chosen by the investigator. For case-control studies, instead of using a ratio of risks (*relative risk*), we use a ratio of odds (*odds ratio*): the odds of a case-patient being exposed, divided by the odds of a control patient being exposed (see Part 2B2, "Therapy, Measures of Association").

When considering both study design and strength of association, we may be ready to interpret a small increase in risk as representing a true harmful effect when the study design is strong (such as in a RCT). A much higher increase in risk might be required of weaker designs (such as cohort or case-control studies), as subtle findings are more likely to be caused by the inevitably higher risk of bias.

Very large values of relative risk or odds ratio represent strong associations that are less likely to be caused by confounding variables or bias.

In addition to showing a large magnitude of relative risk or odds ratio, a second finding will strengthen an inference that we are dealing with a true harmful effect. If, as the quantity or the duration of exposure to the putative harmful agent increases, the risk of the adverse outcome also increases (that is, the data suggest a dose-response gradient), we are more likely to be dealing with a causal relationship between exposure and outcome. The fact that the risk of dying from lung cancer in male physician smokers increases by 50%, 132%, and 220% for 1 to 14, 15 to 24, and 25 or more cigarettes smoked per day, respectively, strengthens our inference that cigarette smoking causes lung cancer.[37]

## How Precise Is the Estimate of the Risk?

Clinicians can evaluate the precision of the estimate of risk by examining the confidence interval around that estimate (see Part 1B1, "Therapy"; see also Part 2B2, "Therapy and Understanding the Results, Confidence Intervals"). In a study in which investigators have shown an association between an exposure and an adverse outcome, the lower limit of the estimate of relative risk associated with the adverse exposure provides a minimal estimate of the strength of the association. By contrast, in a study in which investigators fail to demonstrate an association (a negative study), the upper boundary of the confidence interval around the relative risk tells the clinician just how big an adverse effect may still be present, despite the failure to show a statistically significant association (see Part 2B2, "Therapy and Understanding the Results, Confidence Intervals").

### USING THE GUIDE

**R**eturning to our earlier discussion, the investigators calculated odds ratios (ORs) of the risk of bleeding in those exposed to SSRIs vs those not exposed, but they reported the results as relative risks (RR). Unfortunately, this practice is not unusual. Fortunately, when event rates are low, relative risks and odds ratios closely approximate one another (see Part 2B2, "Therapy, Measures of Association"). The investigators found an association between current use of SSRIs and upper gastrointestinal bleeding (adjusted OR, 3.0; 95% CI, 2.1-4.4). They noted a weak association with nonselective serotonin reuptake inhibitors (adjusted OR, 1.4; 95% CI, 1.1-1.9), but found no association with antidepressant medications that had no action on the serotonin reuptake mechanism. The investigators found that the association between NSAID use and bleeding (adjusted OR, 3.7; 95% CI, 3.2-4.4) was of similar magnitude to the association between bleeding and SSRIs. The current use of SSRIs with prescription NSAID drugs further increased the risk of upper gastrointestinal bleeding (adjusted OR, 15.6; 95% CI, 6.6-36.6). The dose and duration of SSRI use had little influence on the risk of this adverse outcome.

# HOW CAN I APPLY THE RESULTS TO PATIENT CARE?

## Were the Study Patients Similar to the Patient in My Practice?

If possible biases in a study are not sufficient to dismiss the study out of hand, you must consider the extent to which they might apply to the patient in your office. Is the patient before you similar to those described in the study with respect to morbidity, age, sex, race, or other potentially important factors? If not, is the biology of the harmful exposure likely to differ in the patient you are attending (see Part 2B3, "Therapy and Applying the Results, Applying Results to Individual Patients")? Are there important differences in the treatments or exposures between the patients you see and the patients studied? For example, the risk of thrombophlebitis associated with oral contraceptive use described in the 1970s may not be applicable to the patient of the 1990s because of the lower estrogen dose in oral contraceptives used in the 1990s. Similarly, increases in uterine cancer secondary to postmenopausal estrogen replacement do not apply to women who are also taking concomitant progestins tailored to produce monthly withdrawal bleeding with chronic, noncyclic use.

## Was the Duration of Follow-up Adequate?

Let us return for a moment to the study that showed that workers employed in chrysotile asbestos textile operation between 1940 and 1975 showed an increased risk for lung cancer death, a risk that increased from 1.4 to 18.2 in direct relation to cumulative exposure among asbestos workers with at least 15 years since first exposure.[32] The fact that the follow-up was sufficiently long to capture a large proportion of the lung cancers destined to occur enhances our confidence in application of the results to patients in our practice. By contrast, excessively short follow-up may fail to detect harmful effects that emerge with longer observation.

## What Was the Magnitude of the Risk?

The relative risk and the odds ratio do not tell us how frequently the problem occurs; they tell us only that the observed effect occurs more or less often in the exposed group compared to the unexposed group. Thus, we need a method for assessing clinical importance. In our discussion of therapy (see Part 1B1, "Therapy"; see also Part 2B2, "Therapy and Understanding the Results, Measures of Association"), we described the way to calculate the number of patients who must be treated to prevent an adverse event. When the issue is harm, we can use data from a randomized trial or cohort study, but not a case-control study, to make an analogous calculation to determine how many people must be exposed to the harmful agent to cause an adverse outcome.

For example, over an average of 10 months of follow-up, investigators conducting the Cardiac Arrhythmia Suppression Trial (CAST), a RCT of antiarrhythmic agents,[38,39] found that the mortality rate was 3.0% for placebo-treated patients and

7.7% for those treated with either encainide or flecainide. The *absolute risk increase* was 4.7%, the reciprocal of which tells us that, on average, for every 21 patients we treat with encainide or flecainide for about a year, we will cause one excess death. This contrasts with our example of the association between NSAIDs and upper gastrointestinal bleeding. Of 2000 unexposed patients, two will suffer a bleeding episode each year. Of 2000 patients taking NSAIDs, three will suffer such an episode each year. Thus, if we treat 2000 patients with NSAIDs, we can expect a single additional bleeding event.[7]

## Should I Attempt to Stop the Exposure?

After evaluating the evidence that an exposure is harmful and after establishing that the results are potentially applicable to the patient in your practice, determining subsequent actions may not be simple. There are at least three aspects to consider in making a clinical decision.

First is the strength of inference: how strong was the study or studies that demonstrated harm in the first place? Second, what is the magnitude of the risk to patients if exposure to the harmful agent continues? Third, what are the adverse consequences of reducing or eliminating exposure to the harmful agent—that is, the magnitude of the benefit that patients will no longer receive?

Clinical decision making is simple when both the likelihood of harm and its magnitude are great. Because the evidence of increased mortality from encainide and flecainide came from a randomized trial,[38] we can be confident of the causal connection. Since treating only 21 people will result in an excess death, it is no wonder that clinicians quickly curtailed their use of these antiarrhythmic agents when the study results became available.

The clinical decision is also made easier when an acceptable alternative for avoiding the risk is available. For example, beta blockers prescribed for the treatment of hypertension can result in symptomatic increase in airway resistance in patients with asthma or chronic airflow limitation. This risk mandates the use of an alternative drug, such as a thiazide diuretic, in susceptible patients.[40]

Even if the evidence is relatively weak, the availability of an alternative can result in a clear decision. The early case-control studies demonstrating the association between aspirin use and Reye syndrome, for example, were relatively weak and left considerable doubt about the causal relationship. Although the strength of inference was not great, the availability of a safe, inexpensive, and well-tolerated alternative, acetaminophen, justified use of this alternative agent in children at risk of Reye syndrome.[41]

In contrast to the early studies regarding aspirin and Reye syndrome, multiple well-designed cohort and case-control studies have consistently demonstrated an association between NSAIDs and upper gastrointestinal bleeding; therefore, our inference about harm has been relatively strong. However, the risk of an upper gastrointestinal bleeding episode is quite low, and until recently we have not had safer and equally efficacious anti-inflammatory alternatives available. We were therefore probably right in continuing to prescribe NSAIDs for the appropriate clinical conditions. Depending on both their safety profile after longer experience and cost-effectiveness considerations, COX 2-inhibiting NSAIDs may prove to be an appropriate alternative class of agents.

# Clinical Resolution

To decide on your course of action, you proceed through the three steps of using the medical literature to guide your clinical practice. First, you consider the validity of the study before you. The antidepressant and upper gastrointestinal bleeding study addressed multiple classes of antidepressant agents and the risk of upper gastrointestinal bleeding or ulcer perforation. You decide that the limitations of the case-control design, along with the lack of information about loss to follow-up, leave you uncertain about a causal relationship between SSRIs and gastrointestinal bleeding. Furthermore, this is a single study and, as we have previously mentioned, in other areas of medicine subsequent investigations[11, 12, 42-45] have failed to confirm many apparent harmful associations.[10, 46, 47]

Turning to the results, you note the very strong association between the combined use of SSRIs and NSAIDs. Despite the methodologic limitations of this single study, you believe the association is too strong to ignore. You therefore proceed to the third step and consider the implications of the results for the patient before you.

The primary care database from which the investigators drew their sample suggests that the results are readily applicable to the patient before you. You consider the magnitude of the risk to which you would be exposing this patient if you prescribed an SSRI and it actually did cause bleeding. Using the baseline risk reported by Carson et al in a similar population,[14] you calculate that you would need to treat about 625 patients with SSRIs for a year to cause a single bleeding episode in patients not using NSAIDs, and about 55 patients a year taking NSAIDs along with an SSRI for a year to cause a single bleeding episode.

From previous experience with the patient before you, you know that he is risk averse. When he returns to your office, you note the equal effectiveness of the SSRIs and tricyclic antidepressants that you can offer him, and you describe the side-effect profile of the alternative agents. You note, among the other considerations, the possible increased risk of gastrointestinal bleeding with the SSRIs. The patient decides that, on balance, he would prefer a tricyclic antidepressant and leaves your office with a prescription for nortriptyline.

# References

1. Geddes JR, Freemantle N, Mason J, Eccles MP, Boynton J. SSRIs versus other antidepressants for depressive disorder. *Cochrane Database of Systematic Reviews*. 2000:1-26.

2. Trindale E, Menon D. *Selective Serotonin Reuptake Inhibitors (SSRIs) for Major Depression.* Ottawa: Canadian Coordinating Office for Health Technology Assessment; 1997.

3. Mulrow CD, Williams JW Jr, Trivedi M. *Treatment of Depression: Newer Pharmacotherapies.* San Antonio, Texas: San Antonio Evidence-based Practice Centre; 1999.

4. Hotopf M, Hardy R, Lewis G. Discontinuation rates of SSRIs and tricyclic antidepressants: a meta-analysis and investigation of heterogeneity. *Br J Psychiatry.* 1997;170:120-127.

5. Trindale E, Menon D. Review: selective serotonin reuptake inhibitors differ from tricyclic antidepressants in adverse events. *Evidence Based Mental Health.* 1998;1:50.

6. Goldberg RJ. Selective serotonin reuptake inhibitors: infrequent medical adverse effects. *Arch Fam Med.* 1998;7:78-84.

7. de Abajo FJ, Rodriguez LA, Montero D. Association between selective serotonin reuptake inhibitors and upper gastrointestinal bleeding: population based case-control study. *BMJ.* 1999;319:1106-1109.

8. CAPRIE Steering Committee. A randomised, blinded, trial of clopidogrel versus aspirin in patients at risk of ischaemic events (CAPRIE). *Lancet.* 1996;348:1329-1339.

9. Bennett CL, Connors JM, Carwile JM, et al. Thrombotic thrombocytopenic purpura associated with clopidogrel. *N Engl J Med.* 2000;342:1773-1777.

10. Silverstein FE, Graham DY, Senior JR, et al. Misoprostol reduces serious gastrointestinal complications in patients with rheumatoid arthritis receiving nonsteroidal anti-inflammatory drugs: a randomized, double-blind, placebo-controlled trial. *Ann Intern Med.* 1995;123:241-249.

11. Merck and Co. VIGOR Study Summary. Paper presented at: Digestive Disease Week Congress; May 24, 2000; San Diego.

12. Langman MJ, Jensen DM, Watson DJ, et al. Adverse upper gastrointestinal effects of rofecoxib compared with NSAIDs. *JAMA.* 1999;282:1929-1933.

13. Kristensen P, Irgens LM, Daltveit AK, Andersen A. Perinatal outcome among children of men exposed to lead and organic solvents in the printing industry. *Am J Epidemiol.* 1993;137:134-143.

14. Carson JL, Strom BL, Soper KA, et al. The association of nonsteroidal anti-inflammatory drugs with upper gastrointestinal tract bleeding. *Arch Intern Med.* 1987;147:85-88.

15. Walter SD. Determination of significant relative risks and optimal sampling procedures in prospective and retrospective comparative studies of various sizes. *Am J Epidemiol*. 1977;105:387-397.

16. Leufkens HG, Urquhart J, Stricker BH, Bakker A, Petri H. Channelling of controlled release formulation of ketoprofen (Oscorel) in patients with history of gastrointestinal problems. *J Epidemiol Community Health*. 1992;46:428-432.

17. Joseph KS. The evolution of clinical practice and time trends in drug effects. *J Clin Epidemiol*. 1994;47:593-598.

18. Leufkens HG, Urquhart J. Variability in patterns of drug usage. *J Pharm Pharmacol*. 1994;46(suppl 1):433-437.

19. Ray WA, Griffin MR, Downey W. Benzodiazepines of long and short elimination half-life and risk of hip fracture. *JAMA*. 1989;262:3303-3307.

20. Jollis JG, Ancukiewicz M, DeLong ER, Pryor DB, Muhlbaier LH, Mark DB. Discordance of databases designed for claims payment versus clinical information systems: implications for outcomes research. *Ann Intern Med*. 1993;119:844-850.

21. Herbst AL, Ulfelder H, Poskanzer DC. Adenocarcinoma of the vagina: association of maternal stilbestrol therapy with tumor appearance in young women. *N Engl J Med*. 1971;284:878-881.

22. Spitzer WO, Suissa S, Ernst P, et al. The use of beta-agonists and the risk of death and near death from asthma. *N Engl J Med*. 1992;326:501-506.

23. MacMahon B, Yen S, Trichopoulos D, Warren K, Nardi G. Coffee and cancer of the pancreas. *N Engl J Med*. 1981;304:630-633.

24. Baghurst PA, McMichael AJ, Slavotineck AH, Baghurst KI, Boyle P, Walker AM. A case-control study of diet and cancer of the pancreas. *Am J Epidemiol*. 1991;134:167-179.

25. Zheng W, McLaughlin JK, Gridley G, et al. A cohort study of smoking, alcohol consumption and dietary factors for pancreatic cancer. *Cancer Causes Control*. 1993;4:477-482.

26. Lenz W. Epidemiology of congenital malformations. *Ann NY Acad Sci*. 1965; 123:228-236.

27. Soverchia G, Perri PF. Two cases of malformation of a limb in infants of mothers treated with an antiemetic in a very early phase of pregnancy. *Pediatr Med Chir*. 1981;3:97-99.

28. Holmes LB. Teratogen update: Bendectin. *Teratology*. 1983;27:277-281.

29. Kellermann AL, Rivara FP, Rushforth NB, Banton JG, et al. Gun ownership as a risk factor for homicide in the home. *N Engl J Med*. 1993;329:1084-1091.

30. Ray WA, Griffin MR, Schaffner W, et al. Psychotropic drug use and the risk of hip fracture. *N Engl J Med*. 1987;316:363-369.

31. Hiatt RA, Fireman B. The possible effect of increased surveillance on the incidence of malignant melanoma. *Prev Med*. 1986;15:652-660.

32. Dement JM, Harris RL Jr, Symons MJ, Shy CM. Exposures and mortality among chrysotile asbestos workers. Part II: mortality. *Am J Ind Med*. 1983;4:421-433.

33. Jick H, Jick SS, Derby LE. Validation of information recorded on general practitioner based computerised resource in the United Kingdom. *BMJ*. 1991;302:766-768.

34. Garcia Rodriguez LA, Perez Gutthann S. Use of the UK general practice research database for pharmacoepidemiology. *Br J Clin Pharmacol*. 1998;45:419-425.

35. Jick H, Terris B, Derby LE, Jick SS. Further validation of information recorded on a general practitioner database resource in the United Kingdom. *Pharmacoepidemiol Drug Saf*. 1992;1:347-349.

36. Browner WS, Li J, Mangano DT. In-hospital and long-term mortality in male veteran following noncardiac surgery. *JAMA*. 1992;268:228-232.

37. Doll R, Hill AB. Mortality in relation to smoking: ten years' observation of British doctors. *BMJ*. 1964;1:1399-1410, 1460-1467.

38. Echt DS, Liebson PR, Mitchell LB, et al. Mortality and morbidity in patients receiving encainide, flecainide, or placebo: the Cardiac Arrhythmia Suppression Trial. *N Engl J Med*. 1991;324:781-788.

39. The Cardiac Arrhythmia Suppression Trial II Investigators. Effect of the antiarrhythmic agent moricizine on survival after myocardial infarction. *N Engl J Med*. 1992;327:227-233.

40. Ogilvie RI, Burgess ED, Cusson JR, Feldman RD, Leiter LA, Myers MG. Report of the Canadian Hypertension Society Consensus Conference, 3: pharmacologic treatment of essential hypertension. *Can Med Assoc J*. 1993;149:575-584.

41. Soumerai SB, Ross-Degnan D, Kahn JS. Effects of professional and media warnings about the association between aspirin use in children and Reye's syndrome. *Milbank Q*. 1992;70:155-182.

42. Danesh J, Appleby P. Coronary heart disease and iron status: meta-analyses of prospective studies. *Circulation*. 1999;99:852-854.

43. Klebanoff MA, Read JS, Mills JL, Shiono PH. The risk of childhood cancer after neonatal exposure to vitamin K. *N Engl J Med*. 1993;329:905-908.

44. Passmore SJ, Draper G, Brownbill P, Kroll M. Case-control studies of relation between childhood cancer and neonatal vitamin K administration: retrospective case-control study. *BMJ*. 1998;316:178-184.

45. Parker L, Cole M, Craft AW, Hey EN. Neonatal vitamin K administration and childhood cancer in the north of England. *BMJ*. 1998;316:189-193.

46. Salonen JT, Nyyssonen K, Korpela H, Tuomilehto J, Seppanen R, Salonen R. High stored iron levels are associated with excess risk of myocardial infarction in eastern Finnish men. *Circulation*. 1992;86:803-811.

47. Golding J, Greenwood R, Birmingham K, Mott M. Childhood cancer, intramuscular vitamin K, and pethidine given during labour. *BMJ*. 1992;305:341-346.

# THE PROCESS
# OF DIAGNOSIS

W. Scott Richardson, Mark Wilson, and Gordon Guyatt

The following EBM Working Group members also made substantive contributions to this section: Peter Wyer, Jonathan Craig, Roman Jaeschke, Jeroen Lijmer, Luz Maria Letelier, Virginia Moyer, C. David Naylor, and Deborah Cook

## IN THIS SECTION

# CLINICAL SCENARIO

## Generating a Differential Diagnosis

It is another busy day in the emergency department and one of your nurse colleagues tells you that a 60-year-old man has presented with a severe cough of 1 day's duration. Immediately, you think, "upper respiratory tract infection; perhaps pneumonia." When you enter the room, you find the patient appears short of breath and is in more distress than you were expecting. Other possible diagnoses spring to mind: could the patient be suffering from acute airflow obstruction, myocardial infarction with pulmonary edema, a pneumothorax, or a pulmonary embolus? You sit down beside the patient and begin taking a history. You ask the nurse to place him on cardiac and pulse oximetry monitors, to start an intravenous line, and to obtain a 12-lead electrocardiogram and a portable chest radiograph.

The patient appears moderately tachypneic but is able to speak in complete sentences. Vital signs show a regular heart rate of 96 bpm, a blood pressure of 140/90 mm Hg, and a respiratory rate of 24/min. In view of his tachypnea, you request a rectal temperature. Oximetry shows a saturation of 93% and you ask that he receive 4 L/minute of oxygen by nasal cannula.

The patient reports that he was previously in excellent health, but began to suffer from a cough about 24 hours previously. There was no preceding or accompanying fever, runny nose, sore throat, headache, or muscular discomfort. However, he did experience several hours of central chest discomfort at the time of the onset of the cough, a discomfort that subsequently resolved. The cough has been productive of only small amounts of clear sputum which, during the past 2 hours, has been flecked with small amounts of bright red blood. During the past 12 hours, the patient has felt increasingly short of breath on minimal activity and now feels short of breath at rest.

Cardiac auscultation reveals no extra heart sounds or murmurs. Abnormal findings on physical examination are limited to decreased breath sounds and crackles at the left base on chest auscultation. The electrocardiogram confirms mild sinus tachycardia, but is otherwise normal, and the chest radiograph shows only a small left pleural effusion with minimal associated opacification. The nurse reports the patient's temperature to be 38.1°C. You draw arterial blood gases and arrange for an urgent ventilation-perfusion scan. The room air blood gas results show a normal $PCO_2$ and a $PO_2$ of 70 mm Hg with a saturation of 93%.

While waiting for the results of the ventilation-perfusion scan, you consider how likely the diagnosis of pulmonary embolism is, given the available information. On the one hand, the patient lacks risk factors, cough is a very prominent symptom, and highly suggestive findings for clinical examination (such as pleuritic chest pain) or further investigation (such as a typical electrocardiographic pattern) are absent. On the other hand, you believe you have ruled out a number of competing diagnoses, including asthma, pulmonary edema, and pneumothorax, and the clinical picture is not typical of pneumonia. You ultimately decide the probability is intermediate, and you mentally commit yourself to a 30% likelihood of pulmonary embolus. When the ventilation-perfusion scan reveals an unmatched segmental defect that you know is associated with a likelihood ratio of 18,[1] you use your likelihood ratio card (see Part 1C2, "Diagnostic Tests") to generate a posttest probability of approximately 90%, and you begin anticoagulation.

# THE DIAGNOSTIC PROCESS

Making a diagnosis is a complex cognitive task that involves both logical reasoning and pattern recognition.[2,3] Although the process happens largely at an unconscious level, we can identify two essential steps.

Step 1. In the first step, you enumerate the diagnostic possibilities and estimate their relative likelihood.[4] Experienced clinicians often group the findings into meaningful clusters, summarized in brief phrases about the symptom, body location, or organ system involved, such as "generalized pruritus," "painless jaundice," and "constitutional symptoms." These clusters, or clinical problems, may be of biologic, psychologic, or sociologic origin, and they are the object of the differential diagnosis. In the opening scenario, we considered a previously healthy 60-year-old man with a clinical problem encompassing a day-long history of cough and dyspnea. The differential diagnosis included a respiratory infection, acute airflow obstruction, myocardial infarction with pulmonary edema, a pneumothorax, and pulmonary embolus.

Step 2. In the second step in the diagnostic process, you incorporate new information to change the relative probabilities, rule out some of the possibilities, and, ultimately, choose the most likely diagnosis. For each diagnostic possibility, the additional information increases or decreases the likelihood. In our scenario, the absence of manifestations that usually accompany an infectious process reduces the likelihood of an upper respiratory tract infection or pneumonia. The central chest discomfort increased the possibility that we could be observing an atypical presentation of a myocardial infarction and prompted the timely electrocardiogram. Physical examination made heart failure a much less likely possibility; pneumonia and pulmonary embolus remained as the competing diagnoses. The chest radiograph failed to provide definitive evidence of pneumonia, necessitating an additional test, the ventilation-perfusion scan.

Thus, with each new finding, we moved, albeit intuitively and implicitly, from one probability, the *pretest probability,* to another probability—the *posttest probability*. Some findings, such as the absence of any sign of pneumothorax on the chest radiograph, eliminated one of the possibilities (a posttest probability of 0). Prior to the last test, our approach became explicitly quantitative: we committed to a pretest likelihood of 30% and subsequently used information from the literature to arrive at a final, 90% posttest likelihood of pulmonary embolus.

If we know the properties of each of piece of information (and, in the case of pulmonary embolism, if we have strong data for many elements of the diagnostic workup; see Part 2C, "Diagnosis, Examples of Likelihood Ratios"), we can be highly quantitative in our sequential move from pre- to posttest probability. Later in this section, we will show you how.

Because the properties of the individual items of history and physical examination often are not available, you must rely on clinical experience and intuition to predict the extent to which many pieces of information modify your differential diagnosis. For some clinical problems, including the diagnosis of pulmonary embolism, clinicians' intuition has proved remarkably accurate.[1]

## CHOICES IN THE DIAGNOSTIC PROCESS

When considering a patient's differential diagnosis, how can you decide which disorders to pursue? If you were to consider all known causes to be equally likely and test for them all simultaneously (the possibilistic approach), then the patient would undergo unnecessary testing. Instead, the experienced clinician is selective, considering first those disorders that are more likely (a probabilistic approach), more serious if left undiagnosed and untreated (a prognostic approach), or more responsive to treatment if offered (a pragmatic approach).

Wisely selecting a patient's differential diagnosis involves all three considerations (probabilistic, prognostic, and pragmatic). Your single best explanation for the patient's clinical problem(s) can be termed the leading hypothesis or working diagnosis. In the opening scenario, a respiratory infection was the leading diagnosis until the final test result became available. A few (usually one to five) other diagnoses, termed active alternatives, may be worth considering at the time of initial workup because of their likelihood, seriousness if undiagnosed and untreated, or responsiveness to treatment. In the scenario, pulmonary embolus entered the differential diagnosis early because of its seriousness and responsiveness to treatment.

Additional causes of the clinical problem(s), termed other hypotheses, may be too unlikely to consider at the time of initial diagnostic workup, but remain possible and could be considered further if the working diagnosis and active alternatives are later disproved. In our scenario, remote possibilities such a pulmonary hemorrhage or collagen vascular disease never entered the active differential diagnosis, but might eventually have done so if we had not confirmed one of the active alternatives.

# DIAGNOSTIC AND THERAPEUTIC THRESHOLDS

Consider a patient who presents with a painful eruption of grouped vesicles in the distribution of a single dermatome. In an instant, an experienced clinician would make a diagnosis of herpes zoster and would consider whether to offer the patient therapy. In other words, the probability of herpes zoster is so high (near 1.0, or 100%) that it is above a threshold where no further testing is required.

Next, consider a previously healthy athlete who presents with lateral rib cage pain after being accidentally struck by an errant baseball pitch. Again, an experienced clinician would recognize the clinical problem (posttraumatic lateral chest pain), identify a leading hypothesis (rib contusion) and an active alternative (rib fracture), and plan a test (radiograph) to exclude the latter. If asked, the clinician could also list disorders that are too unlikely to consider further (such as myocardial infarction). In other words, while not as likely as rib contusion, the probability of a rib fracture is above a threshold for testing, while the probability of myocardial infarction is below the threshold for testing.

These cases illustrate how you can estimate the probability of disease and then compare disease probabilities to two thresholds (Figure 1C-1). The probability above which the diagnosis is sufficiently likely to warrant therapy defines the upper threshold. That is, if a clinician believes that the diagnosis is sufficiently likely that she is ready to recommend treatment, she has crossed the upper threshold. This threshold is termed the *treatment threshold*.[5] In the case of shingles described above, the clinician judged the diagnosis of herpes zoster to be above this treatment threshold of probability. In our scenario, with the results of the ventilation-perfusion scan we crossed the treatment threshold only after we arrived at a probability of 90% for one of the competing causes, pulmonary embolus.

**FIGURE 1C-1**

## Test and Treatment Thresholds in the Diagnostic Process

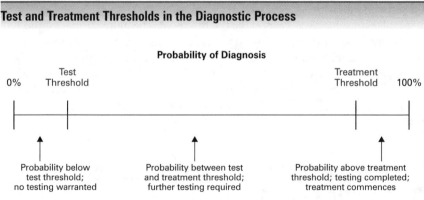

The probability below which the clinician decides a diagnosis warrants no further consideration defines the lower threshold. This threshold is termed the no test-test threshold or, simply, the *test threshold*. In the case of posttraumatic torso pain described above, the diagnosis of rib fracture fell above the test threshold and the diagnosis of myocardial infarction fell below it. In our opening scenario, heart failure dropped below the diagnostic threshold when we received the results of the chest radiograph; we did not, for instance, order an echocardiogram. Immune-mediated pulmonary hemorrhage remained below the test threshold throughout the entire investigation.

For a disorder with a pretest probability above the treatment threshold, a confirming test that raises the probability further would not assist diagnostically. On the other end of the scale, for a disorder with a pretest probability below the test threshold, an exclusionary test that lowers the probability further would not help diagnostically. When the clinician believes the pretest probability is high enough to test for and not high enough to warrant beginning treatment (ie, when probability is between the two thresholds), testing will be diagnostically useful, and it will be most valuable if it moves the probability across either threshold.

What determines our treatment threshold? The greater the adverse effects of treating, the more we will be inclined to choose a high treatment threshold. For instance, because a diagnosis of pulmonary embolus involves long-term anticoagulation with appreciable risks of hemorrhage, we are very concerned about falsely labeling patients. The invasiveness of the next test we are considering will also impact our threshold. If results from the next test (such as a ventilation-perfusion scan) are benign, we will be ready to choose a high treatment threshold. We will be more reluctant to institute an invasive test associated with risks to the patient, such as pulmonary angiogram, and this will drive our treatment threshold downward. That is, we will be more inclined to accept a risk of a false-positive diagnosis because a higher treatment threshold implies putting some patients through the test unnecessarily.

Similar considerations bear on the test threshold. The more serious a missed diagnosis, the lower we will set our test threshold. Since a missed diagnosis of a pulmonary embolus could be fatal, we would be inclined to set our diagnostic threshold low. However, this is again counterbalanced by the risks associated with the next test we are considering. If the risks are low, we will be comfortable with our low diagnostic threshold. The higher the risks, the more it will push our threshold upward.

# USING SYSTEMATIC RESEARCH TO AID IN THE DIAGNOSTIC PROCESS

How do clinicians generate differential diagnoses and arrive at pretest estimates of disease probability? They remember prior cases with the same clinical problem(s), so that disorders diagnosed frequently have higher probability than diagnoses made less frequently. Remembered cases are easily and quickly available, and they are calibrated to our local practices. Yet our memories are imperfect, and the probabilities that result are subject to bias and error.[6-8]

Two sorts of systematic investigations can inform the process of generating a differential diagnosis. One type of study addresses the manifestations with which a disease or condition presents (see Part 2C, "Diagnosis, Clinical Manifestations of Disease"). The second—and more important—type of study directly addresses the underlying causes of a presenting symptom, sign, or constellation of symptoms and signs (see Part 1C1, "Differential Diagnosis"). In our opening scenario, the question would be: When patients present with acute cough and shortness of breath, what are the ultimate diagnoses and the relative frequency of these diagnoses?

Having generated an initial differential diagnosis with associated pretest probabilities, how can you incorporate additional information to arrive at an ultimate diagnosis? For each finding, you must implicitly ask: How frequently will this result be seen in patients with one particular diagnostic possibility (or target condition) in relation to the frequency with which it is seen in the competing diagnostic conditions? Once again, you may intuitively refer to your own past experience. Alternatively, you may use data from research studies focusing on test properties. For instance, in our scenario, the Prospective Investigation of Pulmonary Embolism Diagnosis (PIOPED) study of ventilation-perfusion scanning in the diagnosis of pulmonary embolism[1] provided the likelihood ratio that allowed calculation of the posttest probability of 90% (see Part 1C2, "Diagnostic Tests").

Some articles provide evidence about differential diagnosis as well as diagnostic test properties. For example, in a study of diagnostic tests for anemia in aged persons, investigators compared blood tests with bone marrow results in 259 elderly persons, finding iron deficiency in 94 (36%).[9] The investigators also reported a diagnosis of anemia in the remaining 165 patients. Thus, although this study focused on evaluating tests for iron deficiency, it also provides information about disease frequency.

In the following sections of the book, we provide guidelines for you to assess the validity of both types of formal investigations related to diagnosis: studies that focus on a constellation of presenting symptoms or signs and determine patients' ultimate diagnoses, and studies that explore the properties of a diagnostic test. In each case, we suggest that validity will depend on the answers to questions regarding two key design features: Did the investigators enroll the right group of patients; and did they undertake the appropriate investigations to determine the true diagnosis? As we deal in sequence with each of the three types of study, we will explain how you can use the results to improve the accuracy of diagnosis in your clinical practice. As for therapy, prognosis, and harm, the systematic reviews of all diagnostic test articles addressing a particular issue will provide the strongest inferences (see Part 1E, "Summarizing the Evidence"). To understand and interpret such reviews, we must use the principles of assessing primary diagnostic studies.

# References

1. The PIOPED Investigators. Value of the ventilation/perfusion scan in acute pulmonary embolism. Results of the Prospective Investigation of Pulmonary Embolism Diagnosis (PIOPED). *JAMA*. 1990;263:2753-2759.

2. Sox HC, Blatt MA, Higgins MC, Marton KI. *Medical Decision Making*. Boston: Butterworths; 1988.

3. Glass RD. *Diagnosis: A Brief Introduction*. Melbourne: Oxford University Press; 1996.

4. Barondess JA, Carpenter CCJ, eds. *Differential Diagnosis*. Philadelphia: Lea & Febiger; 1994.

5. Pauker SG, Kassirer JP. The threshold approach to clinical decision making. *N Engl J Med*. 1980;302:1109-1117.

6. Schmidt HG, Norman GR, Boshuizen HP. A cognitive perspective on medical expertise: theory and implication. *Acad Med*. 1990;65:611-621.

7. Bordage G. Elaborated knowledge: a key to successful diagnostic thinking. *Acad Med*. 1994;69:883-885.

8. Regehr G, Norman GR. Issues in cognitive psychology: implications for professional education. *Acad Med*. 1996;71:988-1001.

9. Guyatt GH, Patterson C, Ali M, et al. Diagnosis of iron-deficiency anemia in the elderly. *Am J Med*. 1990;88:205-209.

# DIFFERENTIAL DIAGNOSIS

W. Scott Richardson, Mark Wilson, Jeroen Lijmer, Gordon Guyatt, and Deborah Cook

The following EBM Working Group members also made substantive contributions to this section: Peter Wyer, C. David Naylor, Jonathan Craig, Luz Maria Letelier, and Virginia Moyer

## IN THIS SECTION

## CLINICAL SCENARIO

### A 33-Year-Old Man With Palpitations: What Is the Cause?

You are a primary care physician seeing a patient from your practice, a 33-year-old man who presents with heart palpitations. He describes the new onset as episodes of fast, regular chest pounding that come on gradually, last from 1 to 2 minutes, and occur several times per day. He reports no relationship of symptoms to activities and no change in exercise tolerance. You have previously noted that this patient tends to suffer from anxiety, and he now tells you that he fears heart disease. He has no other symptoms, no personal or family history of heart disease, and he takes no medications. You find his heart rate is 90 bpm and regular, and physical examinations of his eyes, thyroid gland, and lungs are normal. His heart sounds also are normal, without click, murmur, or gallop. His 12-lead ECG is normal, without arrhythmia or signs of preexcitation.

You suspect that anxiety explains this patient's palpitations, that they are mediated by hyperventilation, and that they may be part of a panic attack. Also, although there are no findings to suggest cardiac arrhythmia or hyperthyroidism, you wonder if these disorders are common enough in this sort of patient to warrant serious consideration. You reject pheochromocytoma as too unlikely to consider further. Thus, you can list causes of palpitations, but you want more information about the frequency of these causes to choose a diagnostic workup. You ask the question, "In patients presenting with heart palpitations, what is the frequency of underlying disorders?"

# FINDING THE EVIDENCE

Your office computer networks with the medical library, where MEDLINE is on CD-ROM. In the MEDLINE file for current years, you enter three text words: "palpitations" (89 citations), "differential diagnosis" (7039 citations), and "cause or causes" (71,848 citations). You combine these sets, yielding 17 citations. Reviewing the titles and abstracts onscreen, you see a paper by Weber and Kapoor that explicitly addresses the differential diagnosis in patients presenting with palpitations.[1] With a keystroke and a mouse click, you review this article's full text.

# ARE THE RESULTS VALID?

Table 1C-1 summarizes the guides for an article about the diagnostic possibilities.

**TABLE 1C–1**

## Users' Guide for an Article About Differential Diagnosis

**Are the results valid?**

- Did the investigators enroll the right patients? Was the patient sample representative of those with the clinical problem?
- Was the definitive diagnostic standard appropriate? Was the diagnostic process credible?
- For initially undiagnosed patients, was follow-up sufficiently long and complete?

**What are the results?**

- What were the diagnoses and their probabilities?
- How precise are the estimates of disease probability?

**How can I apply the results to patient care?**

- Are the study patients similar to the one being considered in my own practice?
- Is it unlikely that the disease possibilities or probabilities have changed since this evidence was gathered?

## Did the Investigators Enroll the Right Patients? Was the Patient Sample Representative of Those With the Clinical Problem?

This question asks about two related issues: defining the clinical problem and ensuring a representative population.

First, how do the investigators define the clinical problem under study? The definition of the clinical problem determines the population from which the study patients should be drawn. Thus, investigators studying hematuria might include patients with microscopic and gross hematuria, with or without symptoms. On the other hand, investigators studying asymptomatic, microscopic hematuria would exclude those with symptoms or with gross hematuria.

Differing definitions of the clinical problem will yield different frequencies of underlying diseases. Including patients with gross hematuria or urinary symptoms will raise the frequency of acute infection as the underlying cause relative to those without symptoms. Assessing the validity of an article about differential diagnosis begins with a search for a clear definition of the clinical problem.

Having defined the target population by clinical problem statement, investigators next assemble a patient sample. Ideally, the sample mirrors the target population in all important ways, so that the frequency of underlying diseases in the sample approximates that of the target population. We call a patient sample that mirrors the underlying target population *representative.* The more representative the sample, the more accurate the resulting disease probabilities.

Investigators seldom use the strongest method of ensuring representativeness, which is to obtain a random sample of the entire population of patients with the clinical problem. The next strongest methods are either (1) to include all patients with the clinical problem from a defined geographic area or (2) to include a consecutive series of all patients with the clinical problem who receive care at the investigators' institution(s). To the extent that a nonconsecutive case series opens the study to the differential inclusion of patients with different underlying disorders, it compromises study validity.

You can judge the representativeness of the sample by examining the setting from which patients come. Patients with ostensibly the same clinical problem can present to different clinical settings, resulting in different services seeing different types of patients. Typically, patients in secondary or tertiary care settings have higher proportions of more serious or more uncommon diseases than patients seen in primary care settings. For instance, in a study of patients presenting with chest pain, a higher proportion of referral practice patients had coronary artery disease than the primary care practice patients, even in patients with similar clinical histories.[2]

To further evaluate representativeness, you can note investigators' methods of identifying patients, how carefully they avoided missing patients, and whom they included and excluded. The wider the spectrum of patients in the sample, the more representative the sample should be of the whole population and, therefore, the more valid the results will be. For example, in a study of *Clostridium difficile* colitis in 609 patients with diarrhea, the patient sample consisted of adult inpatients whose diarrheal stools were tested for cytotoxin, thereby excluding any patients whose clinicians chose not to test.[3] Including only those tested is likely to raise the probability of *C difficile* in relation to the entire population of patients with diarrhea.

Weber and Kapoor[1] defined palpitations broadly as any one of several patient complaints (eg, fast heartbeats, skipped heartbeats, etc) and included patients with new and recurring palpitations. They obtained patients from three clinical settings (emergency department, inpatient floors, and a medical clinic) in one university medical center in a middle-sized North American city. Of the 229 adult patients presenting consecutively for care of palpitations at their center during the study period, 39 refused participation; the investigators included the remaining 190 patients, including 62 from the emergency department. No important subgroups appear to have been excluded, so these 190 patients probably represent the full spectrum of patients presenting with palpitations.

## Was the Definitive Diagnostic Standard Appropriate? Was the Diagnostic Process Credible?

Articles about differential diagnosis will provide valid evidence only if the investigators arrive at a correct final diagnosis. To do so, they must develop and apply explicit criteria when assigning each patient a final diagnosis. Their criteria should include not only the findings needed to confirm each diagnosis, but also those findings useful for rejecting each diagnosis. For example, published diagnostic criteria for infective endocarditis include both criteria for verifying the infection and criteria for rejecting it.[4,5] Investigators can then classify study patients into diagnostic groups that are mutually exclusive, with the exception of patients whose symptoms stem from more than one etiologic factor. This allows clinicians to understand which diagnoses remain possible for any undiagnosed patients.

Diagnostic criteria should include a search that is sufficiently comprehensive to ensure detection of all important causes of the clinical problem. The more comprehensive the investigation, the smaller the chance that investigators will reach invalid conclusions about disease frequency. For example, a retrospective study of stroke in 127 patients with mental status changes failed to include a comprehensive search for all causes of delirium, and 118 cases remained unexplained.[6] Since the investigators did not describe a complete and systematic search for causes of delirium, the disease probabilities appear less credible.

The goal of developing and applying explicit, credible criteria is to ensure a reproducible diagnosis, and the ultimate test of reproducibility is a formal agreement evaluation. Your confidence in investigators will increase if, as in a study of causes of dizziness,[7] investigators formally demonstrate the extent to which they achieved agreement in diagnosis (see Part 2C, "Diagnosis, Measuring Agreement Beyond Chance").

While reviewing the diagnostic criteria, keep in mind that "lesion finding" is not necessarily the same thing as "illness explaining." In other words, using explicit and credible criteria, investigators may find that patients have two or more disorders that might explain the clinical problem, causing some doubt as to which disorder is the culprit. Better studies of disease probability will include some assurance that the disorders found actually did account for the patients' illnesses. For example, in a sequence of studies of syncope, investigators required that the symptoms occur simultaneously with an arrhythmia before that arrhythmia was judged to be the cause.[8] In a study of chronic cough, investigators gave cause-specific therapy and used positive responses to this to strengthen the case for these disorders actually causing the chronic cough.[9]

Explicit diagnostic criteria are of little use unless they are applied consistently. This does not mean that every patient must undergo every test. Instead, for many clinical problems, the clinician takes a detailed yet focused history and performs a problem-oriented physical examination of the involved organ systems, along with a few initial tests. Then, depending on the diagnostic clues from this information, further inquiry proceeds down one of multiple branching pathways. Ideally, investigators would evaluate all patients with the same initial workup and then follow the clues, using prespecified testing sequences. Once a definitive test result confirms a final diagnosis, then further confirmatory testing is unnecessary and unethical.

You may find it easy to decide whether patients' illnesses have been well investigated if they were evaluated prospectively using a predetermined diagnostic approach. When clinicians do not standardize their investigation, this becomes harder to judge. For example, in a study of precipitating factors in 101 patients with decompensated heart failure, although all patients underwent a history and physical examination, the lack of standardization of subsequent testing makes it difficult to judge the accuracy of the disease probabilities.[10]

In the Weber and Kapoor study,[1] the investigators developed a priori explicit and credible criteria for confirming each possible disorder causing palpitations and listed their criteria in an appendix, along with supporting citations. They evaluated study patients prospectively and assigned final diagnoses using two principal means: a structured interview completed by one of the investigators and the combined diagnostic evaluation (ie, history, examination, and testing) chosen by the individual physician seeing the patient at the index visit. In addition, all patients completed self-administered questionnaires designed to assist in detecting various psychiatric disorders. Electrocardiograms were obtained in a majority of patients (166 of 190), and a large number underwent other testing for cardiac disease as well. Whenever relevant, the investigators required that the palpitations occurred at the same time as the arrhythmias before they would attribute the symptoms to that arrhythmia. However, they did not report on agreement for the ultimate decisions about the diagnoses attributed to each patient.

Thus, the diagnostic workup was reasonably comprehensive—although not exhaustive—for common disease categories. Since the subsequent testing ordered by the individual physicians was not fully standardized, some inconsistency may have been introduced, although it does not appear likely to have distorted the probabilities of common disease categories, such as psychiatric or cardiac causes.

### For Initially Undiagnosed Patients, Was Follow-up Sufficiently Long and Complete?

Even when investigators consistently apply explicit and comprehensive diagnostic criteria, some patients' clinical problems may remain unexplained. The higher the number of undiagnosed patients, the greater the chance of error in the estimates of disease probability. For example, in a retrospective study of various causes of dizziness in 1194 patients in an otolaryngology clinic, about 27% remained undiagnosed.[11] With more than a quarter of patients' illnesses unexplained, the disease probabilities for the overall sample might be inaccurate.

If the study evaluation leaves patients undiagnosed, investigators can follow these patients over time, searching for additional clues leading to eventual diagnoses and observing the prognosis. The longer and more complete this follow-up is, the greater will be our confidence in the benign nature of the condition in patients who remain undiagnosed yet unharmed at the end of the study. How long is long enough? No single answer would correctly fit all clinical problems, but we would suggest 1 to 6 months for symptoms that are acute and self-limited and 1 to 5 years for chronically recurring or progressive symptoms.

---

## USING THE GUIDE

**R**eturning to our earlier discussion, Weber and Kapoor[1] identified a diagnosable etiology of palpitations in all but 31 (16.3%) of 190 patients included in their study. The investigators followed nearly all of the study patients (96%) for at least a year, during which time one additional diagnosis (symptomatic correlation with ventricular premature beats) was made in those initially undiagnosed. None of the 31 undiagnosed patients had a stroke or died.

---

# WHAT ARE THE RESULTS?

## What Were the Diagnoses and Their Probabilities?

In many studies of disease probability, the authors display the main results in a table listing the diagnoses made, along with the numbers and percentages of patients found with those diagnoses. For some symptoms, patients may have more than one underlying disease coexisting with and, presumably, contributing to the clinical problem. In these situations, authors often identify the major diagnosis for such patients and separately tabulate contributing causes. Alternatively, authors sometimes identify a separate, multiple-etiology group.

Weber and Kapoor[1] present a table that tells us that 58 patients (31%) were diagnosed with psychiatric causes and 82 (43%) had cardiac disorders, while thyrotoxicosis was found in five (2.6%), and none had pheochromocytoma. This distribution differed across clinical settings. For instance, cardiac disorders were more than twice as likely to occur in patients presenting to the emergency department, compared to patients presenting to the outpatient clinic.

## How Precise Are the Estimates of Disease Probability?

Even when valid, these disease probabilities are only estimates of the true frequencies. You can examine the precision of these estimates using the confidence intervals (CIs) presented by the authors. If the authors do not provide them for you, you can calculate them yourself using the following formula:

$$95\% \text{ CI} = P + 1.96 \sqrt{[P(1-P)]/n,}$$

where $P$ is the proportion of patients with the etiology of interest and $n$ is the number of patients in the sample. This formula becomes inaccurate when the number of cases is 5 or fewer, and approximations are available for this situation.

For instance, consider the category of psychiatric causes of palpitations in the Weber and Kapoor[1] study. Using the above formula, we would start with $P = 0.31$, $(1 - P) = 0.69$, and $n = 190$. Working through the arithmetic, we find the CI to be $0.31 \pm 0.066$. Thus, although the most likely true proportion is 31%, it may range between 24.4% and 37.6%.

Whether you will deem the confidence intervals sufficiently precise depends on where the estimated proportion and confidence intervals fall in relation to your test or treatment thresholds. If both the estimated proportion and the entire 95% confidence interval are on the same side of your threshold, then the result is precise enough to permit firm conclusions about disease probability for use in planning tests or treatments. Conversely, if the confidence limit around the estimate crosses your threshold, the result may not be precise enough for definitive conclusions about disease probability. You might still use a valid but imprecise probability result, while keeping in mind the uncertainty and what it might mean for testing or treatment.

## USING THE GUIDE

Weber and Kapoor do not provide the 95% CIs for the probabilities they found. However, as we just illustrated, if you were concerned about how close the probabilities were to your thresholds, you could calculate the 95% CIs yourself.

# HOW CAN I APPLY THE RESULTS TO PATIENT CARE?

## Are the Study Patients Similar to Those in My Own Practice?

As mentioned previously, we suggest you ask yourself whether the setting or patients are so different from those in your practice that you should disregard the results.[12] For instance, consider whether the patients in your practice come from areas where one or more of the underlying disorders are endemic, which could make the occurrence of these disorders much more likely in your situation than was found in the study.

## USING THE GUIDE

**W**eber and Kapoor[1] recruited the 190 patients with palpitation from those presenting to the outpatient clinics, the inpatient medical and surgical services, and the emergency department (62 of the 190) in one university medical center in a middle-sized North American city. Thus, these patients are likely to be similar to the patients seen in your hospital emergency department, and you can use the study results to help inform the pretest probabilities for the patient in the scenario.

## Is It Unlikely That the Disease Possibilities or Probabilities Have Changed Since This Evidence Was Gathered?

As time passes, evidence about disease frequency can become obsolete. Old diseases can be controlled or, as in the case of smallpox, eliminated.[13] New diseases or, at least, new epidemics of disease can arise. Such events can so alter the spectrum of possible diseases or their likelihood that previously valid and applicable studies may lose their relevance. For example, consider how dramatically the arrival of human immunodeficiency virus (HIV) transformed the list of diagnostic possibilities for such clinical problems as generalized lymphadenopathy, chronic diarrhea, and unexplained weight loss.

Similar changes can occur as the result of progress in medical science or public health. For instance, in studies of fever of unknown origin, new diagnostic technologies have substantially altered the proportions of patients who are found to have malignancy or whose fevers remain unexplained.[14-16] Treatment advances that improve survival, such as chemotherapy for childhood leukemia, can bring about shifts in disease likelihood because the treatment might cause complications, such as secondary malignancy years after cure of the disease. Public health measures that control such diseases as cholera can alter the likelihood of occurrence of the remaining etiologies of the clinical problems that the prevented disease would have caused—in this example, acute diarrhea.

## USING THE GUIDE

**T**he palpitations study was published in 1996 and the text states that the study period was 8 months during 1991. In this instance, you know of no new developments likely to cause a change in the spectrum or probabilities of disease in patients with palpitations.

# CLINICAL RESOLUTION

Let us return to the patient in your practice. Considering the possible causes of his palpitations, your leading hypothesis is that acute anxiety is the cause of your patient's palpitations. You do not believe that the diagnosis of anxiety is so certain that you can rule out other disorders (ie, the pretest probability is below your threshold for treatment without testing). After reviewing the Weber and Kapoor[1] palpitations study, you decide to include in your list of "active alternatives" some cardiac arrhythmias (as common, serious, and treatable) and hyperthyroidism (as less common but serious and treatable) and you arrange testing to exclude these disorders (ie, these alternatives are above your threshold for treatment without testing). Finally, given that none of the 190 study patients had pheochromocytoma, and since your patient has none of the other clinical features of this disorder, you place it into your "other hypotheses" category (ie, below your test threshold) and decide to delay testing for this condition.

## References

1. Weber BE, Kapoor WN. Evaluation and outcomes of patients with palpitations. *Am J Med*. 1996;100:138–148.

2. Sox HC, Hickam DH, Marton KI, et al. Using the patient's history to estimate the probability of coronary artery disease: a comparison of primary care and referral practices. *Am J Med*. 1990;89:7–14.

3. Katz DA, Bates DW, Rittenberg E, et al. Predicting *Clostridium difficile* stool cytotoxin results in hospitalized patients with diarrhea. *J Gen Intern Med*. 1997;12:57–62.

4. von Reyn CF, Levy BS, Arbeit RD, Friedland G, Crumpacker CS. Infective endocarditis: an analysis based on strict case definitions. *Ann Intern Med*. 1981;94:505–517.

5. Durack DT, Lukes AS, Bright DK, and the Duke Endocarditis Service. New criteria for diagnosis of infective endocarditis: utilization of specific echocardiographic findings. *Am J Med*. 1994;96:200–209.

6. Benbadis SR, Sila CA, Cristea RL. Mental status changes and stroke. *J Gen Intern Med*. 1994;9:485–487.

7. Kroenke K, Lucas CA, Rosenberg ML, et al. Causes of persistent dizziness: a prospective study of 100 patients in ambulatory care. *Ann Intern Med*. 1992;117:898–904.

8. Kapoor WN. Evaluation and outcome of patients with syncope. *Medicine*. 1990;69:160–175.

9. Pratter MR, Bartter T, Akers S, et al. An algorithmic approach to chronic cough. *Ann Intern Med*. 1993;119:977–983.

10. Ghali JK, Kadakia S, Cooper R, Ferlinz J. Precipitating factors leading to decompensation of heart failure: traits among urban blacks. *Arch Intern Med*. 1988;148:2013–2016.

11. Katsarkas A. Dizziness in aging—a retrospective study of 1194 cases. *Otolaryngol Head Neck Surg*. 1994;110:296–301.

12. Glasziou P, Guyatt GH, Dans AL, Dans LF, Straus SE, Sackett DL. Applying the results of trials and systematic reviews to individual patients [editorial]. *ACP Journal Club*. 1998;129:A15–A16.

13. Barquet N, Domingo P. Smallpox: the triumph over the most terrible of the ministers of death. *Ann Intern Med*. 1997;127:635–642.

14. Petersdorf RG, Beeson PB. Fever of unexplained origin: report on 100 cases. *Medicine*. 1961;40:1–30.

15. Larson EB, Featherstone HJ, Petersdorf RG. Fever of undetermined origin: diagnosis and follow up of 105 cases, 1970–1980. *Medicine*. 1982;61:269–292.

16. Knockaert DC, Vanneste LJ, Vanneste SB, Bobbaers HJ. Fever of unknown origin in the 1980s: an update of the diagnostic spectrum. *Arch Intern Med*. 1992;152:51–55.

# 1C2

# DIAGNOSTIC TESTS

Roman Jaeschke, Gordon Guyatt, and Jeroen Lijmer

The following EBM Working Group members also made substantive contributions to this section: Peter Wyer, Virginia Moyer, Deborah Cook, Jonathan Craig, Luz Maria Letelier, John Williams, C. David Naylor, W. Scott Richardson, Mark Wilson, and James Nishikawa

## IN THIS SECTION

## How Accurate is CT Scanning in Suspected Appendicitis?

**A** 32-year-old woman enters the emergency department presenting with right lower quadrant pain. She is single and is employed by a company that sells Internet-related products. She is sexually active, having had three sexual partners during the past year, and her last menstrual period ended 3 weeks ago. Yesterday, she began to feel unwell and lost her appetite. During the past few hours the pain became much worse and she felt febrile, but she did not take her temperature. She has not experienced any vaginal discharge. She came to the emergency department when the pain became so severe that she started to worry whether something serious might be wrong.

On examination, you see a moderately ill woman with a temperature of 38.2° C and otherwise normal vital signs, who displays tenderness and guarding in the right lower quadrant and questionable rebound tenderness. You find no cervical motion tenderness, nor do you see cervical discharge. Laboratory examination findings include a white blood cell count of 11,000/mm³. Your differential diagnosis includes appendicitis, pelvic inflammatory disease, and ectopic pregancy; as you are debating whether to refer directly to surgery or to begin by obtaining a gynecologist's opinion, your colleague, an interventional radiologist, stops by on his way back from performing an emergency pulmonary angiogram. You describe the patient you are attending to and he mentions that up to 15% of needless laparotomies and up to 20% of admissions can be avoided if a computed tomographic (CT) scan is performed in patients like this one. He mentions "a very good paper that you must read, since it was published in the *New England Journal of Medicine*" although the citation and the details of the investigators' methods and study results currently escape him.

The patient is stable and currently comfortable, and the emergency department has quieted down since the morning rush. A colleague is ready to allow you a break and you decide you can afford to invest 30 minutes to look for and examine the paper recommended by the radiologist.

# FINDING THE EVIDENCE

Upstairs in the library, you use the computer to search the PubMed database. You select "diagnosis" and "specificity" from the clinical queries page (www.ncbi.nlm. nih.gov/entrez/query/static/clinical.html) to have a preformatted search for diagnostic test studies. With the key words "CT" and "appendicitis," the search yields 39 citations. When you limit the search to English-language papers with abstracts that were published during the past 5 years, you find that 18 recent articles remain. The 18 abstracts include two narrative reviews, four retrospective studies, two studies focusing on specific imaging signs, and two studies focusing on a selected group of patients. Two of the abstracts provide no quantitative information about the test's performance and one is from a journal your library does not carry. The remaining five abstracts report a high level of accuracy of the test. The title of the most recent article best fits the patient with right lower quadrant tenderness in that it refers to the value of helical CT scanning for differentiating between appendicitis and acute gynecologic conditions.[1] Furthermore, the *New England Journal of Medicine* article is older and seems less relevant in that it analyzes issues related to cost and patient impact, rather than focusing on diagnostic test accuracy. You decide to retrieve the more recent paper.

In the ensuing discussion of the validity, results, and applicability of studies examining the properties of diagnostic tests, we will focus both on the scenario that included the diagnosis of pulmonary embolism using ventilation-perfusion scanning (see Part 1C, "The Process of Diagnosis") and on the article about the value of CT scanning in the diagnosis of appendicitis. Table 1C-2 summarizes our Users' Guide for a study of interpreting test results.

**TABLE 1C–2**

## Users' Guide for an Article About Interpreting Diagnostic Test Results

**Are the results valid?**

- Did clinicians face diagnostic uncertainty?
- Was there a blind comparison with an independent gold standard applied similarly to the treatment group and to the control group?
- Did the results of the test being evaluated influence the decision to perform the gold standard?

**What are the results?**

- What likelihood ratios were associated with the range of possible test results?

**How can I apply the results to patient care?**

- Will the reproducibility of the test result and its interpretation be satisfactory in my clinical setting?
- Are the results applicable to the patient in my practice?
- Will the results change my management strategy?
- Will patients be better off as a result of the test?

# ARE THE RESULTS VALID?

## Did Clinicians Face Diagnostic Uncertainty?

A diagnostic test is useful only to the extent that it distinguishes between conditions or disorders that might otherwise be confused. Almost any test can differentiate healthy persons from severely affected ones; this ability, however, tells us nothing about the clinical utility of a test. The true, pragmatic value of a test is therefore established only in a study that closely resembles clinical practice. Another way to understand this point is to refer back to Figure 1C-1 in Part 1C, "The Process of Diagnosis." Note that the population of interest comprises patients whose predicament falls between the test and treatment thresholds.

A vivid example of how choosing the right population can dash the hopes raised with the introduction of a diagnostic test comes from the story of carcinoembryonic antigen (CEA) testing in patients with colorectal cancer. When measured in 36 people with known advanced cancer of the colon or rectum, CEA was elevated in 35 of them. At the same time, much lower levels were found in people without cancer who suffered from a variety of other conditions.[2] The results suggested that CEA might be useful in diagnosing colorectal cancer— or even in screening for the disease. In subsequent studies of patients with less advanced stages of colorectal cancer (and, therefore, lower disease severity) and patients with other cancers or other gastrointestinal disorders (and, therefore, different but potentially confused disorders), the accuracy of CEA testing as a diagnostic tool plummeted and clinicians abandoned CEA measurement for cancer diagnosis and screening. Carcinoembryonic antigen testing has proved useful only as one element in the follow-up of patients with known colorectal cancer.[3]

In an empiric study of design-related bias in studies of diagnostic tests, Lijmer and colleagues related features of the design to the power of tests.[4] Their findings included a large overestimate of the power of the test to distinguish between target-positive and target-negative patients when the investigators enrolled separate test and normal control populations (relative diagnostic odds ratio, [OR] 3.0; 95% confidence interval [CI], 2.0-4.5).

This example contrasts with the PIOPED study that demonstrated the utility of ventilation-perfusion scanning in the diagnosis of pulmonary embolism.[5] Here, investigators recruited the whole spectrum of patients suspected of having pulmonary embolism, including those who entered the study with high, medium, and low clinical suspicion of the condition. The patient sample in the helical CT study from the scenario related to scanning and appendicitis mentioned earlier in this section was appropriate because it comprised consecutive, nonpregnant women presenting to the emergency department of a large general hospital—ones in whom acute appendicitis or an acute gynecologic condition was suspected.

## Was There a Blind Comparison With an Independent Gold Standard Applied Similarly to the Treatment Group and the Control Group?

The accuracy of a diagnostic test is best determined by comparing it to the "truth." Accordingly, readers must assure themselves that an appropriate *reference standard* (such as biopsy, surgery, autopsy, or long-term follow-up) has been applied to every patient, along with the test under investigation.[6] In the PIOPED study, the investigators used the pulmonary angiogram as the reference standard, and this was as "gold" as could be achieved without sacrificing the patients.

One way a *gold standard* can go wrong is if the test is part of the gold standard. For instance, one study evaluated the utility of measuring both serum and urinary amylase in making the diagnosis of pancreatitis.[7] The investigators constructed a gold standard that relied on a number of tests, including ones for serum and urinary amylase. This incorporation of the test into the gold standard is likely to inflate the estimate of the test's diagnostic power. Thus, clinicians should insist on the independence of the test and gold standard.

In reading articles about diagnostic tests, if you cannot accept the reference standard (within reason, that is—after all, nothing is perfect), then the article is unlikely to provide valid results for your purposes. If you do accept the reference standard, the next question to ask is whether the test results and the reference standard were assessed blindly (that is, by interpreters who were unaware of the results of the other investigation). Clinical experience demonstrates the importance of this independence or *blinding*. Once clinicians see a pulmonary nodule on a CT scan, they can see the previously undetected lesion on the chest radiograph; once they learn the results of an echocardiogram, they hear the previously inaudible cardiac murmur. The Lijmer et al empiric study of diagnostic test bias to which we have referred demonstrated the bias associated with unblinding even though the magnitude was small (relative diagnostic OR, 1.3; 95% CI, 1.0-1.9).[4]

The more likely that knowledge of the reference standard result could influence the interpretation of a new test, the greater is the importance of the blinded interpretation. Similarly, the more susceptible the gold standard is to changes in interpretation as a result of knowledge of the test, the more important is the blinding of the gold standard interpreter. In their study, the PIOPED investigators did not state explicitly that the tests were interpreted blindly. However, one could deduce from the effort they put into ensuring reproducible, independent readings that the interpreters were, in fact, blind; through correspondence with one of the authors, we have confirmed that this was indeed the case.

In the study of the use of CT in the diagnosis of suspected appendicitis, the investigators used surgical and pathologic findings as the reference standard for patients who went to surgery. For patients who did not go to surgery, the findings at clinical follow-up—including outpatient clinic visits and telephone calls during at least a 2-month period after the CT scan—provided the gold standard. The researchers did not report blinding of the physicians for the results of the helical CT scan. Particularly for patients in whom the diagnosis was made by long-term follow-up, knowledge of the CT result could have created a bias toward making the test look better than it really was.

## Did the Results of the Test Being Evaluated Influence the Decision to Perform the Reference Standard?

The properties of a diagnostic test will be distorted if its results influence whether patients undergo confirmation by the reference standard. This situation, sometimes called *verification bias*[8,9] or *workup bias,*[10,11] applies when, for example, patients with suspected coronary artery disease whose exercise test results are positive are more likely to undergo coronary angiography (the gold standard) than those whose exercise test results are negative. The Lijmer et al study showed a large magnitude of bias associated with use of different reference tests for positive and negative results.[4]

Verification bias proved a problem for the PIOPED study as well. Patients whose ventilation-perfusion scans were interpreted as "normal/near normal" and "low probability" were less likely to undergo pulmonary angiography (69%) than those with more positive ventilation-perfusion scans (92%). This is not surprising, since clinicians might be reluctant to subject patients with a low probability of pulmonary embolism to the risks of angiography.

Most articles would stop here, and readers would have to conclude that the magnitude of the bias resulting from different proportions of patients with high- and low-probability ventilation-perfusion scans undergoing adequate angiography is uncertain but perhaps large. However, the PIOPED investigators applied a second reference standard to the 150 patients with low-probability or normal/near normal scans who failed to undergo angiography (136 patients) or in whom angiogram interpretation was uncertain (14 patients): they would be judged to be free of pulmonary embolism if they did well without treatment. Accordingly, the PIOPED investigators followed each of these patients for 1 year without treating them with anticoagulant drugs. Clinically evident pulmonary embolism developed in none of these patients during this time, from which we can conclude that clinically important pulmonary embolism (if we define clinically important pulmonary embolism as requiring anticoagulation therapy to prevent subsequent adverse events) was not present at the time they underwent ventilation-perfusion scanning.

In the helical CT study, the investigators established the reference standard in all patients. However, the test results probably influenced which reference standard—surgery or follow-up—was chosen. As we have mentioned previously, to the extent that CT results influenced the decision regarding the final diagnosis, the study provides an excessively optimistic picture of the test properties.

# WHAT ARE THE RESULTS?

## What Likelihood Ratios Were Associated With the Range of Possible Test Results?

The starting point of any diagnostic process is the patient presenting with a constellation of symptoms and signs. Consider two patients with nonspecific chest pain and shortness of breath without findings suggesting diagnoses such as pneumonia, airflow obstruction, or heart failure, in whom the clinician suspects pulmonary embolism. One is a 78-year-old woman 10 days after surgery and the other is a 28-year-old man experiencing a high level of anxiety. Our clinical hunches about the probability of pulmonary embolism as the explanation for these two patients' complaints—that is, their pretest probabilities—are very different. In the older woman, the probability is high; in the young man, it is low. As a result, even if both patients have intermediate-probability ventilation-perfusion scans, subsequent management is likely to differ in each. One might well treat the elderly woman immediately with heparin but order additional investigations in the young man.

Two conclusions emerge from this line of reasoning. First, regardless of the results of the ventilation-perfusion scan, they do not tell us whether pulmonary embolism is present. What they do accomplish is to modify the pretest probability of that condition, yielding a new posttest probability. The direction and magnitude of this change from pretest to posttest probability are determined by the test's properties, and the property of most value is the likelihood ratio.

As depicted in Table 1C-3, constructed from the results of the PIOPED study, there were 251 people with angiographically proven pulmonary embolism and 630 people whose angiograms or follow-up excluded that diagnosis. For all patients, ventilation-perfusion scans were classified into four levels: high probability, intermediate probability, low probability, and normal or near-normal. How likely is a high-probability scan among people who do have pulmonary embolism? Table 1C-3 shows that 102 of 251 (or 0.406) people with the condition had high-probability scans. How often is the same test result, a high-probability scan, found among people in whom pulmonary embolism was suspected but has been ruled out? The answer is 14 of 630 (or 0.022) of them. The ratio of these two likelihoods is called the *likelihood ratio* (LR); for a high probability scan, it equals 0.406 ÷ 0.022 (or 18.3). In other words, a high-probability ventilation-perfusion scan is 18.3 times as likely to occur in a patient with—as opposed to without—a pulmonary embolism.

**TABLE 1C–3**

## Test Properties of Ventilation Perfusion (V/Q) Scanning

| | Pulmonary Embolism | | | | | |
|---|---|---|---|---|---|---|
| | Present | | Absent | | | |
| Scan Results | Number | Proportion | Likelihood Number | Proportion | | Ratio |
| High probability | 102 | 102/251 = 0.406 | 14 | 14/630 = 0.022 | | 18.3 |
| Intermediate probability | 105 | 105/251 = 0.418 | 217 | 217/630 = 0.344 | | 1.20 |
| Low probability | 39 | 39/251 = 0.155 | 273 | 273/630 = 0.433 | | 0.36 |
| Normal/near normal | 5 | 5/251 = 0.020 | 126 | 126/630 = 0.200 | | 0.10 |
| Total | 251 | | 630 | | | |

In a similar fashion, we can calculate the likelihood ratio for each level of the diagnostic test results. Each calculation involves answering two questions: First, how likely it is to obtain a given test result (say, a low-probability ventilation-perfusion scan) among people with the target disorder (pulmonary embolism)? Second, how likely it is to obtain the same test result (again, a low-probability scan) among people without the target disorder? For a low-probability ventilation-perfusion scan, these likelihoods are 39/251 (0.155) and 273/630 (0.433), respectively, and their ratio (the likelihood ratio for low-probability scan) is 0.36. Table 1C-3 provides the results of the calculations for the other scan results.

What do all these numbers mean? The Likelihood ratios indicate by how much a given diagnostic test result will raise or lower the pretest probability of the target disorder. A likelihood ratio of 1.0 means that the posttest probability is exactly the same as the pretest probability. Likelihood ratios >1.0 increase the probability that the target disorder is present, and the higher the likelihood ratio, the greater is this increase. Conversely, likelihood ratios <1.0 decrease the probability of the target disorder, and the smaller the likelihood ratio, the greater is the decrease in probability and the smaller is its final value.

How big is a "big" likelihood ratio, and how small is a "small" one? Using likelihood ratios in your day-to-day practice will lead to your own sense of their interpretation, but consider the following a rough guide:

- Likelihood ratios of >10 or < 0.1 generate large and often conclusive changes from pre- to posttest probability;

- Likelihood ratios of 5–10 and 0.1–0.2 generate moderate shifts in pre- to posttest probability;

- Likelihood ratios of 2–5 and 0.5–0.2 generate small (but sometimes important) changes in probability; and

- Likelihood ratios of 1–2 and 0.5–1 alter probability to a small (and rarely important) degree.

Having determined the magnitude and significance of the likelihood ratios, how do we use them to go from pretest to posttest probability? We cannot combine likelihoods directly, the way we can combine probabilities or percentages; their formal use requires converting pretest probability to odds, multiplying the result by the Likelihood ratio, and converting the consequent posttest odds into a posttest probability. Although it is not too difficult (see Part 2B2, "Therapy and Understanding the Results, Measures of Association"), this calculation can be tedious and off-putting; fortunately, there is an easier way.

A *nomogram* proposed by Fagan[12] (Figure 1C-2) does all the conversions and allows an easy transition from pretest to posttest probability. The left-hand column of this nomogram represents the pretest probability, the middle column represents the likelihood ratio, and the right-hand column shows the posttest probability. You obtain the posttest probability by anchoring a ruler at the pretest probability and rotating it until it lines up with the likelihood ratio for the observed test result.

**FIGURE 1C–2**

## Likelihood Ratio Nomogram

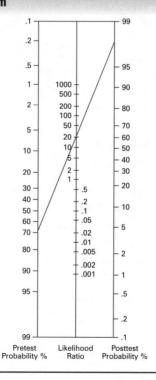

Pretest Probability % — Likelihood Ratio — Posttest Probability %

Recall the elderly woman mentioned earlier with suspected pulmonary embolism after abdominal surgery. Most clinicians would agree that the probability of this patient having the condition is quite high—about 70%. This value then represents the pretest probability. Suppose that her ventilation-perfusion scan was reported as being within the realm of high probability. Figure 1C-2 shows how you can anchor a ruler at her pretest probability of 70% and align it with the Likelihood ratio of 18.3 associated with a high-probability scan. The results: her posttest probability is >97%. If, by contrast, her ventilation-perfusion scan result is reported as intermediate (Likelihood ratio, 1.2), the probability of pulmonary embolism hardly changes (it increases to 74%), whereas a near-normal result yields a posttest probability of 19%.

The pretest probability is an estimate. We have already pointed out that the literature dealing with differential diagnosis can help us in establishing the pretest probability (see Part 1C, "The Process of Diagnosis"). Clinicians can deal with residual uncertainty by examining the implications of a plausible range of pretest probabilities. Let us assume the pretest probability in this case is as low as 60%, or as high as 80%. The posttest probabilities that would follow from these different pretest probabilities appear in Table 1C-4.

**TABLE 1C–4**

**Pretest Probabilities, Likelihood Ratios of Ventilation-Perfusion Scan Results, and Posttest Probabilities in Two Patients With Suspected Pulmonary Embolism**

| Pretest Probability %/(Range)* | Scan Result (LR) | Posttest Probability %/(Range)* |
|---|---|---|
| **78-Year-Old Woman With Sudden Onset of Dyspnea Following Abdominal Surgery** | | |
| 70 (60-80) | High Probability (18.3) | 97 (96-99) |
| 70 (60-80) | Intermediate Probability (1.2) | 74 (64-83) |
| 70 (60-80) | Low Probability (0.36) | 46 (35-59) |
| 70 (60-80) | Normal/Near Normal (0.1) | 19 (13-29) |
| **28-Year-Old Man With Dyspnea and Atypical Chest Pain** | | |
| 20 (10-30) | High Probability (18.3) | 82 (67-89) |
| 20 (10-30) | Intermediate Probability (1.2) | 23 (12-34) |
| 20 (10-30) | Low Probability (0.36) | 8 (4-6) |
| 20 (10-30) | Normal/Near Normal (0.1) | 2 (1-4) |

* The values in parentheses represent a plausible range of pretest probabilities. That is, although the best guess as to the pretest probability is 70%, values of 60% to 80% would also be reasonable estimates.

LR indicates Likelihood ratio.

We can repeat this exercise for our second patient, the 28-year-old man. Let us consider that his presentation is compatible with a 20% probability of pulmonary embolism. Using our nomogram (see Figure 1C-2), the posttest probability with a high-probability scan result is 82%; with an intermediate-probability result, it is 23%; and with a near-normal result, it is 2%. The pretest probability (with a range of possible pretest probabilities from 10% to 30%), likelihood ratios, and posttest probabilities associated with each of the four possible scan results also appear in Table 1C-4.

The investigation of women with possible appendicitis showed that the CT scan was positive in all 32 in whom that diagnosis was ultimately confirmed. Of the 68 who did not have appendicitis, 66 had negative scan results. These data translate into a Likelihood ratio of 0 associated with a negative test and a Likelihood ratio of 34 for a positive test. These numbers effectively mean that the test is extremely powerful. A negative result excludes appendicitis, and a positive test makes appendicitis highly likely.

Having learned to use likelihood ratios, you may be curious about where to find easy access to the Likelihood ratios of the tests you use regularly in your own practice. The Rational Clinical Examination[13] is a series of systematic reviews of the diagnostic properties of the history and physical examination that have been published in *JAMA*. Black and colleagues have summarized much of the available information about diagnostic test properties in the form of a medical text.[14] In addition, we provide our own summary of the likelihood ratios of some common tests in another section of this book (see Part 2C, "Diagnosis, Examples of Likelihood Ratios").

Sensitivity and Specificity. Readers who have followed the discussion to this point will understand the essentials of interpretation of diagnostic tests. In part because they remain in wide use, it is also helpful to understand two other terms in the lexicon of diagnostic testing: sensitivity and specificity.

You may have noted that our discussion of likelihood ratios omitted any talk of "normal" and "abnormal" tests. Instead, we presented four different ventilation-perfusion scan interpretations, each with its own Likelihood ratio. However, this is not the way the PIOPED investigators presented their results. They relied on the older (but less useful) concepts of sensitivity and specificity.

*Sensitivity* is the proportion of people with the target disorder in whom a test result is positive and *specificity* is the proportion of people without the target disorder in whom a test result is negative. To use these concepts, we have to divide test results into normal and abnormal categories; in other words, we must create a two-column x two-column table. Table 1C-5 presents the general form of a 2 x 2 table that we use to understand sensitivity and specificity. Look again at Table 1C-5 and observe that we could transform a 4 x 2 table such as Table 1C-4 into any of three such 2 x 2 tables, depending on what we call normal or abnormal (or depending on what we call negative and positive test results). Let us assume that we call only high-probability scans abnormal (or positive).

**TABLE 1C-5**

## Comparison of the Results of a Diagnostic Test With the Results of Reference Standard Using a 2 x 2 Table*

| | Reference Standard | |
| --- | --- | --- |
| Test Results | Disease Present | Disease Absent |
| Disease present | True Positive (*a*) | False Positive (*b*) |
| Disease absent | False Negative (*c*) | True Negative (*d*) |

| | |
| --- | --- |
| * Sensitivity (Sens) | $= \dfrac{a}{a + c}$ |
| Specificity (Spec) | $= \dfrac{d}{b + d}$ |
| Likelihood ratio for positive test (LR+) | $= \dfrac{sens}{1 - spec} = \dfrac{a/(a + c)}{b/(b + d)}$ |
| Likelihood ratio for negative test (LR–) | $= \dfrac{1 - sens}{spec} = \dfrac{c/(a + c)}{d/(b + d)}$ |

Table 1C-6 presents a 2 x 2 table comparing the results of a ventilation perfusion scan with the results of pulmonary angiogram as a reference standard.

**TABLE 1C–6**

## Comparison of the Results of Diagnostic Test (Ventilation-Perfusion Scan) With the Results of Reference Standard (Pulmonary Angiogram) Assuming Only High-Probability Scans Are Positive (Truly Abnormal)*

| | Angiogram | |
| --- | --- | --- |
| Scan Category | Pulmonary Embolism Present | Pulmonary Embolism Absent |
| High probability | 102 | 14 |
| Others | 149 | 616 |
| Total | 251 | 630 |

* Sensitivity, 41%; specificity, 98%; Likelihood ratio of a high-probability test result, 18.3; Likelihood ratio of other results, 0.61.

To calculate sensitivity from the data in Table 1C-6, we look at the number of people with proven pulmonary embolism (251) who were diagnosed as having the target disorder on ventilation-perfusion scan (102) characterized by a sensitivity of 102/251, or approximately 41% (a/a+c). To calculate specificity, we look at the number of people without the target disorder (630) whose ventilation-perfusion scan results were classified as normal (616), yielding a specificity of 616/630, or 98% (d/b+d). We can also calculate likelihood ratios for the positive and negative test results using this cutpoint: 18.3 and 0.61, respectively.

Let us see how the test performs if we decide to put the threshold of positive vs negative in a different place in the table. For example, let us call only the normal/near-normal ventilation perfusion scan result negative. As shown in the 2 x 2 table depicted in Table 1C-7, the sensitivity is now 246/251, or 98% (among 251 people with pulmonary embolism, 246 are diagnosed on ventilation-perfusion scan), but what has happened to specificity? Among 630 people without pulmonary embolism, test results in only 126 are negative (specificity, 20%). The corresponding likelihood ratios are 1.23 and 0.1. Note that with this cut we not only lose the diagnostic information associated with the high-probability scan result, but we also interpret intermediate- and low-probability results as if they increase the likelihood of pulmonary embolism, when in fact they decrease the likelihood. You can generate the third 2 x 2 table by setting the cutpoint in the middle. If your sensitivity and specificity values are 82% and 63%, respectively, and associated Likelihood ratios of a positive and a negative test are 2.25 and 0.28, you have it right.

**TABLE 1C-7**

**Comparison of the Results of Diagnostic Test (Ventilation-Perfusion Scan) With the Results of Reference Standard (Pulmonary Angiogram) Assuming Only Normal/Near-Normal Scans Are Negative (Truly Normal)\***

|  | Angiogram | |
| --- | --- | --- |
| Scan Category | Pulmonary Embolism Present | Pulmonary Embolism Absent |
| High, intermediate, and low probability | 246 | 504 |
| Near normal/normal | 5 | 126 |
| **Total** | **251** | **630** |

\* Sensitivity, 98%; specificity, 20%; Likelihood ratio of high, intermediate, and low probability, 1.23; Likelihood ratio of near normal/normal, 0.1.

In using sensitivity and specificity you must either discard important information or recalculate sensitivity and specificity for every cutpoint. We recommend the Likelihood ratio approach because it is much simpler and much more efficient.

## USING THE GUIDE

Thus far, we have established that the results are likely true for the people who were included in the PIOPED study, and we have ascertained the Likelihood ratio associated with different results of the test. We have concluded that the helical CT scanning study may have overestimated the power of the test, but not so seriously as to completely invalidate the results. How useful are the tests likely to be in our clinical practice?

# HOW CAN I APPLY THE RESULTS TO PATIENT CARE?

## Will the Reproducibility of the Test Result and Its Interpretation Be Satisfactory in My Clinical Setting?

The value of any test depends on its ability to yield the same result when reapplied to stable patients. Poor reproducibility can result from problems with the test itself (eg, variations in reagents in radioimmunoassay kits for determining hormone levels). A second cause of different test results in stable patients arises whenever a test requires interpretation (eg, the extent of ST-segment elevation on an electrocardiogram). Ideally, an article about a diagnostic test will address the reproducibility of the test results using a measure that corrects for agreement by chance (see Part 2C, "Diagnosis, Measuring Agreement Beyond Chance"). This is especially important when expertise is required in performing or interpreting the test. You can confirm this by recalling the clinical disagreements that arise when you and one or more colleagues examine the same ECG, ultrasound, or CT scan, even when all of you are experts.

If the reproducibility of a test in the study setting is mediocre and disagreement between observers is common, and yet the test still discriminates well between those with and without the target condition, it is very useful. Under these circumstances, the likelihood is good that the test can be readily applied to your clinical setting. If reproducibility of a diagnostic test is very high and observer variation is very low, either the test is simple and unambiguous or those interpreting it are highly skilled. If the latter applies, less skilled interpreters in your own clinical setting may not do as well.

## USING THE GUIDE

The helical CT study made no reference to reproducibility, other than to say that the residents initially interpreted the scans and the consultants agreed in all but one case. The authors did not describe the degree of experience of the radiologists, but the residents' involvement suggests that unusual expertise is not mandatory for accurate interpretation of the images.

## Are the Results Applicable to the Patient in My Practice?

Test properties may change with a different mix of disease severity or with a different distribution of competing conditions. When patients with the target disorder all have severe disease, likelihood ratios will move away from a value of 1.0 (sensitivity increases). If patients are all mildly affected, likelihood ratios move toward a value of 1.0 (sensitivity decreases). If patients without the target disorder have competing conditions that mimic the test results seen in patients who do have the target disorder, the likelihood ratios will move closer to 1.0 and the test will appear less useful (specificity decreases). In a different clinical setting in which fewer of the disease-free patients have these competing conditions, the likelihood ratios will move away from 1.0 and the test will appear more useful (sensitivity increases).

The phenomenon of differing test properties in different subpopulations has been demonstrated most strikingly for exercise electrocardiography in the diagnosis of coronary artery disease. For instance, the more extensive the severity of coronary artery disease, the larger are the likelihood ratios of abnormal exercise electrocardiography for angiographic narrowing of the coronary arteries.[15] Another example comes from the diagnosis of venous thromboembolism, where compression ultrasound for proximal-vein thrombosis has proved more accurate in symptomatic outpatients than in asymptomatic postoperative patients.[16]

Sometimes, a test fails in just the patients one hopes it will best serve. The likelihood ratio of a negative dipstick test for the rapid diagnosis of urinary tract infection is approximately 0.2 in patients with clear symptoms and thus a high probability of urinary tract infection, but is over 0.5 in those with low probability,[17] rendering it of little help in ruling out infection in the latter. If you practice in a setting similar to that of the investigation and if the patient under consideration meets all the study inclusion criteria and does not violate any of the exclusion criteria, you can be confident that the results are applicable. If not, a judgment is required. As with therapeutic interventions, you should ask whether there are compelling reasons why the results should not be applied to the patients in your practice, either because of the severity of disease in those patients or because the mix of competing conditions is so different that generalization is unwarranted. The issue of generalizability may be resolved if you can find an overview that pools the results of a number of studies.[18]

## USING THE GUIDE

The participants in the PIOPED study were a representative sample of patients with suspected pulmonary embolism from a number of large general hospitals. Therefore, the results are readily applicable to most clinical practices in North America. There are groups such as critically ill patients to whom we might be reluctant to generalize the results; such patients were excluded from the study and are likely to have had a different spectrum of competing conditions than other patients.

The patients enrolled in the study of CT scanning in acute appendicitis constitute a representative sample of women presenting to the emergency department with right lower quadrant pain. The patient before you, in whom the differential diagnosis includes appendicitis and pelvic inflammatory disease, meets study eligibility criteria. Thus, you can be confident that the results will apply in her case.

## Will the Results Change My Management Strategy?

It is useful, when making, learning, teaching, and communicating management decisions, to link them explicitly to the probability of the target disorder. As we have described, for any target disorder there are probabilities below which a clinician would dismiss a diagnosis and order no further tests—the test threshold. Similarly, there are probabilities above which a clinician would consider the diagnosis confirmed and would stop testing and initiate treatment—the treatment threshold. When the probability of the target disorder lies between the test and treatment thresholds, further testing is mandated[19] (see Part 1C, "The Process of Diagnosis").

Once we decide what our test and treatment thresholds are, posttest probabilities have direct treatment implications. Let us suppose that we are willing to treat those patients with a probability of pulmonary embolism of 80% or higher (knowing that we will be treating 20% of them unnecessarily). Furthermore, let us suppose we are willing to dismiss the diagnosis of pulmonary embolism in those with a posttest probability of 10% or less. You may wish to apply different numbers here; the treatment and test thresholds are a matter of judgment and they differ for different conditions depending on the risks of therapy (if risky, you want to be more certain of your diagnosis) and the danger of the disease if left untreated (if the danger of missing the disease is high—such as in pulmonary embolism—you want your posttest probability to be very low before abandoning the diagnostic search). In the 28-year-old man discussed earlier in this section, a high-probability scan results in a posttest probability of 82% and may dictate treatment (or, at least, further investigation) and an intermediate probability scan (23% posttest probability) will dictate further testing (perhaps bilateral leg venography, ultrasound, or pulmonary angiography), whereas a low-probability or normal scan (probabilities of less than 10%) will exclude the diagnosis of pulmonary embolism. In the elderly woman, a high-probability scan dictates treatment (97% posttest probability of pulmonary embolism) and an intermediate result (74% posttest probability) may be compatible with either treatment or further testing (likely a pulmonary angiogram), whereas any other result mandates further testing.

If most patients have test results with Likelihood ratios near 1.0, the test will not be very useful. Thus, the usefulness of a diagnostic test is strongly influenced by the proportion of patients suspected of having the target disorder whose test results have very high or very low Likelihood ratios. In the patients suspected of having pulmonary embolism in our ventilation-perfusion scan example, a review of Table 1C-3 allows us to determine the proportion of patients with extreme results (either high probability with an Likelihood ratio of over 10, or normal/near-normal scans with an Likelihood ratio of 0.1). The proportion can be calculated as (102+14+5+126)/881, or 247/881 = 28%. Clinicians who have been frustrated by frequent intermediate- or low-probability results in patients with suspected pulmonary embolism will already know that this proportion (28%) is far from optimal. Thus, despite the high Likelihood ratio associated with a high-probability scan and the low Likelihood ratio associated with a normal/near-normal result, ventilation perfusion scanning is of limited usefulness in patients with suspected pulmonary embolism.

A final comment has to do with the use of sequential tests. We have demonstrated how each item of history—or each finding on physical examination—represents a diagnostic test. We generate pretest probabilities that we modify with each new finding. In general, we can also use laboratory tests or imaging procedures in the same way. However, if two tests are very closely related, application of the second test may provide little or no information, and the sequential application of likelihood ratios will yield misleading results. For example, once one has the results of the most powerful laboratory test for iron deficiency, serum ferritin, additional tests such as serum iron or transferrin saturation add no further useful information.[20] *Clinical prediction rules* deal with the lack of independence of a series of tests that can be applied to a diagnostic dilemma and provide the clinician with a way of combining their results (see Part 2C, "Diagnosis, Clinical Prediction Rules"). For instance, the clinician in the scenario that opened this section could have used a rule that incorporates respiratory symptoms, heart rate, leg symptoms, oxygen saturation, electrocardiographic findings, and other aspects of history and physical examination to accurately classify patients with suspected pulmonary embolism as being characterized by high, medium, and low probability.[21]

## USING THE GUIDE

**G**iven the extreme likelihood ratios of helical CT scanning in women with abdominal pain, CT results are very likely to change management. For any patient with an intermediate likelihood of appendicitis, a positive scan will suggest immediate surgery, and a negative scan will mandate continued observation with treatment of alternative diagnostic possibilities (in this case, pelvic inflammatory disease).

## Will Patients Be Better Off as a Result of the Test?

The ultimate criterion for the usefulness of a diagnostic test is whether the benefits that accrue to patients are greater than the associated risks.[22] How can we establish the benefits and risks of applying a diagnostic test? The answer lies in thinking of a diagnostic test as a therapeutic maneuver (see Part 1B1, "Therapy"). Establishing whether a test does more good than harm will involve (1) randomizing patients to a diagnostic strategy that includes the test under investigation or to one in which the test is not available and (2) following patients in both groups forward in time to determine the frequency of patient-important target outcomes.

When is demonstrating accuracy sufficient to mandate the use of a test, and when does one require a randomized controlled trial? The value of an accurate test will be undisputed when the target disorder is dangerous if left undiagnosed, if the test has acceptable risks, and if effective treatment exists. This is the case for both of the tests we have considered in detail in this section. A high probability or normal/near-normal results of a ventilation-perfusion scan may well eliminate the need for further investigation and may result in anticoagulant agents being appropriately given or appropriately withheld (with either course of action having a substantial positive influence on patient outcome).

The researchers who conducted the investigation of helical CT scanning in women with abdominal pain asked clinicians to formulate management plans before CT results were available and compared the plan to the one that clinicians followed after receiving the CT result. Of 100 patients, clinicians sent home 43 patients whom they would otherwise have admitted for observation, and they sent 13 others, whom they would otherwise have observed, to the operating room for immediate appendectomy. The evident benefits for patients and for the health care system—patients prefer to be at home than in a hospital, along with the fact that delayed appendectomy risks additional complications—eliminate the need for a randomized trial of CT scanning vs standard diagnostic approaches in women presenting to the emergency department with abdominal pain.

In other clinical situations, tests may be accurate and management may even change as a result of their application, but their impact on patient outcome may be far less certain. Consider one of the issues we raised in our discussion of framing clinical questions (see Part 1A1, "Finding the Evidence"). We presented a patient with apparently resectable non-small-cell carcinoma of the lung and wondered whether the clinician should order a CT scan and base further management on the results, or whether an immediate mediastinoscopy should be undertaken. For this question, knowledge of the accuracy of CT scanning is insufficient. A randomized trial of CT-directed management or mediastinoscopy for all patients is warranted—and indeed, investigators have conducted such a trial.[23] Other examples include catheterization of the right side of the heart for critically ill patients with uncertain hemodynamic status, bronchoalveolar lavage for critically ill patients with possible pulmonary sepsis, bronchial provocation testing for patients with asthma, and the incremental value of magnetic resonance imaging over CT for a wide variety of problems. For these and many other tests, confidence in the right management strategy must await the conduct of well-designed and adequately powered randomized trials.

# CLINICAL RESOLUTION

You are sufficiently impressed by the information in the article about helical CT scanning that you decide to bypass the gynecologic consultation. Your radiologist colleague facilitates an emergent scan and soon calls you back, triumphantly announcing that the results are characteristic of appendicitis. The surgeons are soon having the patient whisked to the operating room, and you later hear that the patient is recovering uneventfully after the removal of her inflamed appendix.

# References

1. Rao PM, Feltmate CM, Rhea JT, Schulick AH, Novelline RA. Helical computed tomography in differentiating appendicitis and acute gynecologic conditions. *Obstet Gynecol*. 1999;93:417-421.

2. Thomson DM, Krupey J, Freedman SO, Gold P. The radioimmunoassay of circulating carcinoembryonic antigen of the human digestive system. *Proc Natl Acad Sci U S A*. 1969;64:161-167.

3. Bates SE. Clinical applications of serum tumor markers. *Ann Intern Med*. 1991;115:623-638.

4. Lijmer JG, Mol BW, Heisterkamp S, et al. Empirical evidence of design-related bias in studies of diangostic tests. *JAMA*. 1999;282:1061-1066.

5. The PIOPED investigators. Value of ventilation/perfusion scan in acute pulmonary embolism. Results of the prospective investigation of pulmonary embolism diagnosis (PIOPED). *JAMA*. 1990;263:2753-2759.

6. Sackett DL, Haynes RB, Guyatt GH, Tugwell P. *Clinical Epidemiology, A Basic Science for Clinical Medicine*. 2nd ed. Boston: Little, Brown and Company; 1991:53-57.

7. Kemppainen EA, Hedstrom JI, Puolakkainen PA, et al. Rapid measurement of urinary trypsinogen-2 as a screening test for acute pancreatitis. *N Engl J Med*. 1997;336:1788-1793.

8. Begg CB, Greenes RA. Assessment of diagnostic tests when disease verification is subject to selection bias. *Biometrics*. 1983;39:207-215.

9. Gray R, Begg CB, Greenes RA. Construction of receiver operating characteristic curves when disease verification is subject to selection bias. *Med Decis Making*. 1984;4:151-164.

10. Ransohoff DF, Feinstein AR. Problems of spectrum and bias in evaluating the efficacy of diagnostic tests. *N Engl J Med*. 1978;299:926-930.

11. Choi BC. Sensitivity and specificity of a single diagnostic test in the presence of work-up bias. *J Clin Epidemiol*. 1992;45:581-586.

12. Fagan TJ. Nomogram for Bayes's theorem. *N Engl J Med*. 1975;293:257.

13. Sackett DL, Rennie D. The science and art of the clinical examination. *JAMA*. 1992;267:2650-2652.

14. Black ER, Bordley DR, Tape TG, Panzer RJ. *Diagnostic Strategies for Common Medical Problems*. 2nd ed. Philadelphia: American College of Physicians; 1999.

15. Hlatky MA, Pryor DB, Harrell FE. Factors affecting sensitivity and specificity of exercise electrocardiography. *Am J Med*. 1984;77:64-71.

16. Ginsberg JS, Caco CC, Brill-Edwards PA, et al. Venous thrombosis in patients who have undergone major hip or knee surgery: detection with compression US and impedance plethysmography. *Radiology*. 1991;181:651-654.

17. Lachs MS, Nachamkin I, Edelstein PH, et al. Spectrum bias in the evaluation of diagnostic tests: lessons from the repid dipstick test for urinary tract infection. *Ann Intern Med*. 1992;117:135-140.

18. Irwig L, Tosteson AN, Gatsonis C, et al. Guidelines for meta-analyses evaluating diagnostic tests. *Ann Intern Med*. 1994;120:667-676.

19. Sackett DL, Haynes RB, Guyatt GH, Tugwell P. *Clinical Epidemiology, a Basic Science for Clinical Medicine*. 2nd ed. Boston: Little, Brown and Company; 1991:145-148.

20. Guyatt GH, Oxman A, Ali M, et al. Laboratory diagnosis of iron-deficiency anemia: an overview. *J Gen Intern Med*. 1992;7:145-153.

21. Wells PS, Ginsberg JS, Anderson DR, et al. Use of a clinical model for safe management of patients with suspected pulmonary embolism. *Ann Intern Med*. 1998;129:997-1005.

22. Guyatt GH, Tugwell PX, Feeny DH, Haynes RB, Drummond M. A framework for clinical evaluation of diagnostic technologies. *CMAJ*. 1986;134:587-594.

23. Canadian Lung Oncology Group. Investigation for mediastinal disease in patients with apparently operable lung cancer. *Ann Thorac Surg*. 1995;60:1382-1389.

# 1D

# PROGNOSIS

Adrienne Randolph, Heiner Bucher, W. Scott Richardson, George Wells, Peter Tugwell, and Gordon Guyatt

The following EBM Working Group members also made substantive contributions to this section: Deborah Cook, Jonathan Craig, and Jeremy Wyatt

## IN THIS SECTION

## CLINICAL SCENARIO

### Age 71, a Prior Stroke: What Is the Prognosis?

You are a Swiss internist seeing a 71-year-old man recovering from a right lower lobe pneumonia. The patient, who suffered a right hemispheric stroke 1 year ago, has little function of his left arm but is able to walk with a crutch. He is in sinus rhythm. For at least 15 years, he had hypertension that probably was poorly controlled. His echocardiogram has revealed left ventricular hypertrophy and mild left ventricular dysfunction. A Doppler examination of his carotid arteries shows nonsignificant stenosis of less than 50% bilaterally. He takes aspirin 300 mg per day, an angiotensin-converting enzyme (ACE) inhibitor, and a thiazide diuretic now control his hypertension.

From a lively discussion with the patient, you learn that he is a connoisseur of French wines and that since his early retirement he spends several months each year in Southern France, where he owns a little cottage. The patient grumbles that since the stroke, "things are not going the way they should" and you try to console him. Later on, speaking to the patient's wife, you find she is concerned about her husband's difficulty accepting his disability. She feels that owning two residences, with all of the commuting between them, is too much for both of them. The back-and-forth driving and the care for the two houses has completely become her burden, and she states that the pneumonia was the "proof for her husband's exhaustion." She feels that information about his risks of a recurrent stroke and death could help him and his family to "settle things." Because your knowledge about the prognosis of survivors of stroke is vague, you tell the patient's wife that you will obtain specific information to address her concerns, and you promise to report back to her and to the patient.

# FINDING THE EVIDENCE

Your hospital does not offer access to Best Evidence or the Cochrane Library, but at least you have an Internet connection. During a break, you connect to the Internet and to MEDLINE at the US National Library of Medicine Web site via PubMed. You enter the term "stroke" and, using the thesaurus, you find the correct Medical Subject Heading (MeSH) term, "cerebral infarction." Combining the search with the terms "epidemiology," "recurrence," and "prognosis" yields a number of relevant results. You identify one interesting article, "Long-Term Risk of Recurrent Stroke After a First-ever Stroke," from the Oxfordshire Community Project and obtain a copy from the library.[1]

Clinicians help patients in three broad ways: by diagnosing what is wrong with them, by administering treatment that does more good than harm, and by giving them an indication of what the future is likely to hold. Clinicians require studies of patient *prognosis*—those examining the possible outcomes of a disease and the probability with which they can be expected to occur—to achieve the second and third goals. Although they strive to restore health, sometimes clinicians can only offer relief of discomfort and preparation for death or long-term disability by means of presenting the expected future course of the patient's illness.

To estimate a patient's prognosis, we examine outcomes in groups of patients with a similar clinical presentation—patients in the first year after stroke, for example. We may then refine our prognosis by looking at subgroups and deciding into which subgroup the patient falls. We may define these subgroups by such demographic variables as age (younger patients may fare better than older ones), by disease-specific variables (patients' outcome may differ depending on whether the stroke was hemorrhagic or thrombotic), or by comorbid factors (those with underlying hypertension, even if treated, may have worse outcomes). When these variables or factors really do predict which patients do better or worse, we call them *prognostic factors*.

Authors often distinguish between prognostic factors and *risk factors,* which are those patient characteristics associated with the development of the disease in the first place. For example, smoking is an important risk factor for the development of lung cancer, but it is not as important a prognostic factor as tumor stage in someone who has lung cancer. The issues in studies of prognostic factors and risk factors are identical, both for assessing validity and for using the results in patient care.

Knowledge of a patient's prognosis can help clinicians make the right diagnostic and treatment decisions. If a patient will get well anyway, clinicians should not recommend high-risk invasive procedures or waste money on expensive or potentially toxic treatments. If a patient is at low risk of adverse outcomes, even beneficial treatments may not be worthwhile. For example, stress ulcer prophylaxis to prevent gastrointestinal bleeding may not be worthwhile in nonintubated patients without a coagulopathy who are at extremely low risk of clinically important hemorrhage.[2] In another example, young nonsmoking patients with mild hypercholesterolemia without hypertension or a family history of coronary disease may conclude that their risk of adverse cardiovascular outcomes during the coming decade or two is so low that they will not take lipid-lowering medication. On the other hand, patients may be destined to have poor outcomes despite whatever treatment we offer. Aggressive therapy in such individuals may only prolong suffering and waste resources.

Knowledge of prognosis is also useful for resolution of issues broader than the care of the individual patient. Organizations may attempt to compare the quality of care across clinicians, or institutions, by measuring the outcomes of care. However, differences in outcome may be caused by the variability in the underlying severity of illness rather than by the treatments, clinicians, or health care institutions under study. If we know patients' prognoses, we may be able to compare populations and adjust for differences in prognosis to obtain a more accurate indication of how management is affecting outcome (see Part 2B, "Therapy and Harm, Outcomes of Health Services").

Certain issues are common to all these reasons for determining prognosis—communicating to patients their likely fate, guiding our treatment decisions, and comparing outcomes in populations to make inferences about quality of care—and some differ. In this section of the book, we focus on how to use articles that may contain valid prognostic information that will be useful in counseling patients (Table 1D-1).

---

**TABLE 1D-1**

## Users' Guides to an Article About Prognosis

**Are the results valid?**

- Was the sample of patients representative?
- Were the patients sufficiently homogeneous with respect to prognostic risk?
- Was follow-up sufficiently complete?
- Were objective and unbiased outcome criteria used?

**What are the results?**

- How likely are the outcomes over time?
- How precise are the estimates of likelihood?

**How can I apply the results to patient care?**

- Were the study patients and their management similar to those in my practice?
- Was the follow-up sufficiently long?
- Can I use the results in the management of patients in my practice?

---

Using the same methodology as investigators addressing issues of harm (see Part 1B2, "Harm"), investigators addressing issues of prognosis use cohort and case-control designs in their studies to explore the determinants of outcome. Implicitly, randomized controlled trials also address issues of prognosis. The results reported for both the treatment group and the control group provide prognostic information: the control group results tell us about the prognosis in patients who did not receive treatment, and the treatment group results tell us about the prognosis in patients receiving the intervention. In this sense, each arm of a randomized trial represents a cohort study. If the randomized trial meets criteria we will describe later in this section, it can provide extremely useful information about patients' likely fate.

For issues of harm, the choice of appropriate treatment and control groups is crucial. For issues of prognosis, if there is a control group at all (and for populations in which patients all have more or less the same prognosis, this need not be the case), the controls are patients with different prognostic factors. In the same way that articles addressing issues of diagnosis evaluate tests that distinguish between those with and without a target condition or disease, prognostic studies may suggest factors that differentiate between those at low and high risk for a target outcome or adverse event. Issues in evaluating prognostic studies, however, are sufficiently different from those related to harm or diagnosis that clinicians may find the following guides helpful.

# ARE THE RESULTS VALID?

## Was the Sample of Patients Representative?

*Bias* has to do with systematic differences from the truth. A prognostic study is biased if it yields a systematic overestimate or underestimate of the likelihood of adverse outcomes in the patients under study. When a sample is systematically different from the underlying population—and is therefore likely to be biased because patients will have a better or worse prognosis than those in that population—that sample as "unrepresentative."

How can you recognize an unrepresentative sample? First, look to see if patients pass through some sort of filter before entering the study. If they do, the result is likely to be from a sample that is systematically different from the underlying population of interest (such as patients who have suffered a myocardial infarction or stroke, or with new-onset diabetes). One such filter is the sequence of referrals that leads patients from primary to tertiary centers. Tertiary centers often care for patients with rare and unusual disorders or increased illness severity. Research describing the outcomes of patients in tertiary centers may not be applicable to the general patient suffering from the disorder in the community.

For example, when children are admitted to the hospital with febrile seizures, parents want to know the risk that their child will have more seizures in the future. This risk is much lower in population-based studies (reported risks range from 1.5% to 4.6%) than in clinic-based studies (reported risks are 2.6% to 76.9%).[3] Those in clinic-based studies may have other neurologic problems predisposing them to have higher rates of recurrence. For you to adequately counsel parents, you need to know how similar your patient is to the patients in the various samples.

Failure to clearly define the patients who entered the study increases the risk that the sample is unrepresentative. To help you decide about the representativeness of the sample, look for a clear description of which patients were included and excluded from a study. The way the sample was selected should be clearly specified, along with the objective criteria used to diagnose the patients with the disorder.

## Were the Patients Sufficiently Homogeneous With Respect to Prognostic Risk?

Prognostic studies are most useful if individual members of the entire group of patients being considered are similar enough that the outcome of the group is applicable to each group member. This will be true only if patients are at a similar well-described point in their disease process. The point in the clinical course need not be early, but it does need to be consistent. For instance, in a study of the prognosis of children with acquired brain injury, researchers looked not at the entire population, but at a subpopulation who remained unconscious after 90 days.[4]

After ensuring that the stage of the disease process is not a variable influencing outcome (because investigators held it constant), it is important to consider other factors that might influence patient outcome. For instance, consider the example of acquired brain injury. A study examining neurologic outcome that pooled patients with and without head trauma without distinguishing between them may not be very useful if these two groups have different prognoses. If the overall mortality rate reported in a study is 50% but the patient population is made up of identifiable subgroups, one of which has a mortality rate near zero and the other of which has a mortality rate near 100%, the 50% estimate will be valid for the whole group but not valid for any individual in that group. If the patients are heterogeneous with respect to risk of adverse outcome, the study will be much more useful if the investigators define subgroups that are at lower and higher risk than the overall group.

For example, Pincus and colleagues followed a cohort of patients with rheumatoid arthritis for 15 years.[5] They separated the patients into a number of cohorts depending on their demographic characteristics, disease variables, and functional status. They found that older patients and those with greater impairment of functional status (eg, modified walking time and activities of daily living) died earlier than others. In another example, the authors of the study of children with acquired brain injury found that patients with posttraumatic injuries did much better than those with anoxic injuries. Of 36 patients with closed head trauma, 23 (64%) regained enough social function to be able to express their wants and needs and nine (25%) eventually regained the capacity to walk independently. Of 13 children with anoxic injuries, none regained important social or cognitive function.[4]

Not only must investigators consider all important prognostic factors, but they must also consider them in relation to one another. Consider the Framingham study, in which investigators examined (among many other things) risk factors for stroke.[6] They reported that the rate of stroke in patients with atrial fibrillation and rheumatic heart disease was 41 per 1000 person-years, which was very similar to the rate for patients with atrial fibrillation but without rheumatic heart disease. However, patients with rheumatic heart disease were, on average, much younger than those who did not have rheumatic heart disease. To properly understand the impact of rheumatic heart disease, investigators in these circumstances must consider separately (1) the relative risk of stroke in young people with and without rheumatic disease, and (2) the risk of stroke in elderly people with and without rheumatic disease. We call this separate consideration an *adjusted analysis.* Once adjustments were made for age (and also for gender and hypertensive status of the patients), the investigators found that the rate of stroke was sixfold greater in patients with rheumatic heart disease and atrial fibrillation than in patients with atrial fibrillation who did not have rheumatic heart disease. If a large number of variables have a major impact on prognosis, investigators should use sophisticated statistical techniques to determine the most powerful predictors (see Part 2D, "Prognosis, Regression and Correlation"). Such an analysis may lead to a clinical decision rule that guides clinicians in simultaneously considering all the important prognostic factors (see Part 2C, "Diagnosis, Clinical Prediction Rules").

How can you decide if the groups are sufficiently homogeneous with respect to their risk? On the basis of your clinical experience—and your understanding of the biology of the condition being studied—can you think of factors that the investigators have neglected that are likely to define subgroups with very different prognoses? To the extent that the answer is "yes," the validity of the study is compromised.

## Was Follow-up Sufficiently Complete?

A high patient dropout rate threatens the validity of a study of prognosis. As the number of patients who do not return for follow-up increases, the likelihood of bias also increases (eg, those who are followed may be at systematically higher or lower risk than those not being followed). How many patients lost to follow-up is too many? The answer depends on the relationship between the proportion of patients who are lost and the proportion of patients who have suffered the adverse outcome of interest. The larger the number of patients whose fate is unknown relative to the number who have suffered an event, the greater is the threat to the study's *validity.*

For instance, let us assume that 30% of a particularly high-risk group (such as elderly patients with diabetes) have suffered an adverse outcome (such as cardiovascular death) during long-term follow-up. If 10% of the patients have been lost to follow up, the true rate of patients who had died may be as low as approximately 27% or as high as 40%. Across this range, the clinical implications would not change appreciably, and the loss to follow-up does not threaten the validity of the study. However, in a much lower-risk patient sample (otherwise healthy middle-aged men, for instance) the observed event rate may be 1%. In this case, if we assumed that all 10% of the patients lost to follow up had died, the event rate of 11% might have very different implications.

A large loss to follow-up constitutes a more serious threat to validity when the patients who are lost may be different from those who are easier to find. In one study, for example, after much effort, 180 of 186 patients treated for neurosis were followed.[7] The death rate was 3% among the 60% who were easily traced. Among those who were more difficult to find, however, the death rate was 27%. If a differential fate for those followed and those lost is plausible (and in most prognostic studies, it will be), loss to follow-up that is large in relation to the proportion of patients suffering the adverse outcome of interest constitutes an important threat to validity.

## Were Objective and Unbiased Outcome Criteria Used?

Outcome events can vary from those that are objective and easily measured (eg, death), to those requiring some judgment (eg, myocardial infarction), to those that may require considerable judgment and are challenging to measure (eg, disability or quality of life). Investigators should clearly specify and define their target outcomes before the study and, whenever possible, they should base their criteria on objective measures. In addition, they should specify the intensity and frequency of monitoring. As the subjectivity of the outcome definition increases, it becomes more important that individuals determining the outcomes are blinded to the presence of prognostic factors.

The study of children with acquired brain injury mentioned earlier in this section provides a good example of the issues involved in measuring outcome.[4] The examiners found that patients' families frequently optimistically interpreted interactions with the patients. The investigators therefore required that development of a social response in the affected children needed verification by study personnel, and they made the date that consciousness returned dependent on the date of the next outpatient visit. For instance, for a child who remained unconscious 1 year after injury and who was conscious on the next clinic visit 16 months after the original injury, the duration of unconsciousness would be recorded as being 1 year.

Returning to the patient scenerio, and the article describing the prognosis of stroke patients, the Oxfordshire Community Stroke Project prospectively registered all 675 patients with a first-ever stroke at the time they entered one of the participating hospitals.[1] Thus, patients were recruited at a common, early starting point. Since the study was community based, the population may be representative for a unselected cohort of British first-ever stroke patients. Their mean age was 72 years and 47% were male. In 81% of the patients, cerebral infarction was the cause of stroke; 10% had primary intracerebral hemorrhage; and 5% had subarachnoid hemorrhage—a pattern common to other stroke natural history studies.

One might speculate that a number of risk factors could influence the risk of subsequent stroke, including initial stroke severity, the patient's age, type of stroke, and presence of diabetes, heart failure, or blood pressure. The investigators analyzed all but the first of these factors and found no difference in prognosis across subgroups.

The investigators succeeded in achieving 100% follow-up by a study nurse who evaluated patients at 1 month, 6 months, 1 year after their event, and annually thereafter. The authors provided a detailed definition of what they meant by a stroke (for instance, they excluded asymptomatic new lesions on CT scans). However, they made no attempt to blind the nurse to possible prognostic factors.

# WHAT ARE THE RESULTS?

## How Likely Are the Outcomes Over Time?

The quantitative results from studies of prognosis or risk are the number of events that occur over time. We will use the example of a man asking a physician about the prognosis of his elderly mother who has dementia to illustrate common expressions of this relationship that provide complementary information about prognosis.

The patient's son asks, "What are the chances that my mother will still be alive in 5 years?" A high-validity study of the prognosis of patients with dementia provides a simple and direct answer in absolute terms.[8] Five years after presentation to the clinic, about one half of the patients (50%) had died. Thus, there is about a 50:50 chance that his mother will be alive in 5 years.

The patient's son might then indicate that the only person he knows with Alzheimer disease is a 65-year-old uncle who was diagnosed 10 years ago and is still living. He is surprised that his mother's chance of dying in the next 5 years is so high. This gives the clinician the opportunity to discuss some of the prognostic factors for death in patients with Alzheimer disease. The high-validity study examining the prognosis of demented patients suggested that older patients, those with more severe dementia, those with behavioral problems, and those with hearing loss died earlier.

The son might then ask whether his mother's chance of survival is expected to change over time. That is, although she may be at low risk for the next 2 years, will the risk jump sharply after that? Neither the absolute nor relative expressions of results address this question. For this answer we should turn to a *survival curve*, a graph of the number of events over time (or conversely, the chance of being free of these events over time) (see Part 2B2, "Therapy and Understanding the Results, Measures of Association"). The events must be discrete (eg, death, stroke, or recurrence of cancer) and the time at which they occur must be precisely known.

Figure 1D-1 shows two survival curves—one of survival after a myocardial infarction[9] and the other depicting the results of hip replacement surgery in terms of when patients needed a revision because something had gone wrong after the initial surgery.[10] Note that the chance of dying after a myocardial infarction is highest shortly after the event (reflected by an initially steep downward slope of the curve, which then becomes flat), whereas very few hip replacements require revision until much later (this curve, by contrast, starts out flat and then steepens). The study of patients with dementia provided a survival curve that suggests that the chance of dying is more or less constant during the first 7 years after referral to the clinic for dementia (Figure ID-2)[8].

**FIGURE 1D–1**

## Survival Curves

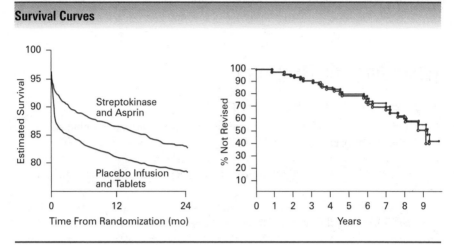

**Left,** survival after myocardial infarction. **Right,** results of hip replacement surgery, proportion of patients who survived without needing a new procedure (revision) after their initial hip replacement.

Reproduced with permission from The Lancet Publishing Group (left) and *The Journal of Bone and Joint Surgery* (right).

## How Precise Are the Estimates of Likelihood?

The more precise the estimate of prognosis a study provides, the less we need be uncertain around the estimated prognosis and the more useful it is to us. Usually, risks of adverse outcomes are reported with their associated 95% confidence intervals (CIs). If the study is valid, the 95% CI defines the range of risks within which it is highly likely that the true risk lies (see Part 2B2, "Therapy and Understanding the Results, Confidence Intervals"). For example, the study of the prognosis of patients with dementia provides the 95% CI around the 49% esti-mate of survival at 5 years after presentation, ie, 39% to 58%. Note that in most survival curves, the earlier follow-up periods usually include results from more patients than do the later periods (owing to losses to follow-up and because patients are not enrolled in the study at the same time). This means that the survival curves are more precise in the earlier periods, which should be indicated by narrower confidence bands around the left-hand parts of the curve.

**FIGURE 1D–2**

## Kaplan-Meier Graph of Overall Survival

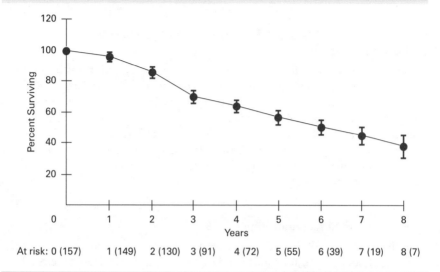

At risk: 0 (157)    1 (149)    2 (130)    3 (91)    4 (72)    5 (55)    6 (39)    7 (19)    8 (7)

Note standard errors of the entire cohort and the number of patients at risk each year.

Reproduced with permission from Wiley-Liss, Inc, a subsidiary of John Wiley & Sons, Inc.

## USING THE GUIDE

The Oxfordshire study found that the absolute risk of death during the first year after a stroke was 31% (95% CI, 27%-34%) and the absolute risk of dying over the next 4 years averaged approximately 4% per year. For patients who survived, the risk of a recurrent stroke was 8.6% (95% CI, 6.5%-10.7%) in the first 6 months, 4.6% (95% CI, 2.6%-6.6%) in the next 6 months, and 6.7% (95% CI, 2.7%-7.3%), 5.0% (95% CI, 1.0%-5.6%), 3.3%, and 1.3%, respectively, in the second, third, fourth, and fifth years (the authors do not accurately report the confidence intervals for the fourth and fifth years). In patients with recurrent strokes, 61% were sufficiently severe that they led to disability in activities of daily living that continued for more than 7 days while 24% led to symptoms that resolved within a week.

The investigators examined whether certain factors—sex, age, smoking, or the presence of diabetes, atrial fibrillation, cardiac failure, a transient ischemic attack, angina or myocardial infarction, intermittent claudication, or hypertension—influenced the risk of recurrent stroke. Of these factors, only smoking influenced the risk—smokers had an increased risk (OR, 1.66; 95% CI, 1.10 -2.51).

# How Can I Apply the Results to Patient Care?

## Were the Study Patients and Their Management Similar to Those in My Practice?

The authors should describe the study patients in enough detail that you can make a comparison with patients in your practice. The patients' characteristics and the way they are defined should be described explicitly. One factor rarely reported in prognostic studies that could strongly influence outcome is therapy. Therapeutic strategies often vary markedly among institutions and change over time as new treatments become available or old treatments regain popularity. To the extent that our interventions are therapeutic or detrimental, overall patient outcome could improve or become worse.

## Was Follow-up Sufficiently Long?

Since the presence of illness often precedes the development of an outcome event by a long period, investigators must follow patients for long enough to detect the outcomes of interest. For example, recurrence in some women with early breast cancer can occur many years after initial diagnosis and treatment.[11] A prognostic study may provide an unbiased assessment of outcome over a short period of time if it meets the validity criteria in Table 1D-1, but it may be of little use if a patient is interested in prognosis over a long period of time.

## Can I Use the Results in the Management of Patients in My Practice?

Prognostic data often provide the basis for sensible decisions about therapy (see Part 2B3, "Therapy and Applying the Results, Applying Results to Individual Patients"). Knowing the expected clinical course of a patient's condition can help you judge whether treatment should be offered at all. For example, warfarin markedly decreases the risk of stroke, in patients with nonrheumatic atrial fibrillation and is indicated for many patients with this disorder.[12] However, in one study, the frequency of stroke in patients with "lone" atrial fibrillation (patients 60 years of age or younger with no associated cardiopulmonary disorders) was 1.3% over a 15-year period.[13] Most patients with a prognosis this good are likely to feel that, for them, the risks of anticoagulant therapy outweigh the benefits.

Even if the prognostic result does not help with selection of appropriate therapy, it can help you in counseling a concerned patient or relative. Some conditions, such as asymptomatic hiatal hernia or asymptomatic colonic diverticulae, have such a good overall prognosis that they have been termed "nondisease."[14] On the other hand, a prognostic result of uniformly bad prognosis provides the clinician with a starting place for a discussion with the patient and family, leading to counseling about end-of-life concerns.

# CLINICAL RESOLUTION

Returning to the opening scenario, our review of the validity criteria suggests that the investigators obtained an unbiased assessment of recurrent stroke risk in their cohort study.[1] The 71-year-old patient introduced at the beginning of this section resembles the majority of those in the cohort study in terms of age and type of stroke, and we can readily generalize the results to his care. The minimum follow-up in the study was 2 years and certain patients were followed up to 6.5 years, allowing investigators to provide estimates for patients up to 5 years.

Given that he has survived the first year after his stoke, the patient's risk of dying within the next 4 years is approximately 16%, and there is another 16% risk of recurrent stroke. Given their relatively narrow confidence intervals, we can be reasonably secure using these estimates. Since aspirin administration likely reduces the risk of recurrent stroke by approximately 25%, we would need to treat 25 patients like the man under consideration for 4 years to prevent a single stroke; the number needed to treat (NNT) = 100 / (16% – 12%). Given the low toxicity of low-dose daily aspirin, we can confidently recommend that therapy to our patient.

Despite his complaints about his state of health, the patient tends to take an optimistic view of life. He is pleased to know that in 4 years his chance of being alive and no more disabled than he is at present is almost 70%. He uses this fact to help persuade his wife to maintain the dual residences, at least for the time being.

## References

1. Burn J, Dennis M, Bamford J, Sandercock P, Wade D, Warlow C. Long-term risk of recurrent stroke after a first-ever stroke: the Oxfordshire Community Project. *Stroke*. 1994;25:333-337.

2. Cook DJ, Fuller HD, Guyatt GH, et al. Risk factors for gastrointestinal bleeding in critically ill patients. *N Engl J Med*. 1994;330:377-381.

3. Ellenberg JH, Nelson KB. Sample selection and the natural history of disease: studies of febrile seizures. *JAMA*. 1980;243:1337-1340.

4. Kriel RL, Krach LE, Jones-Saete C. Outcome of children with prolonged unconsciousness and vegetative states. *Pediatr Neurol*. 1993;9:362-368.

5. Pincus T, Brooks RH, Callahan LF. Prediction of long-term mortality in patients with rheumatoid arthritis according to simple questionnaire and joint count measures. *Ann Intern Med*. 1994;120:26-34.

6. Dawber TR, Kannel WB, Lyell LP. An approach to longitudinal studies in a community: The Framingham study. *Ann NY Acad Sci*. 1963;107:539.

7. Sims AC. Importance of high tracing-rate in long-term medical follow up studies. *Lancet*. 1973;2:433.

8. Walsh JS, Welch G, Larson EB. Survival of outpatients with Alzheimer-type dementia. *Ann Intern Med*. 1990;113:429-434.

9. ISIS-2 (Second International Study of Infarct Survival) Collaborative Group. Randomised trial of intravenous streptokinase, oral aspirin, both, or neither among 17,187 cases of suspected acute myocardial infarction: ISIS-2. *Lancet*. 1988;2:349-360.

10. Dorey F, Amstutz H. The validity of survivorship analysis in total joint arthroplasty. *J Bone J Surg AM*. 1989;71A(4):544-548.

11. Early Breast Cancer Trialists' Collaborative Group. Systemic treatment of early breast cancer by hormonal, cytotoxic, or immune therapy: 133 randomised trials involving 31000 recurrences and 24000 deaths among 75000 women. *Lancet*. 1992;339:1-15.

12. Segal JB, McNamara RL, Miller MR, et al. Prevention of thromboembolism in atrial fibrillation: a meta-analysis of trials of anticoagulants and antiplatelet drugs. *J Gen Intern Med*. 2000;15:56-67.

13. Kopecky SL. The natural history of lone atrial fibrillation: a population-based study over three decades. *N Engl J Med*. 1987;317:669-674.

14. Meador CK. The art and science of nondisease. *N Engl J Med*. 1965;272:92.

# SUMMARIZING THE EVIDENCE

Andrew Oxman, Gordon Guyatt, Deborah Cook, and Victor Montori

The following EBM Working Group members also made substantive contributions to this section: Rose Hatala, Ann McKibbon, Trisha Greenhalgh, Jonathan Craig, and Roman Jaeschke

## IN THIS SECTION

## CLINICAL SCENARIO

### Should We Offer Thrombolytic Drugs to Patients Presenting With Acute Thrombotic Stroke?

**Y**ou are one of a group of neurologists working at an academic medical center. Your institution is not currently administering thrombolytic therapy to patients who present with acute thrombotic stroke. Some of your colleagues, convinced that thrombolysis will reduce ultimate mortality and morbidity in patients with acute thrombotic stroke, are enthusiastic about offering these patients tissue plasminogen activator (tPA) if they present within a few hours of symptom onset. Other members of your group are much more reluctant to initiate a policy of offering thrombolysis. You are undecided.

Your group has decided to address the issue formally. You join a subcommittee charged with collecting the evidence and generating an initial summary. The subcommittee decides to begin by looking for a systematic review.

# FINDING THE EVIDENCE

You start by looking in the Cochrane Library 2000, Issue 1. You enter the terms "stroke" and "tissue plasminogen activator," locate a relevant review in the Cochrane Database of Systematic Reviews, and find that the latest update was in July 1999.[1]

For most of their questions, clinicians can find more than one relevant study. In the same way that it is important to use rigorous methods in primary research to protect against bias and random error, it is also important to use rigorous methods when summarizing the results of several studies. Traditional literature reviews, commonly found in journals and textbooks, typically provide an overview of a disease or condition. This overview may include a discussion of one or more aspects of disease etiology, diagnosis, prognosis, or management and will address a number of clinical, background, and theoretical questions.

For example, a review article or a chapter from a textbook on asthma might include sections on etiology, diagnosis, and prognosis and examine a wide variety of options for the treatment and prevention of asthma. Typically, authors of traditional reviews make little or no attempt to be systematic in the formulation of the questions they are addressing, the search for relevant evidence, or the summary of the evidence they consider. Medical students and clinicians looking for background information nevertheless often find these reviews very useful in obtaining a broad picture of a clinical condition or area of inquiry (see Part 1A1, "Finding the Evidence").

Unfortunately, expert reviewers often make conflicting recommendations and their advice frequently lags behind or is inconsistent with the best available evidence.[2] One important reason for this phenomenon is the use of unsystematic approaches to collecting and summarizing the evidence. Indeed, in one study, self-rated expertise was inversely related to the methodologic rigor of the review.[3]

In this section of the book, we focus on reviews that address specific clinical questions (eg, foreground information). Clinicians seeking to address focused management issues in providing patient care will find such reviews particularly useful (see Part 1A1, "Finding the Evidence").

Authors sometimes use the terms overview, systematic review, and meta-analysis interchangeably. We use the term *overview* for any summary that attempts to address a focused clinical question, *systematic review* for any summary that attempts to address a focused clinical question using methods designed to reduce the likelihood of bias; and *meta-analysis* describes reviews that use quantitative methods to summarize the results. Investigators must make a host of decisions in preparing a systematic review, including determining the focus; identifying, selecting, and critically appraising the relevant studies (which we will call the *primary studies*); collecting and synthesizing (either quantitatively or nonquantitatively) the relevant information; and drawing conclusions. To avoid errors in systematic reviews requires an organized approach; enabling users to assess the validity of the results requires explicit reporting of the methods.

During the past decade, rapid expansion has occurred in the literature in terms of describing the methods used in systematic reviews, including studies that provide an empiric basis for guiding decisions about the methods used in summarizing evidence.[4-6] Here, we emphasize key points from the perspective of a clinician needing to make a decision about patient care.

In applying the Users' Guides, you will find it useful to have a clear understanding of the process of conducting a systematic review. Figure 1E-1 demonstrates how the process begins with the definition of the question, which is synonymous with specifying selection criteria for deciding which studies to include in a review. These criteria define the population, the exposures or interventions, and the outcomes of interest (see Part 1A1, "Finding the Evidence"). A systematic review will also restrict the included studies to those that meet minimal methodologic standards. For example, systematic reviews that address a question of therapy will often include only randomized controlled trials.

**FIGURE 1E-1**

## The Process of Conducting a Systematic Review

**Define the Question**

- Specify inclusion and exclusion criteria
  Population
  Intervention or exposure
  Outcome
  Methodology
- Establish a priori hypotheses to explain heterogeneity

**Conduct Literature Search**

- Decide on information sources: databases, experts, funding agencies, pharmaceutical companies, hand-searching, personal files, registries, citation lists of retrieved articles
- Determine restrictions: time frame, unpublished data, language
- Identify titles and abstracts

**Apply Inclusion and Exclusion Criteria**

- Apply inclusion and exclusion criteria to titles and abstracts
- Obtain full articles for eligible titles and abstracts
- Apply inclusion and exclusion criteria to full articles
- Select final eligible articles
- Assess agreement on study selection

**Create Data Abstraction**

- Data abstraction: participants, interventions, comparison interventions, study design
- Results
- Methodologic quality
- Assess agreement on validity assessment

**Conduct Analysis**

- Determine method for pooling of results
- Pool results (if appropriate)
- Decide on handling missing data
- Explore heterogeneity
  Sensitivity and subgroup analysis
- Explore possibility of publications bias

Having specified their selection criteria, reviewers must conduct a comprehensive search that yields a large number of potentially relevant titles and abstracts. They then apply the selection criteria to the titles and abstracts, arriving at a smaller number of articles that they can retrieve. Once again, the reviewers apply the selection criteria, this time to the complete reports. Having completed the culling process, they assess the methodologic quality of the articles and abstract data from each study. Finally, they summarize the data, including, if appropriate, a quantitative synthesis or meta-analysis. The analysis includes an examination of differences among the included studies, an attempt to explain differences in results (exploring heterogeneity), a summary of the overall results, and an assessment of their precision and validity. Guidelines for assessing the validity of reviews and using the results correspond to this process (Table 1E-1).

**TABLE 1E-1**

**Users' Guides for How to Use Review Articles**

**Are the results valid?**

- Did the review explicitly address a sensible clinical question?
- Was the search for relevant studies detailed and exhaustive?
- Were the primary studies of high methodologic quality?
- Were assessments of studies reproducible?

**What are the results?**

- Were the results similar from study to study?
- What are the overall results of the review?
- How precise were the results?

**How can I apply the results to patient care?**

- How can I best interpret the results to apply them to the care of patients in my practice?
- Were all clinically important outcomes considered?
- Are the benefits worth the costs and potential risks?

# ARE THE RESULTS VALID?

## Did the Review Explicitly Address a Sensible Clinical Question?

Consider a systematic review that pooled results from all cancer therapeutic modalities for all types of cancer to generate a single estimate of the impact on mortality. Next, consider a review that pooled results of the effects in patients suffering from clinically manifest atherosclerosis (whether in the heart, head, or lower extremities) of all doses of all antiplatelet agents (including aspirin, sulfin-pyrazone, and dipyridamole) on major thrombotic events (including myocardial infarctions, strokes, and acute arterial insufficiency in the leg) and mortality. Finally, reflect on a review that addressed the impact of a wide range of aspirin doses to prevent thrombotic stroke in patients who had experienced a transient ischemic attack (TIA) in the carotid circulation.

Clinicians would not find the first of these reviews useful; they would conclude it is too broad. Most clinicians are uncomfortable with the second question, still considering it excessively broad. For this second question, however, a highly credible and experienced group of investigators found the question reasonable and published the results of their meta-analysis in a leading journal.[7-9] Most clinicians are comfortable with the third question, although some express concerns about pooling across a wide range of aspirin doses.

What makes a systematic review too broad or too narrow? Elsewhere in this book, we have argued that identifying the population, the interventions or exposures, and the outcomes of interest is a useful way of structuring a clinical question (see Part 1A1, "Finding the Evidence"). When deciding if the question posed in the review is sensible, clinicians need to ask themselves whether the underlying biology is such that they would expect; that is, the same treatment effect across the range of patients. They should ask the parallel question about the other components of the study question. For example, is the underlying biology such that, across the range of interventions and outcomes included, they expect more or less the same treatment effect? Clinicians can also construct a similar set of questions for other areas of clinical inquiry. For example, across the range of patients, ways of testing, and criterion or gold standard for diagnosis, does one expect more or less the same likelihood ratios associated with studies examining a diagnostic test (see Part 1C2, "Diagnostic Tests")?[10]

The reason that clinicians reject a systematic review that pools across all modes of cancer therapy for all types of cancer is that they know that some cancer treatments are effective in certain cancers, whereas others are harmful. Combining the results of these studies would yield a meaningless estimate of effect that would not be applicable to any of the interventions.

Clinicians who reject the second review might also argue that the biologic variation in antiplatelet agents is likely to lead to important differences in treatment effect. Further, they may contend that there are important differences in the biology of atherosclerosis in the vessels of the heart, head, and legs. Moreover, because clinicians need to make specific decisions about specific patients, they may be inclined to seek a summary of the evidence for the intervention they are considering in patients who most resemble the patient before them.

Those who would endorse the second review would argue the similar underlying biology of antiplatelet agents—and atherosclerosis in different parts of the body—and thus anticipate a similar magnitude of treatment effects. Moreover, they would point out that the best estimate of effect for an individual patient will often come from a broader review rather than a narrower one. There are three reasons for this.

First, focusing on a narrow group of patients (eg, the most severe, or least severe), interventions (such as a single aspirin dose in our cerebrovascular disease example), or studies (eg, those only in the English language)—in each case, a subgroup of those one might have chosen—increases the risk of chance producing a spurious result.[11,12] Second, focusing on a subgroup introduces a risk of false conclusions owing to bias, if the criterion used to select the subgroup is confounded with another determinant of treatment effect. For example, a reviewer may select studies based on the type of patient even though the quality of studies of those patients is methodologically weaker than other studies, resulting in a spurious overestimate of treatment effect. Third, review of all potentially relevant data facilitates exploration of the possible explanations for variability in study results—the patients, the interventions, and the ways of measuring outcome. Thus, a broadly focused review provides a better basis for estimating the effect of a specific agent for a specific manifestation; it also provides a better basis for determining whether to believe a subgroup analysis, rather than a narrowly focused review that risks an inappropriate subgroup analysis (see Part 2E, "Summarizing the Evidence, When to Believe a Subgroup Analysis").

Turning to the third question, most clinicians would accept that the biology of aspirin action is likely to be similar in patients whose TIA reflected right-sided or left-sided brain ischemia, in patients older than 75 years and in younger patients; in men and women, across doses, over periods of follow-up ranging from 1 to 5 years, and in patients with stroke who have been identified by the attending physician and those identified by a team of expert reviewers. The similar biology is likely to result in a similar magnitude of treatment effect. Nonetheless, even within this more narrowly focused question, there is still variation in the types of patients and the types of interventions, as well as possible differences in the types of outcome measures and methods of the included studies. Thus, there will still be a need to examine possible sources of variation in the results (see Part 2E, "Summarizing the Evidence, Evaluating Differences in Study Results"). As a result, the question about whether it is sensible to pool across studies cannot, in general, be resolved until one has looked at the results. If the effect was similar across studies, the results support pooling; if not, they raise questions about any inferences one can make from the pooled results.

The task of the clinician, then, is to decide whether, across the range of patients, interventions or exposures, and outcomes, it is plausible that the intervention will have a similar impact. Doing so requires a precise statement of what range of patients, exposures, and outcomes the reviewer has decided to consider; in other words, explicit selection criteria for studies included in the review are necessary. In addition, criteria are necessary that specify what types of studies were considered relevant. Generally these should be similar to the primary validity criteria we have described for original reports of research in other parts of this book (see Table 1E-2). Explicit eligibility criteria not only facilitate the user's decision regarding whether the question was sensible, but also make it less likely that the authors will preferentially include studies that support their own prior conclusions.

**TABLE 1E-2**

## Guides for Selecting Articles That Are Most Likely to Provide Valid Results[3]

| | |
|---|---|
| **Therapy** | • Were patients randomized?<br>• Was follow-up complete? |
| **Diagnosis** | • Was the patient sample representative of those with the disorder?<br>• Was the diagnosis verified using credible criteria that were independent of the clinical manifestations under study? |
| **Harm** | • Did the investigators demonstrate similarity in all known determinants of outcome, or adjust for differences in the analysis?<br>• Was follow-up sufficiently complete? |
| **Prognosis** | • Was there a representative and well-defined sample of patients at a similar point in the course of disease?<br>• Was follow-up sufficiently complete? |

Bias in choosing articles to cite is a problem for both systematic reviews and original reports of research (in which the discussion section often includes comparisons with the results of other studies). Gøtzsche, for example, reviewed citations in reports of trials of new nonsteroidal anti-inflammatory drugs in rheumatoid arthritis.[13] Among 77 articles in which the authors could have referenced other trials with and without outcomes favoring the new drug, nearly 60% (44) cited a higher proportion of the trials with favorable outcomes. In 22 reports of controlled trials of cholesterol lowering, Ravnskov found a similar bias toward citing positive studies.[14] In 26 reports of RCTs in general medical journals, Clarke and Chalmers found only two articles in which the results were discussed in the context of an updated systematic review.[15] Users should exercise caution when interpreting the results of a study outside of the context of a systematic review.

## Was the Search for Relevant Studies Detailed and Exhaustive?

Authors of a systematic review should conduct a thorough search for studies that meet their inclusion criteria. Their search should include the use of bibliographic databases, such as MEDLINE and EMBASE, the Cochrane Controlled Trials Register (containing more than 250,000 RCTs), and databases of current research.[16] They should check the reference lists of the articles they retrieve, and they should seek personal contact with experts in the area. It may also be important to examine recently published abstracts presented at scientific meetings and to look at less frequently used databases, including those that summarize doctoral theses and databases of ongoing trials held by pharmaceutical companies. Listing these sources, it becomes evident that a MEDLINE search alone will not be satisfactory. Unless the authors tell us what they did to locate relevant studies, it is difficult to know how likely it is that relevant studies were missed.

There are two reasons that reviewers should contact experts in the area under consideration. The first is to identify published studies that may have been missed (including studies that are labeled "in press" and those that have not yet been indexed or referenced). The second is to identify unpublished studies and to include them to avoid publication bias.

*Publication bias* occurs when the publication of research depends on the direction of the study results and whether they are statistically significant. Studies in which an intervention is not found to be effective sometimes are not published. Because of this, systematic reviews that fail to include unpublished studies may overestimate the true effect of an intervention.[17-21] (See Part 2E, "Summarizing the Evidence, Publication Bias.")

If investigators include unpublished studies in a review, they should obtain full written reports and they should appraise the validity of both published and unpublished studies. Reviewers may also use statistical techniques to explore the possibility of publication bias and other reporting biases, although the power of these techniques to detect bias is limited.[22] Systematic reviews based on a small number of studies with small sample sizes are the most susceptible to *publication bias,* and users should be cautious about drawing conclusions in such cases. Results that seem too good to be true may well not be true.

Reviewers may go even farther than simply contacting the authors of primary studies. They may recruit these investigators as collaborators in their review, and in the process they may obtain individual patient records. Access to individual patient records facilitates powerful analysis and strengthens the inferences from a systematic review.

## Were the Primary Studies of High Methodologic Quality?

Even if a review article includes only RCTs, knowing whether they were of good quality is important. Unfortunately, peer review does not guarantee the validity of published research (see Part 1B1, "Therapy").[23] For exactly the same reason that the guides for using original reports of research begin by asking if the results are valid, it is essential to consider the validity of primary articles in systematic reviews.

Differences in study methods might explain important differences among the results.[24-26] For example, less rigorous studies tend to overestimate the effectiveness of therapeutic and preventive interventions.[27] Even if the results of different studies are consistent, determining their validity still is important. Consistent results are less compelling if they come from weak studies than if they come from strong studies.

Consistent results from observational studies are particularly suspect. Physicians may systematically select patients with a good prognosis to receive therapy, and this pattern of practice may be consistent over time and geographic setting. Observational studies summarized in a systematic review,[28] for instance, have consistently shown average relative risk reductions in major cardiovascular events of about 50% with hormone replacement therapy. The only large RCT addressing this issue found no effect of hormone replacement therapy on cardiovascular risk.[29]

There is no one correct way to assess the quality of studies, although in the context of a systematic review the focus should be on validity and users should be cautious about the use of scales to assess the quality of studies.[30, 31] Some investigators use long checklists to evaluate methodologic quality, whereas others focus on three or four key aspects of the study. When considering whether to trust the results of a review, check to see whether the authors examined criteria similar to those we have presented in other sections of this book (see Part 1B1, "Therapy"; Part 1C, "The Process of Diagnosis"; Part 1B2, "Harm"; and Part 1D, "Prognosis"). Reviewers should apply these criteria both in selecting studies for inclusion and in assessing the validity of the included studies (see Figure 1E-1 and Table 1E-2).

## Were Assessments of Studies Reproducible?

As we have seen, authors of systematic review articles must decide which studies to include, how valid they are, and what data to extract. These decisions require judgment by the reviewers and are subject to both mistakes (ie, random errors) and bias (ie, systematic errors). Having two or more people participate in each decision guards against errors; if there is good agreement beyond chance between the reviewers, the clinician can have more confidence in the results of the systematic review (see Part 2C, "Diagnosis, Measuring Agreement Beyond Chance").

### USING THE GUIDE

Returning to our opening scenario, the Cochrane review you located included trials enrolling patients with acute ischemic stroke in whom CT excluded hemorrhage.[1] These patients were randomized to receive or not receive thrombolytic therapy, and an intention-to-treat analysis had been or could be conducted (see Part 2B1, "Therapy and Validity, The Principle of Intention-to-Treat"). (An intention-to-treat analysis examines outcomes for study participants based on the treatment arm to which they were originally randomized rather than the treatment they actually received.) You are concerned that the impact of treatment might differ substantially in patients who present early or late, in those with major or minor deficits, in those who received different thrombolytic agents, and in studies with different ways of measuring functional status or different durations of follow-up. Nevertheless, you are uncertain about the extent to which these variables might affect outcome, and you suspect that combining results across all patients, interventions, and outcomes might prove informative.

The reviewers searched the Cochrane Registry of Controlled Trials and EMBASE. In addition, they hand-searched a number of Japanese-language journals; contacted 321 pharmaceutical companies; contacted principal investigators in Europe, the United States, Japan, and China; attended a number of international stroke treatment symposia; and searched references quoted in the articles they found. It is likely they obtained all the relevant trials.

Of the 17 trials included, seven used centralized randomization of patients to treatment or control groups to ensure concealment. In 13 studies, participants and health care personnel were then blinded to allocation by using sealed, prepacked, and identical-looking thrombolytic and placebo infusions. Because of bleeding complications of thrombolytic therapy, blinding of participants and health care personnel may be difficult to ensure, underscoring the importance of blinding the outcome assessors; long-term outcome assessors were blinded to allocation in only four of the studies. The reviewers do not report on the proportion of patients lost to follow-up in any trial.

One of the review's authors decided whether potentially eligible trials met inclusion criteria. A different author extracted the data but then verified them with the principal investigators and corrected any errors. In 10 trials, the authors of the systematic review were able to obtain scores on a measure of functional status, the Rankin instrument, on individual patients. Scores of up to two out of five on this functional status measurement instrument indicate that patients are still able to look after themselves,[32] so the investigators classified scores of three to five on this instrument as characterizing a poor outcome. In another two trials for which they could not obtain individual data, scores of two or greater represented a poor outcome.

Overall, the methods of the systematic review—and the methodologic quality of the trials included in the systematic review—were strong.

# WHAT ARE THE RESULTS?

## Were the Results Similar From Study to Study?

Most systematic reviews document important differences in patients, exposures, outcome measures, and research methods from study to study. As a result, the most common answer to the initial question about whether we can expect similar results across the range of patients, interventions, and outcomes is "perhaps."

Fortunately, one can resolve this unsatisfactory situation. Having completed the review, investigators should present the results in a way that allows clinicians to check the validity of the initial assumption. That is, did results prove similar from study to study?

There are two things to consider when deciding whether the results are sufficiently similar to warrant making a single estimate of treatment effects that applies across the populations, interventions, and outcomes studied (see Part 2E, "Summarizing the Evidence, Evaluating Differences in Study Results"). First, how similar are the best estimates of the treatment effect (that is, the *point estimates*) from the individual studies? The more different they are, the more clinicians should question the decision to pool results across studies.

Second, to what extent are differences among the results of individual studies greater than you would expect by chance? Users can make an initial assessment by examining the extent to which the confidence intervals overlap. The greater the overlap, the more comfortable one is with pooling results. Widely separated confidence intervals flag the presence of important variability in results that requires explanation (see Part 2E, "Summarizing the Evidence, Evaluating Differences in Study Results").

Clinicians can also look to formal statistical analyses called tests of heterogeneity, which assess the degree of difference or variance among samples, groups, or populations. When the $P$ value associated with the test of heterogeneity is small (eg, < .05), chance becomes an unlikely explanation for the observed differences in the size of the effect (see Part 2B2, "Therapy, Hypothesis Testing"). Unfortunately, a higher $P$ value (.1, or even .3) does not necessarily rule out important heterogeneity. The reason is that, when the number of studies and their sample sizes are both small, the test of heterogeneity is not very powerful. Hence, large differences between the apparent magnitude of the treatment effect between studies—that is, the point estimates—dictates caution in interpreting the overall findings, even in the face of a nonsignificant test of homogeneity. Conversely, if the differences in results across studies are not clinically important, then heterogeneity is of little concern, even if it is statistically significant (see Part 2E, "Summarizing the Evidence, Evaluating Differences in Study Results").

Reviewers should try to explain between-study variability in findings. Possible explanations include differences between patients (eg, thrombolytic therapy in acute myocardial infarction may be much more effective in patients who present shortly after the onset of chest pain than those who present much later), between interventions (eg, tPA may have a larger treatment effect than streptokinase), between outcome measurement (eg, the effect may differ if the outcome is measured at 30 days rather than at 1 year after myocardial infarction), or methodology (eg, the effect may be smaller in blinded trials or in those with more complete follow-up). Although appropriate and, indeed, necessary, this search for explanations of heterogeneity in study results may be misleading (see Part 2E, "Summarizing the Evidence, When to Believe a Subgroup Analysis"). Furthermore, how is the clinician to deal with residual heterogeneity in study results that remains unexplained? We will deal with this issue in our discussion of the applicability of the study results.

## What Are the Overall Results of the Review?

In clinical research, investigators collect data from individual patients. Because of the limited capacity of the human mind to handle large amounts of data, investigators use statistical methods to summarize and analyze them. In systematic reviews, investigators collect data from individual studies. Investigators must also summarize these data and, increasingly, they are relying on quantitative methods to do so.

Simply comparing the number of positive studies to the number of negative studies is not an adequate way to summarize the results. With this sort of "vote counting," large and small studies are given equal weight, and (unlikely as it may seem) one investigator may interpret a study as positive, whereas another investigator may interpret the same study as negative.[33] For example, a clinically important effect that is not statistically significant could be interpreted as positive in light of clinical importance and negative in light of statistical significance. There is a tendency to overlook small but important effects if studies with statistically nonsignificant (but potentially clinically important) results are counted as negative.[34] Moreover, a reader cannot tell anything about the magnitude of an effect from a vote count even when studies are appropriately classified using additional categories for studies with a positive or negative trend.

Typically, meta-analysts weight studies according to their size, with larger studies receiving more weight. Thus, the overall results represent a weighted average of the results of the individual studies (see Part 2E, "Summarizing the Evidence, Fixed-Effects and Random-Effects Models"). Occasionally studies are also given more or less weight depending on their quality, or poorer-quality studies might be given a weight of zero (excluded) either in the primary analysis or in a secondary analysis that tests the extent to which different assumptions lead to different results (a sensitivity analysis).

You should look to the overall results of a systematic review the same way you look to the results of primary studies. In a systematic review of a therapeutic question, you should look for the relative risk and relative risk reduction or the odds ratio (see Part 2B2, "Therapy and Understanding the Results, Measures of Association"). In systematic reviews regarding diagnosis, you should look for summary estimates of the likelihood ratios (see Part 1C2, "Diagnostic Tests").

Sometimes the outcome measures that investigators have used in different studies are similar but not identical. For example, different trials might measure functional status using different instruments. If the patients and the interventions are reasonably similar, estimating the average effect of the intervention on functional status still might be worthwhile. One way of doing this is to summarize the results of each study as an effect size.[35] The *effect size* is the difference in outcomes between the intervention and control groups divided by the standard deviation. The effect size summarizes the results of each study in terms of the number of standard deviations of difference between the intervention and control groups. Investigators can then calculate a weighted average of effect sizes from studies that measured a given outcome in different ways.

You may find it difficult to interpret the clinical importance of an effect size. For example, if the weighted average effect is one half of a standard deviation, is this effect clinically trivial or is it large? Once again, you should look for a presentation of the results that conveys their practical importance (eg, by translating the summary effect size back into natural units[36]). For instance, clinicians may have become familiar with the significance of differences in walk test scores in patients with chronic lung disease. Investigators can then convert the effect size of a treatment on a number of measures of functional status (eg, the walk test and stair climbing) back into differences in walk test scores.[37]

Although it is generally desirable to have a quantitative summary of the results of a review, it is not always appropriate. When quantitative summaries are inappropriate, investigators should still present tables or graphs that summarize the results of the primary studies.

## How Precise Were the Results?

In the same way that it is possible to estimate the average effect across studies, it is possible to estimate a confidence interval around that estimate, that is, a range of values with a specified probability (typically 95%) of including the true effect (see Part 2B2, "Therapy and Understanding the Results, Confidence Intervals").

## USING THE GUIDE

**R**eturning to our opening scenario, four trials used streptokinase, three trials used urokinase, two used Pro-Urokinase, and eight used tPA. Data from six trials for death during the first 7 to 10 days showed that 16.6% of those receiving thrombolytic agents and 9.8% of the control patients died (OR, 1.85; 95% CI, 1.48-2.32). The $P$ value for the test of heterogeneity showed borderline significance with the value for the tPA trials being lower and non-significant (OR, 1.24; 95% CI, 0.85-1.81). Considering data from 11 trials, investigators found that thrombolytic therapy increased fatal intracranial hemorrhage from 1.0% to 5.4% (OR, 4.15; 95% CI, 2.96-5.84), and the results were consistent across studies.

The final assessment of outcome (at 1 month in six trials, 3 months in nine trials, and 6 months in two trials) showed an increase in deaths from 15.9% to 19% (OR, 1.31; 95% CI, 1.13- 1.52). The results showed considerable heterogeneity ($P < .01$).

Thrombolysis reduced the combined endpoint of death and dependency (55.2% in patients receiving thrombolysis and 59.7% in those allocated to the control group (OR, 0.83; 95% CI, 0.73-0.94). The results were consistent across the trials.

The authors explored possible sources of heterogeneity for differences in death rate. Despite large differences in point estimates (urokinase OR, 0.71; streptokinase OR, 1.43; tPA OR, 1.16), differences among drugs failed to reach statistical significance. Death rate was increased when streptokinase and aspirin were given together in comparison to streptokinase alone. The authors failed to find a relationship between control event rate and mortality, though they note that individual data would be required to properly explore the relationship between stroke severity and thrombolytic benefit and harm. Trials in which some patients were randomized within 3 hours and some were randomized after 3 hours showed no difference in deaths between the two groups.

# HOW CAN I APPLY THE RESULTS TO PATIENT CARE?

## How Can I Best Interpret the Results to Apply Them to the Care of Patients in My Practice?

Even if the true underlying effect is identical in each of a set of studies, chance will ensure that the observed results differ (see Part 2B, "Therapy and Harm, Why Study Results Mislead: Bias and Random Error"). As a result, systematic reviews risk capitalizing on the play of chance. Perhaps the studies with older patients happened, by chance, to be those with the smaller treatment effects. The reviewer may erroneously conclude that the treatment is less effective in elderly patients. The more subgroup analyses the reviewer undertakes, the greater is the risk of a spurious conclusion.

The clinician can apply a number of criteria to distinguish subgroup analyses that are credible from those that are not (see Part 2E, "Summarizing the Evidence, When to Believe a Subgroup Analysis"). Criteria that make a hypothesized difference in subgroups more credible include the following: conclusions drawn on the basis of within-study rather than between-study comparisons; a large difference in treatment effect across subgroups; a highly statistically significant difference in treatment effect (eg, the lower the $P$ value on the comparison of the different effect sizes in the subgroups, the more credible the difference); a hypothesis that was made before the study began and that was one of only a few that were tested; consistency across studies; and indirect evidence in support of the difference (eg, "biologic plausibility"). If these criteria are not met, the results of a subgroup analysis are less likely to be trustworthy and you should assume that the overall effect across all patients and all treatments, rather than the subgroup effect, applies to the patient at hand and to the treatment under consideration.

What are clinicians to do if subgroup analyses fail to provide an adequate explanation for unexplained heterogeneity in study results? Although a number of reasonable possibilities exist, including not to pool findings at all, we suggest that, pending further trials that may explain the differences, clinicians should look to a summary measure from all of the best available studies for the best estimate of the impact of the intervention or exposure.[38-40]

## Were All Clinically Important Outcomes Considered?

Although it is a good idea to look for focused review articles because they are more likely to provide valid results, this does not mean that you should ignore outcomes that are not included in a review. For example, the potential benefits of hormone replacement therapy include a reduced risk of fractures and a reduced risk of coronary heart disease, and potential downsides include an increased risk of breast cancer and endometrial cancer. Focused reviews of the evidence are more likely to provide valid results of the impact of hormone replacement therapy on each one of these four outcomes, but a clinical decision requires considering all of them.

Systematic reviews frequently do not report the adverse effects of therapy. One reason is that the individual studies often measure these adverse effects either in different ways or not at all, making pooling, or even effective summarization, difficult. Costs are an additional outcome that you will often find absent from systematic reviews.

### Are the Benefits Worth the Costs and Potential Risks?

Finally, either explicitly or implicitly, the clinician and patient must weigh the expected benefits against the costs and potential risks (see Part 1F, "Moving From Evidence to Action"). Although this is most obvious for deciding whether to use a therapeutic intervention or a preventive one, providing patients with information about causes of disease or prognosis also can have both benefits and risks. For example, informing city dwellers about the health risks of air pollution exposures might result in their reducing their risk of exposure, with potential benefits; however, it might also cause anxiety or make their lives less convenient. Informing an asymptomatic woman with newly detected cancer about her prognosis might help her to plan better, but it might also label her, cause anxiety, or increase the period during which she is "sick."

A valid review article provides the best possible basis for quantifying the expected outcomes, but these outcomes still must be considered in the context of your patient's values and concerns about the expected outcomes of a decision. Ultimately, trading off benefits and risks will involve value judgments (see Part 1F, "Moving From Evidence to Action"), and in individual decision making, these values should come from the patient (see Part 2F, "Moving From Evidence to Action, Incorporating Patient Values").

# CLINICAL RESOLUTION

Returning to the opening scenario, the committee decides it can confidently reach two conclusions on the basis of the systematic review. First, thrombolytic therapy increases the odds of intracranial hemorrhage by a factor of between approximately 3 and 6, with the best estimate being approximately 4. In absolute terms, thrombolytic therapy will cause one intracranial hemorrhage for every 23 patients who are treated. Second, thrombolytic therapy reduces the odds of the combined outcome of death and dependency after approximately 3 months by approximately 5% to 30%, the best estimate being an OR of 0.83 (17%). In absolute terms, 22 patients need to be treated to prevent one patient from dying or becoming seriously dependent after 3 months. A third conclusion also seems likely: the concomitant administration of aspirin increases the risk of intracranial hemorrhage.

The committee concludes that many areas of uncertainty remain. They include questions about whether the risk of death during the 3-month period after stroke is lower for tPA than the combined estimate suggests, as well as the relative effect on both hemorrhage and death and disability, according to the severity and nature of symptoms at initial presentation. Given the extent and nature of the uncertainties, the committee agrees that administration of thrombolytic therapy should be restricted to highly selected patients who are ready to risk an increase in the likelihood of early death to achieve a subsequent reduction in morbidity.

# References

1. Wardlaw JM, del Zoppo G, Yamaguchi T. Thrombolysis for acute ischaemic stroke. *Cochrane Database Syst Rev.* 2000;2:CD000213.

2. Antman EM, Lau J, Kupelnick B, Mosteller F, Chalmers TC. A comparison of results of meta-analyses of randomized control trials and recommendations of clinical experts: treatments for myocardial infarction. *JAMA.* 1992;268:240-248.

3. Oxman AD, Guyatt GH. The science of reviewing research. *Ann N Y Acad Sci.* 1993;703:125-133; discussion 133-134.

4. Clarke M, Olsen KL, Oxman AD, eds. The Cochrane Review Methodology Database. In: *The Cochrane Library.* Oxford: Update Software; 2000, issue 1.

5. Clarke M, Oxman AD, eds. Cochrane Reviewers' Handbook 4.0 [updated July 1999]. In: *The Cochrane Library.* Oxford: Update Software; 2000, issue 1.

6. Egger M, Davey Smith G, Altman DG, eds. *Systematic Reviews in Health Care: Meta-Analysis in Context.* 2nd ed. London: BMJ Books; 2000.

7. Antiplatelet Trialists' Collaboration. Collaborative overview of randomised trials of antiplatelet therapy, I: prevention of death, myocardial infarction, and stroke by prolonged antiplatelet therapy in various categories of patients. *BMJ.* 1994;308:81-106.

8. Antiplatelet Trialists' Collaboration. Collaborative overview of randomised trials of antiplatelet therapy, II: maintenance of vascular graft or arterial patency by antiplatelet therapy. *BMJ.* 1994;308:159-168.

9. Antiplatelet Trialists' Collaboration. Collaborative overview of randomised trials of antiplatelet therapy, III: reduction in venous thrombosis and pulmonary embolism by antiplatelet prophylaxis among surgical and medical patients. *BMJ.* 1994;308:235-246.

10. Irwig L, Tosteson AN, Gatsonis C, et al. Guidelines for meta-analyses evaluating diagnostic tests. *Ann Intern Med.* 1994;120:667-676.

11. Counsell CE, Clarke MJ, Slattery J, Sandercock PA. The miracle of DICE therapy for acute stroke: fact or fictional product of subgroup analysis? *BMJ.* 1994;309:1677-1681.

12. Clarke MJ, Halsey J. D.I.C.E. 3: the need for cautious interpretation of meta-analyses. Paper presented at: First Symposium on Systematic Reviews: Beyond the Basics; January 1998; Oxford.

13. Gøtzsche PC. Reference bias in reports of drug trials. *Br Med J (Clin Res Ed)*. 1987;295:654-656.

14. Ravnskov U. Cholesterol lowering trials in coronary heart disease: frequency of citation and outcome. *BMJ*. 1992;305:15-19.

15. Clarke M, Chalmers I. Discussion sections in reports of controlled trials published in general medical journals: islands in search of continents? *JAMA*. 1998;280:280-282.

16. The *meta*Register of Controlled Trials (*m*RCT). Current Controlled Trials. Available at: *www.controlled-trials.com/*. Accessed January 31, 2001.

17. Dickersin K. The existence of publication bias and risk factors for its occurrence. *JAMA*. 1990;263:1385-1389.

18. Dickersin K, Min Y, Meinert CL. Factors influencing publication of research results. *JAMA*. 1992;267:374-378.

19. Dickersin K. How important is publication bias? A synthesis of available data. *AIDS Educ Prev*. 1997;9(suppl 1):15-21.

20. Stern JM, Simes RJ. Publication bias: evidence of delayed publication in a cohort study of clinical research projects. *BMJ*. 1997;315:640-645.

21. Ioannidis JP. Effect of the statistical significance of results on the time to completion and publication of randomized efficacy trials. *JAMA*. 1998;279:281-286.

22. Egger M, Davey Smith G, Schneider M, Minder C. Bias in meta-analysis detected by a simple, graphical test. *BMJ*. 1997;315:629-634.

23. Williamson JW, Goldschmidt PG, Colton T. The quality of medical literature: analysis of validation assessments. In: Bailar JC, Mosteller F, eds. *Medical Uses of Statistics*. 2nd ed. Waltham: NEJM Books; 1992:370-391.

24. Horwitz RI. Complexity and contradiction in clinical trial research. *Am J Med*. 1987;82:498-510.

25. Detsky AS, Naylor CD, O'Rourke K, McGeer AJ, L'Abbe KA. Incorporating variations in the quality of individual randomized trials into meta-analysis. *J Clin Epidemiol*. 1992;45:255-265.

26. Moher D, Pham B, Jones A, et al. Does quality of reports of randomised trials affect estimates of intervention efficacy reported in meta-analyses? *Lancet*. 1998;352:609-613.

27. Kunz R, Oxman AD. The unpredictability paradox: review of empirical comparisons of randomised and non-randomised clinical trials. *BMJ*. 1998;317:1185-1190.

28. Stampfer MJ, Colditz GA. Estrogen replacement therapy and coronary heart disease: a quantitative assessment of the epidemiologic evidence. *Prev Med*. 1991;20:47-63.

29. Hulley S, Grady D, Bush T, et al. Randomized trial of estrogen plus progestin for secondary prevention of coronary heart disease in postmenopausal women. Heart and Estrogen/progestin Replacement Study (HERS) Research Group. *JAMA*. 1998;280:605-613.

30. Moher D, Jadad AR, Nichol G, Penman M, Tugwell P, Walsh S. Assessing the quality of randomized controlled trials: an annotated bibliography of scales and checklists. *Control Clin Trials*. 1995;16:62-73.

31. Juni P, Witschi A, Bloch R, Egger M. The hazards of scoring the quality of clinical trials for meta-analysis. *JAMA*. 1999;282:1054-1060.

32. de Haan R, Limburg M, Bossuyt P, van der Meulen J, Aaronson N. The clinical meaning of Rankin 'handicap' grades after stroke. *Stroke*. 1995;26:2027-2030.

33. Glass GV, McGaw B, Smith ML. *Meta-analysis in Social Research*. Beverly Hills: Sage Publications; 1981:18-20.

34. Cooper HM, Rosenthal R. Statistical versus traditional procedures for summarizing research findings. *Psychol Bull*. 1980;87:442-449.

35. Rosenthal R. *Meta-analytic Procedures for Social Research*. 2nd ed. Newbury Park: Sage Publications; 1991.

36. Smith K, Cook D, Guyatt GH, Madhavan J, Oxman AD. Respiratory muscle training in chronic airflow limitation: a meta-analysis. *Am Rev Respir Dis*. 1992;145:533-539.

37. Lacasse Y, Wong E, Guyatt GH, King D, Cook DJ, Goldstein RS. Meta-analysis of respiratory rehabilitation in chronic obstructive pulmonary disease. *Lancet*. 1996;348:1115-1119.

38. Peto R. Why do we need systematic overviews of randomized trials? *Stat Med*. 1987;6:233-244.

39. Oxman AD, Guyatt GH. A consumer's guide to subgroup analyses. *Ann Intern Med*. 1992;116:78-84.

40. Yusuf S, Wittes J, Probstfield J, Tyroler HA. Analysis and interpretation of treatment effects in subgroups of patients in randomized clinical trials. *JAMA*. 1991;266:93-98.

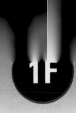

# MOVING FROM EVIDENCE TO ACTION

Gordon Guyatt, Robert Hayward, W. Scott Richardson,
Lee Green, Mark Wilson, Jack Sinclair, Deborah Cook,
Paul Glasziou, Alan Detsky, and Eric Bass

PJ Devereaux also made substantive contributions to this section

## IN THIS SECTION

# CLINICAL SCENARIO

## Warfarin in Atrial Fibrillation:
## Is It the Best Choice for This Patient?

**Y**ou are a primary care practitioner considering the possibility of warfarin therapy in a 76-year-old woman with congestive heart failure and chronic atrial fibrillation who has just entered your practice. Aspirin is the only antithrombotic agent that the patient has received during the 10 years she has had atrial fibrillation. Her other medical problems include stage I hypertension, which she has had since sometime in her fifth decade, and for which she has been taking hydrochlorothiazide and benazepril. Her previous physicians' records suggest that in recent years her systolic blood pressure was 130 to 140 mm Hg and her diastolic pressure was 80 to 90 mm Hg. Current blood pressure is 136/84 mm Hg, with a heart rate of 76 beats per minute, suggesting effective rate control. The patient does not have valvular disease, diabetes, or other comorbidity, and she does not smoke.

The duration of the patient's atrial fibrillation dissuades you from considering cardioversion or antiarrhythmic therapy. The patient lives alone. Although she has never had a significant fall, you are concerned that warfarin would present a risk of intracranial hemorrhage that may prove to be greater than its benefit in terms of stroke prevention. You find she places a high value on avoiding a stroke and a somewhat lower value on avoiding a major bleeding episode. Although she is not fond of medical care, she would accept the inconvenience associated with monitoring anticoagulant therapy.

The question of whether and when to offer anticoagulant therapy to patients with nonvalvular atrial fibrillation arises often in your practice, but there is little agreement on the topic among you and your partners. You are all convinced that warfarin anticoagulant therapy for nonvalvular atrial fibrillation prevents strokes, but some believe that it causes too many bleeding complications. Several patients in the practice with atrial fibrillation have suffered embolic strokes despite aspirin therapy, but two patients suffered serious gastrointestinal bleeding while taking warfarin. Things became even more confusing recently when one of your colleagues, known as a maverick, declared that clopidogrel is the correct agent to use for patients with nonvalvular atrial fibrillation.

You make no change to the patient's medication regimen today, but you make a note to yourself to reconsider when she returns and to raise the issue at a staff meeting next week.

# FINDING THE EVIDENCE

You have little inclination to review the voluminous original literature relating to the benefits of anticoagulant therapy in reducing stroke or its risk of bleeding, but you hope to find an evidence-based recommendation to guide you and your colleagues. You decide to search for two sources of such a recommendation: a practice guideline and a decision analysis.

You bring up your Web browser and go to your favorite search engine, Google.com. Entering the term "practice guidelines," you see that the second item on the results list is "National Guidelines Clearinghouse," at www.guidelines.gov. This looks promising, as you note that the server appears to reside at the US Agency for Healthcare Research and Quality (AHRQ), formerly known as the Agency for Health Care Policy and Research (AHCPR), which you recall created a series of guidelines using formal evidence-based guidelines methodology.[1]

After linking to the clearinghouse, you see a heading labeled "Guidelines Syntheses." The syntheses area is described as containing

" . . . syntheses of selected guidelines that cover similar topic areas.
Key elements of each synthesis include the scope of the guidelines,
the interventions and practices considered, the major recommendations
and the corresponding rating schemes and strength of the evidence,
the areas of agreement, and the areas of disagreement."

This description seems a close fit for the criteria you have for evidence-based guidelines, but unfortunately, atrial fibrillation is not listed among the syntheses completed thus far. Returning to the main page, you enter the term "atrial fibrillation" in the search box, which yields 22 guidelines. The first one on the list seems promising: "Fifth ACCP Consensus Conference on Antithrombotic Therapy," from the American College of Chest Physicians, completed in 1998. The guideline is summarized on the Clearinghouse site and has been published in the peer-reviewed literature.[2] You click on "Complete summary" and then print the text that appears. You also send an e-mail message to the hospital librarian asking for a copy of the published article. You look forward with some trepidation to reading the material, as you are aware that many guidelines, even from sources presumably as authoritative as specialty societies, are poorly constructed.[3,4]

Before you leave Google.com you enter the phrase "atrial fibrillation decision analysis" in the search text box and the results include the following link:

www.thelancet.com/newlancet/sub/issues/vol355no9208/body.article956.html.

The article is a recent decision analysis published in *The Lancet* that appears highly suitable.[5]

# TREATMENT RECOMMENDATIONS

Each day, clinicians make dozens of patient management decisions. Some are relatively inconsequential, whereas others are important. Each one involves weighing benefits and risks, gains and losses, and recommending or instituting a course of action judged to be in the patient's best interest. Implicit in each decision is a consideration of the relevant evidence, an intuitive integration of that evidence, and a weighing of the likely benefits and risks in light of the patient's preferences. When making choices, clinicians may benefit from structured summaries of the options and outcomes, systematic reviews of the evidence regarding the relationship between options and outcomes, and recommendations regarding the best choices. This section of the book explores the process of developing recommendations, suggests how the process may be conducted systematically, and introduces a taxonomy for differentiating recommendations that are more rigorous (and, thus, are more likely to be trustworthy) from those that are less rigorous (and, thus, are at greater risk of being misleading).

Traditionally, authors of original, or primary, research into therapeutic interventions include recommendations about the use of these interventions in clinical practice in the discussion section of their papers. Authors of systematic reviews and meta-analyses also tend to provide their impressions of the management implications of their studies. Typically, however, authors of individual trials or overviews do not consider all possible management options, but instead focus on a comparison of two or three alternatives. They may also fail to identify subpopulations in which the impact of treatment may vary considerably. Finally, when the authors of systematic reviews provide recommendations, they typically are not grounded in an explicit presentation of societal or patient preferences.

Failure to consider these issues may lead to variability in recommendations given the same data. For example, various recommendations emerged from different meta-analyses of selective decontamination of the gut using antibiotic prophylaxis for pneumonia in critically ill patients despite very similar results. The recommendations varied from suggesting implementation, to equivocation, to rejecting implementation.[6-9] Varying recommendations reflect the fact that investigators reporting primary studies and meta-analyses often make their recommendations without benefit of an explicit standardized process or set of rules.

When benefits or risks are dramatic and are essentially homogeneous across an entire population, intuition may provide an adequate guide to making treatment recommendations. However, such situations are unusual. In most instances, because of their susceptibility to both bias and random error, intuitive recommendations risk misleading the clinician and the patient.

These considerations suggest that when clinicians examine treatment recommendations, they should critically evaluate the methodologic quality of the recommendations. Our goal in this section is to provide clinicians with the tools to conduct such a critical evaluation.

Although recommendations that impact on health resource allocation may be directed at health policymakers, our focus in this book is to dispense advice for practicing clinicians. We will begin by describing the process of developing a recommendation, and we will introduce two formal processes that clinical investigators, experts, and authoritative bodies use in developing recommendations: decision analysis and clinical practice guidelines. We will then offer criteria for deciding when the process is done well and when it is done poorly, along with a hierarchy of treatment recommendations that clinicians may find useful.

# DEVELOPING RECOMMENDATIONS

Figure 1F-1 presents the steps involved in developing a recommendation, along with the formal strategies for doing so. The first step in clinical decision making is to define the decision. This involves specifying the alternative courses of action and the possible outcomes. Often, treatments are designed to delay or prevent an adverse outcome such as stroke, death, or myocardial infarction. As usual, we will refer to the outcomes that treatment is designed to prevent as *target outcomes*. Treatments are associated with their own adverse outcomes—side effects, toxicity, and inconvenience. In addition, new treatments may markedly increase—or decrease—costs. Ideally, the definition of the decision will be comprehensive—all reasonable alternatives will be considered and all possible beneficial and adverse outcomes will be identified. In patients like the woman described in the opening scenario with nonvalvular atrial fibrillation, options include not treating the condition, giving aspirin, or administering anticoagulant therapy with warfarin. Outcomes include minor and major embolic stroke, intracranial hemorrhage, gastrointestinal hemorrhage, minor bleeding, the inconvenience associated with taking and monitoring medication, and costs to the patient, the health care system, and society.

**FIGURE 1F-1**

## A Schematic View of the Process of Developing a Treatment Recommendation

| Task | Method for Achieving Task |
|---|---|
| Specify options and outcomes | Explicit decision framing |
| ↓ | |
| Use evidence to determine the link between options and outcomes in all relevant patient subgroups | Randomized controlled trials and other evidence ⟶ Systematic review |
| ↓ | |
| Incorporate values to decide on optimal course of action | Values ⟶ Decision analysis or practice guideline |
| ↓ | |
| If necessary, consider local circumstances and modify course of action | Local circumstances ⟶ Local guidelines |
| | Assess local burdens, local barriers, and local resources |

Having identified the options and outcomes, decision makers must evaluate the links between the two. What will the alternative management strategies yield in terms of benefit and harm?[10, 11] How are potential benefits and risks likely to vary in different groups of patients?[11, 12] Once these questions are answered, making treatment recommendations involves value judgments about the relative desirability or undesirability of possible outcomes. We will use the term *preferences* synonymously with *values* or *value judgments* in referring to the process of trading off positive and negative consequences of alternative management strategies.

Recently, investigators have applied scientific principles to the identification, selection, and summarization of evidence—and to the valuing of outcomes. We will briefly review the systematic approach to the identification, selection, and summarization of evidence that we have presented in Part 1E, "Summarizing the Evidence," and will then describe the two strategies used to move from evidence to action—that is, decision analysis and practice guidelines.

## Systematic Reviews

Unsystematic approaches to identification and collection of evidence risk biased ascertainment. That is, treatment effects may be underestimated or, more commonly, overestimated, and side effects may be exaggerated or ignored. Even if the evidence has been identified and collected in a systematic fashion, if reviewers are then unsystematic in the way they summarize the collected evidence, they run similar risks of bias. One result of these unsystematic approaches may be recommendations advocating harmful treatment; in other cases, there may be a failure to encourage effective therapy. For example, experts advocated routine use of lidocaine for patients with acute myocardial infarction when available data suggested the intervention was ineffective and possibly even harmful, and they failed to recommend thrombolytic agents when data showed patient benefit.[13]

*Systematic reviews* deal with this problem by explicitly stating inclusion and exclusion criteria for evidence to be considered, conducting a comprehensive search for the evidence, and summarizing the results according to explicit rules that include examining how effects may vary in different patient subgroups (see Part 1E, "Summarizing the Evidence"). When a systematic review pools data across studies to provide a quantitative estimate of overall treatment effect, we call it a *meta-analysis*. Systematic reviews provide strong evidence when the quality of the primary study design is good and sample sizes are large; they provide weaker evidence when study designs are poor and sample sizes are small. Because judgment is involved in many steps in a systematic review (including specifying inclusion and exclusion criteria, applying these criteria to potentially eligible studies, evaluating the methodologic quality of the primary studies, and selecting an approach to data analysis), systematic reviews are not immune from bias. Nevertheless, in their rigorous approach to identifying and summarizing data, systematic reviews reduce the likelihood of bias in estimating the causal links between management options and patient outcomes.

## Decision Analysis

Rigorous *decision analysis* provides a formal structure for integrating the evidence about the beneficial and harmful effects of treatment options with the values or preferences associated with those beneficial and harmful effects. Decision analysis applies explicit, quantitative methods to analyzing decisions under conditions of uncertainty; it allows clinicians to compare the expected consequences of pursuing different strategies. The process of decision analysis makes fully explicit all of the elements of the decision, so that they are open for debate and modification.[14-16]

We will use the term *clinical decision analyses* to include studies that use formal, mathematical approaches to analyze decisions faced by clinicians in the course of patient care, such as deciding whether to screen for a condition, choosing a testing strategy, or selecting a type of treatment. Although such analyses can be undertaken to inform a decision for an individual patient ("Should I recommend warfarin to this 76-year-old woman with atrial fibrillation?"), they are undertaken more widely to help inform a decision about clinical policy[17] ("Should I routinely recommend warfarin to patients in my practice with atrial fibrillation?"). The study retrieved by the search in our scenario is an example of the latter, whereas an example of a decision analysis for an individual patient is an analysis of whether to recommend cardiac surgery for an elderly woman with aortic stenosis.[18]

Decision analysis can also be applied to more global questions of health care policy that are viewed from the perspective of society or a national health authority. Examples include analyzing whether or not to screen for prostate cancer[19] and comparing different policies for cholesterol screening and treatment.[20] Decision analyses in health services research share many attributes with clinical analyses[21]; however, a discussion of their differences is beyond the scope of this book.

Most clinical decision analyses are built as decision trees, and the articles usually will include one or more diagrams showing the structure of the decision tree used for the analysis. Reviewing such diagrams will help you understand the model. Figure 1F-2 shows a diagram of a very simplified version of the decision tree for the atrial fibrillation problem mentioned at the beginning of this section. The clinician has three options for patients with atrial fibrillation in whom anti-arrhythmic therapy to achieve and maintain sinus rhythm is not a possible management strategy: to offer no prophylaxis, to recommend aspirin, or to recommend warfarin. Regardless of what choice is made, patients may or may not develop embolic events and, in particular, stroke. Prophylaxis lowers the chance of embolism but can cause bleeding in some patients. This simplified model excludes a number of important consequences, including the inconvenience of warfarin monitoring and the unpleasantness of minor bleeding.

**FIGURE 1F–2**

## Simplified Decision Tree for a Patient With Atrial Fibrillation

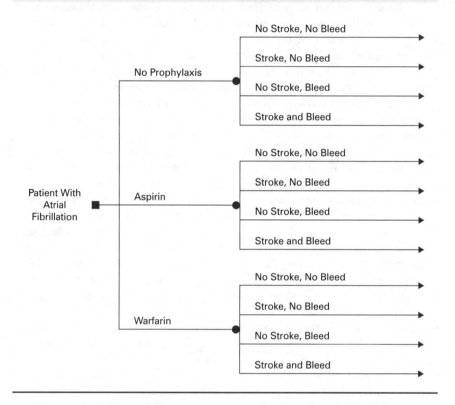

As seen in Figure 1F-2, decision trees are displayed graphically, oriented from left to right, with the decision to be analyzed on the left, the compared strategies in the center, and the clinical outcomes on the right. The decision is represented by a square, termed a *decision node.* The lines emanating from the decision node represent the clinical strategies being compared. Chance events are symbolized by circles, called *chance nodes,* and outcome states are shown (in Figure 1F-2) as triangles or (in other decision trees) as rectangles. When a decision analysis includes costs among the outcomes, it becomes an economic analysis and summarizes tradeoffs between health changes and resource expenditure.[22, 23] (See Part 2F, "Moving From Evidence to Action, Economic Analysis.")

Once a decision analyst has constructed the tree, he or she must generate quantitative estimates of the likelihood of events, or *probabilities.* The scale for probability estimates ranges from 0 (impossible) to 1.0 (absolute certainty). Probabilities must be assigned to each branch emanating from a chance node, and for each chance node, the sum of probabilities must add up to 1.0.

For example, returning to Figure 1F-2, consider the no-prophylaxis strategy (the upper branch emanating from the decision node). This arm has one chance node at which four possible events could occur (the four possible combinations arising from bleeding or not bleeding and from having a stroke or not having a stroke). Figure 1F-3 depicts the probabilities associated with one arm of the decision, the no-prophylaxis strategy (generated by assuming a 1% chance of bleeding and a 10% probability of stroke, with the two events being independent). Patients given no prophylaxis would have a 0.1% chance (a probability of 0.001) of bleeding and having a stroke, a 0.9% chance (a probability of 0.009) of bleeding and not having a stroke, a 9.9% chance (a probability of 0.099) of not bleeding but having a stroke, and an 89.1% chance (a probability of 0.891) of not bleeding and not having a stroke.

**FIGURE 1F–3**

**Decision Tree With Probabilities—No-Prophylaxis Option**

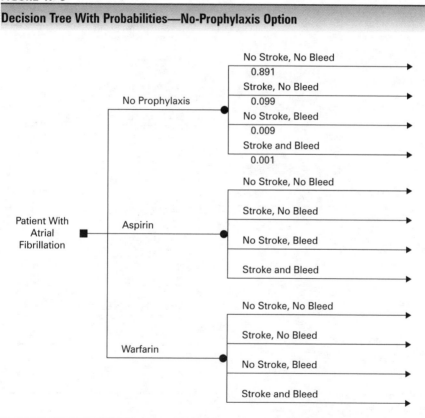

The decision analyst would generate similar probabilities for the other two branches. Presumably, the aspirin branch would have a higher risk of bleeding and a lower risk of stroke. The warfarin branch would have the highest risk of bleeding and the lowest risk of stroke.

These probabilities would not suggest a clear course of action, as the alternative with the lowest risk of bleeding has the highest risk of stroke, and vice versa. Thus, the right choice would depend on the relative value or utility one placed on bleeding and stroke. Decision analysts typically place a utility on each of the final possible outcomes that varies from 0 (death) to 1.0 (full health). Figure 1F-4 presents one possible set of utilities associated with the four outcomes and applied to the no-prophylaxis arm of the decision tree: 1.0 for no stroke or bleeding, 0.8 for no stroke and bleeding, 0.5 for stroke but no bleeding, and 0.4 for stroke and bleeding.

**FIGURE 1F–4**

**Decision Tree With Probabilities and Utilities Included in the No-Prophylaxis Arm of the Tree**

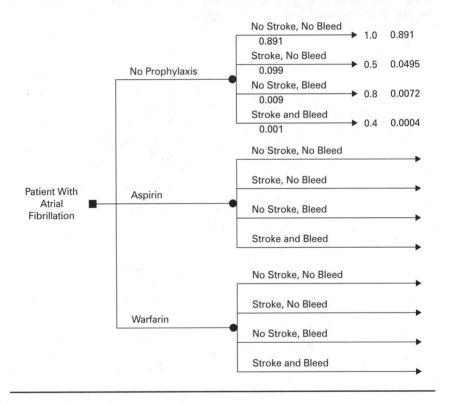

The final step in the decision analysis is to calculate the total value associated with each possible course of action. Given the particular set of probabilities and utilities we have presented, the value of the no-prophylaxis branch would be (0.891 x 1.0) + (0.009 x 0.8) + (0.099 x 0.5) + (0.001 x 0.4), or 0.948. Depending on the probabilities attached to the aspirin and warfarin branches, they would be judged superior or inferior to the no-prophylaxis branch. If the total value of each of these branches were >0.948, they would be judged preferable to the no-prophylaxis branch; if the total value were <0.948, they would be judged less desirable.

The model presented in Figures 1F-2 to 1F-4 is oversimplified in a number of ways, among which are its omission of the time frame of events and the possibility of a patient suffering multiple events. Decision analysts can make use of software programs that model what might happen to a hypothetical cohort of patients over a series of time cycles (say, periods of 1 year's duration). The model allows for the possibility that patients might move from one health state to another. For instance, one unfortunate patient may suffer a mild stroke in one cycle, continue with minimal functional limitation for a number of cycles, suffer a gastrointestinal bleeding episode in a subsequent cycle and, finally, experience a major stroke. These multistate transition models or Markov models permit more sophisticated and true-to-life depictions—and, presumably, more accurate decision analysis.

## Practice Guidelines

Practice guidelines, or "systematically developed statements to assist practitioner and patient decisions about appropriate health care for specific clinical circumstances,"[24] provide an alternative structure for integrating evidence and applying values to reach treatment recommendations.[1, 25-30] Practice guideline methodology places less emphasis on precise quantification than does decision analysis. Instead, it relies on the consensus of a group of decision makers, ideally including experts, front-line clinicians, and patients, who carefully consider the evidence and decide on its implications. The guidelines developers' mandate may be to adduce recommendations for a country, a region, a city, a hospital, or a clinic. Depending on whether the country is the Philippines or the United States, whether the region is urban or rural, whether the institution is a large teaching hospital or a small community hospital, and whether the clinic serves a poor community or an affluent one, guidelines based on the same evidence may differ. For example, clinicians practicing in rural parts of less industrialized countries without resources to monitor its intensity may reject the administration of warfarin to patients with atrial fibrillation.

Both decision analyses and practice guidelines can be methodologically strong or weak and thus may yield either valid or invalid recommendations. In Table 1F-1, we offer four guidelines to assess the validity of a treatment recommendation— one for each step depicted in Table 1F-1—and describe these in detail below.

**TABLE 1F-1**

## Users' Guides for the Validity of Treatment Recommendations

- Did the recommendations consider all relevant patient groups, management options, and possible outcomes?
- Is there a systematic review of evidence linking options to outcomes for each relevant question?
- Is there an appropriate specification of values or preferences associated with outcomes?
- Do the authors indicate the strength of their recommendations?

# ASSESSING RECOMMENDATIONS

## Did the Recommendations Consider All Relevant Patient Groups, Management Options, and Possible Outcomes?

Recommendations pertain to decisions, and decisions involve particular groups of patients, choices for those patients, and the consequences of the choices. Regardless of whether recommendations apply to diagnosis, prevention, therapy, or rehabilitation, they should specify all relevant patient groups, the interventions of interest, and sensible alternative practices. For example, in a decision analysis of the management of suspected herpes encephalitis, the authors included the three strategies available to clinicians at the time: brain biopsy, empiric vidarabine, or neither option.[31] Although this model represented the decision well at the time of publication, acyclovir has subsequently become available and is now widely used for this disorder. Because the original model did not include an acyclovir strategy, it would no longer accurately portray the decision.

To cite another example, in a guideline based on a careful systematic literature review,[32] the American College of Physicians offers recommendations for medical therapeutic options for preventing strokes.[33] Although the authors mention carotid endarterectomy as an alternative in their practice guidelines, the procedure is not included in the recommendations themselves. These guidelines would have been strengthened if medical management for transient ischemic attacks had been placed in the context of the highly effective surgical procedure.[34]

Treatment recommendations often vary for different subgroups of patients. In particular, those at lower risk of target outcomes that treatment is designed to prevent are less likely to benefit from therapy than those who are at higher risk (see Part 2B3, "Therapy and Applying the Results, Applying Results to Individual Patients"). For instance, in a guideline concerning hormone replacement therapy in postmenopausal women, the American College of Physicians provided separate recommendations for women who had undergone a hysterectomy and for those at higher risk of cardiovascular disease or breast cancer than for other women.[35]

Recommendations must consider not only all relevant patient groups and management options, but all important consequences of the options as well. Evidence concerning the effects on morbidity, mortality, and quality of life are all relevant to patients, and efficient use of resources dictates attention to costs. If costs are considered, regardless of whether authors use the perspective of patients, insurers, or the health care system or consider broader issues such as the consequences of time lost from work, they can further affect the conclusions (see Part 2F, "Moving From Evidence to Action, Economic Analysis"). Indeed, a decision analysis that includes economic outcomes is labeled an *economic analysis.*

Making recommendations about screening requires particular attention to identifying all potential outcomes. Attempting to identify disease in asymptomatic individuals may result in a number of negative outcomes that clinicians do not face when diagnosing and treating symptomatic patients. Individuals who screen positive for a disease must live for a longer time with the awareness of their illness and the associated negative psychologic consequences. This is particularly problematic if the condition screened for may remain asymptomatic for long periods of time. For instance, consider a man who screens positive for prostate cancer, but was destined to die of heart disease before the prostate cancer became clinically manifest. Those who screen positive but ultimately prove disease-negative may find the experience traumatic, and people who screen negative but ultimately prove to suffer from the target condition may feel betrayed (see Part 2F, "Moving From Evidence to Action, Recommendations About Screening").

In their guideline on hormone replacement therapy, the American College of Physicians used lifetime probability of developing endometrial cancer, breast cancer, hip fracture, coronary heart disease, and stroke, along with median life expectancy, to estimate risks and benefits for subgroups of women. They acknowledged possible effects of hormone replacement therapy on serum lipoproteins, uterine bleeding, sexual and urinary function, and the need for invasive monitoring, but they did not include these considerations in the model used to synthesize evidence. The effects of hormone replacement therapy on quality of life, which could have a major impact on patient choices, were not explicitly considered.

In a decision analysis concerning anticoagulant therapy for patients suffering from dilated cardiomyopathy,[4] the authors' decision model included all of the clinical events of interest to patients (stroke, other emboli, hemorrhage, etc). The analysts measured outcomes using quality-adjusted life expectancy, a scale that combines information about both the quantity and the quality of life. This metric fit the clinical decision well, for one can expect that warfarin might affect both the quantity and quality of life.

### Is There a Systematic Review of Evidence Linking Options to Outcomes for Each Relevant Question?

Having specified options and outcomes, the next task for decision makers is to estimate the likelihood that each outcome will occur. In effect, they have a series of specific questions. For hormone replacement therapy, the initial question is, "what is the effect of alternative approaches on the incidence of hip fracture, breast cancer, endometrial cancer, myocardial infarction, and sudden coronary death?" Recommendations must consolidate and combine all of the relevant evidence in an appropriate manner. In carrying out this task, decision makers must avoid bias that will distort the results. This requires access to, or conduct of, a systematic review of the evidence bearing on each question. Part 1E, "Summarizing the Evidence," provides guidelines for deciding how likely it is that collection and summarization of the evidence are free from bias.

The best recommendations define admissible evidence, report how it was selected and combined, make key data available for review, and report randomized trials that link interventions with outcomes. However, such randomized trials may be unavailable, and the authors of overviews may reasonably abandon their project if there are no high-quality studies to summarize. Those making recommendations do not have this luxury. For important but ethically, technically, or economically difficult questions, strong scientific evidence may never become available.

Because recommendations must deal with the best (often inadequate) evidence available, a variety of studies (published and unpublished) and reports of expert and consumer experience may need to be considered. This means that the strength of the evidence in support of the recommendations can vary widely. Thus, even recommendations that are grounded in rigorous collection and summarization of evidence may yield weak recommendations if the quality of the evidence is poor, an issue to which we will return later in this section (see Table 1F-1).

## Is There an Appropriate Specification of Values or Preferences Associated With Outcomes?

Linking treatment options with outcomes is largely a question of fact and a matter of science. Assigning preferences to outcomes, by contrast, is a matter of values. Consider, for example, the relative importance of a possible increased risk of developing breast cancer compared with expectations of decreased risks for fractures in association with hormone replacement therapy. Consequently, it is important that authors report the principal sources of such judgments and the method of seeking consensus.

Clinicians should look for information about who was involved in assigning values to outcomes or who, by influencing recommendations, was implicitly involved in assigning values. Expert panels and consensus groups are often used to determine what a guideline will say. You need to know who the "experts" are, bearing in mind that panels dominated by members of specialty groups may be subject to intellectual, territorial, and even financial biases. Panels that include a balance of experts in research methodology, practicing generalists and specialists, and public representatives are more likely to have considered diverse views in their deliberations than panels restricted to content area experts.

Even with broad representation, the actual process of deliberation can influence recommendations. Therefore, clinicians should look for a report of methods used to synthesize preferences from multiple sources. Informal and unstructured processes may be vulnerable to undue influence by individual panel members, particularly that of the chair of the panel. Explicit strategies for describing and dealing with dissent among judges, or frank reports of the degree of consensus, strengthen the credibility of the recommendations.

Knowing the extent to which patient preferences were considered is particularly important. Many guideline reports, by their silence on the matter of patient preferences, assume that guideline developers adequately represent patients' interests. Although they are reported rarely, it also would be valuable for you to know which principles—such as patient autonomy, nonmaleficence, or distributive justice—were given priority in guiding decisions about the value of alternative interventions. Excellent guidelines will state whether the guideline is intended to optimize values for individual patients, for reimbursement agencies, or for society as a whole. Ideally, guidelines will state the underlying value judgments on which they are based.

For instance, in the guideline on medical therapies to prevent stroke, the American College of Physicians recommended that aspirin be considered the drug of choice in patients with transient ischemic attacks and suggested that ticlopidine be reserved for patients who do not tolerate aspirin.[24] The best estimate of the effect of ticlopidine relative to aspirin in patients with transient ischemic attacks is a 15% reduction in relative risk, a benefit that would translate into the prevention of one stroke for every 70 patients treated in a group of patients with a 10% risk of stroke. The recommendation that aspirin, rather than ticlopidine, be the drug of choice for patients with transient ischemic attack is made, at least in part, on the basis of the increased cost of ticlopidine and the need for checking the white blood cell count in patients receiving ticlopidine. This implicit value judgment could be questioned, and the guideline would be strengthened if the authors had made explicit the values underlying their judgment.

Clinicians using a decision analysis will not face the huge problem of implicit and hidden value judgments that afflict practice guidelines. The reason, as Figure 1F-4 demonstrates, is that decision analysis requires explicit and quantitative specification of values. These values, expressed as utilities, represent measurements of the value to the decision maker of the various outcomes of the decision. Several methods are available to measure these values directly[5, 7, 24, 25] (see Part 2B2, "Therapy and Understanding the Results, Quality of Life"); the issue of which of these methods is best remains controversial.

Regardless of the measurement method used, the authors should report the source of the ratings. In a decision analysis built for an individual patient, the most (and probably only) credible ratings are those measured directly from that patient. For analyses built to inform clinical policy, credible ratings could come from three sources. First, they may come from direct measurements from a large group of patients with the disorder in question and to whom results of the decision analysis could be applied. Second, ratings may come from other published studies of quality-of-life judgments by such patients, as was done in a recent analysis of strategies for chronic atrial fibrillation.[26] Third, they may come from ratings made by an equally large group of people representing the general public. Whoever provides the rating must understand the outcomes they are asked to rate; the more the raters know about the condition, the more credible are their utility ratings.

## Do the Authors Indicate the Strength of Their Recommendations?

Multiple considerations should inform the strength or grade of recommendations: the quality of the sources contributing to the systematic review or reviews that bring together the relevant evidence, the magnitude and consistency of the intervention effects in different studies, the magnitude of adverse effects, the burden to the patient and the health care system, the costs, and the relative value placed upon different outcomes. Thus, recommendations may vary from those that rely on evidence from a systematic review of randomized controlled trials that show large treatment effects on patient-important outcomes with minimal side effects, inconvenience, and costs (yielding a very strong recommendation), to those that rely on evidence from observational studies showing a small magnitude of treatment effect with appreciable side effects and costs (yielding a very weak recommendation).

There are two ways that those developing recommendations can indicate their strength. One, most appropriate for practice guidelines, is to formally grade the strength of a recommendation. The other, most appropriate for decision analyses, is to vary the assumptions about the effect of the management options on the outcomes of interest. In this latter approach, a sensitivity analysis, investigators explore the extent to which varying assumptions might impact the ultimate recommendation. We will discuss the two approaches in turn.

### Grades of Recommendation

The Canadian Task Force on the Periodic Health Examination proposed the first formal taxonomy of levels of evidence[36-38] focusing on individual studies. We have modified this framework, taking into account that practice guidelines must rest on systemic reviews that bring together evidence from the best available individual studies (Table 1F-2).

The letter grades in Table 1F-2 (A, B, C+, and C) reflect a hierarchy of methodologic strength that ranges from overviews of randomized trials with consistent results to overviews of observational studies with inconsistent results. Randomized trials yield the strongest evidence (grade A). Since inferences about the health effects of interventions are weakened when there are unexplained major differences in effects in different studies, guidelines based on randomized trials are stronger when the results of individual studies are similar, and guidelines are weaker when major differences between studies, or heterogeneity, are present (grade B). Recommendations from observational studies yield weaker evidence (grade C).

We now identify two situations in which evidence from RCTs directly addressing the question of interest is unavailable, but the evidence is nevertheless strong. First, generalization from one group of patients to another may be very secure. For instance, randomized trials show a large reduction of strokes in patients with atrial fibrillation without mitral valve disease. The underlying biology suggests that clinicians are on strong ground generalizing these results to patients with atrial fibrillation who do have mitral valve disease. Second, observational studies may yield a very high level of consistency and a very large magnitude of effect. Insulin therapy for acute diabetic ketoacidosis provides an example of such a situation. We denote the strength of evidence in both these contexts as C+.

If the evidence linking interventions and outcomes comes from systematic reviews of original studies, clinicians can apply the criteria for a valid systematic review and the schema in Table 1F-2 to decide on the strength of evidence supporting recommendations.

The number categories in Table 1F-2 (1 and 2) reflect the balance between benefits and risks of therapy. If the benefits clearly outweigh the risks (or vice versa) and virtually all patients would make the same choice, the recommendation is designated grade 1. When the balance is less certain and different patients may make different choices, we designate the recommendation as grade 2. A number of factors may make for uncertainty in the balance between benefits and risks, including marked variation in patient values and a wide range of confidence intervals around estimates of benefit and risk (see Part 2F, "Moving From

Evidence to Action, Grading Recommendations: A Qualitative Approach,"
and Part 2F, "Moving From Evidence to Action, Grading Recommendations:
A Quantitative Approach").

**TABLE 1F-2**

## An Approach to Grading Treatment Recommendations Based on Systematic Reviews of the Relevant Evidence

| Grade of Recommendation | Clarity of Risk/Benefit | Methodologic Strength of Supporting Evidence | Implications |
|---|---|---|---|
| 1 A | Clear | RCTs without important limitations | Strong recommendation; can apply to most patients in most circumstances without reservation |
| 1 B | Clear | RCTs with important limitations (inconsistent results, methodologic flaws*) | Strong recommendations, likely to apply to most patients |
| 1 C+ | Clear | No RCTs directly addressing the question, but results from closely related RCTs can be unequivocally extrapolated, or evidence from observational studies may be overwhelming | Strong recommendation; can apply to most patients in most circumstances |
| 1 C | Clear | Observational studies | Intermediate-strength recommendation; may change when stronger evidence is available |
| 2 A | Unclear | RCTs without important limitations | Intermediate-strength recommendation; best action may differ depending on circumstances or patient's or societal values |
| 2 B | Unclear | RCTs with important limitations (inconsistent results, methodologic flaws) | Weak recommendation; alternative approaches likely to be better for some patients under some circumstances |
| 2 C | Unclear | Observational studies | Very weak recommendations; other alternatives may be equally reasonable |

\* These situations include RCTs with both lack of blinding and subjective outcomes where the risk of bias in measurement of outcomes is high, RCTs with large loss to follow-up.

NOTE: Since grade B and C studies are flawed, it is likely that most recommendations in these classes will be level 2.

The following considerations will bear on whether the recommendation is grade 1 or 2: the magnitude and precision of the treatment effect, patients' risk of the target event being prevented, the nature of the benefit and the magnitude of the risk associated with treatment, variability in patient preferences, variability in regional resource availability and health care delivery practices, and cost considerations. Inevitably, weighing these considerations involves subjective judgment.

RCT indicates randomized controlled trial

If recommendations are developed on the basis of observational studies or if the estimate of the magnitude of the treatment effect is imprecise, clinicians can conclude that the recommendation is relatively weak. Investigators can deal with this weakness in recommendations by testing the effect of the guideline on patient outcomes in a real-world clinical situation. For instance, Weingarten and colleagues examined the impact of implementation of a practice guideline, suggesting that low-risk patients admitted to coronary care units should receive early discharge.[39] On alternate months during a 1-year period, clinicians either received or did not receive a reminder of the guideline recommendations. During the months in which the intervention was in effect, hospital stay for coronary care unit patients was approximately 1 day shorter and the average cost was reduced by more than $1000.00. Mortality and health status at 1 month after discharge were similar in the two groups. Such a study, if methodologically strong, addresses the weakness in the underlying evidence and dramatically raises the grade of the recommendations.

The guideline on hormone replacement therapy described previously demonstrates the limitations of recommendations based on weak evidence.[35] Although the guideline did not grade its recommendations, they are based largely on observational studies and would be characterized as 2C in the schema presented in Table 1F-2. In particular, the guideline relied to a large extent on a meta-analysis of observational studies of the impact of hormone replacement therapy on coronary heart disease, suggesting a relative risk reduction of 0.35. Subsequently, in the first large randomized trial in women with established coronary disease, no reduction in coronary events was found with hormone replacement therapy.[40] Clearly, clinicians should be cautious in their implementation of grade C recommendations.

### Sensitivity Analysis

Decision analysts use the systematic exploration of the uncertainty in the data, known as *sensitivity analysis*, to see what effect varying estimates for risks, benefits, and values have on expected clinical outcomes and, therefore, on the choice of clinical strategies. Sensitivity analysis asks the question: is the conclusion generated by the decision analysis affected by the uncertainties in the estimates of the likelihood or value of the outcomes? Estimates can be varied one at a time, termed one-way sensitivity analyses, or can be varied two or more at a time, known as multiway sensitivity analyses. For instance, investiagtors conducting a decision analysis of the administration of antibiotic agents for prevention of *Mycobacterium avium-intracellulare* in patients with HIV infection found that the cost-effectiveness of prophylaxis decreased if they either assumed a longer life span for patients or made a less sanguine estimate of the drugs' effectiveness.[41] If they simultaneously assumed both a longer life span and decreased drug effectiveness (a two-way sensitivity analysis), the cost-effectiveness decreased substantially. Clinicians should look for a table that lists which variables the analysts included in their sensitivity analyses, what range of values they used for each variable, and which variables, if any, altered the choice of strategies.

Generally, all of the probability estimates should be tested using sensitivity analyses. The range over which they should be tested will depend on the source of the data. If the estimates come from large, high-quality randomized trials with narrow confidence limits, the range of estimates tested can be narrow. The less valid the methods or the less precise the estimates, the wider the range that must be included in the sensitivity analyses.

Decision analysts should also test utility values with sensitivity analyses, with the range of values again determined by the source of the data. If large numbers of patients or knowledgeable and representative members of the general public gave very similar ratings to the outcome states, investigators can use a narrow range of utility values in the sensitivity analyses. If the ratings came from a small group of raters, or if the values for individuals varied widely, then investigators should use a wider range of utility values in the sensitivity analyses. To the extent that the bottom line of the decision analysis does not change with varying probability estimates and varying values, clinicians can consider the recommendation a strong one. When the bottom-line decision shifts with different plausible probabilities or values, the recommendation becomes much weaker.

Table 1F-3 presents a schema for classifying the methodologic quality of treatment recommendations, emphasizing the three key components: consideration of all relevant options and outcomes, a systematic summary of the evidence, and an explicit or quantitative consideration, or both, of societal or patient preferences.

**TABLE 1F-3**

## A Hierarchy of Rigor in Making Treatment Recommendations

| Level of Rigor | Systematic Summary of Evidence | Considers All Relevant Options and Outcomes? | Explicit Statement of Values | Sample Methodologies |
|---|---|---|---|---|
| High | Yes | Yes | Yes | Practice guideline or decision analysis* |
| Intermediate | Yes | Yes or no | No | Systematic review* |
| Low | No | Yes or no | No | Traditional review; article reporting primary research |

* Sample methodologies may not reflect the level of rigor shown. Exceptions may occur in either direction. For example, if the author of a practice guideline or decision analysis neither systematically collects nor summarizes information and if neither societal nor patients' values are explicitly considered, recommendations will be produced that are of low rigor. Conversely, if the author of a systematic review does consider all relevant options and at least qualitatively considers values, recommendations approaching high rigor can be produced.

## Are Treatment Recommendations Desirable at All?

The approaches we have described highlight the view that patient management decisions are always a function of both evidence and preferences. Values are likely to differ substantially among settings. For example, monitoring of anticoagulant therapy might take on a much stronger negative value in a rural setting where travel distances are large, or in a more severely resource-constrained environment where, for example, there is a direct inverse relationship between the resources available for purchase of antibiotic drugs and those allocated to monitoring levels of anticoagulation.

Patient-to-patient differences in values are equally important. The magnitude of the negative value of anticoagulant monitoring, or the relative negative value associated with a stroke vs a gastrointestinal bleeding episode, will vary widely among individual patients, even in the same setting. If decisions are so dependent on preferences, what is the point of recommendations?

This line of argument suggests that investigators should systematically search, accumulate, and summarize information for presentation to clinicians. In addition, investigators may highlight the implications of different sets of values for clinical action. The dependence of the decision on the underlying values—and the variability of values—would suggest that such a presentation would be more useful than a recommendation.

We find this argument compelling. However, its implementation depends on standard methods of summarizing and presenting information that clinicians are comfortable interpreting and using. In addition, it assumes that clinicians will have the time and the methods to ascertain patient values that they can then integrate with the information from systematic reviews of the impact of management decisions on patient outcomes. These requirements are unlikely to be fully met in the immediate future. Moreover, treatment recommendations are likely to remain useful for providing insight, marking progress, highlighting areas where we need more information, and stimulating productive controversy. In any case, clinical decisions are likely to improve if clinicians are aware of the underlying determinants of their actions and are able to be more critical about the recommendations offered to them. Our taxonomy may help to achieve both goals.

# CLINICAL RESOLUTION

Let us return to the opening clinical scenario. Addressing the validity of the practice guideline on antithrombotic therapy in atrial fibrillation,[2] you begin by considering whether the guideline developers have addressed all important patient groups, treatment options, and outcomes. You note that they make separate recommendations for patients at varying risk of stroke, but not for patients at different risk of bleeding. The latter omission may occur because studies of prognosis have been inconsistent in the apparent risk factors for bleeding they identified. You have ruled out antiarrhythmic therapy (which another decision analysis of which you are aware suggests as the management option of choice[42]) for the patient before you. The guideline addresses the options you are seriously considering, full- and fixed-dose warfarin and aspirin, but does not mention your eccentric colleague's choice of clopidogrel or a related agent, ticlopidine. The guideline addresses the major outcomes of interest, occlusive (embolic) stroke, hemorrhagic stroke, gastrointestinal bleeding, and other major bleeding events, but does not deal specifically with the need for regular blood testing or the frequent minor bruising associated with warfarin therapy.

Moving to the selection and synthesis of the evidence, you find the guideline's eligibility criteria to be appropriate and the supportive literature search, as documented by the clearinghouse, to be comprehensive. The synthesis method is not stated explicitly, but in reading the text it becomes apparent that it is based on calculation and comparison of absolute and relative event rates for both benefits and risks and that it is tied to the guideline's strength of recommendations.

The authors of the guideline make it clear that they believe patient values are crucial to the decision, although they do not explicitly specify the relative value of stroke and bleeding that underlie their recommendations. The guideline comes down clearly on the side of adjusted-dose warfarin therapy for high-risk patients and aspirin for low-risk patients. Since high-risk patients still bleed with warfarin and low-risk patients experience fewer strokes when they take anticoagulant agents, the recommendations express an implicit relative valuing of strokes vs major and minor bleeding episodes and the inconvenience associated with warfarin therapy.

When, as in this case, guideline developers are implicit, clinicians must examine who the people involved in making recommendations are, and the possible influences on their value judgments. The developers are all expert specialists—the authors do not include patients or primary care physicians. Dupont, the makers of warfarin, funded the production of the guidelines, published as a supplement to the journal Chest.[2] This is worth noting, for the funders of any research project may influence its conduct. When, as is often the case in guidelines, investigators are making implicit value judgments, the possible biases that flow from the source of funding are particularly dangerous.

The guideline developers used the predecessor of the grading scheme described earlier in this section, basing all of their recommendations on the results of randomized controlled trials with consistent results, and thus rated them grade A (see Table 1F-2). They classified both of their recommendations that high-risk patients receive warfarin and low-risk patients aspirin as grade 1, meaning they believe that in both cases, the risk-benefit relationship is clear. The patient from the clinical scenario presented earlier in this section falls into the intermediate-risk category. The recommendations suggest that either warfarin or aspirin represents a reasonable option for her. Overall, the guideline meets validity criteria relatively well, and you are inclined to place a high level of trust in the authors' recommendations.

The decision analysis[5] restricts its comparison to warfarin therapy vs no treatment. Its rationale for omitting aspirin is that its efficacy is not proven (although the aspirin effect in other meta-analyses has achieved statistical significance, it has always been on the border). The investigators do not mention any other antiplatelet treatment. They include outcomes of the inconvenience associated with monitoring of anticoagulant therapy, major bleeding episodes, mild stroke, severe stroke, and cost. They omit minor bleeding.

The investigators present their search strategies very clearly. They restrict themselves to the results of computer searches of the published literature but, given this limitation, their searches appear comprehensive. With great clarity, they also describe their rationale for selecting evidence, and their criteria appear rigorous. They note the limitations of one key decision: to choose data from the Framingham study, rather than from randomized controlled trials of therapy for patients with atrial fibrillation, from which to derive their risk estimates.

To generate values, the authors interviewed 57 community-dwelling elderly people with a mean age of 73 years. They used standard gamble methodology (see Part 2B2, "Therapy and Understanding the Results, Quality of Life") to generate utility values. Their key values include utilities, on a 0 to 1.0 scale where 0 is death and 1.0 is full health, of 0.986 for warfarin managed by a general practitioner, 0.880 for a major bleeding episode, 0.675 for a mild stroke, and 0 for a severe stroke.

The investigators conducted a sensitivity analysis that indicated their model was sensitive to variation in patients' utility for being on warfarin. If they assumed utility values for being on warfarin in the upper quartile (1.0; that is, no disutility is suggested for taking warfarin), their analysis suggests that virtually all patients should be receiving warfarin treatment. If they assumed the lower quartile utility, 0.92), the analysis suggests that most patients should not be taking warfarin.

This decision analysis rates high with respect to the validity criteria in Table 1F-1. The utilities in the investigators' core analysis using median patient values and best estimates of risk and risk reduction (their *base case* analysis) match those of the patient in the scenario quite well. The investigators provided tables that suggest the best decision for different patients; when we add the characteristics of the patient being considered in the opening scenario, we find that the verdict is: no benefit from treatment. However, this patient does fit into a cell near the boundary between no benefit and clear benefit, and the investigators' sensitivity analysis suggests that if she places the same value on life taking warfarin as life not taking warfarin, she would benefit from using the drug.

Having reviewed what turns out to be a rigorous guideline and a rigorous decision analysis, you believe that you are in a much stronger position both in your own decision making and in providing guidance to your colleagues. Your residual discomfort stems from the realization that the best decision for many patients, including the patient in the scenario, is critically dependent on the patient's values. You resolve to have a more detailed discussions of the options and the consequences when you see her next (see Part 2F, "Moving From Evidence to Action, Incorporating Patient Values").

# References

1. Eddy DM. *A Manual for Assessing Health Practices and Designing Practice Policies: The Explicit Approach.* Philadelphia: American College of Physicians; 1992.

2. Laupacis A, Albers G, Dalen J, Dunn MI, Jacobson AK, Singer DE. Antithrombotic therapy in atrial fibrillation. *Chest.* 1998;114:579S-589S.

3. Shaneyfelt TM, Mayo-Smith MF, Rothwangl J. Are guidelines following guidelines? The methodological quality of clinical practice guidelines in the peer-reviewed medical literature. *JAMA.* 1999;281:1900-1905.

4. Grilli R, Magrini N, Penna A, Mura G, Liberati A. Practice guidelines developed by specialty societies: the need for a critical appraisal. *Lancet.* 2000;355: 103-106.

5. Thompson R, Parkin D, Eccles M, Sudlow M, Robinson A. Decision analysis and guidelines for anticoagulant therapy to prevent stroke in patients with atrial fibrillation. *Lancet.* 2000;355:956-962.

6. Vandenbroucke-Grauls CMJE, Vendenbroucke JP. Effect of selective decontamination of the digestive tract on respiratory tract infections and mortality in the intensive care unit. *Lancet.* 1991;338:859-862.

7. Selective Decontamination of the Digestive Tract Trialists' Collaborative Group. Meta-analysis of randomised controlled trials of selective decontamination of the digestive tract. *BMJ.* 1993;307:525-532.

8. Heyland DK, Cook DJ, Jaeschke R, Griffith L, Lee HN, Guyatt GH. Selective decontamination of the digestive tract. *Chest.* 1994;105:1221-1229.

9. Kollef MH. The role of selective digestive tract decontamination on mortality and respiratory tract infections. *Chest.* 1994;105:1101-1108.

10. Glasziou PP, Irwig LM. An evidence based approach to individualising treatment. *BMJ.* 1995;311:1356-1358.

11. Sinclair JC, Cook R, Guyatt GH, Pauker SG, Cook DJ. When should an effective treatment be used? Derivation of the threshold number needed to treat and the minimum event rate for treatment. *J Clin Epidemiol.* In press.

12. Smith GD, Egger M. Who benefits from medical interventions? *BMJ.* 1994;308:72-74.

13. Antman EM, Lau J, Kupelnick B, Mosteller F, Chalmers TC. A comparison of results of meta-analyses of randomized control trials and recommendations of clinical experts: treatments for myocardial infarction. *JAMA.* 1992;268:240-248.

14. Keeney RL. Decision analysis: an overview. *Operations Res.* 1982;30: 803-838.

15. Eckman MH, Levine HJ, Pauker SG. Decision analytic and cost-effectiveness issues concerning anticoagulant prophylaxis in heart disease. *Chest.* 1992;102:538S-549S.

16. Kassirer JP, Moskowitz AJ, Lau J, Pauker SG. Decision analysis: a progress report. *Ann Intern Med*. 1987;106:275-291.

17. Eddy DM. Clinical decision making: from theory to practice. Designing a practice policy. Standards, guidelines and options. *JAMA*. 1990;263:3077, 3081, 3084.

18. Wong JB, Salem DN, Pauker SG. You're never too old. *N Engl J Med*. 1993;328:971-974.

19. Krahn MD, Mahoney JE, Eckman MH, Trachtenberg J, Pauker SG, Detsky AS. Screening for prostate cancer: a decision analytic view. *JAMA*. 1994;272: 773-780.

20. Krahn M, Naylor CD, Basinski AS, Detsky AS. Comparison of an aggressive (U.S.) and a less aggressive (Canadian) policy for cholesterol screening and treatment. *Ann Intern Med*. 1991;115:248-255.

21. Goel V. Decision analysis: applications and limitations. *CMAJ*. 1992;147: 413-417.

22. Drummond MF, Richardson WS, O'Brien B, Levine M, Heyland DK, for the Evidence-Based Medicine Working Group. Users' Guides to the Medical Literature XIII. How to use an article on economic analysis of clinical practice. A. Are the results of the study valid? *JAMA*. 1997;277:1552-1557.

23. O'Brien BJ, Heyland DK, Richardson WS, Levine M, Drummond MF, for the Evidence-Based Medicine Working Group. Users' Guides to the Medical Literature XIII. How to use an article on economic analysis of clinical practice. B. What are the results and will they help me in caring for my patients? *JAMA*. 1997;277:1802-1806.

24. Institute of Medicine. *Clinical Practice Guidelines: Directions for a New Program*. Washington, DC: National Academy Press; 1990.

25. AMA/Specialty *Society Practice Parameters Partnership. Attributes to Guide the Development of Practice Parameters.* Chicago: American Medical Association; 1990.

26. American College of Physicians. *Clinical Efficacy Assessment Project: Procedural Manual*. Philadelphia: American College of Physicians; 1986.

27. Gottlieb LK, Margolis CZ, Schoenbaum SC. Clinical practice guidelines at an HMO: development and implementation in a quality improvement model. *QRB*. 1990;16:80-86.

28. Lohr KN, Field MJ. A provisional instrument for assessing clinical practice guidelines. 1991. Unpublished.

29. Woolf SH. Expert Panel on Preventive Services: analytic methodology. 1991. Unpublished.

30. Park RE, Fink A, Brook RH, et al. Physicians' rating of appropriate indications for six medical and surgical procedures. *Am J Public Health*. 1986;76:766-772.

31. Barza M, Pauker SG. The decision to biopsy, treat, or wait in suspected herpes encephalitis. *Ann Intern Med*. 1980;92:641-649.

32. Matchar DB, McCrory DC, Barnett HJM, Feussner JR. Medical treatment for stroke prevention. *Ann Intern Med*. 1994;121:41-53.

33. American College of Physicians. Guidelines for medical treatment for stroke prevention. *Ann Intern Med*. 1994;121:54-55.

34. North American Symptomatic Carotid Endarterectomy Trial Collaborators. Beneficial effect of carotid endarterectomy in symptomatic patients with high-grade carotid stenosis. *N Engl J Med*. 1991;325:445-453.

35. Grady D, Rubin SM, Petitti DB, et al. Hormone therapy to prevent disease and prolong life in postmenopausal women. *Ann Intern Med*. 1992;117:1016-1037.

36. Canadian Task Force on the Periodic Health Examination. The periodic health examination. *CMAJ*. 1979;121:1193-1254.

37. Woolf SH, Battista RN, Anderson GM, Logan AG, Wang E. Assessing the clinical effectiveness of preventive maneuvers: analytic principles and systematic methods in reviewing evidence and developing clinical practice recommendations. *J Clin Epidemiol*. 1990;43:891-905.

38. Sackett DL. Rules of evidence and clinical recommendations on the use of antithrombotic agents. *Arch Intern Med*. 1986;146:464-466.

39. Weingarten SR, Reidinger MS, Conner L, et al. Practice guidelines and reminders to reduce duration of hospital stay for patients with chest pain. *Ann Intern Med*. 1994;120:257-263.

40. Hulley S, Grady D, Bush T, Furberg C, Herrington D, Riggs B, Vittinghoff E. Randomized trial of estrogen plus progestin for secondary prevention of coronary heart disease in postmenopausal women. Heart and Estrogen/progestin Replacement Study (HERS) Research Group. *JAMA*. 1998;280:605-613.

41. Bayoumi AM, Redelmeier DA. Preventing *Mycobacterium avium* complex in patients who are using protease inhibitors: a cost-effectiveness analysis. *AIDS*. 1998;12:1503-1512.

42. Catherwood E, Fitzpatrick WD, Greenberg ML, et al. Cost-effectiveness of cardioversion and antiarrhythmic therapy in non-valvular atrial fibrillation. *Ann Intern Med*. 1999;130:625-636.

# Beyond the Basics: Using and Teaching the Principles of Evidence-Based Medicine

202

Part 2 of this book provides detailed, in-depth discussions of the key concepts introduced in Part 1. Each section of Part 2 is therefore linked to Part 1. During your reading of Part 1 you probably noted the cross-references to the expanded concepts in Part 2. These expanded discussions, all of which are also included in the associated CD-ROM, include strategies for explaining difficult concepts that established clinicians and instructors of evidence-based medicine may find particularly useful.

Part 2 begins with expansions on issues raised in the Part 1 section entitled "Philosophy of Evidence-Based Medicine," including critics' attacks on evidence-based medicine. The next section provides a perspective on the fundamental threat to inferences from any primary study: bias and random error. Here, we emphasize the link between addressing issues of therapy and issues of harm.

The largest segment of Part 2 addresses issues of delivering the optimal therapy to patients. This segment includes of examples of randomized controlled trial (RCT) results that have differed from those predicted by biologic rationale or suggested by observational studies. This segment expands on a number of statistical issues, including intention-to-treat analysis, hypothesis testing, confidence intervals, and choosing the best way of expressing the magnitude of a treatment effect ("Measures of Association"). We provide a guide for applying the results of RCTs to individual patients, and we describe how clinicians can definitively determine the best treatment for an individual in "N of 1 Randomized Controlled Trials." We also provide examples of numbers needed to treat (NNT) for a number of therapies, emphasizing how the NNT will vary in patients with differing baseline risks.

Part 2 emphasizes the care clinicians should take when therapy clearly affects biologic variables, but may not affect patient-important outcomes ("Surrogate Outcomes"). On the other hand, we provide a deeper understanding of outcomes that RCTs have tended to neglect, namely, patients' quality of life. Part 2 provides clinicians with a strategy for deciding whether to generalize results across a class of drugs, or to conclude that a particular drug in a class is superior to other drugs in that same class. We also offer insights into two particular types of studies: studies addressing computer decision aids and qualitative studies focusing on patients' experience of illness and of health care.

Issues related to diagnostic tests on which Part 2 expands include studies related to describing the clinical manifestations of particular diseases and those that generate or test clinical prediction rules. Part 2 provides a guide to help understand how chance can inflate apparent agreement (for instance, agreement between physicians assessing an element of physical examination) and chance-corrected measures of agreement that help deal with this problem. Next, we provide some examples of likelihood ratios, the ultimate output of studies of diagnostic tests. The related section on prognosis, "Regression and Correlation," deals with concepts of statistical analysis.

Readers of the next segment of Part 2 will deepen their understanding of systematic reviews by considering questions such as the following: what interpretations are possible when studies addressing a similar question yield discrepant results ("Evaluating Differences in Study Results")?; and when should clinicians believe an analysis that suggests that a drug is effective in one group of patients but not in another group, or that differing doses have appreciably different effects on outcome ("When to Believe a Subgroup Analysis")? This segment also discusses the difficulties that unpublished studies present for systematic reviews, along with the issues involved in choosing the optimal strategy for statistical analysis.

Part 2 concludes with an expanded discussion of how to use evidence to arrive at a management approach for an individual patient. Clinicians reading this segment will gain insight into approaches to grade the strength of expert recommendations and will learn how to make sense of a study that examines the economic implications of alternative treatments. We provide a detailed discussion of studies of screening interventions and of studies that examine the quality of clinical care. Finally, we address what is perhaps the most important frontier of evidence-based medicine: how can one efficiently and effectively incorporate the values of the specific patient in health care decisions that will influence the subsequent life of that patient?

# Expanded Philosophy of Evidence-Based Medicine

## Parallel but Separate Goals— Evidence-Based Practitioners and Evidence-Based Care

Gordon Guyatt, Brian Haynes, Roman Jaeschke, Deborah Cook, Trisha Greenhalgh, Maureen Meade, Lee Green, David Naylor, Mark Wilson, Finlay McAlister, and Scott Richardson

The following EBM Working Group members also made substantive contributions to this section: Victor Montori and Heiner Bucher

## IN THIS SECTION

It will not surprise you that we believe high-quality health care implies the practice of medicine that is consistent with the best evidence (evidence-based care). An intuitively appealing way to achieve evidence-based practice is to train clinicians who can independently find, appraise, and judiciously apply the best evidence (evidence-based practitioners). Indeed, our fondest hope for this book is that it will help you become an evidence-based practitioner. However, there are limitations to this strategy for achieving competence in evidence-based care.

In this section we will acknowledge the challenges to developing expertise in evidence-based medicine. Next, we will highlight two complementary alternatives: encouraging physicians to use evidence-based summaries and recommendations and implementing strategies directed specifically at changing physicians' behavior. Finally, we will present some of the reasons you might wish to acquire advanced EBM skills—even though these skills are not prerequisites for practicing evidence-based medicine.

# CHALLENGES TO DEVELOPING EXPERTISE

The skills needed to provide an evidence-based solution to a clinical dilemma include (1) precisely defining the problem, (2) constructing and conducting an efficient search to locate the best evidence, (3) critically appraising the evidence, and (4) considering that evidence—and its implications—in the context of patients' circumstances and values. Although attaining these skills at a basic level is relatively easy, developing expertise allowing efficient and sophisticated critical appraisal requires intensive study and frequent, often time-consuming, application.

We have now had over a decade of experience at McMaster University with an internal medicine residency program explicitly committed to the systematic training of evidence-based practitioners.[1] We have concluded—consistent with prior predictions[2]—that even in this highly facilitative environment, not all trainees are interested in attaining an advanced level of EBM skills. They recognize the time and energy required to gaining an advanced level of skills, and they find they can be quite competent in the practice of medicine without them. Our trainees' responses mirror those of general practitioners in the United Kingdom who often use evidence-based summaries generated by others (72%) and evidence-based practice guidelines or protocols (84%), but who overwhelmingly (95%) believe that "learning the skills of evidence-based medicine" is not the most appropriate method for "moving . . . to evidence-based medicine."[3]

Because of the amount of time required to make evidence-based decisions from scratch, evidence-based practitioners will, in many instances, fail to review the original literature that bears on a clinical dilemma they face. Thus, there are two reasons that training evidence-based practitioners will not, as a sole strategy, necessarily result in the achievement of evidence-based practice at an optimal level of competence. First, many clinicians will not be interested in gaining a high level of sophistication in using the original literature. Second, even those who do have the interest often will not have adequate time to apply these skills.

In our McMaster residency program, however, we have observed that even the trainees who are less interested in evidence-based methods develop a respect for and an ability to track down, recognize, and use secondary sources of preappraised evidence (evidence-based resources) that provide immediately applicable conclusions. Having mastered this more restricted set of EBM skills, these trainees (evidence users) can become highly competent, up-to-date practitioners who deliver evidence-based care. If you have mastered the content of Part 1 of this book, you already have the necessary knowledge to function as an evidence user.

Time limitations dictate that evidence-based practitioners also rely heavily on bottom-line conclusions from preappraised resources. If you have read Part 1A1, "Finding the Evidence," you have already become familiar with such resources, which apply a methodologic filter to original investigations and therefore ensure a minimal standard of validity. These include the Cochrane Library, *ACP Journal Club*, Evidence-Based Medicine, Best Evidence, and an increasing number of computer decision support systems. Producing more comprehensive and more easily accessible preappraised resources constitutes a second strategy for ensuring evidence-based care.

## ANTI-EVIDENCE-BASED MEDICINE FORCES

There are other reasons that the availability of evidence-based resources and recommendations still will be insufficient to produce consistent evidence-based care. Like other physicians, evidence users and practitioners are subject to habit, local practice patterns, and product marketing (in particular, pharmaceutical industry marketing). These forces may often be stronger determinants of practice than current best evidence.

It is unreasonable to expect that most practicing physicians will undertake the continuing education required to become evidence users; in fact, many trainees continue to show little interest. Randomized controlled trials have shown that traditional continuing education has little effect on combating these forces and changing physician behavior.[4]

## COMPLEMENTARY ALTERNATIVE STRATEGIES

On the other hand, approaches that do change targeted clinical behaviors include one-to-one conversations with an expert (pharmaceutical detailing and academic counter-detailing), computerized alerts and reminders, preceptorships, advice from opinion leaders, and targeted audit and feedback.[5-7] Other effective strategies equally removed from practitioners' direct use of the medical literature include the availability of restricted drug formularies and the application of financial incentives[8] and institutional guidelines.[6] Application of a variety of strategies that do not demand even a rudimentary ability to use the original medical literature, in conjunction with a focus on behavior change, constitutes a third strategy for achieving evidence-based care.

# ADVANTAGES OF DEVELOPING ADVANCED EBM SKILLS

We hope that the previous paragraphs have not dissuaded you from continuing to read and study this book. There remain powerful reasons for you to achieve the highest possible skill level in evidence-based practice. First, attempts to change physician practice (in particular, use and interpretation of diagnostic tests, and approaches to patient management) will sometimes be directed to objectives other than evidence-based care such as increasing specific drug utilization or reducing health care costs. Only if you develop advanced skills in interpreting the medical literature will you be able to determine the extent to which these attempts are consistent with the best evidence. Second, a high level of EBM skills will allow you to use the original literature effectively, regardless of whether preappraised synopses and evidence-based recommendations are available.

Third, sophisticated EBM skills are a prerequisite for being an effective leader in the medical community. In a particularly pessimistic assessment of the future of medicine, a colleague of ours has suggested that there will soon be two types of physicians: those who make guidelines and those who follow them. To the extent that this is the case, both content-area expertise and sophisticated EBM training will be necessary to secure a place in the leadership group.

If you are a medical educator, a manager, or a policymaker, take note. As we encourage medical trainees to achieve the highest possible level of EBM skills, two phenomena will be necessary to ensure high levels of evidence-based health care: (1) the widespread availability of comprehensive, preappraised, evidence-based summaries and recommendations, and (2) the widespread implementation of strategies demonstrated to change clinicians' behavior.

# References

1. Evidence-based Medicine Working Group. Evidence-based medicine: a new approach to teaching the practice of medicine. *JAMA*. 1992;268:2420-2425.

2. Sackett DL, Richardson WS, Rosenberg W, Haynes RB. *Evidence-Based Medicine: How to Practice and Teach EBM*. London: Churchill Livingstone; 1997:12-16.

3. McColl A, Smith H, White P, Field J. General practitioners' perceptions of the route to evidence based medicine: a questionnaire survey. *BMJ*. 1998;316: 361-365.

4. Davis DA, Thomson MA, Oxman AD, Haynes RB. Changing physician performance: a systematic review of the effect of continuing medical education strategies. *JAMA*. 1995;274:700-705.

5. Oxman AD, Thomson MA, Davis DA, Haynes RB. No magic bullets: a systematic review of 102 trials of interventions to improve professional practice. *CMAJ*. 1995;153:1423-1431.

6. Grimshaw JM, Russell IT. Achieving health gain through clinical guidelines, II: ensuring guidelines change medical practice. *Qual Health Care*. 1994;3:45-52.

7. Hunt DL, Haynes RB, Hanna SE, Smith K. Effects of computer-based clinical decision support systems on physician performance and patient outcomes: a systematic review. *JAMA*. 1998;280:1339-1346.

8. Chaix-Couturier C, Durand-Zaleski I, Jolly D, Durieux P. Effects of financial incentives on medical practice: results from a systematic review of the literature and methodological issues. *Int J Qual Health Care*. 2000;12(2):133-142.

# EXPANDED PHILOSOPHY OF EVIDENCE-BASED MEDICINE

## Criticisms of Evidence-Based Medicine

Sharon Straus, Finlay McAlister, Deborah Cook, Trisha Greenhalgh, and Gordon Guyatt

The following EBM Working Group members also made substantive contributions to this section: Peter Wyer and Christina Lacchetti

## IN THIS SECTION

When examining evidence-based medicine (EBM), it is useful to distinguish the different ways in which clinicians incorporate evidence into their practices: by critically evaluating original source material, by using preappraised evidence from reliable sources, and by depending on current, ostensibly high-quality, authoritative non-EBM sources (see Part 2A, "Expanded Philosophy of Evidence-Based Medicine, Parallel but Separate Goals—Evidence-Based Practitioners and Evidence-Based Care"). First, clinicians may sometimes function as evidence-based practitioners. In so doing, they will seek original literature, conduct a full critical appraisal of what they find, estimate the magnitude of the benefits and risks associated with alternative options, and work with patients to determine the best course of action (see Part 1A, "Introduction: The Philosophy of Evidence-Based Medicine"). Other times, clinicians may function as evidence users, searching for preappraised evidence from sources that they believe are reliable and applying the bottom-line summaries and recommendations to patients in their own practice.[1] Finally, in yet other situations, clinicians use summaries and recommendations from sources that pay little heed to the tenets of EBM, assuming rightly or wrongly that these authoritative sources are based on high-quality, complete, and current research that has been assessed judiciously and with full consideration of the heterogeneity of patient values.

The increasing attention the medical community is paying to the practice of EBM has led to positive and negative reactions.[2] In this section, we provide our perspective on the most common criticisms. We will discuss those that are universal to the practice of medicine, those that are unique to EBM (and thus represent true limitations of the current practice of EBM), and those that arise from misperceptions about it.

# CHALLENGES TO EVIDENCE-BASED PRACTICE

## The First Principle of EBM: Evidence Is Never Enough

It is easy to confuse limitations in research evidence with the challenges of moving from evidence to action.[3] The first fundamental principle of EBM tells us that evidence alone can never guide our clinical actions; we always will require the application of values or preferences (see Part 1A, "Introduction: The Philosophy of Evidence-Based Medicine"). For instance, although seven meta-analyses of randomized controlled trials examining selective decontamination of the gastrointestinal tract (SDD) to prevent pneumonia in critically ill patients had similar results, showing lower pneumonia rates with SDD, conclusions ranged from support to rejection of this intervention.[4-10] The different recommendations likely arose, at least in part, from the difference in the value the authors of the seven trials placed on the reduction of pneumonia in patients treated with SDD, the possible increase in antibiotic resistance that subsequent patients would face, and the alternative use of societal resources. These different recommendations also reflected varying interpretations of the precision of the estimates.

Problems of coherency and consistency of evidence—and the phenomenon of differing values leading to differing clinical actions despite identical evidence—highlight the importance of EBM training for clinicians who wish to make independent judgments related to the care of patients in their practice. Such judgments require the ability to critically appraise research studies, recognize the uncertainty demonstrated by confidence intervals, and balance benefits and risks within the context of their patients' unique values and expectations.

## The Shortage of Coherent, Consistent Scientific Evidence

Clinicians frequently encounter situations in which there is no direct evidence available from basic or applied research. The exponential growth in clinical research, coupled with international efforts (by groups such as the Cochrane Collaboration) to systematically identify, sort, and rationalize this evidence eventually will close many of these gaps. However, both proponents and critics of EBM agree that evidence from sources lower in the hierarchy—individual clinical experience and physiologic experimentation—"must be applied to traverse the many grey zones of practice."[11] (See Part 1A, "Introduction: The Philosophy of Evidence-Based Medicine.") The available evidence, regardless of its source, often is indirectly related to the immediate dilemma; and clinical reasoning, often based on the principles of basic science (biochemistry, physiology, pharmacokinetics, and so on) is required in its application. For instance, the patient you are currently treating, although similar to those who participated in specific randomized trials, may also yet differ in potentially important ways. To provide another example, randomized controlled trials of prophylactic therapy (beta blockers after myocardial infarction, for instance) may have followed patients for a maximum of 3 years. Clinicians must decide what course to take with patients in their fourth year of taking medication.

Even when evidence from sources higher in the hierarchy exists, frustrations arise when it is inconclusive or inconsistent with previous studies.[12] For example, according to a randomized trial comparing thrombolytic therapy with primary coronary angioplasty in patients with acute myocardial infarction, there was an absolute risk reduction of 0.1% for in-hospital mortality with primary angioplasty.[13] The 95% confidence interval around this absolute risk reduction (−1.6% to +1.8%) indicates an indeterminate result, compatible with both an extra life saved per 56 patients and an additional patient killed per 63 patients treated with angioplasty rather than thrombolysis.

Investigators offered three different interpretations of this result. Although the authors of the study concluded that there was no difference between the two approaches, the author of an accompanying editorial concluded that primary angioplasty was the superior treatment.[14] By contrast, another editorial[15] in the same issue supported thrombolysis. Indeed, few randomized trials (or other studies, for that matter) report their results in light of all of available research. Such piecemeal reporting of research often results in conflicting messages.[16] Systematic reviews provide a solution to the variable reporting of research results.[17,18]

## The Unique Biologic Attributes of the Individual Patient

The universality of biologic variation hampers attempts to extrapolate any evidence, whether from basic or applied research, to individual patients.[3] This is encountered daily when patients do not fit into the mold of textbook descriptions of physiology and disease mechanisms and when their cases vary from applied research reports about the prevention, diagnosis, prognosis, and therapeutic management of their illnesses. This is the reason that we place evidence from the patient before us (see Part 2B1, "Therapy and Validity, N of 1 Randomized Controlled Trials") at the apex of the hierarchy of evidence (see Part 1A, "Introduction: The Philosophy of Evidence-Based Medicine"). The use of N of 1 randomized controlled trials is restricted to treatment of symptomatic chronic conditions in which treatment results occur quickly and in patients who are eager to participate. When N of 1 randomized controlled trials are not available, clinicians must determine the extent to which aggregate results of clinical trials in samples of patients apply to the patients in their practice, taking into account the unique biologic attributes of that individual patient, her personal values, and the sociocultural context. Evidence-based medicine offers guides for making these decisions (see Part 2B3, "Therapy and Applying the Results, Applying Results to Individual Patients"; Part 1F, "Moving From Evidence to Action"; and Part 2F, "Moving From Evidence to Action, Incorporating Patient Values").

## Limited Resources for Health Care

The gap between the demand for health care and the resources available to meet it is growing in many, if not all, countries.[19] Per capita health expenditures have more than doubled during the past two decades, with more than 33% of this rise accounted for by the increased intensity of services.[20] Limited resources inevitably create tension between the best interests of individuals and the best interests of society as a whole. Such conflicts are now universal features of clinical practice. Thus, it is not surprising that in public health care systems, those responsible for resource allocation have increasingly attempted to control escalating health care costs by setting priorities and rationing services.[21] However, curtailing of clinical freedom is a function of resource constraints, rather than of EBM. Indeed, if health care purchasers use EBM principles to guide their decisions, they will eliminate interventions that are harmful or ineffective and preserve funding for efficacious therapies, and they might lobby for funds to institute new, effective treatments. The result may be a net increase in health care resource consumption.

Some critics suggest that EBM exacerbates tensions in health care resource allocation, increasing pressure for clinicians and policymakers to provide expensive services.[22, 23] This pressure, critics charge, could lead to inefficient use of resources as less glamorous interventions with greater benefits for dollars spent are bypassed. These criticisms ignore the high level of attention EBM gives to careful consideration of all the implications of patient management decisions (see Part 1F, "Moving From Evidence to Action"), including costs (see Part 2F, "Moving From Evidence to Action, Economic Analysis") and societal and individual patient values (see Part 2F, "Moving From Evidence to Action, Incorporating Patient Values").

We ruefully acknowledge, however, that when health care rationing decisions are made and defended on the grounds of evidence of effectiveness and cost-effectiveness, the reality of limited health care resources is explicitly exposed. This exposure makes many people uncomfortable, and the EBM movement may get caught in the crossfire. For instance, in the UK, the National Institute for Clinical Excellence was established in 1999 to provide official evidence-based recommendations on whether (and under what clinical circumstances) the government-funded National Health Service should pay for particular drugs, operations, and investigations. During the first few months of its existence, the National Institute for Clinical Excellence advised against the routine extraction of asymptomatic impacted wisdom teeth (a procedure for which dentists had previously been able to claim a generous item-of-service fee). This agency also recommended against the routine use of zanamivir in uncomplicated influenza and the prescription of beta-interferon in all types of multiple sclerosis. In these cases, the media, prompted by various vested interest groups, suggested that the National Institute for Clinical Excellence itself had caused the lack of resources to pay for the therapies. Further, the media conspicuously failed to analyze the evidence behind the recommendations. The events emphasize the need for education of health journalists in principles of EBM.[24]

## The Need to Develop New Skills

Unquestionably, the practice of EBM at its highest level requires the acquisition and development of skills (in literature searching, critical appraisal, and bedside statistics) that are foreign to traditional medical education and clinical training.[25-31] Although skill mastery and application are formidable tasks, many clinicians are interested in mastering them,[25-31] and even most who are not so inclined are nevertheless still interested in achieving competence in the practice of evidence-based medicine.

The problem of skills acquisition can be at least partially overcome in three ways. First, EBM skills can be acquired at any stage in clinical training and practice.[32] Incorporating their acquisition into the routine of grand rounds, postgraduate and undergraduate seminars, and morning reports integrates them with the other skills being developed in these settings.[33] Second, members of clinical teams at various stages of training can collaborate with each other by sharing the searching and appraising tasks. Finally, those uninterested in functioning as evidence-based practitioners can more easily acquire the expertise required to function as evidence users.

## Limited Clinician Time and Technical Resources

Critics of EBM have correctly pointed out that evidence-based practice may require time and resources that are unavailable to the typical busy clinician.[34] The amount of time clinicians have available for accessing and assessing the published literature is very limited.[32] Even clinicians whose lives are graced with the luxury of time may not have quick enough access to the evidence, and they may have to travel several floors, blocks, or miles to their local library.

However, times are changing. Important developments to help overcome barriers of time and inconvenience include systematic reviews of the effects of health care generated by the Cochrane Collaboration, the growing numbers of evidence-based journals of quality-filtered and relevance-filtered secondary publications, and the creation of "best evidence" sections in a number of established journals. Moreover, electronic searching is increasingly available at the point of care, enabling clinicians to access evidence within a few seconds.[35,36]

Two other factors help alleviate the problems of limited time and resources. First, as noted previously, is the division of labor among members of the clinical team. Second, although we can generate several questions about each patient we see, we can pare them down to just one by balancing the question that is most important to our patient's well-being against the question that appears most feasible to answer, is most interesting to us, and is most likely to be raised in other patients we would see subsequently.[32] (See Part 1A1, "Finding the Evidence.")

On an encouraging note, authors of a few observational studies conducted in selected centers have suggested that high-quality research evidence is available to address a substantial proportion of the management issues faced by busy clinicians.[37-42] However, these studies may be subject to publication bias and may not be generalizable to many settings. Moreover, the authors do not address the extent to which the clinical decisions they describe were consistent with patients' values.[43,44] Indeed, the time limitations of clinical practice may challenge the appropriate incorporation of patient values into clinical decisions to an even greater extent than it challenges the incorporation of research evidence (see Part 2F, "Moving From Evidence to Action, Incorporating Patient Values").

# THE IRONY: WHAT IS THE EVIDENCE THAT EVIDENCE-BASED MEDICINE WORKS?

Critics have quite appropriately demanded evidence as to whether EBM improves patient outcomes.[45] What is the precise question being asked when one considers the impact of EBM? One question may be whether application of EBM principles will result in superior, or even different, patient management strategies.

In a classic study, investigators conducted cumulative meta-analyses of therapeutic options for reducing mortality after myocardial infarction.[46] They found that expert recommendations in narrative review articles lagged about a decade behind the accumulated evidence in favor of thrombolysis after myocardial infarction. The delay in expert recommendations for cholesterol reduction was similar. Furthermore, they found that experts advocated routine prophylactic administration of lidocaine and widespread use of calcium antagonists in the face of randomized controlled trial data suggesting a trend toward harm.[46] These findings suggest that evidence-based approaches to summarizing evidence result in recommendations that are more consistent with the evidence than do traditional approaches to making recommendations.

Alternatively, the question may relate to whether therapeutic options shown to be effective in the environment of randomized trials continue to be effective in the setting of routine clinical care. Observational studies have repeatedly documented that those patients who receive proven efficacious therapy have better outcomes than those who do not. For example, myocardial infarction survivors receiving aspirin or beta blockers have lower mortality rates than those not receiving these drugs.[47,48]

Finally, the question may relate to our ability to persuade clinicians and policymakers to adopt evidence-based approaches to health care delivery. Here, the issues relate to how best to teach clinicians EBM principles[49,50] and, more important, how to ensure practice is consistent with the best evidence and with societal and individual patient values. We have already learned a considerable amount about facilitating evidence-based practice.[51-55] Studies have shown that consistently effective methods include educational outreach visits (academic detailing), reminders or prompts (manual or computerized) issued at the time of the consultation, multifaceted interventions (a belt-and-braces combination of two or more methods), and interactive educational meetings.[51,54] Additional effective methods have included audit and feedback (any summary of clinical performance presented to individual clinicians), local opinion leaders, and patient-mediated interventions (such as information leaflets or patient-held prompts).[51,54] Studies have found little or no effect with didactic educational meetings or the distribution of printed guidelines.[51,54] Still, there are no magic bullets, and finding the best ways to implement evidence-based practice remains a major challenge for its proponents.

# MISPERCEPTIONS OF EVIDENCE-BASED MEDICINE

Many criticisms of EBM stem from misperceptions of its purpose and process. We implicitly address these issues in Part 1A, "Introduction: Philosophy of Evidence-Based Medicine"; in the following discussion we will elaborate on some of the points in that section.

Rather than denigrating clinical expertise,[3,55] evidence-based medicine acknowledges expertise as the basis for all clinical practice. Rather than ignoring patient values,[56] the first principle of EBM draws the primacy of patient values to the clinician's attention. Rather than promoting cookbook medicine,[55,57] EBM points out that only through a deep understanding of the evidence, including its strengths and limitations, can the practitioner make independent, valid judgments about the best course of action.

The most common criticism of EBM is that it is an ivory-tower concept.[58] However, surveys and observational studies of front-line clinicians suggest this is not the case.[25-31,37-42] Another misperception is that EBM is limited to doing—as opposed to using—clinical research.[3] The practice of EBM comprises a method for providing care for patients by considering research evidence; it is not a method for performing research.

The final misperception is that only randomized controlled trials or systematic reviews constitute the "evidence" in EBM.[58, 59] Attention to randomized trials will indeed help clinicians avoid the errors they will make if they base treatment and prevention decisions only on physiologic rationale or observational studies (see Part 2B1, "Therapy and Validity, Surprising Results of Randomized Controlled Trials"). However, EBM emphasizes the consideration of evidence from various types of studies appropriate to different clinical questions. For example, EBM suggests that clinicians should seek evidence about the prognosis of a disease or health state from natural history studies (see Part 1D, "Prognosis"). Understanding prevailing practice patterns would require observational studies, surveys, or analyses of administrative databases. Finally, EBM explicitly acknowledges physiologic studies and individual clinical experience as important evidence sources (see Part 1A, "Introduction: Philosophy of Evidence-Based Medicine").

# CONCLUSION

Most criticisms of EBM are based on a different understanding of its philosophy than the one we offer. An accurate understanding of EBM is growing in the medical community, and with this growth, enthusiasm for EBM approaches increases. Evidence-based medicine must now address the challenges to evidence-based practice and teaching by facilitating efficient access to the evidence, by helping clinicians apply that evidence to patient care, and by discovering better ways to integrate patient values into the process of health care provision.

## References

1. Guyatt GH, Meade MO, Jaeschke RZ, Cook DJ, Haynes RB. Practitioners of evidence based care: not all clinicians need to appraise evidence from scratch but all need some skills. *BMJ.* 2000;320:954-955.

2. Straus SE, McAlister FA. Evidence-based medicine: a commentary on common criticisms. *CMAJ.* 2000;163:837-841.

3. Charlton BG. Restoring the balance: evidence-based medicine put in its place. *J Eval Clin Pract.* 1997;3:87-98.

4. Vandenbroucke-Grauls CM, Vendenbroucke JP. Effect of selective decontamination of the digestive tract on respiratory tract infections and mortality in the intensive care unit. *Lancet.* 1991;338:859-862.

5. Selective Decontamination of the Digestive Tract Trialists Collaborative Group. Meta-analysis of randomised controlled trials of selective decontamination of the digestive tract. *BMJ.* 1993;307:525-532.

6. Kollef MH. The role of selective digestive tract decontamination on mortality and respiratory tract infections. *Chest.* 1994;105:1101-1108.

7. Heyland DK, Cook DJ, Jaeschke R, Griffith L, Lee HN, Guyatt GH. Selective decontamination of the digestive tract. *Chest.* 1994;105:1221-1229.

8. Hurley JC. Prophylaxis with enteral antibiotics in ventilated patients: selective decontamination or selective cross-infection? *Antimicrobial Agents Chemother.* 1995;39:941-947.

9. D'Amico R, Pifferi S, Leonetti C, Torri V, Tinazzi A, Liberati A. Effectiveness of antibiotic prophylaxis in critically ill adult patients: systematic review of randomized controlled trials. *BMJ.* 1998;316:1275-1285.

10. Nathens A, Marshall JC. Selective decontamination of the digestive tract in surgical patients. *Arch Surg.* 1999;134:170-176.

11. Naylor CD. Grey zones of clinical practice: some limits to evidence-based medicine. *Lancet.* 1995;345:840-842.

12. Miettinen OS. Evidence in medicine: invited commentary. *CMAJ.* 1998;158: 215-221.

13. Every NR, Parsons LS, Hlatky M, Martin JS, Weaver WD. A comparison of thrombolytic therapy with primary coronary angioplasty for acute myocardial infarction. *N Engl J Med.* 1996;335:1253-1260.

14. Grines CL. Primary angioplasty—the strategy of choice. *N Engl J Med.* 1996;335:1313-1316.

15. Lange RA, Hillis LD. Should thrombolysis or primary angioplasty be the treatment of choice for acute myocardial infarction? Thrombolysis—the preferred treatment. *N Engl J Med.* 1996;335:1311-1312.

16. Clarke M, Chalmers I. Discussion sections in reports of controlled trials published in general medical journals: islands in search of continents? *JAMA.* 1998;280:280-282.

17. Chalmers I, Hetherington J, Elboiurne D, Keirse MJNC, Enkin M. Materials and methods used in synthesizing evidence to evaluate the effects of care during pregnancy and childbirth: provisions for updating and amending overviews (meta-analyses) in the light of new data and criticisms. In: Chalmers I, Enkin M, Keirse MJNC, eds. *Effective Care in Pregnancy and Childbirth*. Oxford: Oxford University Press; 1989.

18. Moher D, Olkin I. Meta-analysis of randomized controlled trials: a concern for standards. *JAMA.* 1995;274:1962-1964.

19. Improving communication between doctors and patients: summary and recommendations of a report of a working party of the Royal College of Physicians. *J R Coll Phy Lond.* 1997;31:258-259.

20. Eddy DM. Health system reform: will controlling costs require rationing services? *JAMA.* 1994;272:324-328.

21. Chisholm J. Viagra: botched test case for rationing. *BMJ.* 1999;318:273-274.

22. Maynard A. Evidence based medicine: an incomplete method for informing treatment choices. *Lancet.* 1997;349:126-128.

23. David DS. Evidence-based medicine. *Am J Med.* 1998;105:361-362.

24. Guyatt GH, Ray J, Gibson N, et al. A journalist's guide for health stories. *Am Med Writers Assoc J.* 1999;14:32-41.

25. McColl A, Smith H, White P, Field J. General practitioners' perceptions of the route to evidence based medicine: a questionnaire survey. *BMJ.* 1998;316: 361-365.

26. Tunis SR, Hayward RS, Wilson MC, et al. Internists' attitudes about clinical practice guidelines. *Ann Intern Med.* 1994;120:956-963.

27. McAlister FA, Graham I, Karr GW, Laupacis A. Evidence-based medicine and the practicing clinician. *J Gen Intern Med.* 1999;14:236-242.

28. Hagdrup N, Falshaw M, Gray RW, Carter Y. All members of primary care team are aware of importance of evidence based medicine. *BMJ.* 1998;317:282.

29. Ghali WA, Saitz R, Eskew AH, Lemaire JB, Gupta M, Hershman WY. Evidence-based medicine: behaviors, skills, and attitudes of medical students. *Ann RCPSC* 1998;31:177-182.

30. Olatunbosun OA, Edouard L, Pierson RA. Physicians' attitudes toward evidence based obstetric practice: a questionnaire survey. *BMJ.* 1998;316:365-366.

31. Mayer J, Piterman L. The attitudes of Australian GPs to evidence-based medicine: a focus group study. *Fam Pract.* 1999;16:627-632.

32. Sackett DL, Straus SE, Richardson WS, Rosenberg WMC, Haynes RB. *Evidence-Based Medicine: How to Practice and Teach EBM.* London: Churchill Livingstone; 2000.

33. Reilly B, Lemon M. Evidence-based morning report: a popular new format in a large teaching hospital. *Am J Med.* 1997;103:419-426.

34. Jacobson LD, Edwards AG, Granier SK, Butler CC. Evidence-based medicine and general practice. *Br J Gen Pract.* 1997;47:449-452.

35. Sackett DL, Straus SE. Finding and applying evidence during clinical rounds: the "evidence cart." *JAMA.* 1998;280:1336-1338.

36. Sauve JS, Lee HN, Meade MO, et al. The critically-appraised topic (CAT): a resident-initiated tactic for applying users' guides at the bedside. *Ann R Coll Phys Surg.* 1995;28:396-398.

37. Ellis J, Mulligan I, Rowe J, Sackett DL. Inpatient general medicine is evidence based. *Lancet.* 1995;346:407-410.

38. Geddes JR, Game D, Jenkins NE, Peterson LA, Pottinger GR, Sackett DL. What proportion of primary psychiatric interventions are based on randomised evidence? *Qual Health Care.* 1996;5:215-217.

39. Gill P, Dowell AC, Neal RD, Smith N, Heywood P, Wilson AK. Evidence based general practice: a retrospective study of interventions in our training practice. *BMJ.* 1996;312:819-821.

40. Kenny SE, Shankar KR, Rintala R, Lamont GL, Lloyd DA. Evidence-based surgery: interventions in a regional paediatric surgical unit. *Arch Dis Child.* 1997;76:50-53.

41. Baraldini V, Spitz L, Pierro A. Evidence-based operation in paediatric surgery. *Pediatr Surg Int.* 1998;13:331-335.

42. Howes N, Chagla L, Thorpe M, McCulloch P. Surgical practice is evidence based. *Br J Surg.* 1997;84:1220-1223.

43. Slawson DC, Shaughnessy AF, Bennett JH. Becoming a medical information master: feeling good about not knowing everything. *J Fam Pract.* 1994;28: 505-513.

44. Greenhalgh T. Is my practice evidence-based? *BMJ.* 1996;313:957-958.

45. Miles A, Bentley P, Polychronis A, Grey J. Evidence-based medicine: why all the fuss? This is why. *J Eval Clin Pract.* 1997;3:83-85.

46. Antman EM, Lau J, Kupelnick B, Mosteller F, Chalmers TC. A comparison of results of meta-analyses of randomized control trials and recommendations of clinical experts: treatments for myocardial infarction. *JAMA.* 1992;268:240-248.

47. Krumholz HM, Radford MJ, Ellerbeck EF, et al. Aspirin for secondary prevention after acute myocardial infarction in the elderly: prescribed use and outcomes. *Ann Intern Med.* 1996;124:292-298.

48. Krumholz HM, Radford MJ, Wang Y, Chen J, Heiat A, Marciniak TA. National use and effectiveness of beta-blockers for the treatment of elderly patients after acute myocardial infarction. National Cooperative Cardiovascular Project. *JAMA.* 1998;280:623-629.

49. Norman GR, Shannon SI. Effectiveness of instruction in critical appraisal (evidence-based medicine) skills: a critical appraisal. *CMAJ.* 1998;158:177-181.

50. Bordley DR, Fagan M, Theige D. Evidence-based medicine: a powerful educational tool for clerkship education. *Am J Med.* 1997;102:427-432.

51. Oxman AD, Thomson MA, Davis DA, Haynes RB. No magic bullets: a systematic review of 102 trials of interventions to improve professional practice. *CMAJ.* 1995;153:1423-1431.

52. Davis DA, Thomson MA, Oxman AD, Haynes RB. Changing physician performance: a systematic review of the effect of continuing medical education strategies. *JAMA.* 1995;274:700-705.

53. Grimshaw JM, Russell IT. Achieving health gain through clinical guidelines, II: ensuring guidelines change medical practice. *Qual Health Care.* 1994; 3:45-52.

54. Hunt DL, Haynes RB, Hanna SE, Smith K. Effects of computer-based clinical decision support systems on physician performance and patient outcomes: a systematic review. *JAMA.* 1998;280:1339-1346.

55. Horwitz RI. The dark side of evidence-based medicine. *Cleve Clin J Med.* 1996;63:320-323.

56. Cohn JN. Evidence-based medicine: what is the evidence? *J Card Fail.* 1996;2:159-161.

57. Charlton BG, Miles A. The rise and fall of EBM. *QJM.* 1998;12:371-374.

58. Hampton JR. Evidence-based medicine, practice variations and clinical freedom. *J Eval Clin Pract.* 1997;3:123-131.

59. Swales JD. Evidence-based medicine and hypertension. *J Hypertens.* 1999;17:1511-1516.

# THERAPY AND HARM

## Why Study Results Mislead— Bias and Random Error

Gordon Guyatt

The following EBM Working Group members also made substantive contributions to this section: Sharon Straus, Deborah Cook, and Peter Wyer

## IN THIS SECTION

# RANDOM ERROR

Our clinical questions have a correct answer that corresponds to an underlying reality or truth. For instance, there is a true underlying magnitude of the impact of beta blockers on mortality in patients with heart failure, of the impact of inhaled steroids on exacerbations in patients with asthma, and of the impact of carotid endarterectomy on incidence of strokes in patients with transient ischemic attacks. Unfortunately, however, we will never know what that true impact really is. Why is this so?

Consider a perfectly balanced coin. Every time we flip the coin, the probability of its landing with head up or tail up is equal—50%. Assume that we, as investigators, do not know that the coin is perfectly balanced—in fact, we have no idea how well balanced it is, and we would like to find out. We can state our question formally: what is the true underlying probability of a resulting head or tail on any given coin flip? Our first experiment addressing this question is a series of 10 coin flips. The result: eight heads and two tails. What are we to conclude? Taking our result at face value, we infer that the coin is very unbalanced (that is, biased in such a way that it yields heads more often than tails) and that the probability of heads on any given flip is 80%.

Few would be happy with this conclusion. The reason for our discomfort is that we know that the world is not constructed so that a perfectly balanced coin will always yield five heads and five tails in any given set of 10 coin flips. Rather, the result is subject to the play of chance—otherwise known as *random error*. Some of the time, 10 flips of a perfectly balanced coin will yield eight heads. On occasion, nine of 10 flips will turn up heads. On rare occasions, we will find heads on all 10 flips.

What if the 10 coin flips yield five heads and five tails? Our awareness of the play of chance makes us very hesitant to conclude that the coin is a true one. We know that not only might we get eight heads and two tails when the real probability of a head is 0.5, but also that a series of 10 coin flips in a very biased coin (a true probability of heads of 0.8, for instance) could yield five heads and five tails.

Let us say that a funding agency, intrigued by the results of our first small experiment, provides us with resources to conduct a larger study. This time, we increase the sample size of our experiment markedly, conducting a series of 1000 coin flips. When we end up with 500 heads and 500 tails, are we ready to conclude that we are dealing with a true coin? Not quite. We know that, were the true underlying probability of heads 51%, we would sometimes see 1000 coin flips yield the very same result we have just observed.

Application. We can apply the above logic to the results of experiments addressing health care issues in human beings. A randomized controlled trial shows that 10 of 100 treated patients die in the course of treatment and that 20 of 100 control patients who do not receive treatment die. Does treatment really reduce the death rate by 50%? Maybe, but awareness of chance will leave us with considerable uncertainty about the magnitude of the treatment effect—and perhaps about whether treatment helps at all. To use a real-world example, in a study of cardiac insufficiency, 228 (17%) of 1320 patients with moderate to severe heart failure allocated to receive placebo died, as did 156 (12%) of 1327 allocated to receive bisoprolol.[1] Although the true underlying reduction in the relative risk of dying is likely to be in the vicinity of the 34% suggested by the study, we must acknowledge that considerable uncertainty remains about the true magnitude of the effect. Let us remember the question with which we started: why is it that, no matter how powerful and well-designed our experiment, we will never be sure of the true treatment effect? The answer is accounted for by chance.

# BIAS

What do we mean when we say that a study is valid, believable, or credible? *Validity* is the degree to which a study appropriately answers the question being asked or appropriately measures what it intends to measure. In this book, we use validity as a technical term that relates to the magnitude of *bias*. In contrast to random error, bias leads to systematic deviations (ie, the error has direction) from the underlying truth. In studies of treatment or harm, bias leads to either an underestimate or an overestimate of the underlying beneficial or harmful effect.

Bias may intrude as a result of differences, other than the experimental intervention, between patients in treatment and control groups at the time they enter a study. Alternatively, it may reflect differences that develop after the study begins. At the start of a study each patient, if left untreated, is destined to do well—or poorly. To do poorly means to have an adverse event—say, a stroke—during the course of the study. We often refer to the adverse event that is the focus of a study as the *target outcome* or event.

There are a host of factors that are associated with—or causally related to— the likelihood of a patient suffering the target outcome. Consider a trial in which patients at risk of a cerebrovascular event are studied. If patients' underlying disease (atherosclerosis) is severe, if they have reached advanced age, if their blood pressure is high, or if they are male, they are more likely than others to have a stroke.[2] We call each of these patient characteristics *prognostic factors* or *determinants of outcome*. These prognostic factors determine patients' destiny with respect to whether or not they will suffer the target adverse event.

We can contrast these patient characteristics with such other characteristics as eye color or shoe size. Eye color and shoe size differ from the first set of characteristics in that they are seldom, if ever, related to the likelihood of having a stroke. Patients with blue eyes are no more or less likely to suffer a stroke than those with brown eyes. Those with size 12 shoes are at no greater or lesser risk than those with size 8 shoes.

Prognostic Differences Between Treatment and Control Patients. Bias will intrude if treated and control patients who are not treated differ in substantive outcome-associated ways at the start of the study. Differences in eye color or shoe size will not create bias because they are not associated with the target outcome, but differences in important prognostic factors will lead to bias. For example, if treated patients have more severe atherosclerosis or are older than their control counterparts, their destiny will be to suffer a greater proportion of adverse events than those in the control group, and the results of the study will be biased against the treatment group. That is, the study will yield a systematically lower estimate of the treatment effect than would be obtained were the study groups alike prognostically. Thus, the study results would not reflect the underlying truth.

What if the control group has a higher mean blood pressure, or a greater proportion of men, than the treatment group? In these cases, the bias will be in the opposite direction (ie, it will be against the control group). If control patients begin the study with a greater stroke risk, study results will be biased in favor of the treatment group, and treatment will appear to benefit patients more than it really does. Thus, one source of bias is prognostic differences between treated and control patients at the start of a study.

Placebo Effect. Even if treated and control patients can begin the study with the same fate or destiny, the study may still produce a biased estimate of the treatment effect. For example, patients who believe they are receiving treatment may anticipate that they will do better. As it turns out, such anticipation may have a profound effect on how patients actually do feel and, furthermore, on how they function. This *placebo effect* may bias the results toward suggesting a greater biologic effect of treatment than is really the case.

Differential Administration of Interventions. Another potential source of bias is differential administration of interventions (other than that under study) to patients in the treatment and control groups. For example, in a study of a new treatment for stroke in which a larger proportion of patients in the treatment group receive aspirin or clopidogrel than those in the control group, the results will overestimate the treatment effect. This will not be true if a larger proportion of patients in the treatment group receive saline eye drops or antacid medications. The reason is that saline eye drops and antacids have no impact on the frequency of stroke, whereas aspirin[3] and clopidogrel[4] reduce stroke incidence. *Cointervention* is a technical term used to describe a situation when treatments that do affect the incidence of the target outcome are differentially administered to treatment and control groups.

Note some parallels: we are not concerned about imbalance of eye color or shoe size when patients start the study (which we often call *baseline characteristics*), nor are we concerned about imbalance of saline eye drops or antacid administration once the study starts. What we are concerned about is imbalance in disease severity in the treatment and control patients, and about differential administration of aspirin to the two groups, because they may affect the likelihood of patients having a stroke. Study results will be biased if factors that affect prognosis, either baseline characteristics or subsequent treatment, are unequal in the groups being compared. A *confounding variable* is any prognostic factor or effective treatment that is not equal in the groups being compared. For a study to be unbiased, the groups must start the same (with respect to their likelihood of suffering the target outcome) and stay the same.

Differential Measurement of the Target Outcome. Differential measurement of the target outcome can also introduce bias. For instance, whether a patient has suffered a transient ischemic attack or a small stroke may be a matter of judgment. If all such events are identified and recorded as strokes in the control group and as transient ischemic attacks in the intervervention group, the study will overestimate the effect of treatment on stroke reduction.

Loss to Follow-up. Another way that a study may introduce bias related to measurement of outcome is when large numbers of patients are *lost to follow-up*. If rates of adverse outcomes differ in patients lost to follow-up, the necessity of relying on data from patients who were followed will result in findings that differ from the underlying truth.

# DIFFERENTIATING DEGREES OF BIAS AND RANDOM ERROR

Students of EBM face conceptual challenges and challenges of nomenclature. When asked to say what makes a study valid, students often respond, "large sample size." Small sample size does not produce bias (and, thus, compromised validity), but it can increase the likelihood of a misleading result through *random error*. You may find the following exercise helpful in clarifying notions of bias and random error.

Consider a set of studies with identical design and sample size that recruit from the same patient pool. Just as an experiment of 10 coin flips will not always yield five heads and five tails, the play of chance will ensure that despite their identical design, each study will have a different result.

Consider four sets of such studies. Within each set, the design and sample size of each individual trial are identical. Two of the four sets of studies have small sample sizes, and two have large sample sizes.

Two sets include only randomized controlled trials (RCTs) in which patients, caregivers, and those assessing outcome are all blinded. Two sets use only an observational design (eg, patients are in treatment or control groups on the basis of their choice, their clinician's choice, or happenstance), which is far more vulnerable to bias. In this exercise we are in the unique position of knowing the true treatment effect. In Figure 2B-1, each of the bull's-eyes in the center of the four components of the figure represents the truth. Each smaller dot represents not a single patient, but the results of one repetition of the study. The farther a smaller dot lies from the central bull's-eye, the larger is the difference between the study result and the underlying true treatment effect.

**FIGURE 2B–1**

## Representation of Four Sets of Identically Conducted Studies Demonstrating Varying Degrees of Bias and Random Error

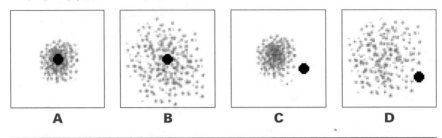

A, A group of randomized controlled trials (large sample size). B, A group of randomized controlled trials (small sample size).
C, A group of observational studies (large sample size). D, A group of observational studies (small sample size).

Each set of studies represents the results of RCTs or observational studies and of studies of large or small sample size. Before reading further, examine Figure 2B-1 and draw your own conclusions about the study designs and number of patients in each of the four (A through D) components.

Figure 2B-1(A) represents the results of a series of randomized trials with large sample size. The results are valid and are thus distributed around the true effect, represented by the central bull's-eye, resulting from the strong study design. The results do not fall exactly on target because of chance or random error. However, the large sample size, which minimizes random error, ensures that the result of any individual study is relatively close to the truth.

Contrast this set of results with those depicted in Figure 2B-1(B). Again, the strong study design results in the individual study results being distributed around the truth. However, because the sample size is small and random error is large, the results of individual studies may be far from the truth.

If we think back to our coin flip experiments, this clarifies the difference between the studies in the Figures 2B-1(A) and 2B-1(B). In a series of experiments in which each study involves 10 flips of a true coin, individual results may fall far from the truth, and findings of 70%, or even 80%, heads (or tails) will not be unusual. This situation is analogous to Figure 2B-1(B). If our experiments each involve 1000 coin flips, analogous to Figure 2B-1(A), we will seldom see distributions more extreme than, say, 540, or a 54% probability of heads or tails. With the smaller sample size, individual results are far from the truth; with the larger sample size, they are all close to the truth.

Figures 2B-1(A) and 2B-1(B) illustrate the rationale for pooling results of different studies, a process called *meta-analysis*. Assume that the available evidence about therapeutic effectiveness comes from a series of small RCTs. However, there is a problem: Chance will ensure that the study results vary widely, and we will not know which one to believe. Because of a strong study design, the distribution of the results is centered around the truth. As a result of this favorable situation we can, by pooling the results of the studies, decrease random error and increase the strength of our inferences from the uncertainty of Figure 2B-1(B) to the confidence of Figure 2B-1(A).

In Figure 2B-1(C), the center of the set of dots is far from the truth. This is because studies with observational designs, even large ones, are vulnerable to bias. Since the studies share an identical design, each one will be subject to the same magnitude and direction of bias. The results are very precise with minimal random error; however, they are incorrect.

One real-world example of this phenomenon is the apparent benefit of vitamin E on reducing mortality from coronary artery disease suggested by the results of a number of large observational studies.[5] By contrast, a subsequent very large, well-conducted RCT failed to demonstrate any impact of vitamin E on coronary deaths.[6]

A second example comes from the many large observational studies suggesting a reduction in the relative risk of coronary death of about 35% in women taking postmenopausal hormone replacement therapy.[7] Notably, the first RCT comparing hormone replacement therapy to placebo in women at high risk of coronary events showed no benefit.[8] In both of these situations, the likely explanation is that people with a lower underlying risk of coronary artery disease are the ones who tend to take vitamin E and hormone replacement therapy. Their lower initial risk resulted in a consistently biased estimate of effectiveness.

The situation depicted in Figure 2B-1(C) is a particularly dangerous one because the large size of the studies instills confidence in clinicians that their results are accurate. For example, many clinicians, fed by the consistent results of very large observational studies, still believe the prevailing dogma of the beneficial effect of hormone replacement therapy on coronary artery disease mortality.

Like Figure 2B-1(C), Figure 2B-1(D) depicts a series of observational studies leading to biased results that are far from the truth. However, because the sample sizes are all small, the results vary widely from study to study. One might be tempted to conduct a meta-analysis of these data. This is dangerous because we risk converting imprecise estimates with large random error to precise estimates with small random error; both, however, are biased.

# STRATEGIES FOR REDUCING BIAS: THERAPY AND HARM

We have noted that bias arises from differences in prognostic factors in treatment and control groups at the start of a study, or from differences in prognosis that arise as a study proceeds. What can investigators do to reduce these biases? Table 2B-1 summarizes the available strategies.

**TABLE 2B-1**

## Ways of Reducing Bias in Studies of Therapy and Harm

| Source of Bias | Therapy: Strategy for Reducing Bias | Harm: Strategy for Reducing Bias |
|---|---|---|
| *Differences noted at the start of the study:* | | |
| Treatment and control patients differ in prognosis | Randomization | Statistical adjustment for prognostic factors in the analysis of data |
| *Differences that arise as the study proceeds:* | | |
| Placebo effects | Blinding of patients | Choice of outcomes (eg, mortality) less subject to placebo effects |
| Cointervention | Blinding of caregivers | Documentation of treatment differences and statistical adjustment |
| Bias in assessment of outcome | Blinding of assessors of outcome | Choice of outcomes (eg, mortality) less subject to observer bias |
| Loss to follow-up | Ensuring complete follow-up | Ensuring complete follow-up |

When studying new treatments, investigators often have a great deal of control. They can reduce the likelihood of differences in the distribution of prognostic features in treated and untreated patients at baseline by randomly allocating patients to the two groups. They can markedly reduce placebo effects by administering placebos that are identical in treatment but biologically inert to control group patients. Blinding clinicians to whether patients are receiving active or placebo therapy can eliminate the risk of important cointervention, and blinding outcome assessors minimizes bias in the assessment of event rates.

In general, investigators studying the impact of potentially harmful exposures have far less control than those investigating the effects of potentially beneficial treatments. They must be content to compare patients whose exposure is determined by their choice or circumstances, and they can address potential differences in patients' fate only by statistical adjustment for known prognostic factors. Blinding is impossible, so their best defense against placebo effects and bias in outcome assessment is to choose endpoints, like death, that are less subject to these biases. Investigators addressing both sets of questions can reduce bias by minimizing loss to follow-up (see Table 2B-1).

These general rules do not always apply. Sometimes, investigators find it difficult or impossible to randomize patients to treatment and control groups. Under such circumstances they choose observational study designs, and clinicians must apply the validity criteria developed for questions of harm to such studies.

Similarly, if the potentially harmful exposure is a drug with beneficial effects, investigators may be able to randomize patients to intervention and control groups. In this case, clinicians can apply the validity criteria designed for therapy questions to the study. Whether for issues of therapy or harm, the strength of inference from RCTs will almost invariably be far greater than the strength of inference from observational studies.

# References

1. CIBIS-II Investigators and Committees. The Cardiac Insufficiency Bisoprolol Study II (CIBIS- II): a randomised trial. *Lancet*. 1999;353:9-13.

2. Goldstein LB, Adams R, Becker K, Furberg CD, Gorelick PB, Hademenos G, et al. Primary prevention of ischaemic stroke: a statement for healthcare professionals from the Stroke Council of the American Heart Association. *Stroke*. 2001;32(1):280-299.

3. Gubitz G, Sandercock P, Counsell C. Antiplatelet therapy for acute ischaemic stroke (Cochrane Review). In: *The Cochrane Library*, 1, 2001. Oxford: Update Software.

4. CAPRIE Steering Committee. A randomized, blinded, trial of clopidogrel versus aspirin in patients at risk of ischaemic events (CAPRIE). *Lancet.* 1996;348(9038): 1329-1339.

5. Knekt P, Reunanen A, Jarvinen R, Seppanen R, Heliovaara M, Aromaa A. Antioxidant vitamin intake and coronary mortality in a longitudinal population study. *Am J Epidemiol*. 1994;139:1180-1189.

6. Yusuf S, Dagenais G, Pogue J, Bosch J, Sleight P. Vitamin E supplementation and cardiovascular events in high-risk patients. The Heart Outcomes Prevention Evaluation Study Investigators. *N Engl J Med*. 2000;342:154-160.

7. Stampfer MJ, Colditz GA. Estrogen replacement therapy and coronary heart disease: a quantitative assessment of the epidemiologic evidence. *Prev Med*. 1991;20:47-63.

8. Hulley S, Grady D, Bush T, et al. Randomized trial of estrogen plus progestin for secondary prevention of coronary heart disease in postmenopausal women. Heart and Estrogen/progestin Replacement Study (HERS) Research Group. *JAMA*. 1998;280:605-613.

# THERAPY AND HARM

## Outcomes of Health Services

C. David Naylor and Gordon Guyatt

The following EBM Working Group members also made substantive contributions to this section: Victor Montori and Christina Lacchetti

## IN THIS SECTION

## CLINICAL SCENARIO

### Transurethral vs Open Prostatectomy: Which Is Safer?

**A** 78-year-old retired internist has been complaining of increasing symptoms of benign prostatic hypertrophy. A patient in your practice, he has long-standing hypertension and coronary artery disease, with a history of a remote anterolateral myocardial infarction and coronary artery bypass graft surgery 10 years ago. His left ventricular ejection fraction was recently documented at 30%, and he has started taking an angiotensin-converting enzyme inhibitor and a beta blocker. Rectal examination confirms a moderately enlarged prostate without irregularities, nodularity, or tenderness. As you discuss management options, the patient insists that transurethral prostate surgery is dangerous and that international studies of thousands of patients have proved that, as he puts it, "old-fashioned open prostatectomy is safer than that keyhole surgery." You prescribe a trial of an alpha blocker, terazosin, and arrange to see him in 4 weeks. However, the retired internist sounds so convinced about the relative safety of the two surgical options that you resolve to examine the evidence about the two forms of prostatectomy.

# FINDING THE EVIDENCE

Later, you sit down in the hospital library computer area to search MEDLINE. You start by entering the phrase "explode prostatic hypertrophy," limiting the search to English-language reports on human subjects and then combining the resulting set with "transurethral" and "mortality" as text words. This yields 15 citations. As you browse through the resulting abstracts, two catch your attention. One, from 1990, appears to underscore your patient's concern, and the other, from 1999, suggests that his concern is misplaced.

The first report, by a Danish group,[1] addresses the long-term outcomes of patients with transurethral vs open (suprapubic or transvesical) prostatectomy using hospitalization data linked to vital status data for the entire Danish male population from 1977 to 1985. The study relies on administrative data and a large population-based sample (38,067 men) and shows excessive mortality among patients undergoing transurethral resection of the prostate (TURP). The other report, by Holman et al,[2] uses similar methods and assesses 10-year survival for 18,464 patients undergoing TURP and 1134 patients undergoing open procedures in Western Australia between 1980 and 1995. In the Australian study, the survival rates appear to be roughly equivalent for each of the two surgical modalities.

# ARE THE RESULTS VALID?

During recent decades, changes in health care delivery have broadened the range of groups interested in the outcomes of medical care. Concern with costs, along with dramatic regional or international differences in practice among clinicians and institutions, have focused the attention of administrators and policymakers on the interplay between the processes and outcomes of health services. The evolution of managed care has sharpened interest in measuring and managing the quality of care delivered by individual practitioners, hospitals, and other institutions.

Implicitly, the questions about quality of care—and the best way to deliver that care—are issues of optimal treatment. For example, once a patient's problem is identified, the primary care physician first determines what intervention, if any, should be undertaken. The physician may then face the quality-related issue of choosing a specialist or institution to offer that service. Decisions about what treatment to provide are best made in light of evidence from randomized controlled trials with complete follow-up (see Part 1B, "Therapy and Harm: An Introduction"; and Part 1B1, "Therapy"). However, investigators generally will be unable to randomize patients to different practitioners or hospitals, and focusing on the outcomes associated with these differences in care will require strategies other than randomized trials. Therefore, investigators increasingly have looked to large administrative or other observational databases to examine the outcomes of care associated with different procedures, practitioners, or institutions.

The situation is analogous to assessing potential harm to patients. For example, since it is impossible to randomize people to cigarette smoking or not smoking, or to exposure to various levels of air pollution, scientists consequently use observational studies or "natural experiments" as sources of insight (see Part 1B2, "Harm"). Investigators comparing outcomes of treatment managed by two or more sets of health care practitioners or delivery systems face the same fundamental challenges. However, the scope and importance of observational studies using administrative databases, which have their own particular challenges, are growing. Therefore, we have written this section of our book to address these issues.

Table 2B-2 revisits our criteria for assessing the validity of an article about harm, listing two questions that are most relevant to studies using large databases to examine the impact of health services on patients.

**TABLE 2B-2**

## Two Core Questions to Ask About a Study That Uses an Observational Design to Examine Sources of Difference in Patients' Outcomes

- Did the investigators demonstrate similarity in all known determinates of outcome or adjust for differences in the analysis?
- Were the outcomes measured in the same way in the groups being compared?

## Did the Investigators Demonstrate Similarity in All Known Determinants of Outcome or Adjust for Differences in the Analysis?

Clinicians and health care managers are interested in a variety of determinants of outcome (Table 2B-3). One type of comparison examines differences that may result from variations in quality of care across individual practitioners or institutions providing services in a specific city or region. State agencies now publish some provider-specific or institution-specific outcomes, and researchers sometimes relate these outcomes to the provider-specific or institution-specific volume of the services under scrutiny. This reflects a belief that "practice makes perfect"—that, all things being equal, centers (and, by inference, physicians or surgeons) with a higher caseload will generally achieve better outcomes than lower-volume centers. For example, various studies suggest that the in-hospital postoperative mortality rates after aortic aneurysm surgery,[3] percutaneous transluminal coronary angioplasty,[4] and coronary artery bypass graft surgery[5,6] are lower for centers or surgeons that manage more patients. Intriguingly, the larger centers also tend to treat the sickest patients and, therefore, may appear at first glance to have outcomes that are no better than those of smaller hospitals. This latter point underscores the importance of assessing differences in the characteristics of patients before drawing any inferences about differences in outcomes from nonrandomized or observational studies.

**TABLE 2B-3**

### Factors That May Systematically Affect Outcomes

- **What** service was provided?*
  For example, consider variations among two or more management strategies with respect to use of drugs, doses, devices, type of procedure, and the like.

- **Who** provided the service?
  For example, consider variations among procedural specialists (eg, nurse practitioners vs family physicians); by level of experience (eg, house staff vs qualified specialists); and by volume of service delivered (eg, high-caseload vs low-caseload practitioners).

- **Where** was the service provided?
  For example, consider variations among hospitals or clinics; among wards in a hospital; between a step-down unit and a conventional intensive care unit; between home and hospital care; by city; by county; and by region or nation.

- **When** was the service provided?
  For example, consider variations in timing of service (eg, during the day vs during the evening; on a weekend vs during the week; the July phenomenon for house staff effects); according to length of stay in the hospital; and across months (seasonal effects) or years (broad temporal trends).

---

* These questions are best addressed using randomized controlled trial methods.

The greater the difference between service settings being compared, the more difficult it is to be sure that patients were similar. It also is difficult to isolate which aspects, if any, of the process of care relate to the outcomes observed. This is especially true when comparisons are made on a broad geographic footing between regions or countries in which populations and processes of care differ in many ways. One such study compared outcomes of Canadian and US patients enrolled in a major trial of thrombolytic therapy for acute myocardial infarction.[7] Rates of revascularization and use of specialist services were much higher in the United States. The investigators observed that in terms of symptoms, functional status, psychological well-being, and health-related quality of life, Canadian patients fared somewhat worse than their US counterparts—a finding of obvious concern to Canadian practitioners. However, some of the difference may exist because the patients recruited by Canadian investigators were destined for worse outcomes regardless of management.

Along with these cross-sectional comparisons, investigators sometimes use observational data on a before/after basis within the same locale to draw inferences about interventions to improve quality of care. A *before-after trial* is an investigation of an intervention in which the investigators compare the status of patients before and after the intervention. For instance, Hannan et al[8] reported on the apparent consequences of a New York program in which two documents were made public: hospital-level mortality outcomes associated with coronary artery bypass surgery and individual surgeon mortality profiles. The authors attributed the reduction in adjusted mortality rate (from 4.17% to 2.45%) to the intervention. O'Connor and colleagues[9] documented a similar reduction in mortality associated with monitoring outcomes and providing an intensive quality improvement program in five New England hospitals.

However, attribution of the reduced mortality rate in these before/after studies to the publicizing of hospital- or surgeon-specific mortality outcomes—or to the introduction of local quality-control programs—assumes that there were no other concurrent changes that could explain the large differences in health outcomes. Ghali et al[10] subsequently examined coronary artery bypass surgery in other states that did not monitor outcomes, release results, or institute large-scale quality-control programs and found mortality reductions over the same time period that were similar to those for the two other studies. These results vividly illustrate that, regardless of whether outcomes are tracked on a large scale with population-based administrative data sets or in smaller clinical studies, a before/after design is a weak source of evidence from which to draw causal inferences.

A third source of variation in outcomes that may occur within similar health systems is the type of treatment provided. This is the sort of comparison that was made in the outcome studies of TURP vs open prostatectomy described in this section's opening clinical scenario. Comparisons of different treatments provided to patients within a single health system avoid broad health system effects and sociocultural or even genetic differences that threaten the comparisons of populations from different health systems. However, it is still possible that differences in the prognostic features of patients receiving the alternative management strategies may be responsible for differences in outcome. Without randomization, patients will inevitably differ in ways other than the treatment being provided to them (a phenomenon known as *selection bias*).

When two alternative procedures are being compared in research, selection bias arises from the exercise of good clinical judgment in routine practice. For example, urologists may choose younger, healthier patients to undergo the more extensive open prostatectomy, and they may select older, sicker patients for TURP (see the discussion of channeling bias in Part 1B2, "Harm"). Conversely, open prostatectomy may be reserved for patients with more severe or acute symptoms, so that TURP, by default, is applied more often in elective surgery on younger patients. In either case, patients end up differing in obvious or subtle ways that affect their likelihood of having a good or bad outcome—a problem epidemiologists call a *confounding variable*, which is a factor that distorts the true relationship of the study variable of interest by also being related to the outcome of interest. The validity of any form of observational research is threatened by case selection biases that create noncomparable groups of patients that confound any comparisons of outcomes.

Researchers must therefore adjust for differences between groups of patients. The sophistication of these so-called risk adjustment methods is growing rapidly.[11] However, researchers and quality-of-care evaluators will not know all the prognostic factors that interact with treatments to affect outcomes. Randomization is important because it distributes these unknown factors in an unbiased manner.

The problem is exacerbated when one considers that not all known prognostic features may have been measured, and if they have been measured, they may not have been measured or recorded accurately. Inaccurate measurement or recording is a particular concern when information comes from administrative databases. For instance, Jollis et al[12] compared information about cardiac risk factors in an administrative database in patients undergoing angiography with information collected prospectively from a clinical database by a cardiac fellow who actually saw the patients. A chance-corrected measure of agreement between the resident's assessment and the information from the database (the kappa value) showed good agreement only for diabetes (83% agreement) and for acute myocardial infarction (76%); agreement was moderate for the presence of hypertension (56%), poor for patients with the presence of heart failure (39%), and no better than chance (9%) for patients with unstable angina. Hannan et al[13] found similar discrepancies in comparing a cardiac surgery registry to an administrative database in the state of New York. These inaccuracies mattered; the ability of evaluators to predict mortality clearly was better with the detailed clinical data than with the administrative database.[13] In a third example, Green and Wintfeld[14] compared hospital administrative records with a chart audit and found errors in principal diagnosis in 9% of the charts, errors in comorbidity in 14.9%, and errors in classification of the urgency of surgery in 45.5%. Furthermore, error rates differed by hospital, suggesting a serious threat to the validity of any attempts to compare hospital performance. Thus, the accuracy, reproducibility, and fairness of adjustments for differences in patients can be undermined by poor data quality.

The problem of limited or inaccurate data in insurance databases or computerized hospital discharge abstracts may be partly ameliorated by supplementing the information with chart audits.[15] This is time consuming and expensive, but it may be the only way to reduce the chances of missing or misconstruing important differences among groups of patients. A more efficient mechanism may be to establish specific registry mechanisms geared to measuring key patient characteristics, process-of-care elements, and relevant outcomes.[16]

How, then, can you best assure yourself that, short of randomization, investigators have made the fairest possible outcome comparison possible? We summarize the steps in Table 2B-4. First, did the researchers convince you, through their review of the literature and on the basis of what you know about the determinants of prognosis, that they measured all of the important prognostic factors? This is more likely to occur if the analysis involves chart audits or, better still, a specific clinical registry, as opposed to reliance on available administrative data. Second, since these measurements are only as good as the data that go into them, you should consider whether these measures of patients' prognostic factors are reproducible and accurate. Third, did they show the extent to which the groups being compared differed on the prognostic factors that they measured? Fourth, did the researchers use some form of *multivariate analysis* wherein they tried to adjust simultaneously not only for the obvious prognostic factors, but also for other more subtle differences that may have confounded the comparisons? And finally, did additional analyses demonstrate the same results as the primary analysis?

**TABLE 2B-4**

**Determining Whether Differences in Prognosis, Rather Than Differences in the Intervention, Explain Differences in Outcomes**

- Were all important prognostic factors measured?
- Were measures of patients' prognostic factors reproducible and accurate?
- To what extent were patients similar with respect to these factors?
- Was multivariate analysis used to adjust for imbalances in prognostic factors?
- Did additional analyses (particularly in low-risk subgroups) demonstrate the same results as the primary analysis?

Localio and colleagues[17] have reported on the consequences of not taking into account all possible prognostic factors. In that study, a large corporation's managed care program sought to determine which of the hospitals serving the corporation's employees delivered better quality of care, as reflected in part by fewer in-hospital deaths. A consultant concluded that the hospitals differed, and this conclusion influenced the company's decisions regarding choice of hospitals. However, an analysis conducted by a group of academic investigators concluded that the difference between even the hospital with the worst record and the rest of the hospitals could be easily attributable to the play of chance. Furthermore, when the investigators included an adjustment for age, a prognostic factor that had been excluded from the consultant's initial analysis, the rank order of the hospitals changed,[18] suggesting that hospitals with worse outcomes may have been selected to receive contracts from the company.

Because observational data are so susceptible to selection biases that may confound the outcome comparisons, researchers should determine whether their results persist when they analyze the data in different ways. For example, if there is a severe imbalance in allocation of patients with a particularly important prognostic factor, it may make sense to eliminate all patients with that factor and then repeat the analyses. Unfortunately, even relative balance on a prognostic factor does not guarantee comparability. One reason is that administrative data and registries tend to use fairly simple categories, such as whether a disease is or is not present. Yet "disease present" may be associated with a wide range of underlying dysfunction and, consequently, equally variable prognosis. Chronic lung disease or chronic heart failure, for instance, can vary from mild to severe, with very different prognostic implications. Thus, apparent balance on the proportion of patients with these diagnoses can mask a situation in which one group has many more severely affected patients than the other group. This is even true for advanced age as a prognostic factor, since elderly persons may vary considerably in their overall robustness.

Because of this problem, a useful double-check mechanism in any outcome comparison is to ensure that the findings are replicable within a relatively low-risk subgroup of the patients being examined. By eliminating patients in categories associated with widely varying physiologic states, we increase the likelihood of a "level playing field" for comparisons. If the results of such an analysis differ from the adjusted analysis taking all patients into consideration, clinicians' skepticism about the results should increase.[19]

How do our two studies of prostate surgery measure up with regard to demonstrating comparability of populations? Andersen et al[1] considered patients' age at surgery, but relied only on diagnoses coded in the computerized hospital records as indicating compromised health status. Even with these limited data, fewer patients with open prostatectomy had high-risk diagnoses. They were also younger and had less heart disease and cancer. In a multivariate analysis to try to adjust for these differences, it did appear that TURP continued to confer a 30% to 40% relative increase in the risk of death over several years of follow-up. Extensive sensitivity analyses were performed, including a specific examination of low-risk patients (described as "healthiest men"). Although low-risk patients also showed an excess risk with TURP, the relative magnitude of the increased risk of death was smaller for low-risk patients than for high-risk patients. As Andersen et al[1] stated: "The extent to which this difference is attributable to the surgical intervention itself remains an open question. The two groups of patients are quite different with regard to age and preoperative health status, and available data may not be sufficient to control such differences through statistical analysis."

Holman et al[2] also used administrative and registry data, linking hospital records, death records, and prostate cancer registrations for the entire state of Western Australia. Like Andersen et al,[1] they characterized patients by using diagnostic codes from hospital discharge abstracts. They also examined hospital bed-days in the year prior to the index prostatectomy as a further measure of comorbid disease. In contrast to the Danish study, the crude mortality ratio significantly favored TURP in this study (relative risk [RR] 0.87; 95% confidence interval [CI], 0.78-0.97). However, because practices shifted dramatically over time, Holman et al[2] found far more TURP patients in the later years of their study, when outcomes in general were better. These patients were younger and more likely to be undergoing prostatectomy electively. After investigators adjusted for these factors, open prostatectomy appeared to be significantly safer. This effect disappeared after adjusting for comorbidity differences between the two populations. This story again demonstrates the vulnerability of observational studies to the adjustment procedures the investigators undertake. In the Holman et al study, the bottom line is that the most sophisticated adjustment suggested no mortality difference between the two procedures.

### Were the Outcomes Measured in the Same Way in the Groups Being Compared?

Many large databases are not designed for clinical research, and just as we have shown that they may mismeasure patients' risk factors, they may also mismeasure outcomes. This further emphasizes that clinicians should note the quality and comprehensiveness of the data source. Ideally, there should be independent cross-checks to ensure that the same outcomes are measured consistently and completely for whatever unit of comparison is used, eg, for verifying that data on ascertainment or cause of death are accurate or for confirming hospital readmission rates after a specific surgical procedure in a quality-of-care study.

How did the two studies of prostate surgery perform in these respects? Andersen et al[1] used vital status data for the entire population of Denmark, whereas Holman et al[2] used vital status data for Western Australia. Therefore, mortality was measured in a reliable and unbiased fashion across all groups for comparison.

# WILL THE RESULTS HELP ME IN CARING FOR PATIENTS IN MY PRACTICE?

A randomized controlled trial must have valid and reliable outcome measures; so must any observational study assessing patients' outcomes. The easiest outcomes for health researchers to measure are those that are defined objectively and that usually are identified in large insurance databases or computerized hospital administrative data, eg, death, routinely coded in-hospital surgical complications, or readmissions. Investigators may also use vital status registries to track out-of-hospital deaths. However, other outcomes, eg, disability, discomfort, distress, and dissatisfaction,[20] are important to patients. Functional status and quality-of-life measures can capture these burdens, but these measures typically are not applied in routine medical care; if they are applied, their results often are not incorporated into administrative databases. Moreover, incorporating these measures into routine care and administrative databases may generate more questions than answers. Researchers have begun to understand some of the factors that predict, say, increased risk of mortality after various types of elective surgery. However, our understanding of the factors that predict functional status and quality of life is far more limited.

Returning to the studies of prostatectomy, the complete resection attained by the open procedure eliminates the need for repeat procedures, as frequently occurs with TURPs. However, neither study compared the two procedures with respect to various other outcomes of interest to patients and physicians, eg, effectiveness in relieving obstructive or irritative symptoms of benign prostatic hypertrophy, overall recovery time, rates of complications such as impotence or incontinence, and so forth. Careful prospective data collection is necessary to capture these outcomes and to provide a more complete tally of the burdens and benefits of the two treatments being compared.

# CLINICAL RESOLUTION

Given the limitations of observational studies using large administrative databases, can we better define the role of this sort of health services research? Observational studies do remain important in the generation of hypotheses about causal pathways from a pathophysiologic standpoint. Furthermore, randomized trials are expensive, are difficult to conduct, and cannot be undertaken for all clinical questions in which practitioners are interested. Observational studies may identify situations in which one type of therapy appears so much better than an alternative that bias would be a very unlikely explanation for the difference. In addition, the hypothesis-generating role of observational studies is illustrated by the example of open prostatectomy. Unfortunately, the convenience of transurethral surgery, together with deeply held beliefs about its safety, probably precludes ever mounting a large-scale trial comparing transurethral surgery and open prostatectomy. Finally, if the outcomes of interest are rare, such as unusual idiosyncratic side effects of a drug, researchers can obtain adequate sample sizes only through the use of administrative databases.

There are other situations in which randomization is not feasible, such as when looking for systematic variations in outcomes of similar procedures provided by different practitioners or institutions ("who" or "where," rather than "what"; see Table 2B-3). It is untenable to assume that all hospitals or clinicians practice equally well, and observational outcome comparisons have a role in assessing quality of care. This is especially applicable for some well-defined services (eg, coronary artery bypass grafts) for which there are validated risk-adjustment algorithms[21-24] and dedicated registries to measure risk factors and outcomes, probably rendering these comparisons meaningful. In general, however, potential harm to patients from poor-quality care must be weighed against the harm to skilled health workers and fine institutions caused by poorly founded inferences about inferior outcomes.

Given the relatively weak inferences possible from most observational studies of outcomes, alternative strategies for ensuring the quality of medical care should always be considered. For some—though certainly not all (see Part 2F, "Moving

From Evidence to Action, Clinical Utilization Review")—processes of care, we can accurately document what occurred and make confident judgments about appropriateness. For example, randomized trials show that preoperative antibiotic and antithrombotic prophylaxis improves patients' outcomes after various surgical procedures.[25-28] The systematic omission of these treatments puts patients at risk and indicates a need for practitioners and institutions to improve their quality of care. Certainly for medical (as opposed to surgical) services, we suggest that in many instances it is most efficient to use randomized trials or meta-analyses of trials to establish optimal management strategies. Furthermore, it is important to ensure that quality of care is maintained by monitoring the process of care so that well-proven practices are consistently applied to eligible patients. The role of observational outcome monitoring as a quality enhancement tool is more important, however, for procedures where a high degree of technical skill is required.

What, then, of the 78-year-old patient? Perhaps predictably, given what we know about the limitations of observational studies, your exploration has been inconclusive. Indeed, had you looked back at other studies, the relevant literature would not have provided a definitive conclusion. Related work[29,30] on elevated mortality after TURP as opposed to open prostatectomy has incorporated extra detail on differences among patients drawn from chart reviews and has failed to eliminate the excess mortality seen with TURP. However, other studies[31-33] using a variety of data sources have shown no increased risk with TURP, and their authors have argued that the apparent excess is an artifact of incomplete adjustment for differences in the populations of patients undergoing the two procedures.

One very small randomized trial from 1987 has shown a trend to excess mortality with TURP.[34] A 1999 report[35] is described in its abstract as a "randomized prospective study." However, the assignment to open prostatectomy vs TURP was made on the basis of the size of the prostate on ultrasonographic examination. The groups appeared balanced prognostically, with the exception of past cerebrovascular accident, which occurred significantly more often in the open prostatectomy group. Overall mortality again was nonsignificantly higher in the TURP group. In conclusion, there has been no definitive trial comparing the two forms of surgery, and TURP remains the predominant procedure for benign prostatic hypertrophy.

The retired internist returns in 4 weeks as planned. "Was I right about the risks of the keyhole method?" he asks. You admit that the abandonment of open prostatectomy may have been premature, but you caution that the severity of his cardiac dysfunction makes him a poor candidate for the more extensive procedure, even if you could find a urologist competent to do it. Hearing your own advice, you again appreciate that similar selection biases may be the real reasons for the apparently higher mortality after TURP. Fortunately, your patient has had an excellent response to the alpha blocker, and the issue of prostatectomy can be set aside for some time. As you usher him from the office, he grumbles: "By the way, did you see that the operative mortalities for all the local heart surgeons are on the front page of the newspaper? Thank heavens I retired."

# References

1. Andersen TF, Bronnum-Hansen H, Sejr T, Roepstorff C. Elevated mortality following transurethral resection of the prostate for benign hypertrophy! But why? *Med Care*. 1990;28:870-881.

2. Holman CD, Wisniewski ZS, Semmens JB, Rouse IL, Bass AJ. Mortality and prostate cancer risk in 19,598 men after surgery for benign prostatic hyperplasia. *BJU Int*. 1999;84:37-42.

3. Hannan EL, Kilburn H Jr, O'Donnell JF, et al. A longitudinal analysis of the relationship between in-hospital mortality in New York State and the volume of abdominal aortic aneurysm surgeries performed. *Health Serv Res*. 1992;27:517-542.

4. Jollis JG, Peterson ED, DeLong ER, et al. The relation between the volume of coronary angioplasty procedures at hospitals treating Medicare beneficiaries and short-term mortality. *N Engl J Med*. 1994;331:1625-1629.

5. Showstack JA, Rosenfeld KE, Garnick DW, Luft HS, Schaffarzick RW, Fowles J. Association of volume with outcome of coronary artery bypass graft surgery: scheduled vs nonscheduled operations. *JAMA*. 1987;257:785-789.

6. Hannan EL, Kilburn H Jr, Bernard H, O'Donnell JF, Lukacik G, Shields EP. Coronary artery bypass surgery: the relationship between inhospital mortality rate and surgical volume after controlling for clinical risk factors. *Med Care*. 1991;29:1094-1107.

7. Mark DB, Naylor CD, Hlatky MA, et al. Use of medical resources and quality of life after acute myocardial infarction in Canada and the United States. *N Engl J Med*. 1994;331:1130-1135.

8. Hannan EL, Kilburn H Jr, Racz M, Shields E, Chassin MR. Improving the outcomes of coronary artery bypass surgery in New York State. *JAMA*. 1994;271:761-766.

9. O'Connor GT, Plume SK, Olmstead EM, et al, for the Northern New England Cardiovascular Disease Study Group. A regional intervention to improve the hospital mortality associated with coronary artery bypass graft surgery. *JAMA*. 1996;275:841-846.

10. Ghali WA, Ash AS, Hall RE, Moskowitz MA. Statewide quality improvement initiatives and mortality after cardiac surgery. *JAMA*. 1997;277:379-382.

11. Daley J, Shwartz M. Developing risk-adjustment methods. In: Iezzoni LI, ed. *Risk Adjustment for Measuring Health Care Outcomes*. Ann Arbor: Health Administration Press; 1994:199-238.

12. Jollis JG, Ancukiewicz M, DeLong ER, Pryor DB, Muhlbaier LH, Mark DB. Discordance of databases designed for claims payment versus clinical information systems: implications for outcomes research. *Ann Intern Med*. 1993;119:844-850.

13. Hannan EL, Kilburn H Jr, Lindsey ML, Lewis R. Clinical versus administrative data bases for CABG surgery: does it matter? *Med Care*. 1992;30:892-907.

14. Green J, Wintfeld N. How accurate are hospital discharge data for evaluating effectiveness of care? *Med Care.* 1993;31:719-731.

15. Malenka DJ, McLerran D, Roos N, Fisher ES, Wennberg JE. Using administrative data to describe casemix: a comparison with the medical record. *J Clin Epidemiol.* 1994;47:1027-1032.

16. Smith SA, Murphy ME, Huschka TR, et al. Impact of a diabetes electronic management system on the care of patients seen in a subspecialty diabetes clinic. *Diabetes Care.* 1998;21:972-976.

17. Localio AR, Hamory BH, Sharp TJ, Weaver SL, TenHave TR, Landis JR. Comparing hospital mortality in adult patients with pneumonia: a case study of statistical methods in a managed care program. *Ann Intern Med.* 1995;122:125-132.

18. Wu AW. The measure and mismeasure of hospital quality: appropriate risk-adjustment methods in comparing hospitals. *Ann Intern Med.* 1995;122:149-150.

19. Wen SW, Hernandez R, Naylor CD. Pitfalls in nonrandomized outcomes studies: the case of incidental appendectomy with open cholecystectomy. *JAMA.* 1995;274:1687-1691.

20. White KL. Improved medical care statistics and the health services system. *Public Health Rep.* 1967;82:847-854.

21. Tu JV, Jaglal SB, Naylor CD, and the Steering Committee of the Provincial Adult Cardiac Care Network of Ontario. Multicenter validation of a risk index for mortality, intensive care unit stay, and overall hospital length of stay after cardiac surgery. *Circulation.* 1995;91:677-684.

22. O'Connor GT, Plume SK, Olmstead EM, et al, for the Northern New England Cardiovascular Disease Study Group. Multivariate prediction of in-hospital mortality associated with coronary artery bypass graft surgery. *Circulation.* 1992;85:2110-2118.

23. Higgins TL, Estafanous FG, Loop FD, Beck GJ, Blum JM, Paranandi L. Stratification of morbidity and mortality outcome by preoperative risk factors in coronary artery bypass patients: a clinical severity score. *JAMA.* 1992;267:2344-2348.

24. Edwards FH, Clark RE, Schwartz M. Coronary artery bypass grafting: the Society of Thoracic Surgeons National Database experience. *Ann Thorac Surg.* 1994;57:12-19.

25. Gadallah MF, Ramdeen G, Mignone J, Patel D, Mitchell L, Tatro S. Role of preoperative antibiotic prophylaxis in preventing postoperative peritonitis in newly placed peritoneal dialysis catheters. *Am J Kidney Dis.* 2000;36(5):1014-1019.

26. Dent CD, Olson JW, Farish SE, Bellome J, Casino AJ, Morris HF, et al. The influence of preoperative antibiotics on success of endosseous implants up to and including state II surgery: a study of 2,641 implants. *J Oral Maxillofac Surg.* 1997;55(12 Suppl 5):19-24.

27. Zibari GB, Gadallah MF, Landreneau M, McMillan R, Bridges RM, Costley K, et al. Preoperative vancomycin prophylaxis decreases incidence of postoperative hemodialysis vascular access infections. *Am J Kidney Dis.* 1997;30(3):343-348.

28. Plares A, Vochelle N, Darmon JY, Fagola M, Bellaud M, Huet Y. Risk of deep-venous thrombosis after hospital discharge in patients having undergone total hip replacement: double-blind randomized comparison of enoxaparin versus placebo. *Lancet.* 1996;348(9022):224-228.

29. Roos NP, Wennberg JE, Malenka DJ, et al. Mortality and reoperation after open and transurethral resection of the prostate for benign prostatic hyperplasia. *N Engl J Med.* 1989;320:1120-1124.

30. Malenka DJ, Roos N, Fisher ES, et al. Further study of the increased mortality following transurethral prostatectomy: a chart-based analysis. *J Urol.* 1990;144:224-228.

31. Concato J, Horwitz RI, Feinstein AR, Elmore JG, Schiff SF. Problems of comorbidity in mortality after prostatectomy. *JAMA.* 1992;267:1077-1082.

32. Koshiba K, Egawa S, Ohori M, Uchida T, Yokoyama E, Shoji K. Does transurethral resection of the prostate pose a risk to life? 22-year outcome. *J Urol.* 1995;153:1506-1509.

33. Crowley AR, Horowitz M, Chan E, Macchia RJ. Transurethral resection of the prostate versus open prostatectomy: long-term mortality comparison. *J Urol.* 1995;153:695-697.

34. Meyhoff HH. Transurethral versus transvesical prostatectomy: clinical, urodynamic, renographic and economic aspects. A randomized study. *Scand J Urol Nephrol Suppl.* 1987;102:1-26.

35. Shalev M, Richter S, Kessler O, Shpitz B, Fredman B, Nissenkorn I. Long-term incidence of acute myocardial infarction after open and transurethral resection of the prostate for benign prostatic hyperplasia [published erratum appears in *J Urol.* 1999;161:1287]. *J Urol.* 1999;161:491-493.

# 2B1

# THERAPY AND VALIDITY

## Surprising Results of Randomized Controlled Trials

### Christina Lacchetti and Gordon Guyatt

The following EBM Working Group members also made substantive contributions to this section: Deborah Cook, Thomas Newman, Peter Wyer, and Jonathan Craig

## IN THIS SECTION

Surrogate Endpoints and Observational Studies Provide Weaker Evidence Than Randomized Controlled Trials of Patient-Important Endpoints

When Randomized Controlled Trial Results Have Contradicted Those of Studies of Physiologic or Surrogate Endpoints

When Randomized Controlled Trial Results Have Contradicted Those of Observational Studies of Patient-Important Endpoints

Conclusion

# SURROGATE ENDPOINTS AND OBSERVATIONAL STUDIES PROVIDE WEAKER EVIDENCE THAN RANDOMIZED CONTROLLED TRIALS OF PATIENT-IMPORTANT ENDPOINTS

Ideally, evidence of the effectiveness of diagnostic, preventive, or therapeutic interventions will come from rigorous randomized controlled trials (RCTs) measuring effects on patient-relevant outcomes. Historically, however, clinicians have often relied on weaker evidence. Evidence may be weaker in two ways. First, the methodology may be pristine—as is the case in rigorous RCTs—but the participants may not be identical to those of interest or the outcomes may not be important to patients. For instance, demonstrating that a type of therapy hastens the resolution of experimentally induced renal failure in rats is provocative, but it provides weak evidence for administration of that therapy to human beings. Similarly, demonstrating the effect of an intervention on cardiac output or pulmonary capillary wedge pressure may herald the introduction of a beneficial drug for patients with heart failure, but trials examining quality of life, frequency of hospitalization, and mortality are imperative before clinicians can confidently offer the medication to patients.

Evidence is also weak if investigators examine the apparent effect of a drug, device, procedure, or program on patient-important outcomes such as stroke, myocardial infarction, or death, but do so using observational study designs. Evidence may suffer from both limitations. Investigators have used observational study designs to test the effects of interventions on other species, or on physiologic (but not patient-important) outcomes in human beings.

Our message is not to dismiss weaker forms of evidence. Physiologic or observational studies may occasionally provide such compelling results that they mandate clinical use of an intervention. Often, they provide the best evidence we have available. We do emphasize, however, that when clinicians rely on weak evidence, they acknowledge the risk of administering useless or even harmful interventions. Our concern arises from examples of conclusions clinicians have drawn based on physiologic or observational studies subsequently refuted by RCTs.

# WHEN RANDOMIZED CONTROLLED TRIAL RESULTS HAVE CONTRADICTED THOSE OF STUDIES OF PHYSIOLOGIC OR SURROGATE ENDPOINTS

In the following sections we present examples of instances in which RCT results contradicted those of prior studies. We have categorized the examples according to whether prior evidence came from studies of surrogate or substitute endpoints—either from randomized trials or observational studies (Table 2B1-1)—or whether investigators focused on patient-important endpoints but used observational study designs (Table 2B1-2). Both tables suggest the same message: clinician, beware! We begin with demonstrating the limitations of physiologic evidence, or use of surrogate endpoints. Note that values, relative risk (RR), odds ratio (OR), confidence interval (CI), and hazard ratio, are expressed here as originally reported in the primary source.

**TABLE 2B1-1**

## Prior Evidence From Studies of Physiologic or Surrogate Endpoints*

| Question | Evidence From Different Endpoints | RCT Evidence of Clinically Important Endpoints |
| --- | --- | --- |
| In patients with chronic heart failure, what impact does beta-adrenergic blockade have on mortality? | In a before/after study of 8 patients scheduled for cardiac catheterization, patients received intravenous propranolol through pulmonary artery catheter. Results in 4 patients, all of whom had advanced coronary artery disease with previous myocardial infarction, demonstrated declines in ejection fraction (range, 0.05-0.22) and increases in end-diastolic volume (range, 30-135 mL). Furthermore, abnormalities of wall motion after propranolol developed in 2 of 4 patients. Investigators suggested that "results are consistent with the thesis that beta adrenergic blocking drugs may inhibit compensatory sympathetic mechanisms."[1] | Authors of a meta-analysis of 18 RCTs of beta-blockers in patients with heart failure found a 32% reduction in the RR of death (95% CI, 12%-47%; $P$=.003) and a 41% reduction in the RR of hospitalization for heart failure (95% CI, 26%-52%; $P$<.001) in patients treated with a beta blocker. When morbidity and mortality were combined, there was a 37% reduction in risk (95% CI, 24%-49%; $P$<.001). In addition, patients assigned to a beta blocker were 32% more likely to experience an improvement in NYHA class (95% CI, 1%-74%; $P$=.04) and 30% less likely to experience worsening of NYHA class (95% CI, 4%-50%; $P$=.03).[2] |
| What effect does treatment with dopamine have on acute renal failure? | Investigators randomized rats to receive or not receive dopamine at the time of initiation of anoxic acute renal failure. Results suggested dopamine partially reduced the severity of acute renal failure, as evidenced by a reduction in blood urea and serum creatinine ($P$<.05) as well as an increase in glomerular filtration rate ($P$<.05).[3] | An RCT exploring the relationship between low-dose dopamine and outcomes in acute renal failure in 256 patients found the RR of death associated with the administration of low-dose dopamine was 1.11 (95% CI, 0.66-1.89). The RR of death or dialysis associated with the administration of low-dose dopamine was 1.10 (95% CI, 0.71-1.71). Researchers conclude that "there is insufficient evidence that low-dose dopamine improves survival or obviates the need for dialysis in persons with acute renal failure. The routine use of low-dose dopamine should be discouraged."[4] |

| Question | Evidence From Different Endpoints | RCT Evidence of Clinically Important Endpoints |
|---|---|---|
| What impact does clofibrate have on mortality in men without clinically evident ischemic heart disease? | A before/after study of the effects of clofibrate on total and beta-cholesterol found, after a 4-week treatment regimen with 750–1500 mg of clofibrate, a significant reduction in total cholesterol in 86% of patients (30/35), and a significant decrease in beta-cholesterol in 91% of patients (21/23). Furthermore, in every case, the tolerance to clofibrate was excellent and no side effects could be observed.[5] | An RCT of men without clinical ischemic heart disease classified participants into three equal groups according to serum cholesterol levels. Participants in the upper third of the cholesterol distribution were randomly allocated to clofibrate therapy or placebo. Fifty percent of the men in the lower third constituted a second control group, which also received placebo. All others were not studied. After a mean observation of 9.6 years, there were 20% fewer incidents of ischemic heart disease in the clofibrate group compared with those in the high-cholesterol control group (P<.05). However, there were 25% more deaths in the clofibrate-treated group than in the comparable high serum cholesterol control group (P<.01).[6] |
| In patients at risk for cardiovascular disease, what effect do multifactorial prevention approaches have on mortality? | An RCT of 19,390 male Belgian industrial workers, aged 40-59 years, paired and randomized 30 industries to receive a health counseling program (directed at such risk factors as serum cholesterol, smoking, hypertension, obesity, and sedentary habits) or to receive no such program. Results: high-risk intervention subjects averaged a drop of 7.8% and 3.9% in systolic blood pressure and serum cholesterol, respectively, compared with a 3.4% drop and a 0.4% increase, respectively, in controls (P<.001). Ultimately, the overall coronary risk profile after 2 years for high-risk subjects was decreased by an average of 20% in the intervention group, compared with an average increase of 12.5% in the control group (P<.001).[7] | An RCT randomly assigned 1222 healthy businessmen with cardiovascular disease risk factors to either receive treatment with dietetic-hygienic measures and, frequently, with hypolipidemic and antihypertensive drugs or to receive no treatment. Results: total coronary events were reduced by 46% in the intervention group as compared with the controls. However, total mortality was 10.9% in the intervention group and 7.5% in the control group (RR, 1.45; 95% CI, 1.01-2.08; P=.048). Furthermore, mortality attributed to coronary artery disease was 5.6% and 2.3% in the intervention and control groups, respectively (RR, 2.42; 95% CI, 1.31-4.46; P=.001).[8] |

| Question | Evidence From Different Endpoints | RCT Evidence of Clinically Important Endpoints |
|---|---|---|
| What impact do steroids have on the mortality of patients with sepsis? | An experiment, making use of a methylprednisolone sodium succinate (MPSS) and gentamicin sulfate (GS) regimen that prevented death in baboons given a 2-hour infusion of *E coli,* attempted to determine survival of baboons if MPSS and GS treatment was delayed until all organisms were infused and severe hypotension had ensued. Results: all nontreated baboons died, whereas 6 (86%) of 7 treated animals survived. Baboons with delayed MPSS, however, demonstrated diminished perfusion and recovered more slowly than those with earlier MPSS treatment. Investigators concluded that "primates in septic shock are clearly protected with delayed steroid/antibiotic therapy."[9] | A meta-analysis of 9 RCTs of corticosteroid therapy for sepsis and septic shock among critically ill adults showed a trend toward increased mortality, with an RR of 1.13 (95% CI, 0.99-1.29). Data also suggested no beneficial effect in patients with septic shock (RR, 1.07; 95% CI, 0.91-1.26). Although no difference in secondary infection rates was demonstrated in corticosteroid-treated patients with sepsis or septic shock, there was a trend toward increased mortality from secondary infections in patients receiving corticosteroids (RR, 1.70; 95% CI, 0.79-1.73).[10] |
| Do the antiarrhythmic drugs encainide and flecainide affect mortality from ventricular arrhythmias in patients after myocardial infarction? | A before/after study of patients with symptomatic, recurrent, previously drug-refractory ventricular tachycardia found encainide completely eliminated recurrence of ventricular tachycardia in 54% of patients for 6 months of therapy and in 29% of patients for 18-30 months of therapy. Investigators concluded that "encainide is a safe, well-tolerated antiarrhythmic agent."[11] | An RCT evaluating the effect of encainide and flecainide in survivors of acute myocardial infarction with ventricular ectopy found a RR of 2.64 (95% CI, 1.60-4.36) for cardiac deaths and cardiac arrests among patients on active drug vs those on placebo.[12] |
| In patients with congestive heart failure, does spironolactone alter mortality when combined with an angiotensin-converting enzyme (ACE) inhibitor? | Authors of a before/after study of 5 patients on treatment regimens of potassium-sparing diuretics and potassium supplements for hypertension or congestive heart failure and captopril, an ACE inhibitor, found a statistically significant increase in serum potassium levels (*P*<.05) once captopril was added to the regimen. Furthermore, laboratory-diagnosed hyperkalemia occurred in 60% of patients.[13] | Investigators randomized 1663 patients with severe heart failure who were being treated with an ACE inhibitor, a loop diuretic, and, in most cases, digoxin to receive 25 mg of spironolactone daily or placebo. Results showed an RR of death among patients in the spironolactone group of 0.70 (95% CI, 0.60-0.82; *P*<.001). The frequency of hospitalization for worsening heart failure was 35% lower in the spironolactone group than in the placebo group (RR, 0.65; 95% CI, 0.54-0.77; *P*<.001).[14] |

| Question | Evidence From Different Endpoints | RCT Evidence of Clinically Important Endpoints |
|---|---|---|
| In patients with chronic heart failure, does treatment with milrinone alter mortality? | A before/after study of the effects of milrinone on the hemodynamic responses to treadmill exercise in 12 patients with congestive heart failure found 4 weeks' treatment with 20 mg daily milrinone produced an improvement in left ventricular function during exercise, as reflected by significant changes in cardiac index, stroke volume index, and pulmonary capillary wedge pressure ($P<.001$). Systemic oxygen consumption also increased ($P<.05$), as did maximum exercise capacity ($P<.001$). The beneficial effects of milrinone on exercise hemodynamics and tolerance were sustained throughout the 4-week treatment period. No drug-related side effects occurred.[15] | In an RCT of 1088 patients with severe chronic heart failure and advanced left ventricular dysfunction, milrinone treatment (as compared with placebo) was associated with a 28% relative increase in overall mortality (95% CI, 1%-61%; $P = .038$) and a 34% increase in cardiovascular mortality (95% CI, 6%-69%; $P = .016$). The effect of milrinone was adverse in all predefined subgroups, including those defined by left ventricular fraction, cause of heart failure, functional class, serum sodium and creatinine levels, age, sex, angina, cardiothoracic ratio, or ventricular tachycardia.[16] |
| What is the relationship between ibopamine, ejection fraction, and mortality? | The effects of ibopamine were studied in 8 patients with idiopathic dilatative cardiomyopathy. After 2 hours, ibopamine increased cardiac output (+16%, $P<.05$), stroke volume (+12%, $P<.05$), and ejection fraction (+10%, $P<.01$). Patients were then randomly treated with placebo or ibopamine according to a double-blind crossover design for two periods of 15 days each. At the end of each period, cardiac output and stroke volume were higher after ibopamine than after placebo ($P<.05$). Treatment was well tolerated.[17] | Investigators conducted an RCT to assess the effect of ibopamine on survival in patients with advanced heart failure. Patients with advanced severe heart failure and evidence of severe left-ventricular disease, who were already receiving optimum treatment for heart failure, were randomly allocated to oral ibopamine or placebo. After 1906 patients had been recruited, the trial was stopped early because of an excess of deaths among patients in the ibopamine group (RR, 1.26; 95% CI, 1.04-1.53; $P=.017$).[18] |
| What effect does atrial natriuretic peptide (anaritide) have on renal function? | An experiment evaluated alpha human atrial natriuretic peptide (alpha-hANP) for its potentially beneficial effects in experimental ischemic renal failure, induced by renal artery occlusion, in renally intact rats. After ischemia, a 4-hour intrarenal infusion of alpha-hANP restored 14C-inulin clearances in the animals ($P<.001$). Histologically, there was a progressive decrease in medullary hyperemia and prevention of intratubular cell shedding and granulocyte margination as a result of the alpha-hANP infusion such that after 24 and 48 hours the histologic appearance of the tissue was essentially normal.[19] | A multicenter, RCT studied administration of anaritide in 504 critically ill patients with acute tubular necrosis. Results: in the prospectively defined subgroup of 120 patients with oliguria, dialysis-free survival was 8% in the placebo group and 27% in the anaritide group ($P=.008$). Conversely, among the 378 patients without oliguria, dialysis-free survival was 59% in the placebo group and 48% in the anaritide group ($P=.03$).[20] |

| Question | Evidence From Different Endpoints | RCT Evidence of Clinically Important Endpoints |
|---|---|---|
| In patients with heart failure, what is the impact of treatment with vesnarinone on morbidity and mortality? | A before/after study of 11 patients with moderate congestive heart failure receiving the drug OPC-8212 found, after 8 hours, that cardiac and stroke work indexes increased by 11% ($P<.01$) and 20% ($P<.005$), respectively, with concomitant decreases in the diastolic pulmonary artery (25%; $P<.005$) and right atrial (33%; $P<.01$) pressures. Furthermore, an inotropic effect of the agent was confirmed by a shift of the function curve upward and to the left. Investigators concluded that "OPC-8212 clearly improves rest hemodynamics . . . and it may be particularly useful for the treatment of mild to moderate cardiac failure."[21] | An RCT evaluated the effects of daily doses of 60 mg or 30 mg of vesnarinone, as compared with placebo, on mortality and morbidity. Results demonstrated 18.9%, 21.0%, and 22.9% death rates in the placebo, 30-mg, and 60-mg vesnarinone groups, respectively. The hazard ratio for sudden death was 1.35 (95% CI, 1.08-1.69) in the 60-mg group and 1.17 (95% CI, 0.91-1.15) in the 30-mg group as compared with the placebo group. The increase in mortality with vesnarinone was attributed to an increase in sudden death, presumably from arrhythmia.[22] |
| In patients with heart failure, is xamoterol a safe and effective treatment? | A single-blind trial assessed the efficacy of xamoterol in 14 patients with mild to moderate heart failure over a period of 18 months. At both 1 month and 18 months, xamoterol, when compared with placebo, produced a significant increase in endurance ($P<.005$) and the amount of work achieved ($P<.05$), plus a decrease in maximum exercise heart rate ($P<.005$).[23] | Investigators randomized 516 patients with class III and IV heart failure to xamoterol 200 mg or placebo twice daily for 13 weeks. Results: there was no significant difference in the amount of work done on exercise testing or on the duration of the exercise between the 2 groups. Furthermore, on intention-to-treat analysis, 9.2% of patients in the xamoterol group and 3.7% of patients in the placebo group died within 100 days of randomization ($P = .02$), yielding a hazard ratio of 2.54 (95% CI, 1.04–6.18).[24] |
| Does active compression-decompression (ACD) CPR vs standard CPR improve the outcome of patients in cardiac arrest? | Patients in cardiac arrest were randomized to receive 2 minutes of either standard CPR or ACD CPR followed by 2 minutes of the alternate technique. Results showed that mean end-tidal carbon dioxide was $4.3\pm3.8$ mm Hg with standard CPR and $9.0\pm0.9$ mm Hg with ACD CPR ($P<.0001$). Systolic arterial pressure was $52.5\pm14.0$ mm Hg and $88.9\pm24.7$ mm Hg with standard and ACD CPR, respectively ($P<.003$). Furthermore, the velocity time integral increased from $7.3\pm2.6$ cm to $17.5\pm5.6$ cm with standard and ACD CPR, respectively ($P<.0001$), and diastolic filling times increased from $0.23\pm0.09$ seconds with standard CPR to $0.37\pm0.12$ seconds with ACD CPR ($P<.004$).[25] | An RCT allocated 1784 adults in cardiac arrest to receive either standard CPR or ACD CPR throughout resuscitation and found, in patients who arrested in the hospital, no significant difference between the standard and ACD CPR groups in survival for 1 hour (35.1% vs 34.6%; $P=.89$) or in survival until hospital discharge (11.4% vs 10.4%; $P=.64$). For patients who collapsed outside of the hospital, there were no significant differences in survival between the standard and ACD CPR groups for 1 hour (16.5% vs 18.2%; $P=.48$) or in the percentage who survived until the time of hospital discharge (3.7% vs 4.6%; $P=.49$).[26] |

| Question | Evidence From Different Endpoints | RCT Evidence of Clinically Important Endpoints |
|---|---|---|
| In patients with myocarditis, does treatment with immuno-suppressive therapy improve mortality over conventional therapy? | Authors of a before/after study of 16 patients with endomyocardial biopsy-proven myocarditis receiving immunosuppressive therapy (azathioprine and prednisolone) in addition to standard measures found a significant fall in cardiothoracic ratio from 62.3±4.7% to 50.6±1.5% at 6-12 months of therapy ($P<.0001$), mean pulmonary artery pressure from 34.3±13.05 mm Hg to 20.0±2.75 mm Hg at 6-12 months ($P<.01$) and mean pulmonary wedge pressure from 26.0±9.1 mm Hg to 13.2±4.6 mm Hg at 6-12 months ($P<.001$). Furthermore, the left ventricular ejection fraction improved from 24.3±8.4% to 49.8±18.2% at 6-12 months of therapy ($P<.0001$).[27] | An RCT assigned 111 patients with a histopathologic diagnosis of myocarditis to receive conventional therapy either alone or combined with a 24-week regimen of immuno-suppressive therapy (prednisolone plus cyclosporine or azathioprine). Results showed the mean change in the left ventricular ejection fraction at 28 weeks did not differ significantly between the group of patients who received immunosuppressive therapy (gain, 0.10; 95% CI, 0.07-0.12) and the control group (gain, 0.07; 95% CI, 0.03-0.12). Furthermore, there was no significant difference in survival between the two groups (RR, 0.98; 95% CI, 0.52-1.87; $P=.96$).[28] |

* Note: Data are expressed here as reported in the original literature.

RR indicates relative risk; CI, confidence interval; NYHA, New York Heart Association.

# WHEN RANDOMIZED CONTROLLED TRIAL RESULTS HAVE CONTRADICTED THOSE OF OBSERVATIONAL STUDIES OF PATIENT-IMPORTANT ENDPOINTS

Table 2B1-1 has provided a clear indication that physiologic rationale is often an inadequate guide for therapeutic decisions. Table 2B1-2 demonstrates that the same is true of the results of observational studies.

**TABLE 2B1-2**

### Prior Evidence From Studies of Same Endpoints*

| Question | Evidence From Same Endpoints | RCT Evidence |
| --- | --- | --- |
| In patients with cerebral malaria, what effect does treatment with dexamethasone have on morbidity and mortality? | A case report of a 40-year-old man with cerebral malaria in a coma for 24 hours suggested dexamethasone had a dramatic and probably life-saving effect and that "dexamethasone should be given routinely, together with antimalarial therapy, to patients with cerebral malaria."[29] | A double-blind controlled clinical trial involving 100 comatose patients, with both patients and caregivers blinded to the allocation of compared high-dose dexamethasone with placebo and demonstrated that, although there was no significant difference in total deaths between the treatment and placebo groups, dexamethasone prolonged coma among the survivors ($P=.02$). Furthermore, complications, including pneumonia and gastrointestinal bleeding, occurred in 52% patients given dexamethasone and 22% given placebo (RR, 2.4; $P=.004$).[30] |
| Does extracranial to intracranial (EC/IC) bypass surgery alter the risk of ischemic stroke? | A before/after study examined stroke rates of 110 patients with cerebrovascular disease undergoing EC/IC arterial bypass. Results: stroke rate was 4.3% in the 70 patients with transient ischemic attacks (TIAs). This compares to an expected TIA rate of 13% to 62% in patients cited in the literature who have not undergone surgery. Stroke rate was 5% in the entire group of 110 patients followed for more than 3 years. Researchers concluded that "there appears to be a dramatic improvement in the symptomatology of virtually all patients" undergoing this bypass procedure.[31] | An RCT of 1377 patients, studying whether EC/IC bypass surgery benefits patients with symptomatic atherosclerotic disease of the internal carotid artery, found a 14% increase in the RR of fatal and nonfatal stroke during the entire trial for the group receiving surgery over those treated with best medical care (90% CI, 3%-34%).[32] |

| Question | Evidence From Same Endpoints | RCT Evidence |
|---|---|---|
| In patients with hypertension and renal artery stenosis, what effect does balloon angioplasty have on blood pressure? | A before/after study of 65 patients with renovascular hypertension found that both mean systolic and diastolic blood pressure fell immediately after percutaneous transluminal dilation (P<.001) and remained significantly lower for a period of up to 5 years. Furthermore, after a mean control period of 21.6 months, improvement in blood pressure values was observed in 32% of patients with fibromuscular dysplasia and in 48% of patients with atherosclerotic stenosis. Researchers concluded that ". . . percutaneous transluminal dilation should be the favored procedure in patients with renovascular hypertension."[33] | Investigators randomized 106 patients with hypertension and atherosclerotic renal artery stenosis to percutaneous transluminal renal angioplasty or drug therapy. Results showed that at 3 months, systolic and diastolic blood pressures were 169±28 and 99±12 mm Hg, respectively, in the angioplasty group and 176±31 and 101±14 mm Hg, respectively, in the drug therapy group (P=.25 and P=.36 for systolic and diastolic pressure, respectively). According to intention-to-treat analysis, at 12 months there were no significant differences between the angioplasty and drug therapy groups in systolic and diastolic blood pressure, daily drug doses, or renal function.[34] |
| Does lowering cholesterol level alter the risk of stoke? | A cohort study looked at potential risk factors for stroke among 789 men during 18.5 years of follow-up. Results showed a mean level of serum cholesterol of 275 mg/dL and 269 mg/dL for stroke victims and among other participants, respectively (P=.40). Analyses did not confirm serum cholesterol level as a risk factor for the incidence of stroke.[35] | An overview of 16 RCTs of statin drugs conducted to determine whether cholesterol lowering with statin drugs reduces the risks of stroke and total mortality showed an RR of 0.73 (95% CI, 0.61-0.88) and 0.79 (95% CI, 0.68-0.92) for stroke and death, respectively, among recipients of statin drugs vs those receiving control treatment.[36] |
| In patients in need of a pacemaker to correct symptomatic bradycardia, what impact does physiologic (AAI) and ventricular (VVI) pacing have on risks of cardiovascular morbidity and death? | Authors of a cohort study of the effect of AAI vs VVI pacing with respect to cardiovascular morbidity and mortality found, after an average follow-up of 4 years in 168 patients, significantly higher incidence of permanent physiologic fibrillation in patients treated with VVI pacing (47%) compared to AAI pacing (6.7%) (RR, 7.0; P<.0005). Congestive heart failure occurred significantly more often in the VVI group than in the AAI group (37% vs 15%; RR, 2.5; P<.005). Analysis of survival data showed a higher overall mortality rate in the VVI group (23%) than in the AAI group (8%) (RR, 2.9; P<.05).[37] | Investigators randomized 2568 patients to a VVI or AAI pacemaker and found that the type of pacemaker had virtually no effect on the annual rate of death from all causes, which was 6.3% among the AAI group and 6.6% among the VVI group (RRR, 0.9%; 95% CI, 18.1-16.8; P=.92). There was no significant difference in the incidence of hospitalization for congestive heart failure between the two groups (AAI group, 3.1% vs VVI group, 3.5%; RRR, 0.79%; 95% CI, 1 8.5%-28.3%; P=.52). The annual stroke rate was 1.1% in the VVI group and 1.0% in the AAI group. Furthermore, there were significantly more perioperative complications with AAI pacing than with VVI pacing (9.0% vs 3.8%, respectively; P<.001).[38] |

| Question | Evidence From Same Endpoints | RCT Evidence |
|---|---|---|
| What effect does plasma exchange have in patents with dermatomyositis and polymyositis? | Authors of a before/after study of 38 patients who had undergone plasma exchanges between 1980 and 1986 found that, based on changes in muscle force, 24 patients (63%) improved (10 appreciably and 14 moderately) and 14 remained unchanged. Plasma exchange was well tolerated in 23 patients.[39] | An RCT of 39 patients with definite polymyositis or dermatomyositis assigned to receive plasma exchange, leukapheresis, or sham apheresis found no significant differences among the 3 treatment groups in final muscle strength or functional capacity; investigators concluded that leukapheresis and plasma exchange are no more effective than sham apheresis.[40] |
| What is the impact of sodium fluoride on vertebral fractures? | In a before/after study utilizing quantitative CT to measure trabecular vertebral body density (TVBD) in the lumbar spine of 18 female patients with osteoporosis, TVBD was significantly greater in the experimental group than mean TVBD for an age-matched group of untreated female patients with osteoporosis ($P < .001$). Only 1 of the 18 fluoride-treated patients with osteoporosis continued to have spinal fractures during therapy, accounting for 4 fractures per 87.2 patient years of observation, a value that is significantly lower than the published incidence of 76 fractures per 91 patient years for untreated osteoporotic patients ($P < .001$).[41] | An RCT studied patients receiving either sodium fluoride or placebo, in addition to daily supplements of calcium. Results: as compared with the placebo group, the treatment group had increases in median bone mineral density of 35% ($P < .0001$) in the lumbar spine, 12% ($P < .0001$) in the femoral neck, and 10% ($P < .0001$) in the femoral trochanter. However, although the number of new vertebral fractures was similar in the two groups (163 and 136, respectively; $P = .32$), the fluoride-treated patients had nonvertebral fractures 3.2 times more often than patients given placebo (95% CI, 1.8-5.6; $P < .01$).[42] |
| Does estrogen replacement therapy alter the risk of coronary heart disease events in postmenopausal women with established coronary disease? | A meta-analysis of 16 cohort studies with internal controls and 3 cross-sectional angiography studies (including studies of women with established coronary heart disease) demonstrated an RR of 0.5 (95% CI, 0.44–0.57) for coronary heart disease among estrogen users. Investigators concluded that ". . . the preponderance of the evidence strongly suggests women taking postmenopausal estrogen therapy are at a decreased risk for CHD."[43] | A randomized controlled secondary prevention trial did not find a reduction in the overall rate of coronary heart disease events in postmenopausal women with established coronary disease (relative hazard of myocardial infarction or coronary heart disease, 0.99; 95% CI, 0.80-1.22).[44] |

| Question | Evidence From Same Endpoints | RCT Evidence |
|---|---|---|
| In patients with diabetes who have isolated systolic hypertension (ISH), does diuretic-based antihypertensive treatment affect mortality? | In a cohort analytic study of 759 participants aged 35 to 69 years with normal serum creatinine levels, cardiovascular mortality in individuals with diabetes, after adjusting for differences in risk factors, was 3.8 times higher in patients treated with diuretics alone than in patients with untreated hypertension (*P*<.001). Investigators concluded that "there is an urgent need to reconsider its continued usage in this population."[45] | Authors of an RCT of diuretic treatment vs placebo in 4736 patients aged 60+ with ISH found an RR in 5-year major cardiovascular death rate of 34% for active treatment compared with placebo, both for patients with diabetes (95% CI, 6%-54%) and for those without diabetes (95% CI, 21%-45%). Absolute risk reduction with active treatment compared with placebo was twice as great for patients with vs without diabetes (101/1000 vs 51/1000 randomized participants, respectively, at the 5-year follow-up), reflecting the higher risk on the part of patients with diabetes.[46] |
| Does a diet low in fat and high in fiber alter the risk of colorectal adenomas? | Authors of a cohort study, prospectively examining the risk of colorectal adenoma of 7284 male health professionals according to quintiles of nutrient intake, found that dietary fiber was inversely associated with the risk of adenoma (*P*<.0001); RR for men in the highest vs the lowest quintile was 0.36 (95% CI, 0.22-0.60). Furthermore, for subjects on a high-saturated-fat, low-fiber diet, the RR was 3.7 (95% CI, 1.5-8.8) compared with those on a low-saturated-fat, high-fiber diet.[47] | Investigators randomly allocated 2079 subjects, who had had 1 or more histologically confirmed colorectal adenomas removed within 6 months, to one of two groups: an intervention group (given intensive counseling and assigned to follow a low-fat, high-fiber diet) and a control group (given a standard brochure on healthy eating and assigned to follow their usual diet). Results showed 39.7% of subjects in the intervention group and 39.5% in the control group had at least one recurrent adenoma (RR, 1.00; 95% CI, 0.90-1.12). Moreover, among subjects with recurrent adenomas, the mean number of such lesions was 1.85±0.08 and 1.84±0.07 in the intervention and control groups, respectively (*P*=.93).[48] |
| Does supplementation with beta-carotene alter the risk of major coronary events? | An analysis of a cohort from the Lipid Research Clinics Coronary Primary Prevention Trial and Follow up Study (LRC-CPPT) found that, after adjustment for known CHD risk factors including smoking, serum carotenoids were inversely related to CHD events. Men in the highest quartile of serum carotenoids had an adjusted RR of 0.64 (95% CI, 0.44-0.92) compared with the lowest quartile for CHD. For men who never smoked, this RR was 0.28 (95% CI, 0.11-0.73).[49] Authors of approximately 8 other observational studies found similar results. | An RCT, the Physicians' Health Study involving 22,071 male physicians, showed no statistically significant benefit or harm from beta-carotene with respect to the number of myocardial infarctions (RR, 0.96; 95% CI, 0.84–1.09), strokes (RR, 0.96; 95% CI, 0.83–1.11), deaths due to cardiovascular causes (RR, 1.09; 95% CI, 0.93–1.27), all important cardiovascular events (RR, 1.00; 95% CI, 0.91–1.09), or deaths from all causes (RR, 1.02; 95% CI, 0.93–1.11). Moreover, there was no significant trend toward greater benefit or harm with an increasing duration of treatment, even 5 or more years after randomization.[50] |

| Question | Evidence From Same Endpoints | RCT Evidence |
|---|---|---|
| Does dietary supplementation with vitamin E alter the risk of major coronary events? | A cohort of 5133 Finnish men and women showed an inverse association between dietary vitamin E intake and coronary mortality in both men and women with relative risks of 0.68 (*P* for trend = .01) and 0.35 (*P* for trend <.01), respectively, between the highest and lowest tertiles of intake.[51] Approximately 12 other observational or experimental studies have shown similar results. | Authors of an RCT of 2545 women and 6996 men at high risk for cardiovascular events found an RR of 1.05 (95% CI, 0.95–1.16) for myocardial infarction, stroke, and death among patients assigned to vitamin E vs placebo. There were no significant differences in the numbers of deaths from cardiovascular causes (RR, 1.05; 95% CI, 0.90-1.22), myocardial infarction (RR, 1.02; 95% CI, 0.90-1.15), or stroke (RR, 1.17; 95% CI, 0.95-1.42).[52] |
| In patients with severe congestive heart failure, does epoprostenol therapy alter mortality? | Authors of an observational study, utilizing historic controls, evaluated the effects of long-term intravenous infusion of prostacyclin in patients with primary pulmonary hypertension. Results: on average, patients could walk more than 100 m farther at 6 and 18 months after prostacyclin therapy was initiated, compared with baseline capability (*P*<.001 and *P*=.02, respectively). The cardiac index increased 18% (*P*=.02); and mean pulmonary artery pressure and total pulmonary resistance decreased 9% (*P*=.03) and 26% (*P*=.02), respectively, compared with baseline. The hazard ratio for death was 0.34 (95% CI, 0.13-1.0; *P*=.045).[53] | An RCT assigned 471 patients with congestive heart failure and decreased left ventricular ejection fraction to either epoprostenol infusion or standard care. The trial terminated early because of a strong trend toward decreased survival in patients treated with epoprostenol. The RR of death was 1.25 (95% CI, 0.84-1.85) and 1.29 (95% CI, 0.92-1.80) at 3 months and 6 months, respectively, for the epoprostenol group vs those receiving conventional therapy.[54] |
| In patients with heart failure, does digitalis alter the risk of morbidity and mortality? | In a case-control study, clinical indicators and incidence of sudden death were examined among 1000 consecutive patients with myocardial infarction. Results: univariate analysis revealed a statistically significant difference in the administration of digitalis and diuretics between the sudden-death group and the cardiac and other patient groups. Multivariate analysis revealed that digitalis treatment was a major contributing factor to sudden death. The odds ratio of sudden death with digitalis therapy was 9.59.[55] | Authors of an RCT investigated the effect of digoxin on mortality and hospitalization. Results: 6% fewer hospitalizations occurred overall in the digoxin group than in the placebo group, and fewer patients were hospitalized for worsening heart failure (RR, 0.72; 95% CI, 0.66-0.79; *P*<.001). Mortality (overall and from cardiovascular causes) did not differ between groups (*P*=.8).[56] |

| Question | Evidence From Same Endpoints | RCT Evidence |
|---|---|---|
| In critically ill patients, does treatment with growth hormone alter the mortality risk? | Authors of a before/after study of 53 patients who had failed standard ventilator weaning protocols and who were subsequently treated with human growth hormone (HGH) found that 81% of the previously unweanable patients were eventually weaned from mechanical ventilation with an overall survival of 76%. Furthermore, predicted mortality of the study group was significantly greater than the actual mortality rate ($P<.05$). Researchers concluded that ". . . this study presents clinical evidence supporting the safety and efficacy of HGH in promoting respiratory independence in a selected group of surgical ICU patients."[57] | Two multicenter RCTs were carried out in patients in intensive care units. The patients received either HGH or placebo until discharge from intensive care or for a maximum of 21 days. Results showed that the in-hospital mortality rate was higher in the patients who received HGH than in those who did not ($P<.001$ for both studies). The RR of death for patients receiving HGH was 1.9 (95% CI, 1.3-2.9) in the Finnish study and 2.4 (95% CI, 1.6-3.5) in the multinational study. Among the survivors, the length of stay in ICU and in the hospital and the duration of mechanical ventilation were prolonged in the HGH group.[58] |
| In patients with deep venous thrombosis (DVT), what is the effect of vena cava filters (vs no filter) on pulmonary embolism and recurrent DVT? | A before/after study followed the insertion of 61 vena cava filters (47 permanent and 14 temporary) in patients with DVT. Results: mortality among the patients was nil, and clinically evident pulmonary embolism was not observed in any patient in whom a vena cava filter was inserted. Researchers concluded that "vena cava filters represent an effective prevention of pulmonary embolism together with medical and surgical treatment."[59] | Investigators randomized 400 patients with proximal DVT who were at risk for pulmonary embolism to receive a vena caval filter or no filter. Results showed an OR of 0.22 (95% CI, 0.05-0.90) for pulmonary embolism at 12 days. However, this reduction of pulmonary embolism risk was counterbalanced by an excess of recurrent DVT (OR, 1.87; 95% CI, 1.10-3.20) at 2 years, without any significant differences in mortality.[60] |
| Is low-dose aspirin as effective as high-dose aspirin for reducing stroke, myocardial infarction, and death? | An observational investigation, resulting from a secondary analysis of data from an RCT of low-and high-dose aspirin for patients undergoing carotid endarterectomy, found an association between perioperative stoke and death and the amount of aspirin taken before surgery. The risk of perioperative stroke and death was 1.8% for patients taking 650-1300 mg daily, compared with 6.9% for patients taking 0-325 mg daily.[61] | An RCT allocated 4 different doses of aspirin to 2849 patients scheduled for carotid endarterectomy. Results demonstrated the combined RR of stoke, myocardial infarction, or death at 3 months was 1.34 (95% CI, 1.03-1.75; $P=.03$) with high-dose aspirin. Efficacy analysis (excluding patients receiving aspirin before randomization) showed a combined RR of 2.21 (95% CI, 1.33-3.65; $P=.002$) at 30 days and 2.36 (95% CI, 1.48-3.75; $P=.0002$) at 3 months for the high-dose aspirin group compared to the low-dose group.[61] |

| Question | Evidence From Same Endpoints | RCT Evidence |
|----------|------------------------------|--------------|
| Do educational and community interventions modify the risk of adolescent pregnancy? | A meta-analysis of observational studies demonstrated a statistically significant delay in initiation of intercourse (OR, 0.64; 95% CI, 0.44-0.93) and a reduction in pregnancy (OR, 0.74; 95% CI, 0.56-0.98) with educational and community interventions.[62] | A meta-analysis of randomized trials provided no support for the effect of educational or community interventions on initiation of intercourse (OR, 1.09; 95% CI, 0.90-1.32) or pregnancy (OR, 1.08; 95% CI, 0.91-1.27).[62] |

\* Note: Data are expressed as reported in the original literature.

RR indicates relative risk; CI, confidence interval.

# CONCLUSION

Physiologic rationale or an observational study usually accurately predicts the results of RCTs. However, this is not always the case. The problem is, one never knows in advance if the particular instance is one in which the preliminary data reflect the truth, or whether they are misleading. Confident clinical action must generally await the results of RCTs.

## References

1. Coltart J, Alderman EL, Robison SC, Harrison DC. Effect of propranolol on left ventricular function, segmental wall motion, and diastolic pressure-volume relation in man. *Br Heart J*. 1975;37:357-364.

2. Lechat P, Packer M, Chalon S, Cucherat M, Arab T, Boissel JP. Clinical effects of beta-adrenergic blockade in chronic heart failure: a meta-analysis of double-blind, placebo-controlled, randomized trials. *Circulation*. 1998;98:1184-1191.

3. Iaina A, Solomon S, Gavendo S, Eliahou HE. Reduction in severity of acute renal failure (ARF) in rats by dopamine. *Biomedicine*. 1977;27:137-139.

4. Chertow GM, Sayegh MH, Allgren RL, Lazarus JM. Is the administration of dopamine associated with adverse or favorable outcomes in acute renal failure? Auriculin Anaritide Acute Renal Failure Study Group. *Am J Med*. 1996;101:49-53.

5. Delcourt R, Vastesaeger M. Action of Atromid on total and ∃-cholesterol. Symposium on Atromid. *J Atheroscler Res* 1963;3:533-537.

6. A co-operative trial in the primary prevention of ischaemic heart disease using clofibrate. Report from the Committee of Principal Investigators. *Br Heart J*. 1978;40:1069-1118.

7. Kornitzer M, De Backer G, Dramaix M, Thilly C. The Belgian heart disease prevention project: modification of the coronary risk profile in an industrial population. *Circulation*. 1980;61:18-25.

8. Strandberg TE, Salomaa VV, Naukkarinen VA, Vanhanen HT, Sarna SJ, Miettinen TA. Long-term mortality after 5-year multifactorial primary prevention of cardiovascular diseases in middle-aged men. *JAMA*. 1991;266:1225-1229.

9. Hinshaw LB, Archer LT, Beller-Todd BK, Benjamin B, Flournoy DJ, Passey R. Survival of primates in lethal septic shock following delayed treatment with steroid. *Circ Shock*. 1981;8:291-300.

10. Cronin L, Cook DJ, Carlet J, et al. Corticosteroid treatment for sepsis: a critical appraisal and meta-analysis of the literature. *Crit Care Med*. 1995;23:1430-1439.

11. Mason JW, Peters FA. Antiarrhythmic efficacy of encainide in patients with refractory recurrent ventricular tachycardia. *Circulation*. 1981;63:670-675.

12. Echt DS, Liebson PR, Mitchell LB, et al. Mortality and morbidity in patients receiving encainide, flecainide, or placebo. The Cardiac Arrhythmia Suppression Trial. *N Engl J Med*. 1991;324:781-788.

13. Burnakis TG, Mioduch HJ. Combined therapy with captopril and potassium supplementation: a potential for hyperkalemia. *Arch Intern Med*. 1984;144:2371-2372.

14. Pitt B, Zannad F, Remme WJ, et al. The effect of spironolactone on morbidity and mortality in patients with severe heart failure. Randomized Aldactone Evaluation Study Investigators. *N Engl J Med*. 1999;341:709-717.

15. Timmis AD, Smyth P, Jewitt DE. Milrinone in heart failure: effects on exercise haemodynamics during short term treatment. *Br Heart J*. 1985;54:42-47.

16. Packer M, Carver JR, Rodeheffer RJ, et al. Effect of oral milrinone on mortality in severe chronic heart failure. The PROMISE Study Research Group. *N Engl J Med*. 1991;325:1468-1475.

17. Gronda E, Brusoni B, Inglese E, Mangiavacchi M, Gasparini M, Ghirardi P. Effects of ibopamine on heart performance: a radionuclide ventriculography study in patients with idiopathic dilatative cardiomyopathy. *Arzneimittelforsch*. 1986;36:371-375.

18. Hampton JR, van Veldhuisen DJ, Kleber FX, et al. Randomised study of effect of ibopamine on survival in patients with advanced severe heart failure. Second Prospective Randomised Study of Ibopamine on Mortality and Efficacy (PRIME II) Investigators. *Lancet*. 1997;349:971-977.

19. Shaw SG, Weidmann P, Hodler J, Zimmermann A, Paternostro A. Atrial natriuretic peptide protects against acute ischemic renal failure in the rat. *J Clin Invest*. 1987;80:1232-1237.

20. Allgren RL, Marbury TC, Rahman SN, et al. Anaritide in acute tubular necrosis. Auriculin Anaritide Acute Renal Failure Study Group. *N Engl J Med*. 1997;336:828-834.

21. Asanoi H, Sasayama S, Iuchi K, Kameyama T. Acute hemodynamic effects of a new inotropic agent (OPC-8212) in patients with congestive heart failure. *J Am Coll Cardiol*. 1987;9:865-871.

22. Cohn JN, Goldstein SO, Greenberg BH, et al. A dose-dependent increase in mortality with vesnarinone among patients with severe heart failure. Vesnarinone Trial Investigators. *N Engl J Med*. 1998;339:1810-1816.

23. Sorensen EV, Faergeman O, Day MA, Snow HM. Long-term efficacy of xamoterol (a beta 1-adrenoceptor partial agonist) in patients with mild to moderate heart failure. *Br J Clin Pharmacol*. 1989;28:86S-88S.

24. Xamoterol in severe heart failure. The Xamoterol in Severe Heart Failure Study Group. *Lancet*. 1990;336:1-6.

25. Cohen TJ, Tucker KJ, Lurie KG, et al. Active compression-decompression: a new method of cardiopulmonary resuscitation. Cardiopulmonary Resuscitation Working Group. *JAMA*. 1992;267:2916-2923.

26. Stiell IG, Hebert PC, Wells GA, et al. The Ontario trial of active compression-decompression cardiopulmonary resuscitation for in-hospital and prehospital cardiac arrest. *JAMA*. 1996;275:1417-1423.

27. Talwar KK, Goswami KC, Chopra P, Dev V, Shrivastava S, Malhotra A. Immunosuppressive therapy in inflammatory myocarditis: long-term follow-up. *Int J Cardiol*. 1992;34:157-166.

28. Mason JW, O'Connell JB, Herskowitz A, et al. A clinical trial of immunosuppressive therapy for myocarditis. The Myocarditis Treatment Trial Investigators. *N Engl J Med*. 1995;333:269-275.

29. Woodruff AW, Dickinson CJ. Use of dexamethasone in cerebral malaria. *BMJ*. 1968;3:31-32.

30. Warrell DA, Looareesuwan S, Warrell MJ, et al. Dexamethasone proves deleterious in cerebral malaria: a double-blind trial in 100 comatose patients. *N Engl J Med*. 1982;306:313-319.

31. Popp AJ, Chater N. Extracranial to intracranial vascular anastomosis for occlusive cerebrovascular disease: experience in 110 patients. *Surgery*. 1977;82:648-654.

32. Failure of extracranial-intracranial arterial bypass to reduce the risk of ischemic stroke: results of an international randomized trial. The EC/IC Bypass Study Group. *N Engl J Med*. 1985;313:1191-1200.

33. Kuhlmann U, Greminger P, Gruntzig A, et al. Long-term experience in percutaneous transluminal dilatation of renal artery stenosis. *Am J Med*. 1985;79:692-698.

34. van Jaarsveld BC, Krijnen P, Pieterman H, et al. The effect of balloon angioplasty on hypertension in atherosclerotic renal-artery stenosis. Dutch Renal Artery Stenosis Intervention Cooperative Study Group. *N Engl J Med*. 2000;342:1007-1014.

35. Welin L, Svardsudd K, Wilhelmsen L, Larsson B, Tibblin G. Analysis of risk factors for stroke in a cohort of men born in 1913. *N Engl J Med*. 1987;317:521-526.

36. Hebert PR, Gaziano JM, Chan KS, Hennekens CH. Cholesterol lowering with statin drugs, risk of stroke, and total mortality: an overview of randomized trials. *JAMA*. 1997;278:313-321.

37. Rosenqvist M, Brandt J, Schuller H. Long-term pacing in sinus node disease: effects of stimulation mode on cardiovascular morbidity and mortality. *Am Heart J*. 1988;116:16-22.

38. Connolly SJ, Kerr CR, Gent M, et al. Effects of physiologic pacing versus ventricular pacing on the risk of stroke and death due to cardiovascular causes. Canadian Trial of Physiologic Pacing Investigators. *N Engl J Med*. 2000;342:1385-1391.

39. Herson S, Lok C, Roujeau JC, et al. Plasma exchange in dermatomyositis and polymyositis: retrospective study of 38 cases of plasma exchange. *Ann Med Interne (Paris)*. 1989;140:453-455.

40. Miller FW, Leitman SF, Cronin ME, et al. Controlled trial of plasma exchange and leukapheresis in polymyositis and dermatomyositis. *N Engl J Med*. 1992;326:1380-1384.

41. Farley SM, Libanati CR, Odvina CV, et al. Efficacy of long-term fluoride and calcium therapy in correcting the deficit of spinal bone density in osteoporosis. *J Clin Epidemiol*. 1989;42:1067-1074.

42. Riggs BL, Hodgson SF, O'Fallon WM, et al. Effect of fluoride treatment on the fracture rate in postmenopausal women with osteoporosis. *N Engl J Med*. 1990;322:802-809.

43. Stampfer MJ, Colditz GA. Estrogen replacement therapy and coronary heart disease: a quantitative assessment of the epidemiologic evidence. *Prev Med*. 1991;20:47-63.

44. Hulley S, Grady D, Bush T, et al. Randomized trial of estrogen plus progestin for secondary prevention of coronary heart disease in postmenopausal women. Heart and Estrogen/progestin Replacement Study (HERS) Research Group. *JAMA*. 1998;280:605-613.

45. Warram JH, Laffel LM, Valsania P, Christlieb AR, Krolewski AS. Excess mortality associated with diuretic therapy in diabetes mellitus. *Arch Intern Med*. 1991;151:1350-1356.

46. Curb JD, Pressel SL, Cutler JA, et al. Effect of diuretic-based antihypertensive treatment on cardiovascular disease risk in older diabetic patients with isolated systolic hypertension. Systolic Hypertension in the Elderly Program Cooperative Research Group. *JAMA*. 1996;276:1886-1892.

47. Giovannucci E, Stampfer MJ, Colditz G, Rimm EB, Willett WC. Relationship of diet to risk of colorectal adenoma in men. *J Natl Cancer Inst*. 1992;84:91-98.

48. Schatzkin A, Lanza E, Corle D, et al. Lack of effect of a low-fat, high-fiber diet on the recurrence of colorectal adenomas. Polyp Prevention Trial Study Group. *N Engl J Med*. 2000;342:1149-1455.

49. Morris DL, Kritchevsky SB, Davis CE. Serum carotenoids and coronary heart disease. The Lipid Research Clinics Coronary Primary Prevention Trial and Follow-up Study. *JAMA*. 1994;272:1439-1441.

50. Hennekens CH, Buring JE, Manson JE, et al. Lack of effect of long-term supplementation with beta carotene on the incidence of malignant neoplasms and cardiovascular disease. *N Engl J Med*. 1996;334:1145-1149.

51. Knekt P, Reunanen A, Jarvinen R, Seppanen R, Heliovaara M, Aromaa A. Antioxidant vitamin intake and coronary mortality in a longitudinal population study. *Am J Epidemiol*. 1994;139:1180-1189.

52. Yusuf S, Dagenais G, Pogue J, Bosch J, Sleight P. Vitamin E supplementation and cardiovascular events in high-risk patients. The Heart Outcomes Prevention Evaluation Study Investigators. *N Engl J Med*. 2000;342:154-160.

53. Barst RJ, Rubin LJ, McGoon MD, Caldwell EJ, Long WA, Levy PS. Survival in primary pulmonary hypertension with long-term continuous intravenous prostacyclin. *Ann Intern Med*. 1994;121:409-415.

54. Califf RM, Adams KF, McKenna WJ, et al. A randomized controlled trial of epoprostenol therapy for severe congestive heart failure: The FIolan International Randomized Survival Trial (FIRST). *Am Heart J*. 1997;134:44-54.

55. Kambara H, Kinoshita M, Nakagawa M, Sakurai T, Kawai C. Sudden death among 1,000 patients with myocardial infarction: incidence and contributory factors. KYSMI Study Group. *J Cardiol*. 1995;25:55-61.

56. The effect of digoxin on mortality and morbidity in patients with heart failure. The Digitalis Investigation Group. *N Engl J Med*. 1997;336:525-533.

57. Knox JB, Wilmore DW, Demling RH, Sarraf P, Santos AA. Use of growth hormone for postoperative respiratory failure. *Am J Surg*. 1996;171:576-580.

58. Takala J, Ruokonen E, Webster NR, et al. Increased mortality associated with growth hormone treatment in critically ill adults. *N Engl J Med*. 1999;341: 785-792.

59. Cotroneo AR, Di Stasi C, Cina A, Di Gregorio F. Venous interruption as prophylaxis of pulmonary embolism: vena cava filters. *Rays*. 1996;21:461-480.

60. Decousus H, Leizorovicz A, Parent F, et al. A clinical trial of vena caval filters in the prevention of pulmonary embolism in patients with proximal deep-vein thrombosis. Prevention du Risque d'Embolie Pulmonaire par Interruption Cave Study Group. *N Engl J Med*. 1998;338:409-415.

61. Taylor DW, Barnett HJ, Haynes RB, et al. Low-dose and high-dose acetylsalicylic acid for patients undergoing carotid endarterectomy: a randomised controlled trial. ASA and Carotid Endarterectomy (ACE) Trial Collaborators. *Lancet*. 1999;353:2179-2184.

62. Guyatt GH, DiCenso A, Farewell V, Willan A, Griffith L. Randomized trials versus observational studies in adolescent pregnancy prevention. *J Clin Epidemiol*. 2000;53:167-174.

**2B1**

# THERAPY AND VALIDITY
## The Principle of Intention-to-Treat

Gordon Guyatt and PJ Devereaux

The following EBM Working Group members also made substantive contributions to this section: Leonila Dans and Peter Wyer

## IN THIS SECTION

How Should Randomized Trials Deal With Treatment Arm Patients Who Do Not Receive Treatment?

A Hypothetical Surgical Randomized Controlled Trial

A Hypothetical Randomized Controlled Trial of Drug Therapy

A Real-World Example

Limitations of the Intention-to-Treat Principle

Misleading Use of "Intention-to-Treat"

# HOW SHOULD RANDOMIZED TRIALS DEAL WITH TREATMENT ARM PATIENTS WHO DO NOT RECEIVE TREATMENT?

In general, one does not need randomized controlled trials (RCTs) to determine the effect of a medication in patients who do not take it. Intuitively, it follows that, in a RCT, one should compare patients in the experimental group who adhered to the treatment with patients in the control group. As it turns out, however, doing so is a mistake. We need to know the outcomes of all the patients in a trial—including, for example, those in the experimental group who do not adhere to or complete therapy.

One argument for incorporating all patients in the final analysis, including those who did not adhere to treatment, has to do with the impact of the treatment on members of the community. If one is interested in knowing the effect of a drug on a given population, one must include all members of that population. When patients do not adhere to a regimen, particularly if side effects have caused nonadherence, reservations will arise about the impact of a medication on a community.

As clinicians, however, we are more interested in the impact of our interventions on individual patients than on populations. Consider the viewpoint of a patient who is determined to adhere to a treatment regimen and is destined to succeed. Let us assume that 50% of treated patients in a trial did not comply with the treatment regimen. Does the motivated patient wish to know the average effect of the treatment in a group of people of whom 50% did not comply? No; she wants the best estimate of the impact the medication will have when she takes it. This would come from a population of other patients who succeeded in adhering to the treatment regimen.

# A HYPOTHETICAL SURGICAL RANDOMIZED CONTROLLED TRIAL

Picture a RCT studying patients with cerebrovascular disease. The trial compares administration of aspirin alone with that of aspirin along with an experimental surgical procedure. Assume that, although the investigators conducting the trial do not know it, the underlying true effect of the surgical procedure is zero, and that patients in the surgical arm of the study do neither better nor worse than those in the aspirin-only arm.

Of 100 patients randomized to surgery, 10 suffer the primary outcome of the trial, a stroke, in the month during which arrangements for surgery are being made. Of the 90 patients who go to surgery, 10 suffer a stroke in the subsequent year (Figure 2B1-1). What will happen to the patients in the control group? Because randomization is supposed to create groups with the same fate or destiny and because we have already established that the surgical procedure has no impact on outcome, we predict that 10 control group patients will suffer a stroke in the month after randomization and another 10 will suffer a stroke in the subsequent year.

**FIGURE 2B1-1**

**Results of a Hypothetical Trial of Surgical Therapy in Patients With Cerebrovascular Disease**

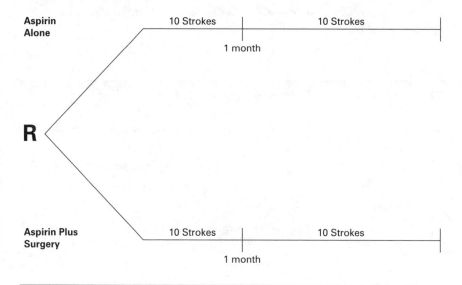

R indicates patients randomized to medical or surgical therapy

The principle that dictates that we count all events in all randomized patients, regardless of whether they received the intended intervention, is the *intention-to-treat principle*. When we apply the intention-to-treat principle in our study of cerebrovascular surgery for stroke, we find 20 events in each group—and, therefore, no evidence of a positive treatment effect. However, if we use the logic that we should not count events in patients in the surgical group who did not receive surgery, the event rate in the experimental groups would be 10/90 (or 11%), in comparison to the 20% event rate in the control group—a reduction in relative risk of close to 50%. These data show how analyses restricted to patients who adhered to assigned treatment (sometimes referred to as as-treated, per-protocol, efficacy, or explanatory analyses) can provide a misleading estimate of surgical therapy's impact.

# A HYPOTHETICAL RANDOMIZED CONTROLLED TRIAL OF DRUG THERAPY

Now consider a trial of a new drug in which 20 of 100 patients are nonadherent (Figure 2B1-2). Under what circumstances would a comparison of the 80 patients who took their active medication with the control group yield an unbiased comparison? This would be true only if the underlying prognosis in the 80 adherent patients were identical to that of the 20 nonadherent patients. If the 20 nonadherent patients were destined to do better than the other members of their group, the per-protocol analysis would provide a misleading underestimate of the true treatment effect. If, as is more usually the case, the nonadherent group were more likely to suffer an adverse outcome, their omission would lead to a spurious overestimate of treatment benefit.

**FIGURE 2B1-2**

## A Schematic View of Per-Protocol and Intention-to-Treat Comparisons

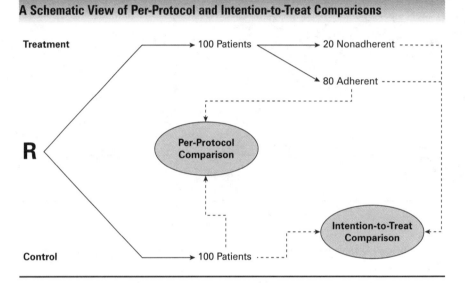

R indicates randomization

To make our demonstration more vivid, we can illustrate with additional hypothetical data. Let us assume that the treatment is once again ineffective and that the true underlying event rate in both treatment and control patients is 20%. Again, the 20 nonadherent patients are sicker but their event rate (60%) is now much higher. Under these circumstances, the nonadherent patients will suffer 12 of the 20 events destined to occur in the treated patients. If one compares only the adherent patients (with an event rate of 8/80, or 10%) with the control group (event rate 20/100, or 20%), one will mistakenly conclude that treatment cuts the event rate in half.

Our hypothetical examples have included a surgical trial and a trial of a medication. The intention-to-treat principle applies regardless of the intervention (surgery, medication, or a behavioral therapy) and regardless of the outcome (mortality, morbidity, or a behavioral outcome such as smoking cessation). Removing patients after randomization always risks introducing bias by creating noncomparable groups.

# A REAL-WORLD EXAMPLE

Perhaps the most dramatic example of how misleading an as-treated analysis can be occurred many years ago in a trial testing the effect of clofibrate, a lipid-lowering agent, in reducing mortality in men between ages 30 and 64 years who had experienced a myocardial infarction.[1] After 5 years of follow-up, slightly fewer (20% of 1103) patients given clofibrate had died than those given placebo (20.9% of 2789; *P* value on the difference, .55). However, the mortality rate in 357 patients treated with clofibrate who took less than 80% of their prescribed treatment was 24.6%, whereas that among those who had taken more than 80% of the medication was 15.0% (*P* value on the difference, .00011). The study found parallel results among placebo-treated patients: the mortality rate in low-adherent patients was 28.2% and in high-adherent patients it was 15.1% (*P* = .0000000000000047). Patients with high adherence both in the experimental group and in the control group clearly represent a prognostically better group. Any inferences about treatment effects based on a selective focus on adherent patients would be extremely misleading. Although a very low *P* value implies that chance is an extremely unlikely explanation of results, the point here is that if we accept the observational design of the clofibrate study, we will conclude erroneously that treatment is effective, and that placebo is even more effective in reducing mortality. Were we to compare adherent patients in the treatment group to the entire control group, we would erroneously conclude that treatment is effective.

# LIMITATIONS OF THE INTENTION-TO-TREAT PRINCIPLE

Even after understanding the logic of the intention-to-treat principle, clinicians may find it unpalatable to count target adverse events in large numbers of patients who did not receive an experimental treatment against the treatment group. After all, the patient we considered at the beginning of this section was interested in the effect the medication would have if she were to take it. The best estimate of this effect would come from a group of patients who all received the experimental intervention, rather than from a group in which some did and some did not receive that intervention.

Indeed, differential nonadherence can produce potentially misleading results, even in an appropriate analysis. Let us say, for instance, that surgery reduces the risk of stroke in patients with cerebrovascular disease by 40%, but 50% of the patients assigned to the no-surgery group receive surgery shortly after randomization. The intention-to-treat analysis will show an apparent treatment effect that is only 50% of what investigators would have observed if all medical patients had adhered to their assigned therapy. The apparent relative risk reduction with surgery will be even less if the patients allocated to medical treatment who nevertheless receive surgery are those at highest risk of adverse events.

Unfortunately, the as-treated analysis cannot solve the problem because we cannot distinguish between treatment effects and bias introduced by baseline differences in prognosis. Our choice in this situation is between a biased estimate of the treatment effect from an as-treated analysis and an unbiased estimate of the effect of the treatment as administered (rather than as intended) from the analysis that attributes events in all patients to the arm to which they were allocated. Such a result may have limited applicability to adherent patients. The best solution to this dilemma is for investigators to design their trials to ensure the highest possible level of adherence and for clinicians to understand the many pitfalls of studies that fail to follow an intention-to-treat approach to analysis of their results.

# MISLEADING USE OF INTENTION-TO-TREAT

We have been careful to talk about the intention-to-treat principle rather than the commonly used term intention-to-treat analysis. The reason is that there is considerable ambiguity in the term *intention-to-treat analysis* and its use can be very misleading.

For instance, picture a trial in which 20% of treated patients and 20% of control patients stop taking medication and investigators elect to terminate their follow-up at that point. At the end of the trial, the investigators count events in all patients of whose status they are aware in the groups to which they are allocated. Technically, they could say they had conducted an intention-to-treat analysis in that they counted all events of which they were aware against the group to which the patient was allocated. Of course, the intention-to-treat analysis has in no way avoided the possible bias introduced by omission of outcome events in patients who discontinued treatment.

One might argue whether investigators should include the patients lost to follow-up in the denominator when calculating the proportion of patients who experienced target outcomes. The danger of including these patients is that if the investigators do not clearly state the proportion lost to follow-up (as is unfortunately often the case), clinicians may get the impression that the study succeeded in following all patients. Whether the denominators include all patients or only those followed ultimately makes little difference, because large loss to follow-up opens the study to major bias. These observations highlight the close conceptual link between biases introduced in an as-treated analysis and those that arise through loss to follow-up.

The problem of misleading statements concerning intention-to-treat analysis in reports of randomized trials is far from theoretical. Hollis and Campbell[2] surveyed all randomized trials published in the *British Medical Journal, The Lancet, JAMA,* and the *New England Journal of Medicine* in 1997. They found that 119 (48%) of the trials used the term "intention-to-treat analysis." Of these 119, 12 explicitly violated the principle of intention-to-treat by excluding patients who did not begin the treatment to which they were allocated. Investigators can justify such a policy if reasons for not starting could not have been affected by allocation. For instance, exclusion of patients allocated to blinded medication who decide they do not want to participate shortly after randomization and before starting treatment is very unlikely to bias study results. Although the approach is potentially justifiable, investigators who use it will mislead if they describe their study as conducting an intention-to-treat analysis.

In another three instances, the investigators' decision to exclude patients from the analyses unequivocally violated intention-to-treat principles.[2] Many of the other trials suffered from the problem we have noted above; the reason for loss to follow-up may have been noncompliance with the intervention to which patients were allocated. Unfortunately, the report by Hollis and Campbell[2] tells us that clinicians must look at the details of what actually happened in the methods sections of the paper, and often in the results as well, rather than accepting statements that the investigators undertook an intention-to-treat analysis.

# References

1. Coronary Drug Project Research Group. Influence of adherence treatment and response of cholesterol on mortality in the Coronary Drug Project. *N Engl J Med*. 1980;303:1038-1041.

2. Hollis S, Campbell F. What is meant by intention to treat analysis? Survey of published randomised controlled trials. *BMJ*. 1999;319:670-674.

# THERAPY AND VALIDITY

## N of 1 Randomized Controlled Trials

Gordon Guyatt, Roman Jaeschke, and Thomas McGinn

## IN THIS SECTION

# INTRODUCTION

The philosophy of evidence-based medicine suggests that clinicians should use the results of randomized controlled trials (RCTs) of groups of patients to guide their clinical care. When deciding which management approach will be best for an individual patient, however, clinicians cannot always rely on the results of RCTs. An RCT addressing the particular issue may not be available (eg, some conditions are so rare that randomized trials are not feasible). Furthermore, even when a relevant RCT generates a clear answer, its result may not apply to an individual patient. First, if the patient does not meet the eligibility criteria, the trial results may not be applicable to that patient (see Part 2B3, "Therapy and Applying the Results, Applying Results to Individual Patients"). Second, regardless of the overall trial results, some patients may benefit from a given therapy, while others receive no benefit. Clinicians may have particularly strong reservations about treatment when randomized trials have shown small treatment effects of questionable importance. Thus, conventional randomized trials have a fundamental limitation: just because a treatment showed a positive effect in a group of other patients does not mean that the patient before us necessarily will benefit.

Under these circumstances, clinicians typically conduct the time-honored *trial of therapy*, in which the patient receives a treatment and the subsequent clinical course determines whether the treatment is judged effective. However, many factors may mislead physicians conducting conventional therapeutic trials. The patient may have gotten better anyway, even without any medication. Or, the physician and the patient may be so optimistic that they may misinterpret the results of the therapeutic trial. Finally, people often feel better when they are taking a new medication even when it does not have any specific activity against their illness (ie, the *placebo effect*), and this may also lead to a misleading interpretation of the value of the new treatment.

To avoid these pitfalls, clinicians must conduct trials of therapy with safeguards that recognize and minimize the effect of these biases. Potential safeguards include repeatedly administering and withdrawing the target treatment, performing quantitative measurement of the target outcomes, and keeping both patients and clinicians blind to the treatment being administered. Investigators routinely use such safeguards in large-scale RCTs involving large numbers of patients.

To maintain the methodologic safeguards provided by RCTs and to determine the best care for an individual patient, RCTs in individual patients (*N of 1 RCTs*) build on the work of experimental psychologists with single-case or single-subject research.[1-3]

In previous publications,[4,5] we have described how N of 1 RCTs may be used in medical practice to determine the optimal treatment for an individual patient, described an "N of 1 service" designed to assist clinicians who wish to conduct such a trial, provided detailed guidelines for clinicians interested in conducting their own N of 1 RCTs, and reviewed our own 3 years of experience in conducting such studies. For each of two conditions (chronic airflow limitation and fibromyalgia), we conducted more than 20 N of 1 RCTs and we have described our experience with these patients in two separate reports.[6,7] The following discussion is based on these experiences. In contrast to most of this book, which provides a guide to using the medical literature, this section provides an approach to applying the principles of of evidence-based medicine to actually conduct an N of 1 RCT in your own practice.

# N OF 1 RANDOMIZED CONTROLLED TRIALS: STUDY DESIGN

Although there are many ways of conducting N of 1 RCTs, the method we have found to be most widely applicable can be summarized as follows:

1. A clinician and patient agree to test a therapy (the *experimental therapy*) for its ability to improve or control the symptoms, signs, or other manifestations (the *treatment targets*) of the patient's ailment.

2. The patient then undergoes pairs of treatment periods organized so that one period of each pair applies the experimental therapy and the other period applies either an alternative treatment or placebo (Figure 2B1-3). The order of these two periods within each pair is randomized by a coin toss or other method that ensures that the patient is equally likely to receive the experimental or control therapy during any treatment period.

**FIGURE 2B1-3**

**Basic Design for N of 1 Randomized Controlled Trial**

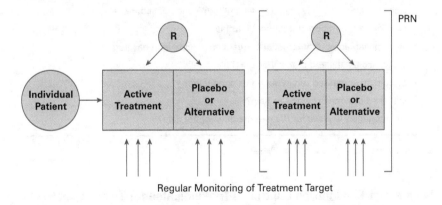

Regular Monitoring of Treatment Target

Circled **R** indicates randomization (ie, the order of placebo and active periods in each pair is determined by random allocation). Bracketed pair with PRN indicates that, beyond the first pair of treatment periods, as many additional pairs of treatment periods as necessary are conducted until patient and physician are convinced of the efficacy—or lack of efficacy—of the trial medication.

Reproduced with permission from McGraw-Hill Companies.

3. Whenever possible, a pharmacist independently prepares medication to ensure that both the clinician and the patient are blind to when the patient is receiving the treatment and alternative therapies (see "Is There a Pharmacist Who Can Help?" later in this section).

4. The clinician monitors the treatment targets, often through a patient diary, to document the effect of the treatment currently being applied.

5. Pairs of treatment periods are replicated until the clinician and patient are convinced that the experimental therapy is effective, is harmful, or has no effect on the treatment targets. This usually requires a minimum of three pairs of treatment periods.

We will now describe an N of 1 RCT in detail. To facilitate its illustration, each step will address a question that must be answered before proceeding to the next step, as summarized in Table 2B1-3. In the remainder of the section, we will provide an overview of a broader perspective on the potential usefulness of N of 1 RCTs.

**TABLE 2B1-3**

## Guidelines for N of 1 Randomized Controlled Trials

**Is an N of 1 Randomized Controlled Trial Indicated for This Patient?**

- Is the effectiveness of the treatment really in doubt?
- If effective, will the treatment be continued on a long-term basis?

**Is an N of 1 Randomized Controlled Trial Feasible in This Patient?**

- Is the patient eager to collaborate in designing and carrying out an N of 1 randomized controlled trial?
- Does the treatment have rapid onset and termination of action?
- Is an optimal duration of treatment feasible?
- What patient-important target(s) of treatment should be measured?
- What dictates the end of the N of 1 RCT?
- Should an unmasked run-in period be conducted?
- Is there a pharmacist who can help?
- Are strategies in place for the interpretation of the data?

## Is an N of 1 Randomized Controlled Trial Indicated for This Patient?

Because N of 1 RCTs are unnecessary for some ailments (such as self-limited illnesses) and unsuited for some treatments (such as surgical procedures or the prevention of distant adverse outcomes such as death, stroke, or myocardial infarction), at the outset it is important to determine whether an N of 1 RCT really is indicated for the patient and treatment in question. If an N of 1 RCT is appropriate, the answers to each of the following questions should be "yes."

### Is the Effectiveness of the Treatment Really in Doubt?

One or several RCTs may have shown that the treatment in question is highly effective. However, if 50% or more of patients in such trials have proved unresponsive, an N of 1 RCT may still be appropriate. Calculations of numbers needed to treat suggest that this will almost always be the case, regardless of whether the treatments are designed to prevent major adverse events or to improve health-related quality of life.[8] Numbers needed to treat of two or less are extremely uncommon.

On the other hand, a patient may have exhibited such a dramatic response to the treatment that both clinician and patient are convinced that it works. N of 1 RCTs are best reserved for the following situations.

- The patient has started taking a medication, but neither patient nor clinician is confident that the treatment is really providing benefit.

- The clinician is uncertain whether a treatment that has not yet been started will work in a particular patient.

- The patient insists on taking a treatment that the clinician believes is useless or potentially harmful—and neither mere words nor logically constructed arguments will change the patient's mind.

- A patient has symptoms that both the clinician and patient suspect—but are not certain—are caused by the side effects of the medications.

- Neither the clinician nor the patient is confident of the optimal dose of a medication the patient is receiving or should receive.

### If Effective, Will the Treatment be Continued on a Long-Term Basis?

If the underlying condition is self-limited and treatment will be continued only over the short term, an N of 1 RCT may not be worthwhile. N of 1 RCTs are most useful when conditions are chronic and maintenance therapy is likely to be prolonged.

## Is an N of 1 Randomized Controlled Trial Feasible in This Patient?

The clinician may wish to determine the efficacy of treatment in an individual patient but the patient, the ailment, or the treatment, may not lend itself to the N of 1 approach.

### Is the Patient Eager to Collaborate in Designing and Carrying Out an N of 1 Randomized Controlled Trial?

N of 1 RCTs are indicated only when patients can fully understand the nature of the experiment and are enthusiastic about participating. The N of 1 RCT is a cooperative venture between clinician and patient.

### Does the Treatment Have Rapid Onset and Termination of Action?

N of 1 RCTs are much easier to carry out when positive treatment effects, if they are indeed present, manifest themselves within a few days. Although it may be possible to conduct N of 1 RCTs with drugs that have longer latency for the development of signs of efficacy (such as gold therapy or penicillamine administration in patients with rheumatoid arthritis, or use of tricyclic antidepressants in patients suffering from depression), the requirement for long treatment periods before the effect can be evaluated may prove prohibitive.

Similarly, treatments whose effects cease abruptly when they are withdrawn are most suitable for N of 1 RCTs. If the treatment continues to act long after it is stopped, a prolonged washout period may be necessary. If this washout period lasts longer than a few days, the feasibility of the trial is compromised. Similarly, treatments that have the potential to cure the underlying condition—or to lead to a permanent change in the treatment target—are not suitable for N of 1 RCTs.

### Is an Optimal Duration of Treatment Feasible?

Although short periods of treatment boost the feasibility of N of 1 RCTs, the trials may need to be long to be valid. For example, if active therapy takes a few days to reach full effect and a few days to cease acting once it is stopped, treatment periods of sufficient duration are required to avoid distortion from these delayed peak effects and washout periods. Thus, our N of 1 RCTs of theophylline in patients with asthma use treatment periods of at least 10 days: 3 days to allow the drug to reach steady state or washout, and 7 days thereafter to monitor the patient's response to treatment.

In addition, since many N of 1 RCTs test a treatment's ability to prevent or mitigate attacks or exacerbations (such as migraines or seizures), each treatment period must be long enough to include an attack or exacerbation. A rough rule of thumb, called the *inverse rule of 3s*, tells us the following: If an event occurs, on average, once every $x$ days, we need to observe $3x$ days to be 95% confident of observing at least one event. For example, applying this rule in a patient with familial Mediterranean fever with attacks that occur, on average, once every 2 weeks, calls for treatment periods of at least 6 weeks' duration.

Finally, the clinician may not want the patient to take responsibility for crossing over from one treatment period to the next—or examination of the patient at the end of each treatment period might be necessary. Thus, other factors such as the clinician's office schedule and the patient's travel considerations may influence or dictate the length of each treatment period.

### What Patient-Important Target(s) of Treatment Should Be Measured?

The targets of treatment, or outcome measures, usually go beyond a set of physical signs (eg, the rigidity and tremor of parkinsonism, or the jugular venous distention and the S3, S4, and pulmonary crackles of congestive heart failure), a laboratory test (eg, serum erythrocyte sedimentation rate or serum blood glucose, uric acid, and creatinine levels), or a measure of patient performance (eg, recordings of respiratory peak flow or results of a 6-minute walk test). Each of these is only an indirect measure of the patient's prognosis or quality of life.

In most situations, it is not only possible but preferable to directly assess the patient's symptoms, feelings of well-being, and quality of life. Principles of measurement of quality of life can be applied in a simple fashion to N of 1 RCTs (see Part 2B2, "Therapy and Understanding the Results, Quality of Life"). To begin with, ask the patient to identify the most troubling symptoms or problems he is experiencing and then decide which of them is likely to respond to the experimental treatment. This responsive subset of symptoms or problems forms the basis of a self-administered patient diary or questionnaire.

For example, a patient with chronic airflow limitation identified his problem as shortness of breath while walking up stairs, bending, or vacuuming.[7] A patient with fibromyalgia (to whom we shall return later) identified fatigue, aches and pains, morning stiffness, and sleep disturbance as problems that should become the treatment targets for her illness.[6]

The questionnaire to record the patient's symptoms can be presented using a number of formats. Figure 2B1-4 shows a typical data sheet for patient symptom recording. For some patients, a daily symptom rating may work best; for others, a weekly summary may be better. The best way of presenting response options to patients is as graded descriptions of symptoms ranging from "none" to "severe." One example of such graded descriptions might be "No shortness of breath," "A little shortness of breath," "Moderate shortness of breath," and "Extreme shortness of breath." Constructing simple symptom questionnaires is not difficult, and completing them allows the patient and the clinician to collaborate in quantifying patient symptoms, on which the analysis of the N of 1 RCT relies.

Regardless of the format chosen by the clinician to measure treatment targets, patients should rate their symptoms at least twice during each study period. The identifying patient information and the ratings on the treatment targets often can be combined on one page. Figure 2B1-4 displays such a form for an N of 1 RCT examining the effectiveness of a new drug, ketanserin, in Raynaud phenomenon.

A final point concerning measurement of a patient's symptoms is that the patient may also record side effects. A patient diary or questionnaire can be used to measure nausea, gastrointestinal disturbances, dizziness, or other common side effects along with symptoms of the primary condition. In N of 1 RCTs designed to determine whether medication side effects are responsible for a patient's symptoms (eg, whether a patient's fatigue is caused by an antihypertensive agent), side effects become the primary treatment targets.

**FIGURE 2B1-4**

# N of 1 Randomized Controlled Trial—Sample Data Sheet

Physician: _____

Patient: _____

Sex: Male    Female    Date of Birth _____ _____ _____

Diagnosis: _____

Occupation: _____

Present Medications: _____

Trial medication: Ketanserin    Dose: _____

Duration of study periods: 2 Weeks

Outcomes: Symptom ratings

Informed consent obtained (Please sign): _____

Answers to symptom questions, Pair 1, Period 1:

1. How many episodes of Raynaud phenomenon did you have in the last week?

   First week (to be completed on _____ _____) _____

   Second week (to be completed on _____ _____) _____

2. On average, in comparison to your usual episodes, how long were the attacks?

   1. Very long; as long as or longer than they have ever been

   2. Very long; almost as long as they have ever been

   3. Longer than usual

   4. As long as usual

   5. Not as long as usual

   6. Not nearly as long as usual

   7. Very short; as brief as or briefer than they have ever been

   Write in the number that best describes your experience for each week.

   First week (to be completed on _____ _____) _____

   Second week (to be completed on _____ _____) _____

3. On average, in comparison to your usual episodes, how severe were the attacks?

   1. Very bad; as severe as or more severe than they have ever been

   2. Very bad; almost as severe as they have ever been

   3. More severe than usual

   4. About as severe as usual

   5. Not as severe as usual

   6. Not nearly as severe as usual

   7. Very mild; as mild as or milder than they have ever been

   Write in the number that best describes your experience for each week.

   First week (to be completed on _____ _____) _____

   Second week (to be completed on _____ _____) _____

## What Dictates the End of the N of 1 RCT?

If the clinician and patient decide not to specify the number of pairs of treatment periods in advance, they can stop anytime they are convinced that the experimental treatment ought to be stopped or continued indefinitely. Thus, if they find dramatic improvement in the treatment target between the two periods of the first pair, both clinician and patient may want to stop the trial immediately. On the other hand, if a minimal difference continues to occur between the two periods of each pair, both the clinician and the patient may need three, four, or even five pairs before confidently concluding that the treatment is or is not effective.

However, if one wishes to conduct a formal statistical analysis of data from the N of 1 RCT, the analysis will be strengthened if the number of pairs is specified in advance. We discuss this issue further in the section concerning strategies for interpretation of N of 1 RCTs (see "Are Strategies for the Interpretation of the N of 1 Trial in Place?").

Regardless of whether one specifies the number of treatment periods in advance, it is advisable to conduct at least two pairs of treatment periods before consulting the code that specfies when the patient has been taking active medication, and when he has been receiving placebo. Too many conclusions drawn after a single pair will be either false-positive judgments (ie, the treatment is deemed effective when it actually is ineffective) or false-negative judgments (ie, the treatment is considered ineffective when it actually is effective). Indeed, we recommend that clinicians resist temptation and refrain from breaking the code until they are quite certain they are ready to terminate the study.

## Should an Unblinded Run-in Period Be Conducted?

A preliminary unblinded run-in period of active therapy, during which both the physician and patient know that the patient is receiving active therapy, could save a lot of time. After all, if there is no hint of response during such an open trial or if intolerable side effects occur, an N of 1 RCT may be fruitless or impossible. For example, we prepared for a double-blind N of 1 RCT of methylphenidate administration in a child with hyperactivity only to find a dramatic increase in agitation during the first 2 days of the first study period (during which the patient was receiving the active drug), mandating an abrupt termination of the study. Finally, the clinician may use an open, or unblinded, run-in period to determine the optimal dose of the medication.

## Is There a Pharmacist Who Can Help?

Conducting an N of 1 RCT that incorporates all the aforementioned safeguards against bias and misinterpretation requires collaboration between the clinician and a pharmacist or pharmacy service. Preparation of placebos identical to the active medication in appearance, taste, and texture is required. Occasionally, pharmaceutical firms can supply such placebos. More often, however, you will want your local pharmacist to repackage the active medication. If it comes in tablet form, the pharmacist can crush and repackage it in capsule form—unless the medication is a modified-release preparation and absorption characteristics would be altered. Thus, a clinician who is interested in the effect of a modified-release preparation may have to sacrifice blinding if the duration of action of the medication is a crucial issue.

If a placebo is judged important, the pharmacist can fill identical-appearing placebo capsules with lactose. Although it is somewhat time consuming, preparation of placebos is not technically difficult. Our average cost for preparing medication for N of 1 studies in which placebos have not been available from a pharmaceutical company has been $200 Canadian.

Nevertheless the expense associated with preparation of identical active and placebo medication can be prohibitive. We have relied on a number of strategies for funding, including use of discretionary research funds or the generosity of a large hospital pharmacy. The large savings that follow from abandoning a useless or harmful treatment that might otherwise be continued indefinitely, along with the reassurance of knowing that long-term treatment really works, emphasize the relatively trivial cost of the N of 1 RCT.

The pharmacist is also charged with preparing the randomization schedule (which requires nothing more than a coin toss for each pair of treatment periods). This allows the clinician, along with the patient, to remain blind to allocation. The pharmacist also may be helpful in planning the design of the trial by providing information regarding the anticipated time to onset of action and the washout period, thus helping with decisions about the duration of study periods. The pharmacist can help monitor compliance and drug absorption. Both tablet counts and serum drug concentration measurements at the end of each treatment period can help ensure that the patient conscientiously takes the study medication throughout the trial.

### Are Strategies for the Interpretation of the Trial Data in Place?

Once you carefully gather data on the treatment targets in your N of 1 trial, how will you interpret them? One approach is to simply plot the data and visually inspect the results. Evaluation of results by visual inspection has a long and distinguished record in the psychology literature concerning single-subject designs.[2,3] Visual inspection is simple and easy. Its major disadvantage is that it is vulnerable to viewer or observer bias.

An alternative approach to analysis of data from N of 1 RCTs is to use a test of statistical significance. The simplest test would be based on the likelihood of a patient's preferring active treatment in each pair of treatment periods. This situation is analogous to the likelihood of heads coming up repeatedly on a series of coin tosses. For example, the likelihood of a patient's preferring active treatment to placebo during three consecutive pairs if the treatment were ineffective would be $1/2 \times 1/2 \times 1/2 = 1/8$, or 0.125. The disadvantage of this approach (which is called the *sign test*[9]) is that it lacks power; five pairs must be conducted before there is any chance of reaching conventional levels of statistical significance.

A second statistical strategy is to use Student $t$ test. The $t$ test offers increased power because not only the direction but also the strength of the treatment effect in each pair is taken into account. The disadvantage of the $t$ test is that it makes additional assumptions about the data that may not be valid. The assumption of greatest concern is that observations are independent of one another, that is, that a patient is equally likely to feel good or bad on a particular day regardless of whether he or she felt good or bad the day before (a phenomenon known as *autocorrelation*). Although some autocorrelation is likely to exist in many N of 1 RCTs, the impact of the autocorrelation can be reduced if one uses the average of all measurements in a given period, rather than the individual observations, in the statistical analysis. Furthermore, the paired design of the N of 1 RCT that we recommend further reduces the impact of any autocorrelation that exists.

If clinicians decide to use statistical tests to interpret data, they face another potential problem. If the clinician and patient use the results from the studies to determine when to stop the trial, the true *P* value may be inflated above the nominal *P* value. Therefore, we recommend that if you plan a statistical test, you specify the number of treatment periods before the study begins.

To conduct a paired *t* test, derive a single score for each pair by subtracting the mean score of the placebo period from the mean score for the active period. These different scores constitute the data for the paired *t*; the number of *degrees of freedom* is simply the number of pairs minus 1. Statistical software programs that will facilitate quick calculation of the *P* value are available.

Table 2B1-4 presents the results of an N of 1 RCT. In this trial, we tested the effectiveness of amitriptyline in a dose of 10 mg at bedtime for a patient with fibrositis.[6] Each week, the patient separately rated the severity of a number of symptoms, including fatigue, aches and pains, and sleep disturbance, on a seven-point scale in which a higher score represented better function. The treatment periods were 4 weeks long, and three pairs were undertaken. Table 2B1-4 presents the mean scores for each of the 24 weeks of the study.

**TABLE 2B1-4**

### Results of an N of 1 Randomized Controlled Trial in a Patient With Fibrositis*

| Treatment | Severity Score | | | | |
|---|---|---|---|---|---|
| | Week 1 | Week 2 | Week 3 | Week 4 | Mean Score |
| *Pair 1* | | | | | |
| Active | 4.43 | 4.86 | 4.71 | 4.71 | 4.68 |
| Placebo | 4.43 | 4.00 | 4.14 | 4.29 | 4.22 |
| | | | | | |
| *Pair 2* | | | | | |
| Active | 4.57 | 4.89 | 5.29 | 5.29 | 5.01 |
| Placebo | 3.86 | 4.00 | 4.29 | 4.14 | 4.07 |
| | | | | | |
| *Pair 3* | | | | | |
| Active | 4.29 | 5.00 | 5.43 | 5.43 | 5.04 |
| Placebo | 3.71 | 4.14 | 4.43 | 4.43 | 4.18 |

* The active drug was amitriptyline hydrochloride. Higher scores represent better function.

The first step in analyzing the results of the study is to calculate the mean score for each period (presented in the far right-hand column of Table 2B1-4). In each pair, the score favored the active treatment. The sign test tells us that the probability of this result occurring by chance if the treatment were ineffective is $1/2 \times 1/2 \times 1/2 = 1/8$ (or $= 0.125$).

However, this analysis ignores the magnitude and consistency of the difference between active and placebo treatments. A paired $t$ test in which data from the same patient during different periods are paired takes these factors into account. We did our $t$ test by entering the data from the pairs of results into a simple statistical program: 4.68 and 4.22; 5.01 and 4.07; 5.04 and 4.18. The program tells us that the $t$ value is 5.07 and there are 2 degrees of freedom; the associated $P$ value is .037. This analysis makes us considerably more confident that the consistent difference in favor of active drug is unlikely to have occurred by chance.

Clinicians and statisticians may remain uncomfortable with the suggested approach to analysis of data from N of 1 RCTs. The use of N of 1 RCTs to improve patient care does not depend on statistical analysis of the results. Even if statistical analysis is not used in the interpretation of the trial, the strategies of randomization, double blinding, replication, and quantifying outcomes, when accompanied by careful visual inspection of the data, still allow a much more rigorous assessment of effectiveness of treatment than is possible in conventional clinical practice.

# ETHICS OF N OF 1 RCTS

Is conducting an N of 1 RCT a clinical task or a research undertaking? If the former, is it the sort of clinical procedure, analogous to an invasive diagnostic test, that requires written informed consent? We would argue that the N of 1 RCT can be—and should be—a part of routine clinical practice.

Nevertheless, a number of ethical issues are important to consider. We believe that patients should be fully informed of the nature of the study in which they are participating and that there should be no element of deception in the use of placebos as part of the study. Written informed consent should be obtained (see Figure 2B1-5 for an example of a consent form). Patients should be aware that they can terminate the trial at any time without jeopardizing their care or their relationship with their physician. Finally, follow-up should be soon enough to prevent any important deleterious consequences of institution or withdrawal of therapy.

**FIGURE 2B1-5**

## Consent Form for N of 1 RCT

We think that it would help you to take part in one of these therapeutic trials of [NAME OF DRUG]. We will conduct a number of pairs of periods. Each period will be [DURATION OF PERIOD]. During one period of each pair you will be taking the active treatment, and during the other you will be using the placebo. The placebo is a pill that looks exactly like the medication, but does not contain the active ingredients. If at any time during the study you are feeling worse, we can consider that treatment period at an end and can go on to the next treatment. Therefore, if you begin to feel worse, just call my office at [INSERT NUMBER], and I will get in touch with you.

If you don't think this new way of conducting a therapeutic trial is a good idea for you, we will try the new drug in the usual way. Your decision will not interfere with your treatment in any way. You can decide to stop the trial at any time along the way, and this will not interfere with your treatment either. All information we collect during the trial will remain confidential.

PATIENT SIGNATURE _____

WITNESS SIGNATURE _____

PHYSICIAN SIGNATURE _____

DATE _____

# THE IMPACT OF N OF 1 RCTS IN CLINICAL PRACTICE

We have reported a series of more than 50 N of 1 RCTs, each one designed to improve the care being delivered to an individual patient.[5] Patients suffered from a wide variety of conditions, including chronic airflow limitation, asthma, fibrositis, arthritis, syncope, anxiety, insomnia, and angina pectoris. In general, these trials were successful in sorting out whether or not the treatment was effective. In approximately a third of the trials, the ultimate treatment differed from that which would have been given had the trial not been conducted. In most of the trials in which treatment differed from that which would have been given had the trial not been conducted, medication that would otherwise have been given over the long term was discontinued. Other clinical groups have reported on their experience with N of 1 RCTs, generally confirming the feasibility and usefulness of the approach.[10-12] Table 2B1-5 presents a set of conditions and therapeutic options that are excellent candidates for N of 1 RCTs.

TABLE 2B1-5

## Examples of N of 1 RCTs

| Type of Condition | Possible Outcome Measures | Example of Intervention |
|---|---|---|
| Chronic headache | Duration, severity, and frequency of headache | Tricyclic antidepressant or beta blockers |
| Low back pain | Pain or function | Cyclobenzaprine or acupuncture* |
| Recurrent syncope | Syncopal episodes | Beta blockers |
| Chronic airway obstruction | Dyspnea, peak flow rates | Aerosolized beta agonists, ipratropium, steroids |
| Fibromyalgia | Aches and pains, fatigue, sleep disruption | Low-dose tricyclic antidepressant |
| Fatigue | Fatigue | Ginseng tablets* |
| Insomnia | Sleep disruption, satisfaction | Low-dose tricyclic antidepressant |
| Anxiety | Anxiety, formal anxiety questionnaire such as Beck | Black cohosh* |
| Hot flashes of menopause | Frequency and severity of hot flashes | Clonidine or soy milk* |

* Alternative therapies with little evidence to support efficacy but frequently used by patients with substantial costs.

These reports do not definitively answer the question about whether patients who undergo N of 1 RCTs are better off than those whose treatment regimen is determined by conventional methods. The most rigorous test of the usefulness of N of 1 RCTs would be a randomized trial. Two such trials, in which patients were randomized to conventional care or to undergo N of 1 RCTs, have been undertaken.[13,14] Both were conducted by the same group of investigators and both studied the use of theophylline in patients with chronic airflow limitation. The investigators found that although using N of 1 RCTs did not affect patients' quality of life or functional status, of patients initially on theophylline, fewer in the N of 1 RCT groups ended up receiving the drug over the long term. Thus, N of 1 RCTs saved patients the expense, inconvenience, and potential toxicity of useless long-term theophylline therapy.

While confirming the potential of N of 1 RCTs, groups with extensive experience with this type of investigation have noted the time and effort required. It is unlikely that full implementation of N of 1 RCTs will become a major part of clinical practice. However, clinicians can incorporate many of the key principles of N of 1 RCTs into their practice without adopting the full rigor of the approach presented here. Medication can be repeatedly withdrawn and reintroduced in an open fashion without the safeguard (and the inconvenience) of blinding.

Symptoms and physical findings can be carefully quantified. However, without the additional feature of double blinding, both the placebo effect and physician and patient expectations can still bias the results.

In summary, the N of 1 approach clearly has potential for improving the quality of medical care and the judicious use of expensive and potentially toxic medication in patients with chronic disease. Using the guidelines offered here, we believe that clinicians will find the conduct of N of 1 RCTs feasible, highly informative, and stimulating.

# References

1. Guyatt GH, Sackett D, Taylor DW, Chong J, Roberts R, Pugsley S. Determining optimal therapy—randomized trials in individual patients. *N Engl J Med*. 1986;314:889-892.

2. Kratchowill TR. *Single Subject Research: Strategies for Evaluating Change*. New York: Academic Press; 1978.

3. Kazdin AE. *Single-Case Research Designs: Methods for Clinical and Applied Settings*. New York: Oxford University Press; 1982.

4. Guyatt GH, Sackett DL, Adachi JD, et al. A clinician's guide for conducting randomized trials in individual patients. *CMAJ*. 1988;139:497-503.

5. Guyatt GH, Keller JL, Jaeschke R, Rosenbloom R, Adachi JD, Newhouse MT. The n-of-1 randomized controlled trial: clinical usefulness. Our three-year experience. *Ann Intern Med*. 1990;112:293-299.

6. Jaeschke R, Adachi JD, Guyatt GH, Keller JL, Wong B. Clinical usefulness of amitriptyline in fibromyalgia: the results of 23 N-of-1 randomized controlled trials. *J Rheumatol*. 1991;18:447-451.

7. Patel A, Jaeschke R, Guyatt G, Newhouse MT, Keller J. Clinical usefulness of n-of-1 randomized controlled trials in patients with nonreversible chronic airflow limitation. *Am Rev Respir Dis*. 1991;144:962-964.

8. Guyatt GH, Juniper EL, Walter SD, Griffith LE, Goldstein RS. Interpreting treatment effects in randomised trials. *BMJ*. 1998;316:690-693.

9. Conover WJ. *Practical Nonparametric Statistics*. New York: John Wiley & Sons; 1971:121-126.

10. Menard J, Serrurier D, Bautier P, Plouin PF, Corvol P. Crossover design to test antihypertensive drugs with self-recorded blood pressure. *Hypertension*. 1988; 11:153-159.

11. Johannessen T. Controlled trials in single subjects, 1: value in clinical medicine. *BMJ*. 1991;303:173-174.

12. Larson EB, Ellsworth AJ, Oas J. Randomized clinical trials in single patients during a 2-year period. *JAMA*. 1993;270:2708-2712.

13. Mahon J, Laupacis A, Donner A, Wood T. Randomised study of n of 1 trials versus standard practice. *BMJ*. 1996;312:1069-1074.

14. Mahon JL, Laupacis A, Hodder RV, et al. Theophylline for irreversible chronic airflow limitation: a randomized study comparing n of 1 trials to standard practice. *Chest*. 1999;115:38-48.

# THERAPY AND VALIDITY

## Computer Decision Support Systems

Adrienne Randolph, Brian Haynes, Jeremy Wyatt, Deborah Cook, and Gordon Guyatt

The following EBM Working Group members also made substantive contributions to this section: Peter Pronovost and Lee Green

## IN THIS SECTION

## Will Computer Decision Support Systems Fulfill Their Promise?

It is 7 AM and medical rounds are starting on University Hospital Ward 3B. During the past 24 hours of your residency, you have transferred two critically ill patients to the intensive care unit, accepted 11 patients to your medical service, examined and revised medication orders for 22 patients, placed nine intravascular catheters, written 35 notes, and reviewed, categorized, and acted on more than 300 new pieces of laboratory and radiologic data. You were planning to ask the infectious disease specialist about a patient, but the consultant appears to be very busy and the broad-spectrum antibiotic regimen you prescribed should cover everything.

Abruptly you are told that you have ordered total parenteral nutrition for the wrong patient. As you investigate to which patient the order really pertains, you realize that the calculations for the amino acid concentration are erroneous. Five minutes into your first patient presentation, the senior physician asks you for details from the past medical history. You wish you could refer to your admission note, but you were unable to access it before rounds because a utilization review clerk had the chart.

Thinking of your present dilemma, you recall that the Chair of Medicine keeps promising to install computers to help manage all of this information, but she is feeling a budget squeeze. She needs proof that computerization will improve patient care to justify such a major expense, and she asks you to help. You remember reading, in the many professional journals piled up at home, about how computers can be used to provide decision support, ultimately leading to improved patient outcomes. If you can show that computers improve patient care, maybe the hospital administrators will see the expense as an investment that could reduce costs.

# FINDING THE EVIDENCE

When you return home that night, you connect to the Internet and decide to search the medical literature for information on computer use in clinical care by searching *Internet Grateful Med* from the US National Library of Medicine. You type "igm.nlm.nih.gov/" into the address bar of your browser, quickly realizing that you do not know which search terms to use. You type in "decision" and then click on "Find MeSH/Meta Terms." From the 31 MeSH terms offered, you choose "Decision-Making, Computer-Assisted," "Therapy, Computer-Assisted," "Diagnosis, Computer-Assisted," and "Drug Therapy, Computer-Assisted," specifying that they are the major topic of the article. You limit your search to English-language randomized controlled trials from the years 1995 through 2000. Browsing through the 135 abstracts emanating from the search, you choose one entitled, "A Randomized Trial of Corollary Orders to Prevent Errors of Omission." The abstract of this article concludes that ". . . physician work stations, linked to a comprehensive electronic medical record, can be an efficient means for decreasing errors of omission and improving adherence to practice guidelines."[1]

You order the full article over the Internet from Loansome Doc. In this study,[1] conducted on the inpatient general medical wards of an inner-city public hospital, six independent services (Red service, Green service, and so forth) care for the inpatients. Each service includes a faculty internist, a senior resident, and two interns. A different physician team rotates onto each service every 6 weeks, and during the course of a year, eight different teams work on each service. At the beginning of the study, the investigators randomly allocated three of the six services to the intervention group, which had access to a computer-based clinical decision support systems (CDSS), and the other three served as controls who lacked CDSS access. The CDSS responded to a specified set of orders called *trigger orders* (orders in response to which the CDSS system would initiate action) by suggesting *corollary orders* needed to detect or ameliorate adverse reactions, and it allowed physicians to accept or reject these suggestions. Examples of corollary orders (also called *response orders*) would be the orders to monitor electrolyte, magnesium, and creatinine levels in patients receiving amphotericin B (the trigger order). Table 2B1-6 shows more examples of these corollary orders and their relevant trigger order.

**TABLE 2B1-6**

## Examples of Trigger and Corollary Orders

| Trigger Orders | Corollary Orders |
|---|---|
| Heparin infusion | 1. Check serum platelet count once before heparin starts, then every 24 hours.<br>2. Ascertain serum activated partial thromboplastin time (APTT) at start, again 6 hours after a dosage change.<br>3. Ascertain serum prothrombin time (PT) once before heparin is started.<br>4. Check serum hemoglobin level at start of therapy, then every morning.<br>5. Test stools for occult blood while on heparin. |
| Intravenus Fluids | 1. Place a saline lock when intravenus fluids are discontinued. |
| Narcotics (class II) | 1. Order a stool softener or laxative. |
| Nonsteroidal agents | 1. Assess serum creatinine level (if not done in previous 10 days); SMA12; blood urea nitrogen (BUN) counted as equivalent to creatinine. |
| Aminoglycosides | 1. Check serum peak and trough levels of the drug after dosage changes and once a week.<br>2. Assess serum creatinine level twice per week (for example, every Monday and Thursday). |
| Warfarin | 1. Check serum prothrombin time each morning. |
| Amphotericin B | 1. Assess serum creatinine level twice per week (every Monday and Thursday).<br>2. Check serum magnesium level (twice per week while on therapy).<br>3. Check serum electrolytes (twice per week while on therapy).<br>4. Give acetaminophen, 650 mg by mouth, 30 minutes before each dose of amphotericin.<br>5. Give diphenhydramine, 50 mg by mouth, 30 minutes before each amphotericin dose. |

Clinicians depend on computers. Laboratory data management software, pharmacy information management systems, applications for tracking patient location through admission and discharge, mechanical ventilators, and oxygen saturation measurement devices are among the many types of computerized systems that have become an integral part of the modern hospital. These devices and systems capture, transform, display, or analyze data for use in clinical decision making. Of the available computer aids, we restrict the term *computer decision support system* (CDSS) to software designed to aid directly in clinical decision making about individual patients.

In computer decision support systems, detailed individual patient data are entered into a computer program and are sorted and matched to programs or algorithms in a computerized database, resulting in the generation of patient-specific assessments or recommendations for clinicians.[2] Table 2B1-7 shows categories of computer decision support systems developed for the following medical purposes: alerting, reminding, critiquing, interpreting, predicting, diagnosing, and suggesting.[3]

**TABLE 2B1-7**

## Functions of Computer-Based Clinical Decision Support Systems

| Function | Example |
|---|---|
| Alerting | Highlighting out-of-range (either too high or too low) laboratory values |
| Reminding | Reminding the clinician to schedule a mammogram |
| Critiquing | Rejecting an inappropriate electronic order for a new drug |
| Interpreting | Analyzing an electrocardiogram |
| Predicting | Calculating risk of mortality from a severity of illness score |
| Diagnosing | Listing a differential diagnosis for a patient with chest pain |
| Assisting | Tailoring the antibiotic choices for patients with liver transplant and renal failure |
| Suggesting | Generating suggestions for adjusting a mechanical ventilator |

Many alerting, reminding, and critiquing systems are based on simple if/then rules or *conditional probabilities* that tell the computer what to do when a certain event occurs. *Alerting* systems monitor a continuous signal or stream of data and generate a message (an alert) in response to items or patterns that might require action on the part of the clinician.[4] An example of an alert is the starred (*) or highlighted items (with the letters H or L denoting values that are either high or low in bold or with color changes on the screen) that alert the clinician to values that are out of range (either too high or too low) on computerized laboratory printouts and display screens. Alerting systems draw attention to events as they occur.

*Reminder* systems notify clinicians of important tasks that need to be done before an event occurs. An outpatient clinic reminder system may generate a list of immunizations required by each patient on the daily schedule. Although the rules behind alerts and reminders are often simple, alerting the right person in a timely fashion is quite complex. Physicians, for instance, may not notice or attend to reminders.

When the computer evaluates a clinician's decision and generates an appropriateness rating or an alternative suggestion, the decision support approach is called *critiquing*. The distinction between assisting and critiquing decision support programs is that assisting programs help formulate the clinical decision, whereas critiquing programs have no part in decision making, but evaluate the entered plan against an algorithm in the computer.[3] Critiquing systems are commonly applied to physician order entry. For example, a clinician entering an order for a blood transfusion may receive a message stating that the patient's serum hemoglobin level is above the transfusion threshold and the clinician must justify the order by stating an indication such as active bleeding.[5] Getting the attention of the person who can take action is one of the most difficult aspects of making alerting, reminding, and critiquing systems effective.

The automated interpretations of electrocardiogram readings[6] and the outcome predictions generated by severity of illness scoring systems[7] are examples of decision support systems used for interpreting and predicting, respectively. These systems filter and abstract detailed clinical data and generate a report characterizing the meaning of the data such as "anterior myocardial infarction."[6]

Computer-aided diagnostic systems also can assist the clinician with the process of differential diagnosis.[8] When an electrocardiogram is not definitive, computer systems that try to distinguish between myocardial infarction and other sources of chest pain can sometimes outperform some clinicians.[9] These types of systems require pertinent patient information such as signs, symptoms, past medical history, laboratory values, and demographic characteristics. The program offers hypotheses, often prompts the user for more information, and ultimately provides a diagnosis or a list of possible diagnoses ranked probabilistically.

Computerized patient management systems are complex programs that make suggestions about the optimal decision based on the information currently known by the system. These types of systems are often integrated into the physician ordering process. After collecting information on specific patient variables, the patient management program tailors the order to the patient based on prior information in the database regarding appropriate dosages—or by implementing specified protocols. For example, the Antibiotic Assistant[10] is a CDSS that implements guidelines to assist physicians in ordering antibiotic agents. This system recommends the most cost-effective antibiotic regimen while taking into account the following: the patient's renal function and drug allergies, the site of infection, the epidemiology of organisms in patients with this infection at the particular hospital during a span of many years, the efficacy of the chosen antibiotic regimen, and the cost of therapy. A system that instructs caregivers on how to manage the ventilation of patients with adult respiratory distress syndrome[11] is another example of a patient management program.

The primary reason to invest in computer support is to improve quality of care. If a computer system purports to aid clinical decisions, enhance patient care, and improve outcomes, then it should be subject to the same rules of testing as for any other health care intervention with similar claims. In this section, we describe how to use articles that evaluate the clinical impact of a CDSS. Although the focus of a CDSS may be restricted to diagnosis or prognosis, we will limit our discussion to the situation in which the system is designed to change clinician behavior and patient outcome.

Many iterative steps are involved in developing, evaluating, and improving a CDSS before it is good enough to move beyond the laboratory environment and pilot-testing phase to have a broader impact on physicians and patients. These steps involve the application of social science methods for evaluating human behavior and computer science methods for evaluating technologic safety and and the ability of the system to deal with different situations. We will limit our discussion to mature systems that have surpassed initial evaluation and are being implemented to change physician behavior and patient outcome.

# ARE THE RESULTS VALID?

In keeping with the approach integrated throughout earlier sections of this book, we will consider three primary questions related to validity of results, nature of results, and clinical application of results (Table 2B1-8). In so doing we will continue to refer back to the article by Overhage et al[1] evaluating the impact of computerized reminders of corollary orders to prevent errors of omission during the ordering process.

**TABLE 2B1-8**

## Using Articles Describing Computer-Based Clinical Decision Support Systems

**Are the Results Valid?**

*Did experimental and control groups begin the study with a similar prognosis?*

- Were patients randomized?
- If not, did the investigators demonstrate similarity in all known determinants of prognosis—or adjust for differences in the analysis?
- Was the control group uninfluenced by the CDSS?

*Did experimental and control groups retain a similar prognosis after the study started?*

- Was follow-up complete?
- Were interventions that affect prognosis similar in the two groups?
- Was outcome assessed uniformly the experimental and control groups?

**What Are the Results?**

- How large was the treatment effect?
- How precise was the estimate of the treatment effect?

**How Can I Apply the Results to Patient Care?**

- Were all clinically important outcomes considered?
- What elements of the CDSS are required?
- Is the CDSS exportable to a new site?
- Is the CDSS likely to be accepted by clinicians in your setting?
- Are the likely treatment benefits worth the potential risks and costs?

When clinicians examine the effect of a CDSS on patient management or outcome, they should use the same criteria that are appropriate for any other intervention, whether it is a drug, a rehabilitation program, or an approach to diagnosis or screening[12] (see Part 1B1, "Therapy"). Thus, you will find that Table 2B1-8, which summarizes our approach to evaluating an article that examines the impact of a CDSS, includes the same validity criteria as our guide to therapy. Table 2B1-8 also includes criteria from our guide to articles concerning harm (see Part 1B2, "Harm"). This is because randomization—and other strategies used to reduce bias in randomized trials—may not be feasible in a CDSS evaluation. Our discussion includes only issues of particular importance in the evaluation of a CDSS.

## Were Study Participants Randomized?

## If Not, Did the Investigators Demonstrate Similarity in All Known Determinants of Prognosis—or Adjust for Differences in the Analysis?

The validity of the observational study designs often used to evaluate a CDSS is limited (see Part 1B, "Therapy and Harm: An Introduction"; see also Part 2B, "Therapy and Harm, Why Study Results Mislead—Bias and Random Error"). The most common observational design, the before/after design, compares outcomes before a technology is implemented (by means of a historic control group) to those after the system is implemented. The validity of this approach is threatened by the risk that changes over time (*secular trends*) in patient mix or in aspects of health care delivery may be responsible for changes in behavior that appear to be attributable to the CDSS.

Consider a CDSS assisting physicians with the ordering of antibiotic drugs[10] that was implemented in the late 1980s and that was associated with improvements in the cost-effectiveness of antibiotic ordering during the subsequent 5 years. Changes in the health care system, including the advent of managed care, were occurring simultaneously during that time period. To control for secular trends, the computerized antibiotic practice guideline study investigators[10] compared antibiotic prescribing practices to those of other US acute-care hospitals for the duration of the study. Of course, these other hospitals differed in many ways aside from the CDSS, limiting the validity of the comparison.

Investigators may strengthen the before/after design by turning the intervention on and off multiple times, a type of *time series* design. Although this makes it less likely that investigators will attribute changes independent of the intervention to the CDSS, random allocation of patients to a concurrent control group remains the strongest study design for evaluating therapeutic or preventive interventions (see Part 1B1, "Therapy"; see also Part 2B1, "Therapy and Validity, Surprising Results of Randomized Controlled Trials"). Investigators have implemented successful randomized controlled trials of more than 70 CDSSs.[13-15]

A special issue for CDSS evaluation is the unit of allocation. Usually, investigators in clinical trials randomize patients. When evaluating the effect of a CDSS on patient care, the intervention is usually aimed at having an impact on the decisions clinicians make. Hence, investigators may randomize individual clinicians or clinician clusters such as health care teams, hospital wards, or outpatient practices.[16] A common mistake made by investigators is to analyze their data as if they had randomized patients rather than clinicians.[17]

To highlight the problem, we will use an extreme example. Investigators randomize study participants to ensure that treatment and control groups are balanced with respect to important predictors of outcome. Randomization often fails to balance groups if sample size is small. Consider a study in which an investigator randomizes one team of clinicians to a CDSS and randomizes another team to standard practice. During the course of the study, each team sees 10,000 patients. If the investigator analyzes the data as if patients were individually randomized, the sample size appears huge. However, it is very plausible, perhaps even likely, that the two teams' performance differed at the start and that this difference persisted throughout the study independent of the CDSS. Because the sample size in this study is only two (two teams), the likelihood of imbalance despite randomization is very large.

Obtaining a sample of sufficient size can be difficult when randomizing physicians and health care teams. If only a few health care teams are available, investigators can pair them according to their similarities on numerous factors and they can randomly allocate the intervention within each matched pair.[18] In addition, investigators can use statistical methods developed specifically for analyzing studies using cluster randomization, which allow investigators to take full advantage of the available data.[19]

There is one other issue regarding randomization to which clinicians should attend. Consider the following: if some clinicians assigned to CDSS fail to receive the intervention, should these clinicians be included in the analysis? The answer, counterintuitive to some, is "yes" (see Part 2B1, "Therapy and Validity, The Principle of Intention-to-Treat"). Randomization can accomplish the goal of balancing groups with respect to both known and unknown determinants of outcome only if patients (or clinicians) are analyzed in the groups to which they are randomized. Deleting or moving patients after randomization compromises or destroys the balance randomization is designed to achieve. The technical term for an analysis in which patients are included in the groups to which they were randomized, whether or not they received the intervention, is intention-to-treat (see Part 2B1, "Therapy and Validity, The Principle of Intention-to-Treat").

During the course of a year, Overhage et al[1] randomized 18 teams to CDSS and 18 to control services. They required house staff to write all orders and used the individual house staff as the unit of analysis. Each service admitted patients in sequence so that all six services received equal numbers of patients. A total of 86 house staff physicians who received more than five corollary orders during the study cared for 2181 different patients during 2955 different admissions.

Random assignment of teams to CDSS and non-CDSS services increases the likelihood that the study yielded valid results. However, although investigators did not randomly assign house staff to services, they conducted their analysis at the individual house staff level, comparing 45 intervention physicians in the intervention group with 41 physicians in the control group. The investigators did not take steps to ensure that the characteristics of house staff on the intervention and control teams were similar, leaving the study open to biases from baseline or intrinsic differences in house staff performance. Moreover, the use of individual house staff instead of the appropriate analysis that takes into account the team as the unit of randomization may have led to false precision in estimating the impact of the intervention (as described above, a falsely inflated sample size).

In this study,[1] the investigators excluded six physicians from the intervention group because they received fewer than five suggestions about corollary orders. This decision violates the intention-to-treat principle and risks introducing bias (after all, similar physicians on the control side would be included). Fortunately, the small number of excluded physicians were mostly off-service physicians covering night calls for one or two nights and not actually service team members, so the contribution of such physicians to the results of the comparison of CDSS intervention group with the no-CDSS control group is small.

## Was the Control Group Uninfluenced by the Computer Decision Support System?

The possibility that the physicians in the control group would have receive all or part of the therapeutic intervention threatens the validity of randomized trials. Computer decision support system evaluations are particularly vulnerable to this problem of *contamination*. As an example, Strickland and Hasson[20] randomly allocated patients to have changes in their level of mechanical ventilator support directed by a computer protocol and either implemented through a physician or directed by the physician independently. Because the same physicians and respiratory therapists using the computer protocol were also managing the care of patients not assigned to the protocol, it is possible clinicians could remember and apply protocol algorithms in control patients. When the control group is influenced by the intervention, the effect of the CDSS may be diluted. Contamination may spuriously decrease, or even eliminate, a true intervention effect.

One method of preventing exposure of the control group to the CDSS is to assign individual clinicians to use or not use the CDSS. This is often problematic because of cross-coverage of patients. Comparing the performance of wards or hospitals that do or do not use the CDSS is another possibility. Unfortunately, it is usually not feasible to enroll a sufficient number of hospitals to avoid the problem that we described earlier: When sample size is small, randomization may fail to ensure prognostically similar groups.

In the Overhage study,[1] physicians whose team was assigned to a control service had the CDSS guidelines available on paper but did not receive assistance when ordering. To control for the risk that cross-coverage of patients could expose the control group to the CDSS, the investigators had the chief medical resident construct the residents' evening call schedule to separate coverage for patients based on their study status. If personnel switches in the schedule were made, physicians in the control group provided call coverage only for non-CDSS patients and intervention physicians covered only CDSS patients. Further, to avoid contamination that could occur if intervention physicians cared for patients assigned to physicians in the control group, the computer suggested orders only when the patient had been assigned to a physician in the CDSS group, and corollary order suggestions were suppressed if the patient was assigned to the control group. If physicians returned for a second rotation and changed study status, the investigators excluded data from their second rotation. All of these efforts were intended to prevent contamination of the control group by the CDSS.

## Were Interventions Similar in the Two Groups?

The results of studies evaluating interventions aimed at therapy or prevention are more believable if patients, their caregivers, and study personnel are blind to the treatment (see Part 1B1, "Therapy"). Blinding also diminishes the placebo effect, which in the case of CDSS may be the tendency of patients to ascribe positive attributes to use of a computer workstation. Although blinding the clinicians, patients, and study personnel to the presence of the computer-based CDSS may prevent this type of bias, blinding is sometimes not possible.

Lack of blinding can result in bias if interventions other than the treatment are differentially applied to the treatment and control groups, particularly if the use of very effective nonstudy treatments is permitted at the physicians' discretion. Clinicians' concerns regarding lack of blinding are ameliorated if investigators describe permissible cointerventions and their differential use or standardize cointerventions,[21] or both, to ensure that their application was similar both in the treatment group and in the control group.

In the study by Overhage et al,[1] although faculty were proscribed from writing orders except during emergencies, the reality is that physicians practice within teams and the faculty influenced the residents through their teaching. Further complicating this situation, faculty could rotate with different house staff on different rotations during the study. To allow for this clustering of physicians within teams, the investigators used a statistical method (generalized estimating equations).

### Was Outcome Assessed Uniformly in the Experimental and Control Groups?

Unblinded study personnel who measure outcomes may provide different interpretations of marginal findings or differential encouragement during performance tests.[22] In some studies, the computer system may be used as a data collection tool to evaluate the outcome in the CDSS group. Using the information system to log episodes in the treatment group and using a manual system in the non-CDSS group can create a *data completeness bias*.[4] If the computer logs more episodes than the manual system, it may appear that the CDSS group had more events, which could bias the outcome in favor of or against the CDSS group. To prevent this bias, investigators should log outcomes similarly in both groups as Overhage and colleagues did by using the computerized order entry system to monitor ordering behavior in both groups.[1]

# WHAT ARE THE RESULTS?

### What Is the Effect of the Computer Decision Support System?

The therapy users' guide (see Part 1B1, "Therapy") provides a discussion of relative risk and relative risk reductions, risk differences and absolute risk reductions, and confidence intervals used to summarize intervention effects. In the Overhage et al study,[1] intervention physicians ordered the corollary orders suggested by the CDSS much more frequently than control physicians spontaneously ordered them. This was true when measured by immediate compliance (46.3% vs 21.9%; relative risk, 2.11; $P < .0001$), 24-hour compliance (50.4% vs 29.0%; relative risk, 1.74; $P < .0001$), or hospital stay compliance (55.9% vs 37.1%; relative risk, 1.51; $P < .0001$). Overhage et al[1] did not report their data in sufficient detail to allow us to calculate the confidence intervals around the risk difference for the increase in compliance. However, because the $P$ values are very small, we know that the confidence interval is relatively narrow (see Part 2B2, "Therapy and Understanding the Results, Confidence Intervals").

Length of stay and hospital charges did not differ significantly between the patients assigned to physicians in the intervention group and the patients assigned to physicians in the control group. However, pharmacists made 105 interventions with the CDSS group of physicians and 156 interventions with physicians in the control group (two-tailed $P = .003$) for errors considered to be life threatening, severe, or significant.

# HOW CAN I APPLY THE RESULTS TO PATIENT CARE?

Many of the issues specific to a CDSS arise in its application. Implementing the CDSS within your own environment may be very challenging.

### What Elements of the Computer Decision Support System Are Required?

It is important to understand what intervention the investigators of a particular CDSS evaluated. They may evaluate two of the major elements comprising a CDSS—the logic that has been incorporated and the computer interface used to present the logic—separately. However, sometimes it is not possible to separate these two elements and achieve the same impact. For example, we mentioned a randomized controlled trial comparing a computerized protocol for managing patients with adult respiratory distress syndrome, which investigators compared to standard clinical care with extracorporeal $CO_2$ removal used as rescue therapy.[11] The computerized protocol group without rescue therapy did as well as the rescue therapy group. Was this caused by the logic in the protocol, the use of the computer, or both interacting together? To test whether the computer is needed requires that one group apply the protocol logic as written on paper and the other group use the same logic implemented in the computer. Sometimes the logic is so complex that use of a computer may be required for implementation.

The CDSS may have a positive impact for unintended reasons. The impact of structured data collection forms and performance evaluations (respectively called the *checklist effect* and the *feedback effect*)[4] on decision making can equal that of computer-generated advice.[23] The CDSS intervention itself may be administered by research personnel or paid clinical staff receiving scant mention in the published report but without whom the impact of the system is seriously undermined.

The CDSS in the Overhage et al study of corollary orders[1] and in the ARDS study[11] had three components: (1) a knowledge base defining which corollary orders were required for each trigger order; (2) a database that stored the trigger orders; and (3) an inference engine that compared the database to the knowledge base when a trigger order was received and sent a list of suggested corollary orders to the computer terminal for display.

## Is the Computer Decision Support System Exportable to a New Site?

For a CDSS to be exported to a new site, it must have the ability to be integrated with existing software. In addition, users at the new site must be able to maintain the system—and they must accept the system. Double-charting occurs when systems require staff (usually nurses) to enter the data once into the computer and once again on a flow sheet. Systems that require double-charting increase staff time devoted to documentation, frustrate users, and divert time that could be devoted to patient care. In general, experience suggests that systems that require double entry of data fail in clinical use, and are ultimately abandoned.

Therefore, it is important to assess how the information necessary to run the decision support gets into the system. In general, successful systems are ones with automatic electronic interfaces to existing data producing systems. Unfortunately, building interfaces to diverse computer systems is often extremely challenging and sometimes is impossible.

The program described in the Overhage et al study[1] was implemented using the Regenstrief Medical Record System developed at Indiana University School of Medicine. This system provides an electronic medical record system and a physician order entry system. Although it may be possible to take the knowledge built into the system and use it in a health care environment where the patients are similar to those enrolled in the study, the inference engine used to compare the rules against the order entered into the database is not easily exported to other locations. If, after critically appraising a study describing the impact of a CDSS, you are convinced that a CDSS for implementing guidelines would be useful, you would need sufficient resources to rebuild the system at your own site.

## Is the Computer Decision Support System Likely to Be Accepted by Clinicians in Your Setting?

Clinicians who differ in important ways from those in the study may not accept the CDSS. The choice of evaluative group may limit the generalizability of the conclusions if recruitment is based on enthusiasm, demographics, or a zest for new technology. Clinicians in a new setting may be surprised when their colleagues do not use a CDSS with the same enthusiasm as the original participants.

The user interface is an important component of the effectiveness of a CDSS. The CDSS interface should be developed on the basis of potential users' capabilities and limitations, the users' tasks, and the environment in which those tasks are performed.[23] One of the main difficulties with alerting systems is getting the information that there is a potential problem (such as an abnormal laboratory value) as rapidly as possible to the individual with decision-making capability. A group of investigators tried a number of different alerting methods, from a highlighted icon on the computer screen to a flashing yellow light placed on the top of the computer.[24] These investigators later gave the nurses pagers to alert them about abnormal laboratory values.[25] The nurses could then decide how to act on the information and when to alert the physician.

To ensure user acceptance, users must believe that they can count on the system to be available whenever they need it. The amount of down time needed for data backup, troubleshooting, and upgrading should be minimal. The response time must be fast, data integrity must be maintained, and data redundancy must be minimized. If systems have been functioning at other sites for a period of time, major problems or software problems may have been eradicated, decreasing down time and improving acceptance. It is also important to assess the amount of training required for users to feel comfortable with the system. If users become frustrated with the system, system performance will be suboptimal.

Many computer programs may function well at the site where the program was developed. Unfortunately, the staff at your own institution may have objections to the approaches taken elsewhere. For example, an expert system for managing patients with ventilators who have adult respiratory distress system may use continuous positive airway pressure trials to wean patients off of the ventilator, whereas clinicians at your institution may prefer pressure support weaning. Syntax, laboratory coding, and phrasing of diagnoses and therapeutic interventions can vary markedly across institutions. Customizing the application to the environment may not be feasible and additional expense may be invoked when mapping vocabulary to synonyms, unless a mechanism to do so has already been incorporated by means of programming. To ensure user acceptance, the needs and concerns of users should be considered and users should be included in the decision-making and implementation stages.

The developers of the Regenstrief Order Entry system[1] based its logic on the expertise of a hospital committee of staff physicians and pharmacists. Although the developers used reference texts, the degree to which the investigators applied an evidence-based approach is not clear. Use of solid evidence[26] from the literature could enhance clinician acceptance by convincing physicians that the rules positively impact patient outcomes. However, evidence-based practices do not ensure acceptance, and you are likely to need a method for gaining consensus in your local culture of care. Further, physicians will need some time to become acquainted with any new system, especially an order entry system.

When the Overhage et al study began, all physicians on the medical wards had been entering all inpatient orders directly into physician workstations for 12 months.[1] Because the order entry program was developed over time and refined by user input, it was tailored to the needs of the clinicians at that hospital. Whether this system would be easily accepted in a new environment by clinicians who had nothing to do with its development is open to question.

## Do the Benefits of the Computer Decision Support System Justify the Risks and Costs?

The real cost of the CDSS is usually much higher than the initial hardware, software, interface, training, maintenance fees, and upgrade costs (which may not be in the report). Often the CDSS is designed and maintained by staff whose actions are critical to the success of the intervention. Your institution might not want to pay for the time of such people in addition to the cost of the computer software and hardware. Indeed, it can be very difficult to estimate the costs of purchasing or building and implementing an integrated CDSS.

Are CDSSs beneficial? Human performance may improve when participants are aware that their behavior is being observed (the *Hawthorne effect*)[27] or evaluated (the *sentinal effect*). The same behavior may not be exhibited when the monitoring of outcomes has stopped. Taking into account the influence of a study environment, a published systematic review of studies assessing CDSSs used in inpatient and outpatient clinical settings by clinicians[2] that was recently updated[15] showed that the majority of CDSSs studied were beneficial. The outcomes assessed were patient-related outcomes (eg, mortality, length of stay, and decrease in infections) or health care process measures (eg, compliance with reminders or with evidence-based processes of care). A total of 68 prospective trials using a concurrent control group have reported the effects of using CDSSs related to drug dosing, diagnosis, preventive care, and active medical care. Sixty-six percent of studies (43/65) showed that CDSSs improved physician performance. These included nine of 15 studies on drug dosing systems, one of five studies on diagnostic aids, 14 of 19 studies of preventive care systems, and 19 of 26 studies evaluating CDSSs for active medical care. Forty-three percent of studies (6/14) showed that CDSSs improved patient outcomes, three studies showed no benefit, and the remaining studies lacked sufficient power to detect a clinically important effect.

Investigators evaluate health care processes more often than patient health outcomes because process events occur more frequently than major health outcomes. For example, a trial designed to show a 25% improvement (from 50% to 62.5%) in the proportion of patients who are compliant with a certain medication regimen would need to enroll 246 patients per group. A trial designed to show that this medication reduces mortality by 25% (from 5% to 3.75%) would need to enroll 4177 patients per group. Furthermore, long follow-up periods are required to show that preventive interventions improve patient health outcomes.

Fortunately, evaluation of health care processes will be adequate to infer benefit if the care processes being monitored are already known to improve outcomes.[28] We could conclude that a CDSS was beneficial if it increased the frequency with which aspirin, beta blockers, and angiotensin-converting enzyme inhibitors were administered to appropriate patients after myocardial infarction. The reason is that large, well-designed randomized trials have demonstrated the benefit of these three interventions. Unfortunately, however, the link between processes and outcomes is often unknown or weak.

The study by Overhage et al[1] demonstrated that physician work stations, when linked to an order entry system able to run a series of rules, was an efficient means for decreasing errors of omissions and improving adherence to practice guidelines. It is unclear how many of the rules in the system were based on solid evidence, and thus how likely compliance with rules is to improve outcomes. Therefore, it is unclear whether the benefits are worth the cost of purchasing, configuring, installing, and maintaining the CDSS. Ultimately, decisions about adopting CDSSs will depend on local values and local politics.

# Conclusions and Resolution

A computer-based CDSS evaluation involves the interplay between three complex elements:

- One or more human intermediaries

- An integrated computerized system and its interface

- The knowledge in the decision support

This makes evaluation of a computer-based CDSS a complex undertaking. Systematic reviews of the impact of a CDSS on clinician behavior and patient outcome have shown evidence of benefit.[2, 13-15] Because the evaluation process used in these reviews was not standard, it is difficult to compare the results of these reviews.

In this section, we described a process of evaluating articles that aim to measure the impact of a computer-based CDSS on clinician decisions or patient outcomes. Despite the complexity in evaluation, clinicians can use basic principles of evidence-based care to evaluate a CDSS. A study evaluating a CDSS is more believable if there is a concurrent control group with random allocation of subjects. Randomization of clinicians by clusters can prevent the cross-contamination of the control group by the intervention that could mask the effect of the CDSS. When using multilevel designs (the physician or physician group and their respective patients) it is important to consider the physician or group, rather than the patients, to be the unit of analysis. Because most studies evaluating a CDSS are not blinded, controlling for cointerventions that could bias the outcome is particularly important.

Even if the study is valid and a positive effect is shown, CDSSs have special applicability issues that clinicians and managers must consider. Is the computer essential to deployment of the knowledge in the CDSS? Can the CDSS be exported to a new site? Will clinicians at your site accept the CDSS? And, finally, is it possible to evaluate the cost of the CDSS accurately when assessing risks and benefits?

## References

1. Overhage J, Tierney W, Zhou XH, McDonald C. A randomized trial of "corollary orders" to prevent errors of omission. *JAMA*. 1997;4:364-375.

2. Johnston M, Langton K, Haynes R, Mathieu A. Effects of computer-based clinical decision support systems on clinician performance and patient outcome: a critical appraisal of research. *Ann Intern Med*. 1994;120:135-142.

3. Pryor TA. Development of decision support systems. *Int J Clin Monit Comput*. 1990;7:137-146.

4. Friedman CP, Wyatt JC. *Evaluation Methods in Medical Informatics*. New York: Springer-Verlag; 1997.

5. Lepage E, Gardner R, Laub R, Golubjatnikov O. Improving blood transfusion practice: role of a computerized hospital information system. *Transfusion*. 1992;32:253-259.

6. Weinfurt PT. Electrocardiographic monitoring: an overview. *J Clin Monit*. 1990; 6:132-138.

7. Knaus WA, Wagner DP, Draper EA, et al. The APACHE III prognostic system: risk prediction of hospital mortality for critically ill hospitalized adults. *Chest*. 1991;100:1619-1636.

8. Berner E, Webster G, Shugerman A, et al. Performance of four computer-based diagnostic systems. *N Engl J Med*. 1994;330:1792-1796.

9. Kennedy R, Harrison R, Burton A, et al. An artificial neural network system for diagnosis of acute myocardial infarction (AMI) in the accident and emergency department: evaluation and comparison with serum myoglobin measurements. *Comput Methods Programs Biomed*. 1997;52:93-103.

10. Evans RS, Pestotnik SL, Classen DC, et al. A computer-assisted management program for antibiotics and other antiinfective agents. *N Engl J Med*. 1998; 38:232-238.

11. Morris AH, Wallace CJ, Menlove RL, et al. Randomized clinical trial of pressure-controlled inverse ratio ventilation and extracorporeal $CO_2$ removal for adult respiratory distress syndrome. *Am J Respir Crit Care Med*. 1994;149:295-305.

12. Spiegelhalter DJ. Evaluation of clinical decision-aids, with an application to a system for dyspepsia. *Stat Med*. 1983;2:207-216.

13. Shea S, DuMouchel W, Bahamonde L. A meta-analysis of 16 randomized controlled trials to evaluate computer-based clinical reminder systems for preventive care in the ambulatory setting. *J Am Med Inform Assoc*. 1996;3:399-409.

14. Balas E, Austin S, Mitchell J, Ewigman B, Bopp K, Brown G. The clinical value of computerized information services: a review of 98 randomized clinical trials. *Arch Fam Med*. 1996;5:271-278.

15. Hunt D, Haynes R, Hanna S. Effects of computer-based clinical decision support systems on physician performance and patient outcomes: a systematic review. *JAMA*. 1998;280:1339-1346.

16. Cornfield J. Randomization by group: a formal analysis. *Am J Epidemiol*. 1978:108;100-102.

17. Whiting-O'Keefe Q, Henke C, Simborg D. Choosing the correct unit of analysis in medical care experiments. *Med Care*. 1984;22:1101-1114.

18. Klar N, Donner A. The merits of matching in community intervention trials: a cautionary tale. *Stat Med*. 1997;16:1753-1764.

19. Thompson SG, Pyke SD, Hardy RJ. The design and analysis of paired cluster randomized trials: an application of meta-analysis techniques. *Stat Med*. 1997;16:2063-2079.

20. Strickland JH, Hasson JH. A computer-controlled ventilator weaning system. *Chest*. 1993;103:1220-1226.

21. Morris A, East T, Wallace C, et al. Standardization of clinical decision making for the conduct of credible clinical research in complicated medical environments. *Proceedings/ AMIA Annual Fall Symposium*. 1996:418-422.

22. Guyatt GH, Pugsley SO, Sullivan MJ, et al. Effect of encouragement on walking test performance. *Thorax*. 1984;39:818-822.

23. Adams ID, Chan M, Clifford PC, et al. Computer aided diagnosis of acute abdominal pain: a multicentre study. *BMJ*. 1986;293:800-804.

24. Bradshaw K, Gardner R, Pryor T. Development of a computerized laboratory alerting system. *Comput Biomed Res*. 1989;22:575-587.

25. Tate K, Gardner R, Scherting K. Nurses, pagers, and patient-specific criteria: three keys to improved critical value reporting. In: *Annual Symposium on Computer Applications in Medical Care*. Washington, DC: American Medical Informatics Association; 1995:164-168.

26. Guyatt G, Sackett D, Sinclair J, et al. Users' guides to the medical literature, IX: a method for grading health care recommendations. *JAMA*. 1995;274:1800-1804.

27. Roethligsburger FJ, Dickson WJ. *Management and the Worker.* Cambridge: Harvard University Press; 1939.

28. Mant J, Hicks N. Detecting differences in quality of care: the sensitivity of measures of process and outcome in treating acute myocardial infarction. *BMJ*. 1995;23:793-796.

# THERAPY AND UNDERSTANDING THE RESULTS
## Quality of Life

Gordon Guyatt, C. David Naylor, Elizabeth Juniper,
Daren Heyland, Roman Jaeschke, and Deborah Cook

The following EBM Working Group members also made substantive
contributions to this section: Trisha Greenhalgh, Victor Montori,
and Regina Kunz

## IN THIS SECTION

## CLINICAL SCENARIO

### Methotrexate and Crohn Disease: Are the Benefits Worth the Risks?

**Y**ou are a physician following a 35-year-old man who has had active Crohn disease for 8 years. Four years ago, the symptoms were severe enough to require resectional surgery, and despite treatment with sulfasalazine and metronidazole, the patient has continued to have active disease requiring the use of oral steroids for the past 2 years. Repeated attempts to decrease the dose of prednisone have failed, and at times the patient has required doses of greater than 15 mg per day to control symptoms. You are impressed by both the methodology and results of a recent report documenting that similarly afflicted patients benefit from treatment with oral methotrexate[1] and you suggest to the patient that he consider taking this medication. Not surprisingly, when you explain some of the risks of methotrexate, particularly potential liver toxicity, the patient is hesitant. "How much better," he asks, "am I likely to feel while taking this medication?"

Why do we offer treatment to patients? There are three reasons. We believe that our interventions increase longevity, prevent future morbidity, and make patients feel better. "Feeling better" includes avoiding discomfort (pain, nausea, breathlessness, and so forth), disability (loss of function), and distress (emotional suffering).[2] The first two of these three endpoints are relatively easy to measure. At least in part because of difficulty in measurement, for many years clinicians were willing to substitute physiologic or laboratory tests for the direct measurement of the third endpoint. During the past 20 years, however, clinicians have recognized the importance of direct measurement of how people are feeling and the extent to which they are able to function in daily activities. Investigators have developed increasingly sophisticated methods of making these measurements, which we will describe in the following discussion.

Since, as clinicians, we are most interested in aspects of quality of life that are directly related to health rather than such issues as financial solvency or the quality of the environment, we frequently refer to measurements of how people are feeling as *health-related quality of life (HRQL)*.[3] Investigators measure HRQL using questionnaires that typically include questions about how patients are feeling or what they are experiencing associated with response options such as "yes/no" or seven-point (or any other number) *Likert-type* scales—or *visual analogue* scales. Investigators aggregate responses to these questions into domains or dimensions (such as physical or emotional function) that yield an overall score.

Controversy exists concerning the boundaries of HRQL and the extent to which medical investigators must include individual patients' values in its measurement.[4-6]

Is it sufficient to know that, in general, patients with chronic obstructive lung disease value being able to climb stairs without becoming short of breath, or does one need to establish that the patient before us values climbing stairs without dyspnea? Further controversy exists about how the relative values of items and domains need to be established—and how these values should be determined. Is it enough to know that both dyspnea and fatigue are important to people with lung disease, or does one need to establish their relative importance? If establishing their relative importance is necessary, which of the many available approaches should we use?

In this section, we take a simple approach. We use HRQL to refer to the health aspects of their lives that people generally value, and we are ready to accept patients' statements of what they value without precise determination of ranking of items or domains.

Physicians often have limited familiarity with methods of measuring how patients feel. At the same time, they are reading articles that recommend administering or withholding treatment on the basis of its impact on patients' well-being. This section is designed for clinicians asking the question, "Will this treatment make the patient feel better?" As in other sections of this book, we will use the framework of assessing the validity of the methods, interpreting the results, and applying the results to patients (Table 2B2-1). We preface our discussion with a commentary on when one should and should not be concerned with HRQL measurement. Although this section focuses on using HRQL measures to help with treatment decisions, we hope that it may also improve clinical care by emphasizing certain aspects of patients' experience, including functional, emotional, and social limitations, that clinicians sometimes neglect.

**TABLE 2B2-1**

## Guidelines for Using Articles About Health-Related Quality of Life

**Are the Results Valid?**

*Primary Guides*

- Have the investigators measured aspects of patients' lives that patients consider important?
- Did the HRQL instruments work in the intended way?

*Secondary Guides*

- Are there important aspects of HRQL that have been omitted?
- If there are tradeoffs between quality and quantity of life, or if an economic evaluation has been performed, have the most appropriate measures been used?

**What Are the Results?**

- How can we interpret the magnitude of the effect on HRQL?

**How Can I Apply the Results to Patient Care?**

- Will the information from the study help patients make informed decisions about treatment?
- Did the study design simulate clinical practice?

# Do You Need to Worry About Health-Related Quality of Life?

Until at least 1980, few—if any—treatment studies included measurements of HRQL. When should you be concerned if investigators have not paid adequate attention to how patients feel?

Most patients will agree that, under most circumstances, prolonging their lives is a sufficient reason to accept a course of treatment. Some years ago, investigators showed that 24-hour oxygen administration in patients with severe chronic airflow limitation reduced mortality.[7] The omission of HRQL data from the original article ultimately was not an important one. Since the intervention prolongs life, our enthusiasm for continuous oxygen administration is not diminished by a subsequent report suggesting that more intensive oxygen therapy had little or no impact on HRQL.[8] Similarly, although feeling better is important to patients with heart failure, when interventions either extend[9] or shorten[10] life span, we usually do not need an HRQL assessment to inform our clinical decisions.

There are exceptions to this rule. Although many of our life-prolonging treatments have a negligible impact on or actually improve HRQL, this is not always the case. If treatment leads to deterioration in HRQL, patients may be concerned that small gains in life expectancy come at too high a cost. This concern is vividly illustrated by patient decisions regarding whether to accept toxic cancer chemotherapy that will provide marginal gains in longevity. In the extreme, an intervention such as mechanical ventilation may prolong the life of a patient in a vegetative state, but the patient's family may wonder if their loved one would be better off dead.

When the goal of treatment is to improve how people are feeling (rather than to prolong their lives) and physiologic correlates of patients' experience are lacking, HRQL measurement is imperative. For example, we would pay little attention to studies of antidepressant medications that failed to measure patients' mood—or to trials of antimigraine medication that failed to measure pain.

The difficult decisions occur when the relationship between physiologic or laboratory measures and HRQL outcomes is uncertain. Practitioners have relied on substitute endpoints not because they have not been interested in making patients feel better, but because they assumed a strong link between physiologic measurements and patients' well-being. As we argue in another section of this book (see Part 2B3, "Therapy and Applying the Results, Surrogate Outcomes"), substitute endpoints such as bone density for fractures, cholesterol level for coronary artery disease deaths, and laboratory exercise capacity for capacity to undertake day-to-day activities have often proved misleading. Changes in conventional measures of clinical status show only weak to moderate correlations with changes in HRQL[11, 12] and fail to detect patient-important changes in HRQL.[13] Randomized trials that measure both physiologic endpoints and HRQL may show effects on one but not on the other. For example, trials in patients with chronic lung disease have shown treatment effects on peak flow rates —without improvement in HRQL.[14, 15] We therefore advocate great caution in reliance on surrogate outcomes.

Referring back to our opening scenario, investigators reported the results of a randomized trial of methotrexate in 141 patients with chronically active Crohn disease despite at least 3 prior months of prednisone therapy.[1] Patients who received methotrexate were twice as likely to be in clinical remission after 16 weeks of treatment than those who received placebo (39.4% vs 19.1%; $P = .025$), and actively treated patients received less prednisone and showed less disease activity.

Is additional information regarding HRQL necessary to interpret the results of this study? As depicted in the scenario, the decision to give methotrexate depends on the balance between the benefits and risks, and the patient's question about how much better he is likely to feel on medication may well be relevant to his decision. Without information about the effect of the medication on HRQL, therefore, neither the clinician nor the patient can make a fully informed choice.

# ARE THE RESULTS VALID?

## Have the Investigators Measured Aspects of Patients' Lives That Patients Consider Important?

We have described how investigators often substitute their own endpoints—ones that make intuitive sense to them—for those that patients value. Clinicians can recognize these situations by asking themselves the following question: if the endpoints measured by the investigators were the only thing that changed, would patients be willing to take the treatment? In addition to change in clinical or physiologic variables, patients would require that they feel better or live longer. For instance, if a treatment for osteoporosis increased bone density without preventing back pain, loss of height, or fractures, patients would not be interested in risking the side effects—or incurring the costs and inconvenience—of treatment.

How can clinicians be secure that investigators have measured aspects of life that patients value? Investigators may show that the outcomes they have measured are important to patients by asking them directly. For example, in a study examining HRQL in patients with chronic airflow limitation who were recruited from a secondary-care respiratory care clinic, we used a literature review and interviews with clinicians and patients to identify 123 items reflecting possible ways that patients' illness might impact on their quality of life.[16] We then asked 100 patients to identify the items that were problems for them and to indicate how important those items were. We found that the most important problem areas for patients were their dyspnea during day-to-day activities and their chronic fatigue. An additional area of difficulty was emotional function, including having feelings of frustration and impatience.

If the authors do not present direct evidence that their outcome measures are important to patients, they may cite prior work. For example, researchers conducting a randomized trial of respiratory rehabilitation in patients with chronic lung disease used an HRQL measure based on the responses of patients in the study described just above, and they referred back to that study.[17] Ideally, the report will include a summary of the developmental process that is sufficiently detailed to obviate the need to return to the prior report.

Alternatively, investigators may describe the content of their outcome measures in detail. An adequate description of the content of a questionnaire allows clinicians to use their own experience to decide whether what is being measured is important to patients. For instance, the authors of an article describing a randomized trial of surgery vs watchful waiting for benign prostatic hyperplasia "assessed the degree to which urinary difficulties bothered the patients or interfered with their activities of daily living, sexual function, social activities, and general well-being."[18] Few would doubt the importance of these items and—since patients in primary care often are untroubled by minor symptoms of benign prostatic hyperplasia—the importance of including them in the results of the trial.

In the study of methotrexate for patients with inflammatory bowel disease, patients completed the Inflammatory Bowel Disease Questionnaire (IBDQ), which addresses patients' bowel function, emotional function, systemic symptoms, and social function. Although the authors do not mention this in their paper, the 32 items in the IBDQ were chosen because patients with inflammatory bowel disease labeled them as being the most important ones in their daily lives.[19]

## Did the Health-Related Quality of Life Instruments Work in the Intended Way?

Measuring how people are feeling is not easy. Investigators must demonstrate that their instruments allow strong inferences about the effect of treatment on HRQL. We will now review how an HRQL instrument should perform (its measurement properties) if it is going to be useful.

### Signal and Noise

There are two distinct ways in which investigators use HRQL instruments. They may wish to help clinicians distinguish between people who have a better or worse level of HRQL, or to measure whether people are feeling better or worse over time.[20] For instance, suppose a trial of a new drug for patients with heart failure shows that it works best in patients with the New York Heart Association (NYHA) functional classification class IV symptoms. We could use the NYHA classification for two purposes. First, for treatment decisions, we might use it as a tool by which to discriminate between patients who do and do not warrant therapy. For instance, at the time of writing, a single trial has suggested that spironolactone reduces mortality in NYHA class III and IV patients. One might choose to restrict therapy to this group, in which the intervention has been tested directly.[21] We might also want to determine whether the drug was effective in improving an individual patient's functional status, and in so doing monitor changes in patient's NYHA functional class.

If, when we are trying to discriminate among people at a single point in time, everyone gets the same score, we will not be able to tell who is doing better and who is doing worse. The key differences we are trying to detect—the signal—come from differences in scores among patients. The bigger those differences are, the better off we will be. At the same time, if patients' scores on repeated measurement fluctuate wildly—we call this fluctuation the *noise*—we will not be able to say much about their relative well-being.[22] The greater the noise, which comes from variability within patients, the more difficulty we will have detecting the signal. For instance, consider an instrument in which scores range from 20 to 100. If we measure stable patients once and again 2 weeks later, and if each patient's scores on the two occasions are within five points of one another, we might feel satisfied with an instrument's reproducibility. However, if all patients score between 55 and 60 on the two repetitions, we will be unable to comment on which patients have less HRQL impairment and which have more.

The technical term usually used to describe the ratio of variability between patients—the *signal*—to the total variability—the signal plus the noise—is reliability. If patients' scores change little over time but are very different from patient to patient, reliability will be high. If the changes in score within patients is high in relation to differences among patients, reliablity will be low. The mathematical expression of reliability is the variance (or variability) among patients divided by the variance among patients and the variance within patients.

By contrast, instruments used to evaluate change over time must be able to detect any important changes in the way patients are feeling, even if those changes are small. Thus, the signal comes from the difference in score in patients whose status has improved or deteriorated, and the noise comes from the variability in score in patients whose status has not changed. The term we use for the ability to detect change (the ratio of signal to noise over time) is *responsiveness.*

An unresponsive instrument can result in false-negative results in which the intervention improves how patients feel, yet the instrument fails to detect the improvement. This problem may be particularly salient for questionnaires that have the advantage of covering all relevant areas of HRQL, but the disadvantage of covering each area superficially. With only four categories, a crude instrument such as the NYHA functional classification may work well for stratifying patients, but it may not be able to detect small but important improvement resulting from treatment.

In studies that show no difference in change in HRQL when patients receive a treatment vs a control intervention, clinicians should look for evidence that the instruments have been able to detect small or medium-sized effects in previous investigations. In the absence of this evidence, instrument unresponsiveness becomes a plausible reason for the failure to detect differences in HRQL. For example, researchers who conducted a randomized trial of a diabetes education program reported no changes in two measures of well-being, attributing the result to, among other factors, lack of integration of the program with standard therapy.[23] However, those involved in the educational program, in comparison to a control group that did not experience it, showed an improvement in knowledge and self-care, along with a decrease in feelings of dependence on physicians. Given these changes, another explanation for the negative result—no difference between treatments in well-being—is inadequate responsiveness of the two well-being measures the investigators used.

In the trial of methotrexate in patients with Crohn disease, concern about responsiveness decreases because the study showed statistically significant differences between treatment and control groups.[1] As it turns out, the IBDQ had detected small to medium-sized differences in previous investigations.[13, 24, 25]

## Validity

*Validity* has to do with whether the instrument is measuring what it is intended to measure. The absence of a reference or criterion standard for HRQL creates a challenge for anyone hoping to measure how patients are feeling. We can be more confident that an instrument is doing its job if the items appear to measure what is intended (the instrument's *face validity*), although face validity alone is of limited help. Empirical evidence that it measures the domains of interest allows stronger inferences.

To provide such evidence, investigators have borrowed validation strategies from psychologists who for many years have struggled with determining whether questionnaires assessing intelligence, attitudes, and emotional function really do measure what is intended. Investigators who are interested in underlying attitudes may find apparent differences between individuals that actually reflect variability in the tendency to provide socially acceptable answers, rather than differences in attitudes. For example, when investigators are demonstrating the apparent effects of rehabilitation on HRQL, in reality they may be merely detecting differences in satisfaction with care. Were this so, the instrument would be detecting a signal, but it would be the wrong signal.

Establishing validity therefore involves examining the logical relationships that should exist between assessment measures. For example, we would expect that patients with lower treadmill exercise capacity generally will have more dyspnea in daily life than those with higher exercise capacity, and we would expect to see substantial correlations between a new measure of emotional function and existing emotional function questionnaires. When we are interested in evaluating change over time, we examine correlations of change scores. For example, patients who deteriorate in their treadmill exercise capacity should, in general, show increases in dyspnea, whereas those whose exercise capacity improves should experience less dyspnea; a new emotional function measure should show improvement in patients who improve on existing measures of emotional function. The technical term for this process is testing an instrument's *construct validity*.

Clinicians should look for evidence of the validity of HRQL measures used in clinical studies. Reports of randomized trials using HRQL measures seldom review evidence of the validity of the instruments they use, but clinicians can gain some reassurance from statements (backed by citations) that the questionnaires have been validated previously. In the absence of evident face validity or empirical evidence of validity, clinicians are entitled to skepticism about the study's measurement of HRQL.

In the methotrexate and inflammatory bowel disease study, the investigators refer to the IBDQ as "previously validated" and provide two relevant citations.[13, 17] These papers describe extensive validation of the questionnaire, including correlations of change that document the instruments' usefulness for measuring change over time.

## Are There Important Aspects of Health-Related Quality of Life That Have Been Omitted?

Although investigators may have addressed HRQL issues, they may not have done so comprehensively. Exhaustive measurement may be more or less important in a particular context. One can think of a hierarchy that begins with symptoms, moves on to the functional consequences of the symptoms, and ends with more complex elements such as emotional function. If, as a clinician, you believe your patients' sole interest is in whether a treatment relieves the primary symptoms and most important functional limitations, you will be satisfied with a limited range of assessment. Recent randomized trials in patients with migraine[26, 27] and postherpetic neuralgia[28] restricted themselves primarily to the measurement of pain; studies of patients with rheumatoid arthritis[29, 30] and back pain[31] measured pain and physical function, but not emotional or social function. Depending on the magnitude of effect on pain, the side effects of the medication, and the circumstances of the patient (degree of pain, concern about toxicity, degree of impairment of function, or emotional distress), lack of comprehensiveness of outcome measurement may or may not be important.

Thus, as a clinician, you can judge whether or not these omissions are important to you or, more importantly, to patients. You should consider that although the omissions are unimportant to some patients, they may be critical to others (see Part 2F, "Moving From Evidence to Action, Incorporating Patient Values"). We encourage you to bear in mind the broader impact of disease on patients' lives. Disease-specific measures that explore the full range of patients' problems and experience remind us of domains we might otherwise forget. We can trust these measures to be comprehensive if the developers have conducted a detailed survey of patients suffering from the illness or condition.

If you are interested in going beyond the specific illness and comparing the impact of treatments on HRQL across diseases or conditions, you will require a more comprehensive assessment. None of the measures, whether they are disease-specific, system- or organ-specific, function-specific (such as instruments that examine sleep or sexual function), or problem-specific (such as pain), are adequate for comparisons across conditions. These comparisons require generic measures, covering all relevant areas of HRQL, that are designed for administration to people with any kind of underlying health problem (or no problem at all). One type of generic measure, a *health profile*, yields scores for all domains of HRQL (including, for example, mobility, self-care, and physical, emotional, and social function). There are a number of well-established health profiles, including the Sickness Impact Profile[32] and the short forms of the instruments used in the Medical Outcomes Study,[33, 34] with notable advantages, such as simplicity, self-administration, and the ability to put changes in specific functions in the context of overall HRQL. Inevitably, however, such instruments cover each area superficially. This may limit their responsiveness. Indeed, several randomized trials have found that generic instruments were less powerful in detecting treatment effects than specific instruments.[4, 11, 35-39] Ironically, generic instruments also may suffer from not being sufficiently comprehensive; in certain cases, they may completely omit patients' primary symptoms.

Disease-specific measures may comprehensively sample all aspects of HRQL relevant to a specific illness and also be responsive, but they are unlikely to deal with side effects. For instance, the IBDQ measures all important disease-specific areas of HRQL, including symptoms directly related to the primary bowel disturbance, systemic symptoms, and emotional and social function. Coincidentally, it measures some side effects of methotrexate, including nausea and lethargy, because they also afflict patients with inflammatory bowel disease who are not taking methotrexate, but it fails to measure others such as skin rash or mouth ulcers. The investigators could have administered a generic instrument to tap in to non-IBD-related aspects of HRQL, but once again, they likely would have failed to measure side effects in sufficient detail. Side effect-specific instruments are limited; the investigators chose a checklist approach and documented the frequency of occurrence of adverse events that were both severe enough and not severe enough to warrant discontinuation of treatment.

## If There Are Tradeoffs Between Quality of Life and Quantity of Life, or if an Economic Evaluation Has Been Performed, Have the Most Appropriate Measures Been Used?

Although they provide information about the broad domains of HRQL and therefore permit comparisons across conditions, health profiles are ill-suited for health care policy decisions that involve integrating costs. Such decisions require choices about resource allocation across diseases, conditions, or medical problems, and they inevitably mandate cost considerations (see Part 2F, "Moving From Evidence to Action, Economic Analysis"). Choosing among health care programs requires standardized comparisons that allow one to relate the impact of very different treatment modalities (such as drugs, surgery, or rehabilitation programs) on very different conditions (such as chronic lung disease, renal failure, or Parkinson disease). Inevitably, they involve putting a value on health states; they may thus require sophisticated weighting for patient preferences and may necessitate relating health states to anchors of death and full health. Such measures may aid policymakers in making the right decisions about how public money is allocated.

Most HRQL questionnaires describe the resultant health states of programs and interventions in a way that is sufficient to inform clinicians and patients, but they do not quantify how much individuals or society value specific health states or services. Additional measures (economic ones) of a different dimension are needed to ascertain the value of the health state. Studies that measure both descriptive aspects of HRQL (using generic health indices) and the valuation of that health state in the same patient show that there is poor correlation between how patients describe health states and how they value them.[40] Measures that provide a single number that summarizes all of HRQL are preference-weighted or value-weighted; these have the preferences or values anchored to death and full health and are called *utility measures*. Typically, utility measures use a scale from zero (death) to 1.0 (full health) to summarize HRQL. Since they weight the duration of life according to its quality, their output is often called *quality-adjusted life years (QALY)* or *disability-adjusted life years (DALY)*. Thus, utilities are holistic measures that ask patients to express, in a single value, their strengths of preferences for particular health states.

An instrument called the *standard gamble* provides one way of obtaining the utility a patient attaches to a health state. One might ask the patient to picture himself at age 60 in good health excepting severe osteoarthritis of the right hip, which results in severe pain with movement and marked functional limitation. The patient chooses between two options (Figure 2B2-1). In one option (the lower arm of Figure 2B2-1), the patient will live in the current state of health, limited by pain and disability, for 20 years—and then die. In the other hypothetical option (the upper arm of Figure 2B2-1) the patient will either return to full health and live for 20 years and then die, or he will die immediately. One may start by setting the probability of full health in the gamble arm (*x* in Figure 2B2-1) at 95%, and the probability of immediate death (*y* in Figure 2B2-1) at 5%. If the patient chooses the gamble, one progressively lowers *x* and increases *y* until the patient becomes indifferent. If the patient becomes indifferent at a probability of full health of 90%, he is indicating that the utility he attaches to living with the pain and limitation of hip osteoarthritis is 0.90. If he becomes indifferent when *x* is 60%, he is telling us that the utility associated with living with hip osteoarthritis is 0.60. The standard gamble is only one of a number of ways of measuring patient utilities.

**FIGURE 2B2-1**

## The Standard Gamble

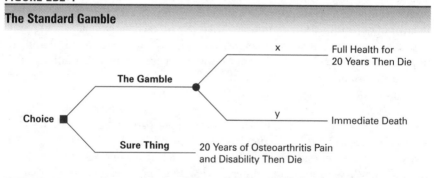

In a classic article, Boyle and colleagues[41] used a utility measure to calculate that treating critically ill infants weighing 1000 to 1499 g at birth cost $3200 per quality-adjusted life-year gained, whereas treating infants with a birth weight of 500 to 999 g cost $22,400 per quality-adjusted life-year gained. Estimates for the cost per quality-adjusted life year for treating patients on renal dialysis have ranged from approximately $30,000 to $50,000.[42,43] Although different weighting schemes yield different results and may therefore be considered arbitrary, a number of increasingly simple utility measures are now available, have provided interesting results in clinical trials, and may facilitate integrating cost into policy decisions. However, the use, measurement, and interpretation of utility measures remain controversial (see Part 2F, "Moving From Evidence to Action, Economic Analysis").[44] The investigators in the methotrexate trial[1] did not use a health profile or a utility measure, limiting use of the data for comparisons across disease states and preventing a formal economic analysis.

# WHAT ARE THE RESULTS?

## How Can We Interpret the Magnitude of Effect on Health-Related Quality of Life?

Understanding the results of a trial involving HRQL involves special challenges. Patients with acute back pain prescribed bed rest had mean scores on the Owestry Back-Disability Index, a measure that focuses on disease-specific functional status, that were 3.9 points worse than those of control patients.[25] Patients with severe rheumatoid arthritis allocated to treatment with cyclosporine had a mean disability score that was 0.28 unit better than that of control patients.[23] Are these differences trivial, are they small but important, are they of moderate magnitude, or do they reflect large and extremely important differences in efficacy among treatments?

These examples show that the interpretability of most HRQL measures is not self-evident. When trying to interpret HRQL results, we must consider that depending on the patient, a different value will be placed on the same change in function or capacity. This explains why in some lines of research (particularly health economics), investigators set aside HRQL measures with multiple domains in favor of holistic measures ("utilities") that rely on each individual patient's preferences (such as the standard gamble). Thus, although we can try to set "minimal important differences," it is likely that for some patients, even smaller differences may be important—or, conversely, that much larger differences are required before they would see a given change in HRQL as worthwhile.

The result is a series of tradeoffs that are often assessed informally in the interaction between physicians and patients. For example, patient A may be desperate for small improvements in a particular domain of HRQL and will be willing to take drugs with severe side effects to achieve that improvement. Patient B, by contrast, may have an altogether different view. Eliciting these preferences is an integral part of practicing evidence-based medicine effectively and sensitively (see "How to Use This Book"; see also Part 1A, "Introduction: The Philosophy of Evidence-Based Medicine," and Part 2F, "Moving From Evidence to Action, Incorporating Patient Values").

However, when reading the literature, clinicians still must arrive at some estimates of how well, in general, a given therapy performs with regard to effecting improvements in HRQL. There are a number of methods available for understanding the magnitude of HRQL effects. Investigators may relate changes in HRQL questionnaire scores to well-known functional measures (such as the NYHA classification), to clinical diagnosis (such as the change in score needed to move people in or out of the diagnostic category of depression), or to the impact of major life events.[45] They may relate changes in HRQL score to patients' global ratings of the magnitude of change they have experienced[46] or to the extent they rate themselves as feeling better or worse than other patients.[47] Regardless of strategy, if investigators do not provide an indication of how to interpret changes in HRQL scores, the findings are of limited use to clinicians.

These strategies lead to estimates of change in HRQL measures that, either for individual patients or for a group of patients, constitute trivial, small, medium, and large differences. For instance, we may establish that 3.9 points on the Owestry Back-Disability Index or 0.28 unit on a rheumatoid arthritis disability index signifies, on average, small but important changes for individuals. This still leaves a problem in interpretation of results from clinical trials. For instance, if the mean change on the Owestry Back-Disability Index is only 2.0, does this mean that we can dismiss the difference as unimportant to patients?

Investigators have gained insight into this issue by examining the distribution of change in HRQL in individual patients and by calculating the proportion of patients who achieved small, medium, and large gains from treatment and the associated numbers needed to treat (NNTs).[48] The investigators who conducted the trial of methotrexate for Crohn disease do not help clinicians interpret the magnitude of difference in HRQL.[1] The mean difference in IBDQ score between treatment and control groups at 16 weeks was 0.59. Other investigations suggest that, for measures structured in the manner of the IBDQ, differences of approximately 0.5 may represent small but important changes to an individual, whereas large improvements correspond to a difference in score of greater than 1.0.[39, 40, 49, 50] Thus, the mean difference between treated and control patients in the methotrexate study is likely to fall within the category of small but important change in HRQL.

The mean difference of 0.59, however, does not mean that every patient achieved a small but important difference. Rather, one would expect a distribution of benefits across patients, some achieving large improvements in HRQL and others showing trivial or absent gains. One can ask the question: how many patients must I treat to achieve an important benefit in a single patient? In other investigations, when mean effects have approximated the minimal important difference, as in this study, investigators have found the NNT to achieve an important improvement in HRQL to range between two and five (see Part 1B1, "Therapy"; see also Part 2B2, "Therapy and Understanding the Results, Measures of Association").[41] That is, for every two to five patients we treat with methotrexate, one will achieve an important improvement in HRQL. As it turns out, even if mean differences between treatment and control are quite small—less, for instance, than the smallest difference important to an individual patient—they can still be associated with single-digit NNTs.[11, 51, 52]

# HOW CAN I APPLY THE RESULTS TO PATIENT CARE?

## Will the Information From the Study Help Patients Make Informed Decisions About Treatment?

People with the same chronic disease often vary markedly in the problems they experience. Even if the problems are the same, the magnitude of the impact of those problems in their lives may differ. Assessment of HRQL will help in the care of an individual patient only if that patient's problems are similar to those of patients in the trial.

Knowing whether HRQL results of a study are relevant for patients in your practice means understanding their experience of illness. Even the most common problems of a chronic disease do not affect all of those who are comparably afflicted. For instance, 92% of patients with inflammatory bowel disease complain of frequent bowel movements, and 82% complain of abdominal cramps.[53] With respect to emotional function, 78% feel frustrated and 76% feel depressed. These percentages come from a study that recruited patients from a secondary care setting[53]; the proportion of patients with these problems is likely to be even smaller if investigators sampled from primary care settings. Furthermore, the patients who experienced these difficulties varied in the extent to which they felt the problems were important. Thinking back to our opening scenario, before answering the question about how the treatment would impact on the patient's life, the clinician would have to be cognizant of the problems the patient was currently experiencing, the importance he attached to those problems, and the value he might attach to having the problems ameliorated (see Part 2F, "Moving From Evidence to Action, Incorporating Patient Values").

Ideally, one would measure the impact of the treatment on the individual patient (see Part 2B1, "Therapy and Validity, N of 1 Randomized Controlled Trials"). However, this is often not feasible, and when the clinician is using data collected from other patients to inform the patient under consideration, HRQL instruments that focus on specific aspects of patients' function and their symptoms may be of more use than global measures—or measures that tell us simply about patients' satisfaction or well-being. For instance, patients with chronic lung disease may find it more informative to know that their compatriots who accepted treatment became less dyspneic and fatigued in daily activity, rather than simply that they judged their quality of life to be improved. Health-related quality of life measures will be most useful when results facilitate their practical use by you and the patients in your practice.

## Did the Study Design Simulate Clinical Practice?

Treatments affect quality of life both by reducing disease symptoms and consequences and by creating new problems: side effects. In fact, side effects may make the cure worse than the disease. Clinicians conducting clinical trials are usually blind to treatment allocation and they try to maintain patients on study medication as long as possible. Patients may therefore soldier on in the face of considerable side effects; ultimately, this may be reflected in their HRQL measure.

This is not how we normally conduct clinical practice. If patients experience significant side effects, we discontinue the medication, particularly if there is a suitable alternative. Thus, the design of the clinical trial may create an artificial situation, with misleading estimates of the impact of treatment on HRQL. This issue is of particular concern for patients receiving treatment with medications such as antihypertensive agents, in which much of the impairment in HRQL may result from the treatment, rather than the medical condition.

The trial of methotrexate in Crohn disease is likely to have simulated clinical practice well. Inflammatory bowel disease is serious enough—and its symptoms troubling enough—that if methotrexate is beneficial, patients are likely to continue with the treatment despite minor side effects. If the patient is experiencing problems similar to those of the trial patients and if those problems are important to him, he is likely to achieve comparable benefit to patients enrolled in the trial.

# CLINICAL RESOLUTION

Returning to our opening clinical scenario, in light of the available information you inform the patient that, on average, the HRQL improvement that patients experienced with methotrexate was small, but it was of a magnitude that most patients would consider important. The patient decides to reflect on what you have told him for the next week, and to return at that time with his decision.

We encourage clinicians to consider the impact of their treatments on patients' HRQL and to look for information regarding this impact in clinical trials. Responsive, valid, and interpretable instruments measuring experiences of importance to most patients should increasingly help guide our clinical decisions.

## References

1. Feagan BG, Rochon J, Fedorak RN, et al. Methotrexate for the treatment of Crohn's disease. *N Engl J Med*. 1995;332:292-297.

2. Fletcher RH, Fletcher SW, Wagner EH. *Clinical Epidemiology: The Essentials*. 3rd ed. Baltimore: Williams & Wilkins; 1996:4-6.

3. Guyatt GH, Feeny DH, Patrick DL. Measuring health-related quality of life. *Ann Intern Med*. 1993;118:622-629.

4. Gill TM, Feinstein AR. A critical appraisal of the quality of quality-of-life measurements. *JAMA*. 1994;272:619-626.

5. Wilson IB, Cleary PD. Linking clinical variables with health-related quality of life: a conceptual model of patient outcomes. *JAMA*. 1995;273:59-65.

6. Guyatt GH, Cook DJ. Health status, quality of life, and the individual. *JAMA*. 1994;272:630-631.

7. Nocturnal Oxygen Therapy Trial Group. Continuous or nocturnal oxygen therapy in hypoxemic chronic obstructive lung disease: a clinical trial. *Ann Intern Med*. 1980;93:391-398.

8. Heaton RK, Grant I, McSweeny AJ, Adams KM, Petty TL. Psychologic effects of continuous and nocturnal oxygen therapy in hypoxemic chronic obstructive pulmonary disease. *Arch Intern Med*. 1983;143:1941-1947.

9. Mulrow CD, Mulrow JP, Linn WD, Aguilar C, Ramirez G. Relative efficacy of vasodilator therapy in chronic congestive heart failure: implications of randomized trials. *JAMA*. 1988;259:3422-3426.

10. Packer M, Carver JR, Rodeheffer RJ, et al, for the PROMISE Study Research Group. Effect of oral milrinone on mortality in severe chronic heart failure. *N Engl J Med*. 1991;325:1468-1475.

11. Juniper EF, Svensson K, O'Byrne PM, et al. Asthma quality of life during 1 year of treatment with budesonide with or without formoterol. *Eur Respir J*. 1999;14:1038-1043.

12. Juniper EF, Norman GR, Cox FM, Roberts JN. Can the standard gamble and rating scale be used to measure quality of life in asthma? Comparison with the AQLQ and SF-36. *Am J Respir Crit Care Med*. Submitted.

13. Juniper EF, Price DB, Stampone P, Creemers JPHM, Mol SJM, Fireman P. Improved asthma-specific quality of life with approximately half the dose of extrafine-BDP compared with conventional-BDP in patients with asthma when pulmonary function remained stable. *J Allergy Clin Immunol*. Submitted for publication.

14. The COMBIVENT Inhalation Solution Study Group. Routine nebulized ipratropium and albuterol together are better than either alone in COPD. *Chest*. 1997;112:1514-1521.

15. Jaeschke R, Guyatt GH, Willan A, et al. Effect of increasing doses of beta agonists on spirometric parameters, exercise capacity, and quality of life in patients with chronic airflow limitation. *Thorax*. 1994;49:479-484.

16. Guyatt GH, Berman LB, Townsend M, Pugsley SO, Chambers LW. A measure of quality of life for clinical trials in chronic lung disease. *Thorax*. 1987;42:773-778.

17. Goldstein RS, Gort EH, Stubbing D, Avendano MA, Guyatt GH. Randomised controlled trial of respiratory rehabilitation. *Lancet*. 1994;344:1394-1397.

18. Wasson JH, Reda DJ, Bruskewitz RC, Elinson J, Keller AM, Henderson WG, for the Veterans Affairs Cooperative Study Group on Transurethral Resection of the Prostate. A comparison of transurethral surgery with watchful waiting for moderate symptoms of benign prostatic hyperplasia. *N Engl J Med*. 1995;332:75-79.

19. Guyatt GH, Mitchell A, Irvine EJ, et al. A new measure of health status for clinical trials in inflammatory bowel disease. *Gastroenterology*. 1989;96:804-810.

20. Kirshner B, Guyatt GH. A methodological framework for assessing health indices. *J Chronic Dis*. 1985;38:27-36.

21. Pitt B, Zannad F, Remme WJ, et al. The effect of spironolactone on morbidity and mortality in patients with severe heart failure. *N Engl J Med*. 1999;341: 709-717.

22. Guyatt GH, Kirshner B, Jaeschke R. Measuring health status: what are the necessary measurement properties? *J Clin Epidemiol*. 1992;45:1341-1345.

23. de Weerdt I, Visser AP, Kok GJ, de Weerdt O, van der Veen EA. Randomized controlled multicentre evaluation of an education programme for insulin-treated diabetic patients: effects on metabolic control, quality of life, and costs of therapy. *Diabet Med*. 1991;8:338-345.

24. Irvine EJ, Feagan B, Rochon J, et al, for the Canadian Crohn's Relapse Prevention Trial Study Group. Quality of life: a valid and reliable measure of therapeutic efficacy in the treatment of inflammatory bowel disease. *Gastroenterology*. 1994;106:287-296.

25. Greenberg GR, Feagan BG, Martin F, et al, for the Canadian Inflammatory Bowel Disease Study Group. Oral budesonide for active Crohn's disease. *N Engl J Med*. 1994;331:836-841.

26. Salonen R, Ashford E, Dahlof C, et al, for the International Intranasal Sumatriptan Study Group. Intranasal sumatriptan for the acute treatment of migraine. *J Neurol*. 1994;241:463-469.

27. Mathew NT, Saper JR, Silberstein SD, et al. Migraine prophylaxis with divalproex. *Arch Neurol*. 1995;52:281-286.

28. Tyring S, Barbarash RA, Nahlik JE, et al, for the Collaborative Famciclovir Herpes Zoster Study Group. Famciclovir for the treatment of acute herpes zoster: effects on acute disease and postherpetic neuralgia: a randomized, double-blind, placebo-controlled trial. *Ann Intern Med*. 1995;123:89-96.

29. Tugwell P, Pincus T, Yocum D, et al, for the Methotrexate-Cyclosporine Combination Study Group. Combination therapy with cyclosporine and methotrexate in severe rheumatoid arthritis. *N Engl J Med*. 1995;333:137-141.

30. Kirwan JR, for the Arthritis and Rheumatism Council Low-Dose Glucocorticoid Study Group. The effect of glucocorticoids on joint destruction in rheumatoid arthritis. *N Engl J Med*. 1995;333:142-146.

31. Malmivaara A, Hakkinen U, Aro T, et al. The treatment of acute low back pain— bed rest, exercises, or ordinary activity? *N Engl J Med*. 1995;332:351-355.

32. Bergner M, Bobbitt RA, Carter WB, Gilson BS. The Sickness Impact Profile: development and final revision of a health status measure. *Med Care*. 1981;19:787-805.

33. Tarlov AR, Ware JE Jr, Greenfield S, Nelson EC, Perrin E, Zubkoff M. The Medical Outcomes Study: an application of methods for monitoring the results of medical care. *JAMA*. 1989;262:925-930.

34. Ware JE Jr, Kosinski M, Bayliss MS, McHorney CA, Rogers WH, Raczek A. Comparison of methods for the scoring and statistical analysis of SF-36 health profile and summary measures: summary of results from the Medical Outcomes Study. *Med Care*. 1995;33(suppl 4):AS264-AS279.

35. Tandon PK, Stander H, Schwarz RP Jr. Analysis of quality of life data from a randomized, placebo-controlled heart-failure trial. *J Clin Epidemiol*. 1989;42:955-962.

36. Smith D, Baker G, Davies G, Dewey M, Chadwick DW. Outcomes of add-on treatment with lamotrigine in partial epilepsy. *Epilepsia*. 1993;34:312-322.

37. Chang SW, Fine R, Siegel D, Chesney M, Black D, Hulley SB. The impact of diuretic therapy on reported sexual function. *Arch Intern Med*. 1991;151:2402-2408.

38. Tugwell P, Bombardier C, Buchanan WW, et al. Methotrexate in rheumatoid arthritis: impact on quality of life assessed by traditional standard-item and individualized patient preference health status questionnaires. *Arch Intern Med*. 1990;150:59-62.

39. Laupacis A, Wong C, Churchill D, for the Canadian Erythropoietin Study Group. The use of generic and specific quality-of-life measures in hemodialysis patients treated with erythropoietin. *Control Clin Trials*. 1991;12(suppl 4):168S-179S.

40. Bosch JL, Hunink MG. The relationship between descriptive and valuational quality-of-life measures in patients with intermittent claudication. *Med Decis Making*. 1996;16:217-225.

41. Boyle MH, Torrance GW, Sinclair JC, Horwood SP. Economic evaluation of neonatal intensive care of very-low-birth-weight infants. *N Engl J Med*. 1983;308:1330-1337.

42. Hornberger JC, Garber AM, Chernew ME. Is high-flux dialysis cost-effective? *Int J Technol Assess Health Care*. 1993;9:85-96.

43. Hornberger JC, for the Renal Physicians Association Working Committee on Clinical Guidelines. The hemodialysis prescription and cost effectiveness. *J Am Soc Nephrol*. 1993;4:1021-1027.

44. Naylor CD. Cost-effectiveness analysis: are the outputs worth the inputs? *ACP Journal Club*. 1996;124:A12-A14.

45. Testa MA, Anderson RB, Nackley JF, Hollenberg NK, for the Quality-of-Life Hypertension Study Group. Quality of life and antihypertensive therapy in men: a comparison of captopril with enalapril. *N Engl J Med*. 1993;328:907-913.

46. Juniper EF, Guyatt GH, Willan A, Griffith LE. Determining a minimal important change in a disease-specific Quality of Life Questionnaire. *J Clin Epidemiol*. 1994;47:81-87.

47. Redelmeier DA, Guyatt GH, Goldstein RS. Assessing the minimal important difference in symptoms: a comparison of two techniques. *J Clin Epidemiol*. 1996;49:1215-1219.

48. Guyatt GH, Juniper EF, Walter SD, Griffith LE, Goldstein RS. Interpreting treatment effects in randomised trials. *BMJ*. 1998;316:690-693.

49. Jaeschke R, Singer J, Guyatt GH. Measurement of health status: ascertaining the minimal clinically important difference. *Control Clin Trials*. 1989;10:407-415.

50. Juniper EF, Guyatt GH, Feeny DH, Ferrie PJ, Griffith LE, Townsend M. Measuring quality of life in children with asthma. *Qual Life Res*. 1996;5:35-46.

51. Juniper EF, Buist AS, for the Study Group. Health-related quality of life in moderate asthma: 400 μg hydrofluoroalkane beclomethasone dipropionate vs 800 μg chlorofluorocarbon beclomethasone dipropionate. *Chest*. 1999;116:1297-1303.

52. Van Cauwenberge P, Juniper EF. Comparison of the efficacy, safety and quality of life provided by fexofenadine hydrochloride 120 mg, loratadine 10 mg and placebo administered once daily for the treatment of seasonal allergic rhinitis. *Clin Exp Allergy*. 2000;30:891-899.

53. Mitchell A, Guyatt G, Singer J, et al. Quality of life in patients with inflammatory bowel disease. *J Clin Gastroenterol*. 1988;10:306-310.

# THERAPY AND UNDERSTANDING THE RESULTS

## Hypothesis Testing

Gordon Guyatt, Roman Jaeschke, Deborah Cook, and Stephen Walter

Rose Hatala also made substantive contributions to this section

## IN THIS SECTION

We have said that there is a true, underlying effect of a treatment that only can be estimated by any individual experiment (see Part 2B, "Therapy and Harm, Why Study Results Mislead—Bias and Random Error"). Investigators use statistical methods to advance their understanding of this true effect. For some time, the essential paradigm for statistical inference in the medical literature has been that of hypothesis testing. The investigator starts with what is called a *null hypothesis* that the statistical test is designed to consider and, possibly, disprove. Typically, the null hypothesis is that there is no difference between treatments being compared. In a randomized trial in which investigators compare an experimental treatment with a placebo control, one can state the null hypothesis as follows: the true difference in effect on the outcome of interest between the experimental and control treatments is zero. For instance, in a comparison of vasodilator treatment in 804 men with heart failure, investigators compared the proportion of enalapril-treated survivors with the proportion of survivors given a combination of hydralazine and nitrates.[1] We start with the assumption that the treatments are equally effective and we adhere to this position unless data make it untenable. In the vasodilator trial, the null hypothesis could be stated more formally as follows: the true difference in the proportion surviving between patients treated with enalapril and those treated with hydralazine and nitrates is zero.

In this hypothesis-testing framework, the statistical analysis addresses the question of whether the observed data are consistent with the null hypothesis. The logic of the approach is as follows: Even if the treatment truly has no positive or negative impact on the outcome (that is, the effect size is zero), the results observed will seldom show exact equivalence; that is, no difference at all will be observed between the experimental and control groups. As the results diverge farther and farther from the finding of "no difference," the null hypothesis that there is no difference between treatment effects becomes less and less credible. If the difference between results of the treatment and control groups becomes large enough, clinicians must abandon belief in the null hypothesis. We will further develop the underlying logic by describing the role of chance in clinical research.

# THE ROLE OF CHANCE

In Part 2B, "Therapy and Harm, Why Study Results Mislead—Bias and Random Error," we considered a balanced coin with which the true probability of obtaining either heads or tails in any individual coin toss is 0.5. We noted that if we tossed such a coin 10 times, we would not be surprised if we did not see exactly five heads and five tails. Occasionally, we would get results quite divergent from the 5:5 split, such as 8:2 or even 9:1. Furthermore, very infrequently the 10 coin tosses would result in 10 consecutive heads or tails.

Chance is responsible for this variability in results, and certain recreational games illustrate the way chance operates. On occasion, the roll of two unbiased dice (dice with an equal probability of rolling any number between 1 and 6) will yield two ones or two sixes. On occasion (much to the delight of the recipient), the dealer at a poker game will dispense a hand consisting of five cards of a single suit. Even less frequently, the five cards will not only belong to a single suit, but will also have consecutive face value.

Chance is not restricted to the world of coin tosses, dice, and card games. If we take a sample of patients from a community, chance may result in unusual distributions of chronic disease. Chance also may be responsible for substantial imbalance in event rates in two groups of patients given different treatments that are, in fact, equally effective. Much statistical inquiry is geared to determining the extent to which unbalanced distributions could be attributed to chance and the extent to which one should invoke other explanations (treatment effects, for instance). As we will demonstrate, the conclusions of statistical inquiry are determined to a large extent by the size of the study.

# THE *P* VALUE

One way that an investigator can err is to conclude that there is a difference between a treatment group and a control group when, in fact, no such difference exists. In statistical terminology, making the mistake of erroneously concluding there is such a difference is called a *type I error* and the probability of making such an error is referred to as the alpha level. Imagine a situation in which we are uncertain whether a coin is biased. That is, we suspect that a coin toss is more likely to result in either heads or tails. One could construct a null hypothesis that the true proportions of heads and tails are equal (that is, the coin is unbiased). With this scenario, the probability of any given toss landing heads is 50%, as is the probability of any given toss landing tails. We could test this hypothesis by an experiment in which we conducted a series of coin tosses. Statistical analysis of the results of the experiment would address the question of whether the results observed were consistent with chance.

Let us conduct a hypothetical experiment in which the suspected coin is tossed 10 times and on all 10 occasions, the result is heads. How likely is this to have occurred if the coin was indeed unbiased? Most people would conclude that it is highly unlikely that chance could explain this extreme result. We would therefore be ready to reject the hypothesis that the coin is unbiased (the null hypothesis) and conclude that the coin is biased. Statistical methods allow us to be more precise by ascertaining just how unlikely the result is to have occurred simply as a result of chance if the null hypothesis is true. The law of multiplicative probabilities for independent events (where one event in no way influences the other) tells us that the probability of 10 consecutive heads can be found by multiplying the probability of a single head (1/2) 10 times over; that is, $1/2 \times 1/2 \times 1/2$, and so on. The probability of getting 10 consecutive heads is then slightly less than one in a thousand. In a journal article, one would likely see this probability expressed as a *P* value, such as $P < .001$. What is the precise meaning of this *P* value? If the coin were unbiased (that is, if the null hypothesis were true) and one were to repeat the experiment of the 10 coin tosses many times, 10 consecutive heads would be expected to occur by chance less than once in a thousand times. The probability of obtaining either 10 heads or 10 tails is approximately 0.002, or two in a thousand.

In the framework of hypothesis testing, the experiment would not be over, for one has to make a decision. Are we willing to reject the null hypothesis and conclude that the coin is biased? This has to do with how much faith we have in concluding that the coin is biased when, in fact, it is not. In other words, what risk or chance of making a type I error are we willing to accept? The reasoning implies a threshold value that demarcates a boundary. On one side of this boundary we are unwilling to reject the null hypothesis; on the other side we are ready to conclude that chance is no longer a plausible explanation for the results. To return to the example of 10 consecutive heads, most people would be ready to reject the null hypothesis when the results observed would be expected to occur by chance alone less than once in a thousand times.

Let us repeat the thought experiment. This time we obtain nine tails and one head. Once again, it is unlikely that the result is because of the play of chance alone. This time the $P$ value is .02. That is, if the coin were unbiased and the null hypothesis were true, results as extreme as—or more extreme than—those observed (that is, 10 heads or 10 tails, nine heads and one tail, or nine tails and one head) would be expected to occur by chance alone two times per hundred repetitions of the experiment.

Given this result, are we willing to reject the null hypothesis? The decision is arbitrary and is a matter of judgment. Statistical convention, however, would suggest that the answer is "yes," because the conventional boundary or threshold that demarcates the plausible from the implausible is five times per hundred, which is represented by a $P$ value of .05. This boundary is dignified by long tradition, although other choices of boundary could be equally reasonable. We call results that fall beyond this boundary (that is, $P$ value <.05) *statistically significant*. The meaning of statistically significant, therefore, is "sufficiently unlikely to be due to chance alone that we are ready to reject the null hypothesis."

Let us repeat our experiment twice more, both times with a new coin. On the first repetition we obtain eight heads and two tails. Calculation of the $P$ value associated with an 8/2 split tells us that, if the coin were unbiased, results as or more extreme than 8/2 (or 2/8) would occur solely as a result of the play of chance 11 times per hundred ($P = .11$). We have crossed to the other side of the conventional boundary between what is plausible and what is implausible. If we accept the convention, the results are not statistically significant and we will not reject the null hypothesis.

On our final repetition of the experiment, we obtain seven tails and three heads. Experience tells us that such a result, although not the most common, would not be unusual even if the coin were unbiased. The $P$ value confirms our intuition: results as extreme as or more extreme than this 7/3 split would occur under the null hypothesis 34 times per hundred ($P = .34$). Again, we will not reject the null hypothesis.

Although medical research is concerned with questions other than determining whether coins are unbiased, the reasoning associated with the $P$ values reported in journal articles is applicable. When investigators compare two treatments, the question they ask is, "How likely is the observed difference due to chance alone?" If we accept the conventional boundary or threshold ($P < .05$), we will reject the null hypothesis and conclude that the treatment has some effect when the answer to this question is that repetitions of the experiment would yield differences as extreme as or more extreme than those we have observed less than 5% of the time.

Let us return to the example of the randomized trial in which investigators compared enalapril to the combination of hydralazine and nitrates in 804 men with heart failure. Results of this study illustrate hypothesis testing using a dichotomous (yes/no) outcome—in this case, mortality.[1] During the follow-up period, which ranged from 6 months to 5.7 years, 132 of 403 patients (33%) assigned to enalapril died, as did 153 of 401 (38%) of those assigned to hydralazine and nitrates. Application of a statistical test that compares proportions (the *chi-square test*) reveals that if there were actually no difference in mortality between the two groups, differences as large or larger than those actually seen would be expected 11 times per 100 ($P = .11$). Using the hypothesis-testing framework and the conventional threshold of $P < .05$, we would conclude that we cannot reject the null hypothesis and that the difference observed is compatible with chance.

# THE RISK OF A FALSE-NEGATIVE RESULT

A clinician might comment on the results of the comparison of treatment with enalapril with that of a combination of hydralazine and nitrates as follows: "Although I accept the 5% threshold and therefore agree that we cannot reject the null hypothesis, I am nevertheless still suspicious that enalapril results in a lower mortality than does the combination of hydralazine and nitrates. The experiment still leaves me in a state of uncertainty." In making these statements, the clinician recognizes a second type of error that an investigator can make: falsely concluding that an effective treatment is useless. A *type II error* occurs when one erroneously dismisses an actual treatment effect—and a potentially useful treatment.

In the comparison of enalapril with hydralazine and nitrates, the possibility of erroneously concluding there is no difference between the two treatments looms large. The investigators found that 5% fewer patients receiving enalapril died than those receiving the alternative vasodilator regimen. If the true difference in mortality really were 5%, we would readily conclude that patients will receive an important benefit if we prescribe enalapril. Despite this, we were unable to reject the null hypothesis.

Why is it that the investigators observed an important difference between the mortality rates and yet were unable to conclude that enalapril is superior to hydralazine and nitrates? The answer is that their study did not enroll enough patients to warrant confidence that the important difference they observed is a real difference. The likelihood of missing an important difference (and, therefore, of making a type II error) decreases as the sample size gets larger. When a study is at high risk of making a type II error, we say it has inadequate power. The larger the sample size, the lower the risk of type II error and the greater the power. Although the 804 patients recruited by the investigators conducting the vasodilator trial may sound like a substantial number, for dichotomous outcomes such as mortality, very large sample sizes often are required to detect small treatment effects. For example, researchers conducting the trials that established the optimal treatment of acute myocardial infarction with thrombolytic agents both anticipated and found absolute differences between treatment and control mortality of less than 5%. Because of these small absolute differences between treatment and control they required—and recruited—thousands of patients to ensure adequate power.

Whenever a trial has failed to reject the null hypothesis (ie, when $P > .05$), the investigators may have missed a true treatment effect, and you should consider whether the power of the trial was adequate. In these negative studies, the stronger the nonsignificant trend in favor of the experimental treatment, the more likely it is that the investigators missed a true treatment effect.[2] Another section in this book describes how to decide if a study is large enough (see Part 2B2, "Therapy and Understanding the Results, Confidence Intervals").

Some studies are not designed to determine whether a new treatment is better than the current one, but, rather, whether a treatment that is less expensive, easier to administer, or less toxic yields more or less the same treatment effect as standard therapy. Such studies are often referred to as *equivalence studies*.[3] In equivalence studies, considering whether investigators have recruited an adequate sample size to make sure they will not miss small but important treatment effects is even more important. If the sample size of an equivalence study is inadequate, the investigator runs the risk of concluding that the treatments are equivalent when, in fact, patients given standard therapy derive important benefits in comparison to the easier, less expensive, or less toxic alternative.

# AN EXAMPLE USING A CONTINUOUS MEASURE OF OUTCOME

To this point, all of our examples have used outcomes such as yes/no, heads or tails, or dying or not dying, all of which we can express as a proportion. Often, investigators compare the effects of two or more treatments using a variable such as spirometric measurements, cardiac output, creatinine clearance, or score on a quality-of-life questionnaire. We call such variables, in which results can take a large number of values with small differences between those values, continuous variables.

The study of enalapril vs hydralazine and nitrates in patients with heart failure described above[1] provides an example of the use of a *continuous variable* as an outcome in a hypothesis test. The investigators compared the effect of the two regimens on exercise capacity. In contrast to the effect on mortality, which favored enalapril, exercise capacity improved with hydralazine and nitrates but not with enalapril. Using a test (the $t$ test) appropriate for continuous variables, the investigators compared the changes in exercise capacity from baseline to 6 months in the patients receiving hydralazine and nitrates to those changes in the enalapril group over the same period of time. Exercise capacity in the hydralazine group improved more, and the differences between the two groups are unlikely to have occurred by chance ($P = .02$).

# TAKING ACCOUNT OF BASELINE DIFFERENCES

Readers will often find that investigators have conducted their hypothesis tests taking account of baseline differences in the groups under study—an *adjusted analysis*. Randomization, a process whereby chance alone dictates to which group a patient is allocated, generally produces comparable groups. If, however, the investigator is unlucky, prognostic factors that determine outcome might have substantially different distributions in the two groups. For example, in a trial in which it is known that older patients have a poorer outcome, a larger proportion of the older patients may be randomly allocated to one of the two treatments being compared. Since older patients are at greater risk of adverse events, an imbalance in age could threaten the validity of an analysis that did not take age into account. The adjusted test yields a $P$ value corrected for differences in the age distribution of the two groups. In this example, readers can consider that investigators are providing them with the probability that would have been generated had the age distribution in the two groups been the same. Investigators can make adjustments for several variables at once, and you can interpret the $P$ value in the same way as we have already explained.

# MULTIPLE TESTS

University students have long been popular subjects for all sorts of experiments. In keeping with this tradition, we have chosen medical students as the subjects for our next hypothetical experiment.

Picture a medical school in which two instructors teach an introductory course on medical statistics. One instructor is more popular than the other instructor. The dean of the medical school has no substitute for the less popular faculty member. She has a particular passion for fairness and decides that she will deal with the situation by assigning the 200 medical students in her first-year class to one instructor or the other by a process of random allocation through which each student has an equal chance (50%) of being allocated to one of the two instructors.

The instructors decide to take advantage of this decision and illustrate some important principles of medical statistics. They therefore ask the question: are there characteristics of the two groups of students that differ beyond a level that could be explained by the play of chance? The characteristics they choose include sex distribution, eye color, height, grade-point average in the last year of college before entering medical school, socioeconomic status, and favorite type of music. The instructors formulate null hypotheses for each of their tests. For instance, the null hypothesis associated with sex distribution is as follows: the students are drawn from the same group of people and, therefore, the true proportion of females in the two groups is identical. You will note that, in fact, the students were drawn from the same underlying population and were assigned to the two groups by random allocation. The null hypothesis in each case is true; therefore, any time in this experiment in which the hypothesis is rejected will represent a false-positive result.

The instructors survey their students to determine their status on each of the six variables of interest. For five of these variables they find that the distributions are similar in the two groups, and all of the $P$ values associated with formal tests of the differences between groups are >.10. The instructors find that for eye color, however, 25 of 100 students in one group have blue eyes, whereas 38 of 100 in the other group have blue eyes. A formal statistical analysis reveals that if the null hypothesis were true (which it is), then differences in the proportion of people with blue eyes in the two groups as large or larger than the difference observed would occur slightly less than five times per 100 repetitions of the experiment. Using the conventional boundary, the instructors would reject the null hypothesis.

How likely is it that in testing six independent hypotheses on the same two groups of students, the instructors would have found at least one that crossed the threshold of 0.05 by chance alone? By *independent* we mean that the result of a test of one hypothesis does not depend in any way on the results of tests of any of the other hypotheses. Since our likelihood of crossing the significance threshold for any one characteristic is 0.05, the likelihood of not crossing the threshold for that same characteristic is 1.0 − 0.05, or 0.95. When two hypotheses are tested, the probability that neither one would cross the threshold would be 0.95 multiplied by 0.95 (or the square of 0.95); when six hypotheses are tested, the probability that not a single one would cross the 5% threshold is 0.95 to the sixth power, or 74%. When six independent hypotheses are tested, the probability that at least one result is statistically significant is therefore 26% (100% − 74%)—or approximately one in four, rather than one in 20. If we wished to maintain our overall standard of 0.05, we would have to divide the threshold $P$ value by six so each of the six tests would use a boundary value of 0.008.

The message here is twofold. First, rare findings do occasionally happen by chance. Even with a single test, a finding with a $P$ value of .01 will happen 1% of the time. Second, one should beware of multiple hypothesis testing that may yield misleading results. Examples of this phenomenon abound in the clinical literature. For example, in a survey of 45 trials from three leading medical journals, Pocock et al found that the median number of endpoints mentioned was six, and most were tested for statistical significance.[2]

We find a specific example of the dangers of use of multiple endpoints in a randomized trial of the effect of rehabilitation on quality of life after myocardial infarction. In this study, investigators randomized patients to receive standard care, an exercise program, or a counseling program, and they obtained patient reports on work, leisure, sexual activity, satisfaction with outcome, compliance with advice, quality of leisure and work, psychiatric symptoms, cardiac symptoms, and general health.[4] For almost all of these variables, there was no difference among the three groups. However, at follow-up after 18 months, patients were more satisfied with the exercise regimen than with the other two regimens, families in the counseling group were less protective than in the other groups, and patients participating in the counseling group worked more hours and had sexual intercourse more frequently. Does this mean that both exercise and rehabilitation programs should be implemented because of the small number of outcomes that changed in their favor, or that they should be rejected because most of the outcomes showed no difference? The authors themselves concluded that their results did not support the effectiveness of rehabilitation in improving quality of life. However, a program's advocate might argue that if even some of the ratings favored treatment, the intervention is worthwhile. The use of multiple instruments opens the door to such potential controversy.

A number of statistical strategies exist for dealing with the issue of testing multiple hypotheses on the same data set. We have illustrated one of these in a previous example: dividing the $P$ value by the number of tests. One can also specify, before the study is undertaken, a single primary outcome on which the major conclusions of the study will hinge. A third approach is to derive a single global test statistic (a pooled effect size, for instance) that effectively combines the multiple outcomes into a single measure. Full discussion of these strategies for dealing with multiple outcomes is beyond the scope of this book, but the interested reader can find a cogent discussion elsewhere.[5]

# LIMITATIONS OF HYPOTHESIS TESTING

At this point, some clinicians may be entertaining a number of questions that leave them uneasy. Why, for example, use a single cutpoint when the choice of a cutpoint is so arbitrary? Why dichotomize the question of whether a treatment is effective into a yes/no issue, when it may be viewed more appropriately as a continuum (eg, from, for instance, very unlikely to be effective to almost certainly effective)?

We believe that clinicians asking these questions are on the right track. They can look to another part of this book (see Part 2B2, "Therapy and Understanding the Results, Confidence Intervals") for an explanation of why we consider an alternative to hypothesis testing a superior approach.

# References

1. Cohn JN, Johnson G, Ziesche S, et al. A comparison of enalapril with hydralazine-isosorbide dinitrate in the treatment of chronic congestive heart failure. *N Engl J Med*. 1991;325:303-310.

2. Detsky AS, Sackett DL. When was a "negative" trial big enough? How many patients you needed depends on what you found. *Arch Intern Med*. 1985;145:709-715.

3. Kirshner B. Methodological standards for assessing therapeutic equivalence. *J Clin Epidemiol*. 1991;44:839-849.

4. Mayou R, MacMahon D, Sleight P, Florencio MJ. Early rehabilitation after myocardial infarction. *Lancet*. 1981;2:1399-1401.

5. Pocock SJ, Geller NL, Tsiatis AA. The analysis of multiple endpoints in clinical trials. *Biometrics*. 1987;43:487-498.

# THERAPY AND UNDERSTANDING THE RESULTS

## Confidence Intervals

Gordon Guyatt, Stephen Walter, Deborah Cook, and Roman Jaeschke

The following EBM Working Group members also made substantive contributions to this section: Mark Wilson and Martin Stockler

## IN THIS SECTION

Hypothesis testing involves estimating the probability that observed results would have occurred by chance if a *null hypothesis*, which most commonly states that there is no difference between a treatment condition and a control condition, were true (see Part 2B2, "Therapy and Understanding the Results, Hypothesis Testing"). Health researchers and medical educators have increasingly recognized the limitations of hypothesis testing; consequently, an alternative approach, estimation, is becoming more popular. A number of authors[1-5] have outlined the concepts that we will introduce here, and you can use the full expanse of their discussions to supplement our presentation. We will illustrate the concepts with an example introduced earlier in this book (see Part 2B2, "Therapy and Understanding the Results, Hypothesis Testing").

# HOW SHOULD WE TREAT PATIENTS WITH HEART FAILURE? A PROBLEM IN INTERPRETING STUDY RESULTS

In a double-blind randomized controlled trial of 804 men with heart failure, investigators compared treatment with enalapril to that with a combination of hydralazine and nitrates.[6] In the follow-up period, which ranged from 6 months to 5.7 years, 132 of 403 patients (33%) assigned to receive enalapril died, as did 153 of 401 patients (38%) assigned to receive hydralazine and nitrates. The *P* value associated with the difference in mortality is .11.

Looking at this study as an exercise in hypothesis testing (see Part 2B2, "Therapy and Understanding the Results, Hypothesis Testing") and adopting the usual 5% risk of obtaining a false-positive result, we would conclude that chance cannot be excluded as an explanation of the study results. We would classify this as a negative study (ie, we would conclude that no important difference existed between the treatment and control groups). The investigators also conducted an analysis that compared not only the proportion of patients surviving at the end of the study, but also the time pattern of the deaths occurring in both groups. This survival analysis, which generally is more sensitive than the test of the difference in proportions (see Part 2B2, "Therapy and Understanding the Results, Measures of Association"), showed a nonsignificant *P* value of .08, a result that leads to the same conclusion as the simpler analysis that focused on results at the end of the study. However, the authors also tell us that the *P* value associated with differences in mortality at 2 years ("a point predetermined to be a major endpoint of the trial") was significant at .016.

At this point, clinicians could be excused for being a little confused. Ask yourself: is this a positive study dictating use of an angiotensin-converting enzyme (ACE) inhibitor instead of the combination of hydralazine and nitrates, or is it a negative study, showing no difference between the two regimens and leaving the choice of drugs open?

# SOLVING THE PROBLEM: WHAT ARE CONFIDENCE INTERVALS?

How can clinicians deal with the limitations of hypothesis testing and resolve the confusion? The solution comes from an alternative approach that does not ask about how compatible the results are with the null hypothesis, or whether the *P* values differ significantly. By contrast, this approach poses two questions: (1) what is the single value most likely to represent the true difference between treatment and control? and (2) given the observed difference between treatment and control, what is the plausible range of differences between them within which the true difference might actually lie? This second question can be answered using *confidence intervals*. Before applying them to resolve the issue of enalapril vs hydralazine and nitrates in patients with heart failure, we will illustrate the use of confidence intervals with a coin-toss experiment.

Suppose that we have a coin that may or may not be balanced. That is, although it may be that the true probability of heads on any individual coin toss is 0.5, it may also be that the true probability is as high as 1.0 in favor of heads (every toss will yield heads) or 1.0 in favor of tails (every toss will yield tails). We now decide to conduct an experiment to determine the true nature of the coin.

We begin by tossing the coin twice, observing one head and one tail. At this point, what is our best estimate of the probability of heads on any given coin toss? Is it the value we have obtained (otherwise known as the *point estimate*), which is 0.5? What is the plausible range within which the true probability of finding a head on any individual coin toss might lie? This range is very wide, and most people would think that the probability might still be as high or higher than 0.9— or as low as or lower than 0.1. In other words, if the true probability of heads on any given coin toss is 0.9, it would still not be terribly surprising if, in any sample of two coin tosses, one were heads and one were tails. Hence, after our two coin tosses we are not much further ahead in determining the true nature of the coin.

We proceed with eight additional coin tosses; after a total of 10 tosses, we have observed five heads and five tails. Our best estimate of the true probability of heads on any given coin toss remains 0.5, the point estimate. The range within which the true probability of heads might plausibly lie has narrowed, however. It is no longer plausible that the true probability of heads is as great as 0.9. That is, if the true probability were 0.9, it would be very unlikely that in a sample of 10 coin tosses, one would observe five tails. People's sense of the range of probabilities that might still be plausible may differ, but most would agree that a probability greater than 0.8 or less than 0.2 is very unlikely.

After 10 coin tosses, values between 0.2 and 0.8 are not all equally plausible. The most likely value for the probability is the point estimate, 0.5, but probabilities close to that point estimate (0.4 or 0.6, for instance) are also quite likely. The further the probability from the point estimate, the less likely it is that the value represents the truth.

Ten coin tosses have still left us with considerable uncertainty about our coin, so we conduct another 40 repetitions. After 50 coin tosses, we have observed 25 heads and 25 tails and our point estimate remains 0.5. We are now beginning to believe that the coin is very unlikely to be extremely biased, and our estimate of the range of probabilities, which is still reasonably consistent with 25 heads in 50 coin tosses, might be 0.35 to 0.65. This range still is quite wide and we may persist with another 50 repetitions. If after 100 tosses we observed 50 heads, we might guess that the true probability is unlikely to be more extreme than 0.40 or 0.60. If we were willing to endure the tedium of 1000 coin tosses and if we observed 500 heads, we would be very confident (but still not certain) that our coin is minimally, if at all, biased.

What we have done through this experiment is to use common sense to generate confidence intervals around an observed proportion, 0.5. In each case, the confidence interval represents the range within which the truth plausibly lies. The smaller the sample size, the wider the confidence interval. As the sample size gets very large, we become increasingly certain that the truth is not far from the point estimate we have calculated from our experiment and the confidence interval is smaller.

It is fortunate that, since people's common sense differs considerably, we can turn to statistical techniques for precise estimation of confidence intervals. To use these techniques, we must first be a little more specific about what we mean by "plausible." In our coin-toss example, we might ask "what is the range of probabilities within which, 95% of the time, the truth would lie?" Table 2B2-2 presents the actual 95% confidence intervals around the observed proportion of 0.5 for our experiment. If we need not be quite so certain, we could ask about the range within which the true value would lie 90% of the time. This 90% confidence interval, also presented in Table 2B2-2, is somewhat narrower.

**TABLE 2B2-2**

## Confidence Intervals Around a Proportion of 0.5 in a Coin-Toss Experiment

| Number of Coin Tosses | Observed Result | 95% Confidence Interval | 90% Confidence Interval |
|---|---|---|---|
| 2 | 1 head, 1 tail | 0.01–0.99 | 0.03–0.98 |
| 10 | 5 heads, 5 tails | 0.19–0.81 | 0.22–0.78 |
| 50 | 25 heads, 25 tails | 0.36–0.65 | 0.38–0.62 |
| 100 | 50 heads, 50 tails | 0.40–0.60 | 0.41–0.59 |
| 1000 | 500 heads, 500 tails | 0.47–0.53 | 0.47–0.53 |

The coin-toss example also illustrates how the confidence interval tells you whether the study is large enough to answer the research question. If you wanted to be reasonably sure that the bias was no greater than 10% (that is, the ends of the confidence interval are within 10% of the point estimate), you would need approximately 100 coin tosses. If you needed greater precision—with 3% in either direction—1000 coin tosses would be required. All you have to do to obtain greater precision is to make more measurements. In clinical research, this involves enrolling more patients or increasing the number of measurements in each patient who is enrolled.

# USING CONFIDENCE INTERVALS TO INTERPRET THE RESULTS OF CLINICAL TRIALS

How do confidence intervals help us interpret the results of the trial of vasodilators in patients with heart failure? The mortality in the ACE inhibitor arm was 33% and in the hydralazine plus nitrate group it was 38%, an absolute difference of 5%. The difference of 5% is the point estimate, our best single estimate of the mortality benefit from using an ACE inhibitor. The 95% confidence interval around this difference works out to –1.2% to 12%.

How can we now interpret the study results? The most likely value for the mortality difference between the two vasodilator regimens is 5%, but the true difference may be as high as 1.2% in favor of the combination of hydralazine and nitrates or as high as 12% in favor of the ACE inhibitor. Values progressively farther from 5% will be less and less probable. We can conclude that patients offered ACE inhibitors will most likely (but not certainly) die later than patients offered hydralazine and nitrates—but the magnitude of the difference may be either trivial or quite large. This way of understanding the results avoids the yes/no dichotomy of hypothesis testing and the possible consequences of spending time and energy deciding about the legitimacy of the authors' focus on mortality at 2 years. It also obviates the need to argue whether the study should be considered positive or negative. One can conclude that, all else being equal, an ACE inhibitor is the appropriate choice for patients with heart failure, but the strength of this inference is weak. Toxicity, expense, and evidence from other studies would all bear on the final treatment decision (see Part 1F, "Moving From Evidence to Action"). Since a number of large randomized trials have now shown a mortality benefit from ACE inhibitors in patients with heart failure,[7] one can confidently recommend this class of agents as the treatment of choice.

# INTERPRETING APPARENTLY "NEGATIVE" TRIALS

Another example of the use of confidence intervals in interpreting study results comes from the results of the Swedish Co-operative Stroke Study, a randomized trial that was designed to determine whether patients with cerebral infarction might have fewer subsequent strokes if they took aspirin.[8,9] The investigators gave placebos to 252 patients, of whom 18 (7%) subsequently had nonfatal stroke. They also gave aspirin to 253 patients, of whom 23 (9%) had recurrent nonfatal stroke. The point estimate from these results is a 2% increase in the incidence of strokes among those patients in the aspirin group.

This trial of more than 500 patients might appear to exclude any possible benefit from aspirin. The 95% confidence interval on the absolute difference of 2% in favor of placebo, however, is from 7% in favor of placebo to 3% in favor of aspirin. Were the truth that 3% of the patients who would otherwise have strokes been spared had they taken aspirin, many patients would want to receive that drug. This would represent a 43% relative risk reduction, suggesting that we would need to treat only 33 patients to prevent a stroke. One can thus conclude that the trial has not excluded a patient-important benefit and, in that sense, was not large enough.

This example emphasizes that many patients must participate if trials are to generate precise estimates of treatment effects. In addition, it illustrates why we recommend that, whenever possible, clinicians turn to systematic reviews that pool data from the most valid studies.[10] In this case, such an overview shows that administration of antiplatelet agents in patients with transient ischemic attack or stroke reduces the relative risk of subsequent events by approximately 25% (with confidence intervals ranging from approximately 19% to 31%).[11] Given these data, many patients whose event rates without treatment would be over 10% (a number needed to treat of 50 or less) or even 5% (a number needed to treat of 100 or less) would be enthusiastic about taking aspirin.

This example also illustrates that when you see an apparently negative trial (one that, in our previous hypothesis-testing framework, fails to exclude the null hypothesis), you can focus on the upper end of the confidence interval (that is, the end that suggests the largest benefit from treatment). If the upper boundary of the confidence interval excludes any important benefit of treatment, you can conclude the trial is definitively negative. If, on the other hand, the confidence interval includes an important benefit, the possibility has not been ruled out that the treatment still might be worthwhile.

This logic of the negative trial is crucial in the interpretation of studies designed to help determine whether we should substitute a treatment that is less expensive, easier to administer, or less toxic for an existing treatment. In such an *equivalence study,* we will be ready to make the substitution only if we are sure that the standard treatment does not have important additional benefit beyond the less expensive or more convenient substitute. We will be confident that we have excluded the possibility of important additional benefit of the standard treatment if the upper boundary of the confidence interval around the difference is below our threshold.

# Interpreting Apparently "Positive" Trials

How can confidence intervals be informative in a positive trial (one that, in the previous hypothesis-testing framework, makes chance an unlikely explanation for observed differences between treatments)? In another double-blind randomized controlled trial of patients with heart failure, treatment with enalapril was compared to that with placebo.[12] Of 1285 patients randomized to the ACE inhibitor, 613 (48%) died or were hospitalized for accelerated heart failure, whereas 736 (57%) of 1284 patients in the placebo group experienced one of these adverse outcomes. The point estimate of the difference in death or hospitalization for heart failure is 10%, and the 95% confidence interval is 6% to 14%. Thus, the smallest effect of the ACE inhibitor that is compatible with the data is a 6% reduction in the number of patients with the adverse outcomes. If you consider it worthwhile to treat 17 patients to prevent one patient from dying or developing heart failure (6% is equivalent to about one in 17), then this represents a definitive trial. If, before treating, you would require a greater reduction than 6% in the proportion of patients who are spared an adverse advent, a larger trial (with a correspondingly narrower confidence interval) would be required.

# Was the Trial Large Enough?

As implied in our discussion to this point, confidence intervals provide a way of answering the question: "Was the trial large enough?" We illustrate the approach in Figure 2B2-2. In this figure, we present the distribution of randomized trial results you would expect from two treatments—one that results in an absolute reduction in mortality of 5% and one that results in an absolute increase in mortality of 1%. The vertical line in the center of the figure represents an absolute risk reduction of zero, when the experimental and control groups have exactly the same mortality. Values to the right of the vertical line represent results in which the treated group had a lower mortality than the control group. Values to the left of the vertical line represent results in which the treated group fared worse and had a higher mortality rate than the control group.

**FIGURE 2B2-2**

**Deciding Whether a Trial Is Definitive: Distributions of the Results of Trials of Two Therapies**

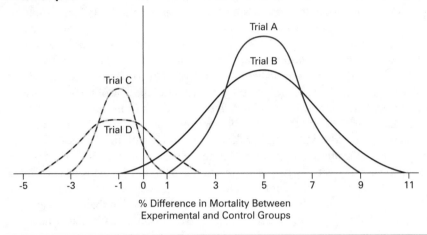

A represents the results of large trials of a therapy with an absolute mortality reduction of 5%; **B** represents the results of smaller trials of a therapy with an absolute reduction in mortality of 5%; **C** represents the results of large trials of a therapy with an absolute mortality increase of 1%; **D** represents the results of smaller trials of a therapy with an absolute reduction in mortality increase of 1%.

Reproduced with permission from the Canadian Medical Association.

For each of the two treatments, we present two distributions of results: one for a set of trials with a relatively small sample size, and one for a set of trials with a relatively large sample size. For each of the four distributions, the highest point of the distribution represents the underlying truth, the actual change in mortality. Distributions A and B come from the trials of the therapy that reduced mortality by 5%, and distributions C and D come from trials of the therapy that increased mortality by 1%.

Now, suppose we assume that absolute reductions in mortality greater than 1% warrant treatment. That is, the benefits outweigh the risks and costs whenever the absolute reduction in risk is 1% or greater (see Part 1F, "Moving From Evidence to Action"; see also Part 2F, "Moving From Evidence to Action, Grading Recommendations—A Quantitative Approach"), whereas reductions less than 1% do not warrant treatment (that is, the risks outweigh the benefits). For instance, if experimental treatment results in a true reduction in mortality from 5% to less than 4%, we would want to use the treatment. If, on the other hand, the true reduction in mortality was 5% to 4.5%, we would consider that the experimental treatment was not worth the associated toxicity and expense. What implications does this have for the way we will interpret the results of studies of this treatment?

In distribution A, more than 95% of the distribution lies above an absolute risk reduction of 1% (distribution A, like the others, depicts a simplified presentation of the situation—probabilities never actually sink to zero). Based on trials of this therapy and on this sample size, 95% confidence intervals would, in most instances, exclude an absolute risk reduction as small as 1%. In such trials, we could be confident that the true treatment effect is above our threshold, 1%, and we have a definitive positive trial. That is, we would be very confident that the true reduction in risk is greater than 1% (and, most likely, is appreciably greater), suggesting that many patients would be interested in receiving the treatment. The sample size in such trials would be adequate to demonstrate that the treatment provides a clinically important benefit.

Distribution B also comes from trials of a therapy that reduces mortality by 5%, but these trials include fewer patients. Whereas some of these trials would exclude the null hypothesis (that is, no difference is assumed between the treatment and control groups), many of the 95% confidence intervals would include mortality reductions less than 1%. When the 95% confidence interval includes values less than 1%, the data are consistent with an absolute risk reduction less than 1%. For such trials, we are left in doubt that the treatment effect is really greater than our threshold. Such trials would still be perceived as positive, but their results would not be definitive. The sample size of these trials would be inadequate to definitively establish the appropriateness of administering the experimental treatment.

Distribution C shows the results of a set of trials, all of which would be negative in that they would not exclude the null hypothesis of "no treatment effect." On average, investigators conducting these trials would observe a mortality rate that was 1% higher in the treatment group than in the control group. Most such trials would generate a narrow 95% confidence interval, all of which would lie to the left of our 1% threshold. The fact that the upper limit of the confidence interval is less than 1% would mean that we can be very confident that, if there is a benefit, it is very small and is unlikely to be appreciably greater than the risks, costs, and inconvenience of therapy. These trials would therefore exclude any patient-important benefit of treatment and they could be considered definitive. We would therefore dismiss the experimental treatment—at least for this type of population.

Distribution D comes from the same therapy as is reflected in distribution C, in which the mortality is 1% higher in the experimental group than in the control group. Distribution D, however, depicts trials with smaller sample size and, consequently, a much wider distribution of results. Because the confidence interval of most of these trials would include an appreciable portion that lies above our 1% threshold, we would conclude that it remains plausible (though unlikely) that the true effect of the experimental treatment is a reduction in mortality greater than 1%. Although we would still refrain from using this treatment (indeed, we would conclude it most likely kills people), we would not totally dismiss it. Most trials from distribution D, therefore, would not be definitive, and we would require larger trials enrolling more patients to exclude a clinically important treatment effect.

# CONCLUSION

We can restate our message as follows: in a positive trial establishing that the effect of treatment is greater than zero, look to the lower boundary of the confidence interval to determine whether sample size has been adequate. If this lower boundary—the smallest plausible treatment effect compatible with the data—is greater than the smallest difference that you consider important, the sample size is adequate and the trial is definitive. If the lower boundary is less than this smallest important difference, the trial is nondefinitive and further trials are required.

In a negative trial, look to the upper boundary of the confidence interval to determine whether sample size has been adequate. If this upper boundary, the largest treatment effect compatible with the data, is less than the smallest difference that you consider important, the sample size is adequate and the trial is definitively negative. If the upper boundary exceeds the smallest important difference, there may still be an important positive treatment effect, the trial is nondefinitive, and further trials are required.

## References

1. Simon R. Confidence intervals for reporting results of clinical trials. *Ann Intern Med.* 1986;105:429-435.

2. Gardner MJ, Altman DG, eds. *Statistics With Confidence: Confidence Intervals and Statistical Guidelines*. London: BMJ Publishing Group; 1989.

3. Bulpitt CJ. Confidence intervals. *Lancet*. 1987;1:494-497.

4. Pocock SJ, Hughes MD. Estimation issues in clinical trials and overviews. *Stat Med*. 1990;9:657-671.

5. Braitman LE. Confidence intervals assess both clinical significance and statistical significance. *Ann Intern Med.* 1991;114:515-517.

6. Cohn JN, Johnson G, Ziesche S, et al. A comparison of enalapril with hydralazine-isosorbide dinitrate in the treatment of chronic congestive heart failure. *N Engl J Med*. 1991;325:303-310.

7. Garg R, Yusuf S. Overview of randomized trials of angiotensin-converting enzyme inhibitors on mortality and morbidity in patients with heart failure. Collaborative Group on ACE Inhibitor Trials. *JAMA*. 1995;273:1450-1456.

8. Britton M, Helmers C, Samuelsson K. High-dose salicylic acid after cerebral infarction: a Swedish co-operative study. *Stroke*. 1997;18:325.

9. Sackett DL, Haynes RB, Guyatt GH, Tugwell P. *Clinical Epidemiology; A Basic Science for Clinical Medicine*. Boston: Little, Brown and Company; 1991:218-220.

10. Oxman AD, Guyatt GH. Guidelines for reading literature reviews. *CMAJ.* 1988;138:697-703.

11. Antiplatelet Trialists' Collaboration. Secondary prevention of vascular disease by prolonged antiplatelet treatment. *BMJ.* 1988;296:320-331.

12. The SOLVD Investigators. Effect of enalapril on survival in patients with reduced left ventricular ejection fractions and congestive heart failure. *N Engl J Med.* 1991;325:293-302.

# Therapy and Understanding the Results

## Measures of Association

Roman Jaeschke, Gordon Guyatt, Alexandra Barratt,
Stephen Walter, Deborah Cook, Finlay McAlister,
and John Attia

Sharon Straus also made substantive contributions to this section

## IN THIS SECTION

When clinicians consider the results of clinical trials, they are interested in the association between a treatment and an outcome. The study under consideration may or may not demonstrate an association between treatment and outcome; for example, it may or may not demonstrate a decrease in the risk of adverse events in patients receiving experimental treatment.

The focus of this section is on yes/no or dichotomous outcomes like death, stroke, or myocardial infarction. In their presentation of the results of studies addressing intervention effects on dichotomous outcomes, authors generally include the proportion of patients in each group who suffered an adverse event. As depicted in Figure 2B2-3, consider three different treatments that reduce mortality administered to three different populations. The first treatment, administered to a population with a 30% risk of dying, reduces the risk to 20%. The second treatment, administered to a population with a 10% risk of dying, reduces the risk to 6.7%. The third treatment reduces the risk of dying from 1% to 0.67%.

**FIGURE 2B2-3**

**Constant Relative Risk With Varying Risk Differences**

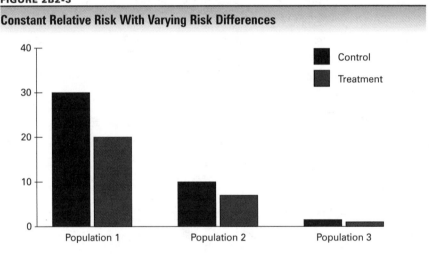

Although all three treatments reduce the risk of dying by a third, this piece of information is not adequate to fully capture the impact of treatment. Expressing the strength of the association as a *relative risk (RR)*, a *relative risk reduction (RRR)*, an *absolute risk reduction (ARR)* or *risk difference (RD)*, an *odds ratio (OR)*, or a *number needed to treat (NNT)* or *number need to harm (NNH)* conveys a variety of different information.

# DICHOTOMOUS AND CONTINUOUS OUTCOMES

A study's primary analysis often is concerned with the proportion of patients who suffer a particular target outcome, endpoint, or event in the treatment and control groups. This is true whenever the outcome captures the presence or absence of negative events like stroke, myocardial infarction, cancer recurrence, or death. It is also true for positive events like ulcer healing or resolution of symptoms. Even if the outcome is not one of these dichotomous variables, investigators sometimes elect to present the results as if this were the case. For example, investigators may present endpoints such as the duration of exercise time before the development of chest pain, the number of episodes of angina per month, the change in pulmonary function, or the number of visits to the emergency department as the mean values in the two groups. Alternatively, they may transform these variables into dichotomous data by specifying a threshold or degree of change that constitutes an important improvement or deterioration and then examine the proportion of patients above and below this threshold. For example, in a study of the use of forced expiratory volume in 1 second ($FEV_1$) in the assessment of the efficacy of oral corticosteroids in patients with chronic stable airflow limitation, investigators defined an event as an improvement in $FEV_1$ over baseline of more than 20%.[1] In another study in patients with chronic lung disease, investigators examined the difference in the proportion of patients who achieved an important improvement in health-related quality of life.[2] The investigators' choice of the magnitude of change required to designate an improvement as "important" can affect the apparent effectiveness of the treatment (although less so for odds ratios, discussed later in this section, than for the other measures of association).

# THE 2 X 2 TABLE

Table 2B2-3 depicts a 2 x 2 table that captures the information for a dichotomous outcome of a clinical trial. For instance, in a randomized trial, investigators compared mortality rates in patients with bleeding esophageal varices controlled either by endoscopic ligation or endoscopic sclerotherapy.[3] After a mean follow-up of 10 months, 18 of 64 participants assigned to ligation died, as did 29 of 65 patients assigned to sclerotherapy (Table 2B2-4).

**TABLE 2B2-3**

## The 2 x 2 Table

|  |  | Outcome | |
|---|---|---|---|
|  |  | Yes | No |
| Exposure | Yes | a | b |
|  | No | c | d |

Relative Risk (RR) $= \dfrac{a/(a+b)}{c/(c+d)}$

Relative Risk Reduction (RRR) $= \dfrac{c/(c+d) - a/(a+b)}{c/(c+d)}$

Absolute Risk Reduction (ARR) $= \dfrac{c}{c+d} - \dfrac{a}{a+b}$

Number Needed to Treat (NNT) $= \dfrac{1}{ARR}$

Odds Ratio (OR) $= \dfrac{a/b}{c/d} = \dfrac{ad}{cb}$

**TABLE 2B2-4**

## Results From a Randomized Trial of Endoscopic Sclerotherapy as Compared With Endoscopic Ligation for Bleeding Esophageal Varices*

|  |  | Outcome | | |
|---|---|---|---|---|
|  |  | Death | Survival | Total |
| Exposure | Ligation | 18 | 46 | 64 |
|  | Sclerotherapy | 29 | 36 | 65 |

Relative Risk (RR) = 0.63

Relative Risk Reduction (RRR) = 0.37

Absolute Risk Reduction (ARR) = 0.165

Number Needed to Treat (NNT ) = 6

Odds Ratio (OR) = 0.49

* Data from reference 3.

# The Absolute Risk

The simplest measure of association to understand is the *absolute risk*. The absolute risk of dying in the ligation group is 28% (18/64, or *a/a+b*), and the absolute risk of dying in the sclerotherapy group is 45% (29/65, or *c/c+d*). We often refer to the risk of the adverse outcome in the control group as the *baseline risk* or *control event rate*.

# The Absolute Risk Reduction

One can relate these two absolute risks by calculating the difference between them. We refer to this difference as the *absolute risk reduction* (ARR) or the risk difference (RD). Algebraically, the formula for calculating the ARR or RD is $[a/(a+c)]-[b/(b+d)]$ (see Table 2B3-3). This measure of effect tells us what proportion of patients are spared the adverse outcome if they receive the experimental therapy, rather than the control therapy. In our example, the ARR is 0.446 − 0.281, or 0.165 (ie, an ARR of 16.5%).

# The Relative Risk

Another way to relate the absolute risks in the two groups is to take the ratio of the two; this is called the *relative risk* or *risk ratio (RR)*. The RR tells us the proportion of the original risk (in this case, the risk of death with sclerotherapy) that is still present when patients receive the experimental treatment (in this case, ligation). Looking at our 2 x 2 tables, the formula for this calculation is $[a/(a+c)]/[b/(b+d)]$ (see Table 2B2-3 and the Appendix). In our example, the RR of dying after receiving initial ligation versus sclerotherapy is 18/64 (the risk in the ligation group) divided by 29/65 (the risk in the sclerotherapy group), or 63%. In other words, we would say the risk of death with ligation is about two thirds of that with sclerotherapy.

# The Relative Risk Reduction

Another measure used when assessing effectiveness of treatment is the *relative risk reduction (RRR)*. An estimate of the proportion of baseline risk that is removed by the therapy, it is calculated by dividing the absolute risk reduction by the absolute risk in the control group (see Table 2B2-3 and the Appendix). In our bleeding varices example, the RRR is 16.5% (the ARR) divided by 44.6% (the risk in the sclerotherapy group), or 0.37. One may also derive the RRR as (1.0 − RR). In the example, we have RRR = 1.0 − 0.63 = 0.37, or 37%. Using nontechnical language, we would say that ligation decreases the relative risk of death by 37% compared to sclerotherapy.

# THE ODDS RATIO

Instead of looking at the risk of an event, we could estimate the odds of having vs not having an event. You might be most familiar with odds in the context of sporting events, when bookies or newspaper commentators quote the chances for and against a horse, a boxer, or a tennis player winning a particular event. When used in medicine, the *odds ratio (OR)* represents the proportion of patients with the target event divided by the proportion without the target event. In most instances in medical investigation, odds and risks are approximately equal—so much so that many authors calculate relative odds and then report the results as if they had calculated relative risks. The following discussion will inform clinicians who wish to understand what an odds ratio is and who wish to be alert to those circumstances when treating an odds ratio as a relative risk will be misleading.

To provide a numerical example: If 1/5 of the patients in a study suffer a stroke, the odds of their having a stroke is (1/5)/(4/5) or 0.20/0.80, or 0.25. It is easy to see that because the denominator is the same in both the top and bottom expressions, it is canceled out, leaving the number of patients with the event (1) divided by the number of patients without the event (4). To convert from odds to risk, divide the odds by 1 plus the odds. For instance, if the odds of a poor surgical outcome is 0.5, the risk is 0.5/1 + 0.5, or 0.33. Table 2B2-5 presents the relationship between risk and odds. Note that the greater the magnitude of the risk, the greater is the divergence between the risk and odds.

**TABLE 2B2-5**

## Risks and Odds*

| Risk | Odds |
|------|------|
| 80% | 4 |
| 60% | 1.5 |
| 50% | 1.0 |
| 40% | 0.67 |
| 33% | 0.50 |
| 25% | 0.33 |
| 20% | 0.25 |
| 10% | 0.11 |
| 5% | 0.053 |

* Risks are equal to odds / 1 + odds. Odds are equal to risk / 1 – risk.

In our example, the odds of dying in the ligation group are 18 (death) vs 46 (survival), or 18 to 46 or 18/46 (*a/b*), and the odds of dying in the sclerotherapy group are 29 to 36 (*c/d*). The formula for the ratio of these odds is (*a/c*)/(*b/d*) (see Table 2B2-3); in our example, this yields (18/46)/(29/36), or 0.49. If one were formulating a terminology parallel to risk (where we call a ratio of risks a relative risk), one would call the ratio of odds a *relative odds*. Epidemiologists, who have been averse to simplifying parallel terminology, have chosen *relative risk* as the preferred term for a ratio of risks and *odds ratio* for a ratio of odds.

Clinicians have a good intuitive understanding of risk and even of a ratio of risks. Gamblers have a good intuitive understanding of odds. No one (with the possible exception of certain statisticians) intuitively understands a ratio of odds.[4,5] Nevertheless, until recently the OR has been the predominant measure of association.[6] The reason is that the OR has a statistical advantage in that it is essentially independent of the arbitrary choice between a comparison of the risks of an event (such as death) or the corresponding nonevent (such as survival), which is not true of the RR.[7]

As clinicians, we would like to be able to substitute the RR—which we intuitively understand—for the OR—which we do not understand. Looking back at our 2 x 2 table (see Table 2B2-3), we see that the validity of this substitution requires that [*a/(a+b)*]/[*c/(c+d)*]—the RR—be more or less equal to (*a/b*)/(*c/d*)— the OR. For this to be the case, *a* must be much less than *b*, and *c* much less than *d*; in other words, the outcome must occur infrequently in both the treatment and the control groups. As we have noted, Table 2B2-5 demonstrates that as the risk falls, the odds and risk come closer together. For low event rates, common in most randomized trials, the OR and RR are very close. The RR and OR will also be closer together when the magnitude of the treatment effect is small (that is, OR and RR are close to 1.0) than when the treatment effect is large.

When event rates are high and effect sizes are large, there are ways of converting the OR to RR.[8,9] Fortunately, clinicians will rarely need to consult such tables. To see why, consider a meta-analysis of ligation vs sclerotherapy for esophageal varices,[10] which demonstrated a rebleeding rate of 47% with sclerotherapy—as high an event rate as one is likely to find in most trials. The OR associated with treatment with ligation was 0.52—a large effect. Despite the high event rate and large effect, the RR is 0.60, which is not very different from the OR. The two are close enough—and this is the crucial point—that choosing one measure or the other is unlikely to have an important influence on treatment decisions.

# RELATIVE RISK AND ODDS RATIO VS ABSOLUTE RELATIVE RISK: WHY THE FUSS?

Having decided that distinguishing between OR and RR will seldom have major importance, introducing hypothetical changes to the 2 x 2 table (see Table 2B2-4) shows us why we must pay much more attention to distinguishing between the OR and RR vs the ARR. Let us assume that the number of patients dying decreased by approximately 50% in both groups. We now have nine deaths among 64 patients in ligation group and 14 deaths among 65 patients in the sclerotherapy group. The risk of death in the ligation group decreases from 28% to 14%, and in the sclerotherapy group, it decreases from 44.6% to 22.3%. The RR becomes 14/22.3 or 0.63, the same as before. The OR becomes (9/55)/(14/51) or 0.60, moderately different from 0.49 and closer to the RR. The absolute risk reduction decreases quite dramatically from 16.5% to approximately 8%. Thus, the decrease in the proportion of those dying in both groups by a factor of two leaves the RR unchanged, results in a moderate increase in the OR, and reduces the ARR by a factor of 2. This (see Figure 2B2-3) shows how the same RR can be associated with quite different ARRs—and that although the RR does not reflect changes in the risk of an adverse event without treatment (or, as in this case, with the inferior treatment), the ARR can change markedly with changes in this baseline risk.

Thus, a RR of 0.67 may represent both a situation in which a treatment reduces the risk of dying from 1% to 0.67%, or from 30% to 20% (see Figure 2B2-3). Assume that the frequency of severe side effects associated with such a treatment were 10%—we might encounter this situation in offering chemotherapy to a patient with cancer, for instance. Under these circumstances we would probably not recommend the treatment to most patients if it reduced the probability of dying by 0.33% (from 1% to 0.67%), but we may well be willing to recommend this treatment if the probability of an adverse outcome drops from 30% to 20%. In the latter situation, 10 patients per 100 would benefit, whereas one would suffer adverse effects—a tradeoff that most would consider worthwhile.

The RRR behaves the same way as the RR and does not reflect the change in the underlying risk in the control population. In our example, the RRR will be of the same magnitude if the frequency of events decreases by approximately half in both groups: (22.3 − 14)/22.3, or 0.37.

# THE NUMBER NEEDED TO TREAT

One can also express the impact of treatment by the number of patients one would need to treat to prevent an adverse event, the *number needed to treat* (*NNT*).[11] Table 2B2-4 shows that the risk of dying in the ligation group is 28.1%, and in the sclerotherapy group, it is 44.6%. If these estimates are accurate, treating 100 patients with ligation rather than sclerotherapy will result in between 15 and 16 patients avoiding death (the ARR, the control event rate minus the intervention event rate). If treating 100 patients results in avoiding 16 events, how many patients do we need to treat to avoid one event? The answer, 100 divided by 16, or approximately 6 (that is, 100 divided by the risk difference expressed as a percentage), is the NNT. One can also arrive at this number by taking the reciprocal of the ARR expressed as a proportion; that is, one can calculate the NNT by the formula 1/ARR (see Table 2B2-3). You may see that both the NNT and the ARR change with the difference in the underlying risk—which is not surprising, because the NNT is the reciprocal of the ARR. Given knowledge of the baseline risk and relative risk reduction, a nomogram presents a third way of arriving at the NNT (see Figure 2B2-4).[12]

**FIGURE 2B2-4**

## Nomogram for Calculating the Number Needed to Treat

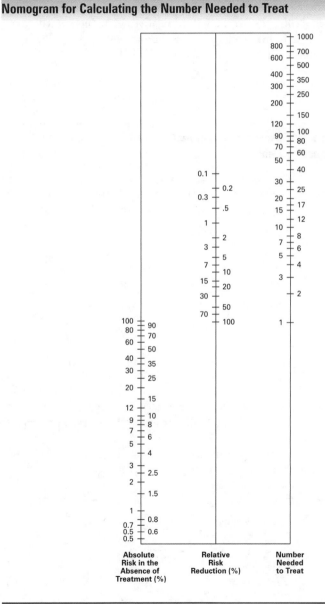

The NNT is inversely related to the proportion of patients in the control group who suffer an adverse event. If the risk of an adverse event doubles, we need treat only half as many patients to prevent an adverse event. If the risk decreases by a factor of 4, we will have to treat four times as many people. In our example, if the frequency of events (the baseline risk) decreases by a factor of 2 while the RRR remains constant, treating 100 patients with ligation would then result in avoiding eight events (22 − 14) and the NNT would double to 12.

The NNT is also inversely related to the RRR. A more effective treatment with twice the RRR will reduce the NNT by half. If the relative risk reduction with one treatment is only a quarter of that achieved by an alternative strategy, the NNT will be four times greater. Table 2B2-6 presents hypothetical data that illustrate these relationships.

**TABLE 2B2-6**

**Relationship Between the Baseline Risk, the Relative Risk Reduction, and the Number Needed to Treat\***

| Control Event Rate | Intervention Event Rate | Relative Risk | Relative Risk Reduction | Risk Difference | NNT |
|---|---|---|---|---|---|
| 0.02 | 0.01 | 50% | 50% | 0.01 | 100 |
| 0.4 | 0.2 | 50% | 50% | 0.2 | 5 |
| 0.04 | 0.02 | 50% | 50% | 0.02 | 50 |
| 0.04 | 0.03 | 75% | 25% | 0.01 | 100 |
| 0.4 | 0.3 | 75% | 25% | 0.1 | 10 |
| 0.01 | 0.005 | 50% | 50% | 0.005 | 200 |

\* Relative risk is equal to the intervention event rate/control event rate; the relative risk reduction is equal to 1− relative risk; the risk difference is equal to control event rate − intervention event rate; the NNT is equal to 1 / risk difference.

Using ARR and its reciprocal, the NNT, incorporates the influence of the changing baseline risk. If all we know is the ARR or the NNT, however, we remain ignorant of the size of the baseline risk. For example, an ARR of 5% (and a corresponding NNT of 20) may represent reduction of the risk of death from 10% to 5% (a RRR of 50%) or from 50% to 45% (a RRR of 10%).

# THE NUMBER NEEDED TO HARM

Clinicians can calculate the *number needed to harm* (NNH) in exactly the same way. If one expects that five of 100 patients will become fatigued when given a beta blocker, one will have to treat 20 patients to cause one to become tired, and the NNH is 20.

In this discussion we have not mentioned the problem that investigators may report odds ratios instead of relative risks. As we have mentioned, the best way of dealing with this situation when event rates are low is to assume the RR will be very close to the OR. The higher the risk, the less secure is the assumption. Tables 2B2-7 and 2B2-8 provide a guide for making an accurate estimate of the NNT and NNH when you know the patient's baseline risk and the investigator has provided only an odds ratio.

**TABLE 2B2-7**

## Deriving the NNT From the Odds Ratio*

| Control Event Rate | Therapeutic Intervention (OR) | | | | | | | | |
|---|---|---|---|---|---|---|---|---|---|
| | 0.5 | 0.55 | 0.6 | 0.65 | 0.7 | 0.75 | 0.8 | 0.85 | 0.9 |
| 0.05 | 41 | 46 | 52 | 59 | 69 | 83 | 104 | 139 | 209 |
| 0.1 | 21 | 24 | 27 | 31 | 36 | 43 | 54 | 73 | 110 |
| 0.2 | 11 | 13 | 14 | 17 | 20 | 24 | 30 | 40 | 61 |
| 0.3 | 8 | 9 | 10 | 12 | 14 | 18 | 22 | 30 | 46 |
| 0.4 | 7 | 8 | 9 | 10 | 12 | 15 | 19 | 26 | 40 |
| 0.5 | 6 | 7 | 8 | 9 | 11 | 14 | 18 | 25 | 38 |
| 0.7 | 6 | 7 | 9 | 10 | 13 | 16 | 20 | 28 | 44 |
| 0.9 | 12 | 15 | 18 | 22 | 27 | 34 | 46 | 64 | 101 |

* Adapted from reference 18.

The formula for determining the NNT is:

$$NNT = \frac{1 - CER(1 - OR)}{CER(1 - CER)(1 - OR)}$$

(CER = control event rate, OR = odds ratio)

**TABLE 2B2-8**

## Deriving the NNH From the Odds Ratio*

| Control Event Rate | Therapeutic Intervention (OR) | | | | | | | | |
|---|---|---|---|---|---|---|---|---|---|
| | 1.1 | 1.2 | 1.3 | 1.4 | 1.5 | 2 | 2.5 | 3 | 3.5 |
| 0.05 | 212 | 106 | 71 | 54 | 43 | 22 | 15 | 12 | 9 |
| 0.1 | 112 | 57 | 38 | 29 | 23 | 12 | 9 | 7 | 6 |
| 0.2 | 64 | 33 | 22 | 17 | 14 | 8 | 5 | 4 | 4 |
| 0.3 | 49 | 25 | 17 | 13 | 11 | 6 | 5 | 4 | 3 |
| 0.4 | 43 | 23 | 16 | 12 | 10 | 6 | 4 | 4 | 3 |
| 0.5 | 42 | 22 | 15 | 12 | 10 | 6 | 5 | 4 | 4 |
| 0.7 | 51 | 27 | 19 | 15 | 13 | 8 | 7 | 6 | 5 |
| 0.9 | 121 | 66 | 47 | 38 | 32 | 21 | 17 | 16 | 14 |

* Adapted from reference 18.

The formula for determining the NNH is:

$$NNH = \frac{CER(OR - 1) + 1}{CER(OR - 1)(1 - CER)}$$

(CER=control event rate, OR=odds ratio)

# BACK TO THE 2 X 2 TABLE

Whichever way of expressing the magnitude of the treatment effect we choose, the 2 x 2 table reflects results at a given point in time. Therefore, our comments on RR, ARR, RRR, OR, and NNT or NNH must be qualified by imposing a time frame on them. For example, we have to say that using ligation rather than sclerotherapy resulted in absolute risk reduction of death of 17% and an NNT of 6 over a mean time of 10 months. The results could be different if the duration of observation was very short (if there was no time to develop an event) or very long (after all, if an outcome is death, after 100 years of follow-up, everybody will die).

# CONFIDENCE INTERVALS

We have presented all of the measures of association of the treatment with ligation vs sclerotherapy as if they represented the true effect. The results of any experiment, however, represent only an estimate of the truth. The true effect of treatment may actually be somewhat greater—or less—than what we observed. The confidence interval tells us, within the bounds of plausibility, how much greater or smaller the true effect is likely to be (see Part 2B2, "Therapy and Understanding the Results, Confidence Intervals"). Statistical programs permit computation of confidence intervals for each of the measures of association we have discussed.

# SURVIVAL DATA

As we pointed out, the analysis of a 2 x 2 table implies an examination of the data at a specific point in time. This analysis is satisfactory if we are looking for events that occur within relatively short periods of time and if all patients have the same duration of follow-up. In longer-term studies, however, we are interested not only in the total number of events, but in their timing as well. For instance, we may focus on whether therapy for patients with a uniformly fatal condition (severe congestive heart failure or unresectable lung cancer, for example) delays death.

When the timing of events is important, investigators could present the results in the form of several 2 x 2 tables constructed at different points of time after the study began. For example, Table 2B2-4 represented the situation after a mean of 10 months of follow-up. Similar tables could be constructed describing the fate of all patients available for analysis after their enrollment in the trial for 1 week, 1 month, 3 months, or whatever time frame we choose to examine. The analysis of accumulated data that takes into account the timing of events is called *survival analysis*. Do not infer from the name, however, that the analysis is restricted to deaths; in fact, any dichotomous outcome will qualify.

The survival curve of a group of patients describes the status of patients at different time points after a defined starting point.[13] In Figure 2B2-5, we show the survival curve from the bleeding varices trial. Because the investigators followed approximately half of the patients for a longer time, the survival curve extends beyond the mean follow-up of 286 days. At some point, prediction becomes very imprecise because there are few patients available to estimate the probability of survival. Confidence intervals around the survival curves capture the precision of the estimate.

Even if the true relative risk, or relative risk reduction, is the same for each duration of follow-up, the play of chance will ensure that the point estimates differ. Ideally then, we would estimate the overall relative risk reduction by applying an average, weighted for the number of patients available, for the entire survival experience. Statistical methods allow just such an estimate. The weighted relative risk over the entire study is known as the *hazard ratio*.

**FIGURE 2B2-5**

**Survival Curves for Ligation and Sclerotherapy**

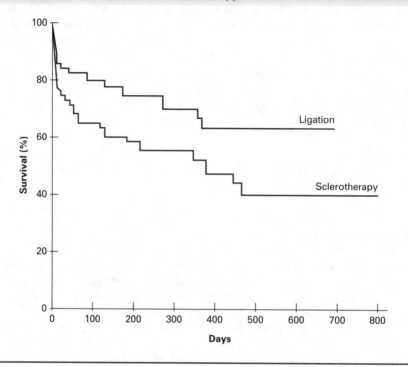

Reproduced with permission from the Massachusetts Medical Society.

Assuming the null hypothesis (ie, that there is no difference between two survival curves), we can generate a *P* value that informs us about the likelihood that chance explains the differences in results. Statistical techniques (most commonly, the *Cox regression model*) allow the results to be adjusted or corrected for differences in the two groups at baseline (see "Part 2B2, Therapy and Understanding the Results, Confidence Intervals"). If one group was older (and, thus, was at higher risk) or had less severe disease (and, thus, was at lower risk), the investigators might focus on an analysis that takes these differences into account. This, in effect, tells us what would have happened had the two groups had comparable risk factors for adverse outcome at the start of the trial.

Another way of reading survival curves is to plot the points at which a chosen percentage of the patients in each group have reached an endpoint. The difference between these points is a reflection of the delay in outcomes in the treatment group. For example, although ACE inhibitors may be associated with an up to 25% decrease in mortality in patients with postmyocardial infarction, this translates into an extra few months of life for patients in the treatment group, a result that may not appear as impressive.[14]

# CASE-CONTROL STUDIES

Up to now, our examples have come from prospective randomized controlled trials. In these trials, we start with a group of patients who are exposed to an intervention and a group of patients who are not exposed to the intervention. The investigators follow the patients over time and record the frequency of events. The process is similar in observational studies termed *prospective cohort studies*, although in this study design the exposure or treatment is not controlled by the investigators. For randomized trials and prospective cohort studies we can calculate risks, absolute risk reductions, and relative risks.

In case-control studies, investigators choose or sample participants not according to whether they have been exposed to the treatment or risk factor, but on the basis of whether they have experienced a target outcome. Participants start the study with or without the event, rather than with or without the exposure or intervention. Investigators compare patients with the adverse outcome—be it stroke, myocardial infarction, or cancer—to controls who have not suffered the outcome. The usual question asked is if there are any factors that seem to be more commonly present in one of these groups than in the other group.

In one case-control study, investigators examined the question of whether sunbeds or sunlamps increase the risk of skin melanoma.[15] They identified 583 patients with melanoma and 608 controls. The control patients and the cases had similar distributions of age, sex, and residence. Table 2B2-9 presents the findings for the men who participated in this study.

**TABLE 2B2-9**

**Results From a Case-Control Study Examining the Association of Cutaneous Melanoma and the Use of Sunbeds and Sunlamps***

|  | Exposure | Cases | Controls |
|---|---|---|---|
| Sunbeds or sunlamps | Yes | 67 | 41 |
|  | No | 210 | 242 |

\* Data from reference 11.

If the information in Table 2B2-9 came from a prospective cohort study or randomized controlled trial, we could begin by calculating the risk of an event in the exposed and control groups. This would not make sense in the case-control study because the number of patients who did not have melanoma was chosen by the investigators. For calculation of relative risk, we need to know the population at risk, and a case-control study does not provide this information.

The OR provides the only sensible measure of association in a case-control study. One can ask whether the odds of having been exposed to sunbeds or sunlamps among people with melanoma were the same as the odds of exposure among the control patients. In the study, the odds of exposure were 67/210 in the melanoma patients and 41/242 in the control patients. The OR is therefore (67/210)/(41/242), or 1.88 (95% CI, 1.20-2.98), suggesting an association between using sunbeds or sunlamps and developing melanoma. The fact that the confidence interval does not overlap or include 1.0 suggests that the association is unlikely to have resulted from chance.

Even if the association were not chance related, it does not necessarily mean that the sunbeds or sunlamps were the cause of melanoma. Potential explanations could include greater recollection of using these devices among people with melanoma (recall bias), longer sun exposure among these people, and different skin color; of these explanations, the investigators addressed many. To be confident that exposure to sunbeds or sunlamps was the cause of melanoma would require additional confirmatory studies.

# WHICH MEASURE OF ASSOCIATION IS BEST?

As evidence-based practitioners, we must decide which measure of association deserves our focus. Does it matter? The answer is "yes." The same results, when presented in different ways, may lead to different treatment decisions.[16-20] For example, Forrow and colleagues[16] demonstrated that clinicians were less inclined to treat patients after presentation of trial results as the absolute change in the outcome compared with the relative change in the outcome. In a similar study, Naylor and colleagues[17] found that clinicians rated the effectiveness of an intervention lower when events were presented in absolute terms rather than using relative risk reduction. Moreover, effectiveness was rated lower when results were expressed in terms of NNT than when the same data were presented as relative or absolute risk reductions. The pharmaceutical industry's awareness of this phenomenon may be responsible for their propensity to present physicians with treatment-associated relative risk reductions.

Patients turn out to be as susceptible as clinicians to the mode in which results are communicated.[12, 21-23] In one study, when researchers presented patients with a hypothetical life-threatening illness, those patients were more likely to choose a treatment described in terms of relative risk reduction than in terms of the equivalent absolute risk reduction.[12]

Aware that they will perceive results differently depending on how they are presented, what are clinicians to do? We believe that the best option is to consider all of the data (either as a 2 x 2 table or as a survival analysis) and then consider both the relative and the absolute figures. As you examine the results, you will find that if you can calculate the ARR and its reciprocal, the NNT, in an individual patient, these will be most useful in deciding whether to institute treatment (see Part 2B3, "Therapy and Applying the Results, Example Numbers Needed to Treat"). The conscientious evidence-based practitioner will use all available information to formulate the likely risks and benefits for the individual patient (see Part 2B3, "Therapy, Applying Results to Individual Patients").

# References

1. Callahan CM, Dittus RS, Katz BP. Oral corticosteroid therapy for patients with stable chronic obstructive pulmonary disease: a meta-analysis. *Ann Intern Med*. 1991;114:216-223.

2. Guyatt GH, Juniper EF, Walter SD, Griffith LE, Goldstein RS. Interpreting treatment effects in randomised trials. *BMJ*. 1998;316:690-693.

3. Stiegmann GV, Goff JS, Michaletz-Onody PA, et al. Endoscopic sclerotherapy as compared with endoscopic ligation for bleeding esophageal varices. *N Engl J Med*. 1992;326:1527-1532.

4. Sinclair JC, Bracken MB. Clinically useful measures of effect in binary analyses of randomized trials. *J Clin Epidemiol*. 1994;47:881-889.

5. Sackett DL. Down with odds ratios! *Evid Based Med*. 1996;1:164-166.

6. Laird NM, Mosteller F. Some statistical methods for combining experimental results. *Int J Technol Assess Health Care*. 1990;6:5-30.

7. Walter SD. Choice of effect measure for epidemiological data. *J Clin Epidemiol*. 2000;53:931-939.

8. Davies HT, Crombie IK, Tavakoli M. When can odds ratios mislead? *BMJ*. 1998;316:989-991.

9. Zhang J, Yu KF. What's the relative risk? A method of correcting the odds ratio in cohort studies of common outcomes. *JAMA*. 1998;280:1690-1691.

10. Laine L, Cook D. Endoscopic ligation compared with sclerotherapy for treatment of esophageal variceal bleeding: a meta-analysis. *Ann Intern Med*. 1995;123:280-287.

11. Laupacis A, Sackett DL, Roberts RS. An assessment of clinically useful measures of the consequences of treatment. *N Engl J Med*. 1988;318:1728-1733.

12. Chatellier G, Zapletal E, Lemaitre D, Menard J, Degoulet P. The number needed to treat: a clinically useful nomogram in its proper context. *BMJ*. 1996;312:426-429.

13. Coldman AJ, Elwood JM. Examining survival data. *CMAJ*. 1979;121:1065-1068, 1071.

14. Tan LB, Murphy R. Shifts in mortality curves: saving or extending lives? *Lancet*. 1999;354:1378-1381.

15. Walter SD, Marrett LD, From L, Hertzman C, Shannon HS, Roy P. The association of cutaneous malignant melanoma with the use of sunbeds and sunlamps. *Am J Epidemiol*. 1990;131:232-243.

16. Forrow L, Taylor WC, Arnold RM. Absolutely relative: how research results are summarized can affect treatment decisions. *Am J Med*. 1992;92:121-124.

17. Naylor CD, Chen E, Strauss B. Measured enthusiasm: does the method of reporting trial results alter perceptions of therapeutic effectiveness? *Ann Intern Med*. 1992;117:916-921.

18. Hux JE, Levinton CM, Naylor CD. Prescribing propensity: influence of life-expectancy gains and drug costs. *J Gen Intern Med*. 1994;9:195-201.

19. Redelmeier DA, Tversky A. Discrepancy between medical decisions for individual patients and for groups. *N Engl J Med*. 1990;322:1162-1164.

20. Bobbio M, Demichelis B, Giustetto G. Completeness of reporting trial results: effect on physicians' willingness to prescribe. *Lancet*. 1994;343:1209-1211.

21. Malenka DJ, Baron JA, Johansen S, Wahrenberger JW, Ross JM. The framing effect of relative and absolute risk. *J Gen Intern Med*. 1993;8:543-548.

22. McNeil BJ, Pauker SG, Sox HC Jr, Tversky A. On the elicitation of preferences for alternative therapies. *N Engl J Med*. 1982;306:1259-1262.

23. Hux JE, Naylor CD. Communicating the benefits of chronic preventive therapy: does the format of efficacy data determine patients' acceptance of treatment? *Med Decis Making*. 1995;15:152-157.

# THERAPY AND APPLYING THE RESULTS

## Applying Results to Individual Patients

Antonio Dans, Finlay McAlister, Leonilla Dans,
W. Scott Richardson, Sharon Straus, and Gordon Guyatt

Thomas McGinn also made substantive contributions to this section

## IN THIS SECTION

### For Which Patients Is Thrombolytic Therapy Indicated in the Philippines?

**Y**ou are the attending physician on duty when a 40-year-old university history professor presents to the emergency department of a general hospital in the Philippines. He has experienced severe chest pain for 2 hours, associated with clammy perspiration. The pain is now settling and the patient is not feeling dyspneic or otherwise in distress. Physical examination reveals a blood pressure of 110/70 mm Hg, a heart rate of 92 bpm, a normal first heart sound, and clear lungs. An electrocardiogram discloses 3-mm ST segment elevation in the inferior leads. As intravenous lines are placed and the patient is prepared for admission to the coronary care unit, you consider the possible benefits and risks of administering thrombolytic therapy. You have recently reviewed the issues for just such a patient, and you now make a quick mental summary of what you learned and how you might apply it to this individual.

# FINDING THE EVIDENCE

Streptokinase is the only thrombolytic agent that the patient before you might afford. You therefore confine your search to this drug, trying to locate the best evidence from an appropriate randomized trial or, if possible, a meta-analysis of many trials. Launching Grateful Med software, you select "myocardial infarction" from the list of Medical Subject Headings (MeSH) used to index articles. On the second subject line, you use the MeSH term "streptokinase." You limit your search to English-language articles; to find quantitative reviews or original studies, you use the terms "meta-analysis" or "randomized controlled trial" to signal the publication type.

You retrieve a systematic meta-analysis of randomized trials that you find deals with effectiveness[1] but not with toxicity. Therefore, you also review a single trial, second International Study of Infarct Survival (ISIS-2),[2] which you choose on the basis of its size (17,000 patients), its strong design (which includes double-blinding), and the wide variety of settings in which the study was undertaken. You apply the criteria you have learned for evaluating the validity of the studies, as well as for interpreting the magnitude and precision of the treatment effects and toxicity. The articles meet the validity criteria and you note that, in the meta-analysis, the treatment reduced the event rate from 17.4% to 12.8%.[1] For the average participant in these trials, this seems to outweigh the potential harm of bleeding requiring transfusion, which occurred in 0.5% of streptokinase-treated patients, compared to 0.2% in the placebo group in the ISIS-2 trial.[2]

When considering how to manage the patient you are treating, you note that Asians composed only a small minority of the patients in the trial in the meta-analysis. Furthermore, you are uncertain about your hospital staff's ability to cope with technical requirements for administering the drug or dealing with complications.

As clinicians look more often to randomized controlled trials (RCTs) to guide their clinical care, they must decide how to apply RCT results to individual patients in their practice setting. Part 1B1, "Therapy," suggested three criteria for deciding on applicability: could you apply the results of the research to the patient before you, did the investigators measure all important outcomes, and what is the balance between the benefits and risks of intervening?

With regard to the first of these three questions, we suggested that clinicians would be wise to apply the results to patients in their practice unless there was a compelling reason to believe the results would differ substantially as a function of the particular characteristics of those patients. Empirical support for this position comes from a number of sources. In general, meta-analyses of therapeutic interventions have suggested that treatment effects are usually similar across subgroups of patients.[3] For example, although beta blockers are prescribed to only a minority of patients with acute myocardial infarction, patients with myocardial infarction who also have concomitant conditions (such as peripheral vascular disease, diabetes mellitus, heart failure, or chronic obstructive pulmonary disease) that might lead clinicians to withhold treatment derive substantial survival benefits from beta-blocker therapy.[4] This is a consistent theme emerging from cardiovascular outcomes research.[5]

Nevertheless, the underlying biologic characteristics of a group of patients may differ from those who composed the majority of participants in clinical trials to the extent that we must call the applicability of the data into question. Clinicians managing patients who differ economically, racially, or culturally from those recruited in typical clinical trials face particular challenges in deciding whether patient groups are sufficiently different that applicability of results is threatened. Examples of such patients include those from the inner cities of North America, from the Native American reservations, or from developing countries.

In this section, we expand on the criteria related to both applying results to the individual and achieving a balance of benefits and risks. Table 2B3-1 summarizes the guides, categorizing them into biologic and socioeconomic issues (ones that help us decide if the treatment can work) and epidemiologic issues (ones that help us decide on the magnitude of the likely benefit and the magnitude of the risks). As we discuss each issue, we will offer sources of information that will help physicians answer their questions.

**TABLE 2B3-1**

## Users' Guides for Applying Study Results to Individual Patients

**How Can I Apply the Results to Patient Care?**

*Biologic Issues*

- Are there pathophysiologic differences in the illness under study that may lead to a diminished treatment response?
- Are there patient differences that may diminish the treatment response?

*Socioeconomic Issues*

- Are there important differences in patient compliance that may diminish the treatment response?
- Are there important differences in provider compliance that may diminish the treatment response?

*Epidemiologic Issues*

- Do patients in my practice have comorbid conditions that significantly alter the potential benefits and risks of the treatment?

**Are the Likely Benefits Worth the Potential Risks and Costs?**

- What is the patient's risk of sustaining adverse events?

# HOW CAN I APPLY THE RESULTS TO PATIENT CARE?

## Biologic Issues

### Are There Pathophysiologic Differences in the Illness Under Study That May Lead to a Diminished Treatment Response?

Diseases with a single name may represent conditions with important pathophysiologic differences. These differences can sometimes lead to diminished treatment responses resulting from either divergence in pathogenetic mechanisms among patients or biologic differences in the causative agent. For example, hypertension in African-Americans or black non-Americans has been observed to be relatively responsive to diuretics and unresponsive to beta blockers.[6] This selective response reflects a state of relative volume excess that investigators now theorize may have served protective functions in their hot and arid ancestral environments.[7]

Malaria provides an example of a condition that may vary because of biologic differences in the causative agent. Malaria treatment protocols vary depending on drug-resistance patterns.[8] In such examples, clinicians should anticipate variation in response to treatment and should temper hasty conclusions regarding the applicability of trial results.

To address our scenario of applicability of streptokinase to the treatment of myocardial infarction in a patient in the Philippines, we reviewed a case series of autopsies done on Filipino patients with myocardial infarction.[9] Pathologic changes in the coronary arteries and myocardium were similar to those noted among North American patients,[10] whereas nonatherosclerotic causes of coronary disease occurred rarely. Clinical surveys have demonstrated that persons of Philippine descent share the same risk factors for coronary artery disease[11] as persons of North American descent.[12] Thus, we can be confident that disease pathogenesis is similar.

**Are There Patient Differences That May Diminish the Treatment Response?**
Between-population differences in response to treatment may arise from differences in drug metabolism, differences in immune response, or differences in environmental factors that affect drug toxicity. Differences in drug metabolism may directly influence the efficacy of a treatment regimen. If they are not identified, patients in whom drugs are metabolized slowly could face the risk of greater toxicity, whereas those in whom drugs are metabolized rapidly might experience a significant decrease in efficacy. Such differences usually are based on genetic polymorphism in the activity of metabolizing enzymes. A well-known example is hepatic $N$-acetyltransferase, an enzyme with increased activity among persons of Asian descent.[13] For this reason, clinicians offer patients higher drug dosages for agents such as isoniazid, hydralazine, and procainamide. Other examples of genetic polymorphism include pseudocholinesterase activity in the metabolism of suxamethonium, and glucose-6-phosphate dehydrogenase activity in the metabolism of sulfonamides and other drugs.[14]

Differences in patients' immune response may also modulate treatment effect. *Haemophilus influenzae* vaccine, for example, has a lower efficacy rate in indigenous Alaskan populations than in nonindigenous populations.[15] Finally, environmental factors may affect response to therapy. For instance, the incidence of thyroid dysfunction from amiodarone differs in low-iodine vs high-iodine environments.[16]

Pharmacokinetic and bioavailability studies may provide evidence regarding differences in treatment response. Such studies generally require small sample sizes and commonly available equipment. Unfortunately, for a wide variety of drugs, technology for assays remains unavailable. Reasonable alternatives include dose ranging and descriptive studies of patients receiving treatment, which can also provide information on immune response to vaccines and environmental factors that may increase or decrease the toxic effects of drugs. Postmarketing surveillance studies and large RCTs require very large sample sizes and long-term follow-up, but may provide definitive information about differential response to therapy, as in the example of the decreased effect of *H influenzae* vaccine in indigenous Alaskan patients.

Although we found no studies evaluating the pharmacokinetic profile of streptokinase when given to Filipino patients, postmarketing studies show that they experience the same reperfusion arrhythmias and bleeding complications as North

Americans when given streptokinase at the same dose.[17] These studies provide some assurance of similarities in the response to adverse effects of treatment.

## Socioeconomic Issues

When satisfied that biologic differences do not compromise treatment applicability, clinicians must examine constraints related to the social environment that may diminish treatment effectiveness.

### Are There Important Differences in Patient Adherence That May Diminish the Treatment Response?

To the extent that groups of people exhibit different levels of adherence to treatment, clinicians may expect variation in treatment effectiveness. Variability in compliance between populations may stem from obvious resource limitations in a particular setting or from less obvious attitudinal or behavioral characteristics. For example, both types of problems may affect the safety of outpatient administration of anticoagulant agents. Neither indigent patients nor their society may be able to afford repeated clinic visits and tests for treatment monitoring. Persons suffering from alcohol or other drug addiction, regardless of their financial situation, may be less likely to comply with monitoring. Inadequate monitoring, regardless of reason, increases bleeding risk from overanticoagulation, shifting the balance between benefit and harm—even to the point where harm outweighs benefit.

Although clinicians are often unable to predict patient compliance, a systematic examination of compliance in individual patients—or groups of patients—is likely to aid in identifying varying compliance patterns. Clinicians may also refer to more general sources of evidence, such as sociologic descriptions of attitudes of specific groups of people (see Part 2B3, "Therapy and Applying the Results, Qualitative Research"). In the Philippines, for example, an attitude called *bahala na* connotes a lack of capacity or will to control one's fate.[18] A near-equivalent would be expressed roughly as, "Let's just wait and see; there's really nothing much we can do about the situation." This external *locus of control*[19] may have an adverse effect on patient adherence. In our scenario, we do not expect patient adherence to be a problem since we give streptokinase intravenously as a single dose.

### Are There Important Differences in Provider Adherence That Might Diminish the Safety and Efficacy of the Treatment?

In this section, the term *provider adherence* or *compliance* refers to a host of diagnostic tests, monitoring equipment, interventional requirements, and other technical specifications that clinicians must use or satisfy to administer a treatment safely and effectively. Financial conditions in a health care center, access to equipment, technologic expertise, and the availability and skill of health care personnel may influence treatment effectiveness. For instance, in randomized trials of asymptomatic patients with carotid endarterectomy, patients at relatively low risk of stroke nevertheless showed benefit from surgery.[20] However, the surgery-associated stroke rate was low, probably because of the high level of experience and expertise of the surgical centers that participated in the trial. The net effect for such low-risk patients in centers with higher surgery-associated stroke rates may be an increase in adverse outcomes.[21] This is particularly worrisome since surgical teams whose complication rates and operative volumes would have rendered them ineligible for the trial do most endarterectomies.[22]

In developing countries, many hospitals and clinics do not have easy access to sophisticated equipment; therefore, problems of provider compliance are common. For example, although rheumatic atrial fibrillation remains a common problem in Asian countries, very few laboratories in rural areas in those countries perform the tests necessary for titration of warfarin dose. This limitation is likely to mean that the critical balance between effectiveness and safety of treatment, instead of favoring treatment, now favors not treating.

Administration of streptokinase carries potential hazards, foremost of which is catastrophic bleeding. Facilities for emergency administration of cryoprecipitate, fresh frozen plasma, or whole blood must be available.[23] In hospitals without efficient blood banking systems, coping with bleeding emergencies may be difficult. This increases the potential hazards of treatment and may tip the balance between benefit and harm.

## Epidemiologic Issues

When satisfied that biologic and socioeconomic differences do not compromise applicability, the clinician must examine patient characteristics that can influence either the magnitude of the benefit or the risks of treatment (and, thus, the trade-off between the two).[24]

### Do Patients in My Practice Have Comorbid Conditions That Significantly Alter the Potential Benefits and Risks of the Treatment?

The presence of other conditions in a particular locality may affect treatment efficiency in two possible ways: as competing diagnostic possibilities or as competing etiologies of outcome. The management of pneumonia in developing countries provides an example of a competing diagnostic possibility.

The acute respiratory infection management protocol includes a symptom-driven algorithm for differentiating pneumonia from nonpneumonia. This protocol identifies children who need antibiotics and has proved effective in reducing mortality from pneumonia among children under 5 years of age.[25] However, similarities exist in the clinical presentation of pneumonia and malaria. In malaria-endemic areas, clinicians may expect an increase in false-positive pneumonias. Patients with such results that mimic pneumonia when malaria is actually present will not respond to antibiotics for pneumonia, and a delay in instituting antimalarial treatment may result. If the drop in accuracy is large enough, the balance between harm and benefit will change. To resolve this issue, investigators have initiated a study to determine if the acute respiratory infection protocol can maintain its effectiveness in malaria-endemic areas.[26]

Competing causes of target events may also affect the magnitude of benefit. An example comes from the management of patients with acute myocardial infarction in some Filipino hospitals. A recent study disclosed 30 in-hospital deaths in a cohort of 149 such patients admitted to a charity hospital.[27] On the basis of results from the meta-analysis discussed previously, clinicians might expect streptokinase to reduce this 20% death rate by 25%.[1] However, a closer look at the local data shows a contrast with the original studies, in which virtually all deaths were a direct result of cardiac ischemia. In the Philippine study, noncardiac causes—mostly pneumonia with sepsis—were responsible for 11 of the 30 deaths. Streptokinase will not reduce mortality in such patients. Adequate antibiotic coverage may result in a greater (and more economic) reduction in mortality for patients who develop pneumonia.

In addition to reducing benefit, other morbidity may affect the magnitude of risk. For example, surgical mortality may increase in malnourished patients, shifting the balance between benefit and risk. On occasion, other morbidity can also work in the opposite direction—by increasing efficiency. For example, a patient with a large infarct for whom the clinician is considering warfarin may also have atrial fibrillation. Since anticoagulation reduces stroke risk in such patients, the presence of atrial fibrillation strengthens the indication for treatment.

In the myocardial infarction clinical scenario, we used data from the local study of 149 charity patients to evaluate the impact of other morbid conditions.[27] As we noted, we can expect streptokinase to prevent approximately five of the 19 cardiac deaths, but none of those from other causes, and the absolute reduction in all-cause mortality among all patients represents a decline from 30 of 149 (20.1%) to 25 of 149 (16.8%).

# ARE THE LIKELY BENEFITS WORTH THE POTENTIAL RISKS AND COSTS?

## What Is the Patient's Risk of Adverse Target Events?

We discuss the relationship between a patient's risk of an adverse event and the magnitude of the treatment impact elsewhere in this book (see Part 1B1, "Therapy"; see also Part 2B2, "Therapy and Understanding the Results, Measures of Association" and Part 2B3, "Therapy and Applying the Results, Example Numbers Needed to Treat"). Because the issue is so important in assessing applicability of randomized controlled trial results, we review it here as well. We assume that readers have achieved a basic understanding of the statistical tools known as relative risk reduction (RRR), absolute risk reduction (ARR), and number needed to treat (NNT).

The NNT is the inverse of the ARR resulting from a particular treatment in a particular group of patients. If a patient's risk without treatment is 20%, then we expect that 20 in 100 untreated patients will suffer an adverse event. When we administer a treatment with a RRR of 10%, we can expect that only 18 treated patients will experience adverse events. Thus, for every 100 patients treated, we prevent two events; therefore, the NNT is 100/2, or 50. If the expected event rate in untreated patients (the *baseline risk* or *expected event rate*) is cut by half to 10% and the RRR remains the same, in treating 100 patients we will prevent only one adverse event and the NNT will double to 100/1, or 100.

This reasoning, and much of what follows, assumes that the relative risk (RR) and, thus, the RRR remain constant across subgroups. For instance, we assume that streptokinase will result in a RRR in mortality by about 25% in all patients, regardless of age or severity of infarct. There are instances in which the assumption will fail, and clinicians should be alert to this possibility[28-31] (see Part 2E, "Summarizing the Evidence, When to Believe a Subgroup Analysis"). In many circumstances, however, both RR and odds ratios (ORs) do not vary greatly across subgroups.[3, 32-36] When the proportion of patients experiencing the adverse outcome (the event rate) is low, the RR and OR are similar; as event rates increase, the RR and OR diverge (see Part 2B2, "Therapy and Understanding the Results, Measures of Association"). Whether it is more often accurate to assume a constant RR or a constant OR across subgroups remains in question. The OR has desirable statistical properties that the RR lacks, but clinicians find it much easier to understand and use the RR and the RRR (see Part 2B2, "Therapy and Understanding the Results, Measures of Association"). It is therefore fortunate that, for most diseases and treatments, assuming constant RR across patient groups will not introduce important inaccuracies in calculating the NNT.

Once assuming that RR is constant across subgroups, the key issue for clinicians in determining the impact of therapy on an individual is that patient's baseline risk. Clinicians can derive estimates of the patient's baseline risk from various sources. First, they can use their intuition, which may sometimes be accurate—at least in terms of the extent to which risk is increased or decreased relative to a typical patient.[37] Second, if the randomized trials report risks in patient subgroups, clinicians can choose the risk that best applies to the patient in their practice. However, most trials are not large enough to allow the generation of precise estimates of baseline risk in patient subgroups; even those that are large enough often do not provide the required information. Systematic reviews that pool data from multiple trials can provide more precise estimates. For example, the atrial fibrillation investigators pooled the individual patient data from all of the randomized trials testing antithrombotic therapy in nonvalvular atrial fibrillation and were able to provide estimates of prognosis for patients in clinically important subgroups.[38]

Clinicians are most likely to find information about risks in easily identifiable subgroups of patients from studies directly targeted at prognosis (see Part 1D, "Prognosis"). For example, analysis of the Malmo Stroke Registry demonstrated that during the three years after a stroke, patients have a 6% risk of recurrent nonfatal stroke and a 43% risk of death.[39] When contemplating stroke-prevention therapies in individual patients, including aspirin, clopidogrel, and carotid endarterectomy, clinicians can take into account that these risks proved even higher in older patients and in those with diabetes mellitus or cardiac disease.[39] Investigators sometimes use data from prognostic studies to construct models that incorporate a number of variables to create clinically helpful risk strata (see Part

2C, "Diagnosis, Clinical Prediction Rules"). When prospectively validated in new populations, these risk stratification systems can provide accurate patient-specific estimates of prognosis.

As we have described elsewhere (see Part 1B1, "Therapy"; see also Part 2B2, "Therapy and Understanding the Results, Measures of Association"), the final step in generating a patient-specific NNT or number needed to harm (NNH) involves calculating the patient-specific ARR and its reciprocal. Although this may sound intimidating, the arithmetic turns out to be relatively simple. Consider, for instance, the decision about whether to recommend carotid endarterectomy for a patient with a previous mild ischemic stroke and high-grade carotid stenosis. The Malmo Stroke Registry study tells us that a 65-year-old patient with diabetes, ipsi-lateral carotid stenosis, and minor stroke faces an 8.4% probability of recurrent stroke within the next 3 years.[39] Carotid endarterectomy will reduce that risk by approximately 49%. Using the formula for NNT (1.0/baseline risk x RRR), we find: 1.0/(0.084 × 0.49) = 24. For clinicians who are more comfortable with whole numbers, an alternative line of reasoning follows: treatment cuts the risk of stroke in half, from 8.4% to 4.2%. The absolute risk reduction is about 4%; and 100/4 is 25. The NNT is therefore approximately 25. For those who prefer to avoid arith-metic altogether, a nomogram allows the clinician armed only with a ruler (or any other straight edge) to proceed from the patient's baseline risk, through the rela-tive risk reduction, to the NNT[40] (see Figure 2B2-4 from Part 2B2, "Therapy and Understanding the Results, Measures of Association"). Another approach depends on starting with knowledge of the NNT for the average or typical patient. For instance, the clinician might be aware that in one RCT, carotid endarterectomy reduced patients' risk of stroke during a 5-year period from 10.3% to 5.3%, an ARR of 5% associated with an NNT of 20 (100/5). If a clinician estimated that risk of stroke in a patient with diabetes was 50% greater than that of the average, one could divide the average NNT of 20 by 1.5 to generate the NNT of approximately 13 for the patient with diabetes.[41]

One can consider the patient's risk of harm from the intervention in exactly the same way. For instance, the risk of perioperative disabling stroke or death in the carotid endarterectomy trial[42] was approximately 1.4%, corresponding to an NNH of 63 (100/1.4). If one is ready to consider benefits and risks equivalent (in this instance, prevention of death equivalent to disabling stroke or death), one can construct a ratio of NNT to NNH to provide an index of the relative likelihood of help vs harm.[43] For the typical patient considering carotid endarterectomy, the likelihood that the patient will benefit (represented by ARR, or 5%) is approxi-mately three times that of the likelihood of harm (the absolute increase in risk with treatment, or 1.4%). As we demonstrate in another section of this book, clini-cians can adjust this likelihood of help versus harm according to the patient's val-ues (see Part 2F, "Moving From Evidence to Action, Incorporating Patient Values").

One source of differences in patients' baseline risk is country of origin and residence. Keys compared the 20-year incidence of deaths from coronary heart disease in the United States, five European countries, and Japan.[44] They found an extremely low incidence of death from coronary heart disease in the Japanese cohort, despite correction for baseline differences in recognized risk factors. Similar results have been observed in preliminary reports of the ongoing Multinational Monitoring of Cardiovascular Disease and Their Determinants (MONICA) project.[45] In this study, involving 39 centers from 26 countries, East Asians showed a much lower incidence of death from coronary heart disease than their Western counterparts. Age-standardized mortality rates for coronary heart disease were lowest in Japan (40/100,000) and highest in North Ireland (414/100,000).

If we consider the NNT, this 10-fold difference in incidence among the Japanese would translate to a 10-fold increase in the NNT for a drug preventing coronary deaths. This decrease in efficiency may warrant a reconsideration of applying the results of a trial to low-risk patients (see Part 1F, "Moving From Evidence to Action").

Returning to our decision about the administration of thrombolytic agents to a patient in the Philippines, a cohort study conducted in nine centers in metropolitan Manila showed that of 424 Filipinos with myocardial infarction eligible for streptokinase but in whom the drug was not administered, 37 (11.1%) suffered cardiac deaths.[27] This provides a good estimate of the expected event rate. If streptokinase had been given, it would have prevented 25% of the deaths, reducing the absolute mortality rate to 8.3%. Thus, 2.8% of those otherwise destined to die would not have died (the ARR), and the NNT is 100/2.8, or approximately 36 patients.

The expected event rates varied in patient subpopulations.[27] Younger patients with small infarcts had a much lower expected mortality (and thus much larger NNTs) than older patients with large infarcts. Using prognostic information from these various subgroups, we constructed Table 2B3-2, which shows the expected mortality according to age and left ventricular wall involvement. Also shown is the corresponding NNT to save one life in each group. As the table shows, NNT can range from as low as 16 (when treatment is applied to patients with a poor prognosis) to as high as 179 (when treatment is applied to patients with a good prognosis).

**TABLE 2B3-2**

**Baseline Mortality Rate Without Treatment and Estimated Number Needed to Treat to Save One Life Using Streptokinase in Filipinos With Acute Myocardial Infarction\***

| Wall Involvement | Age < 60 | | Age > 60 | |
|---|---|---|---|---|
| | MR | NNT | MR | NNT |
| Inferior | 0.02 | 179 | 0.13 | 27 |
| Non-Q wave | 0.04 | 89 | 0.18 | 23 |
| Anterior/lateral | 0.05 | 71 | 0.19 | 20 |
| Massive anterior | 0.14 | 26 | 0.23 | 16 |

\* Tabulated according to age and wall involvement.

MR indicates monthly rate; NNT, number needed to treat.

Varying patient risk will impact on benefit regardless of the environment in which you practice. Even if you work in the Western tertiary care environment in which investigators conducted their original studies, you will still face high- and low-risk patients. The critical tradeoff between risk and benefit may vary in these patient groups, mandating different treatment decisions (see Part 1F, "Moving From Evidence to Action").

## USING THE GUIDES

This section addresses the task of applying the results of clinical trials done on restricted populations to other groups. Although one inspiration for these guides has come from the sufficiently different predicament in patients from developing countries, the guides are relevant to all situations in which clinicians must make decisions regarding applicability. By breaking down the problem into specific questions, we have provided guides for clinicians' daily attempts to strike a balance between making "unjustifiably broad generalizations and being too conservative in one's conclusions."[4]

When clinicians suspect limited applicability, what can they do? This will depend on whether or not the anticipated differences are important—and if they are important, whether or not they are remediable. For example, differences in disease pathophysiology do not always mean that applicability is limited. Management of a cataract, for instance, will probably be the same regardless of the cause. Differences in treatment response can sometimes be accommodated by altering administration of a treatment (such as adjusting the dose of a drug). Education, training, provision of necessary equipment, and other attempts at optimizing compliance may address problems in patient and provider compliance.

For differences in comorbid conditions or expected target event rates, the clinician's response will depend on the difference observed. If an increase in efficiency is anticipated (as when disease prognosis is worse or the incidence of an adverse outcome is greater), a recommendation to treat can be accepted more easily. A decrease in efficiency, on the other hand, should lead clinicians to be more cautious in accepting a treatment recommendation.

When differences in patient populations are important and not easily remediable, clinicians should not assume that the trial results can be readily applied. In these instances, an additional RCT may be warranted.

# CLINICAL RESOLUTION

What should we recommend regarding use of thrombolytic agents for the Filipino patient admitted to the hospital with acute myocardial infarction? There is no reason to believe that Filipinos have a different disease pathogenesis or a different response to treatment with thrombolytic agents. Patient compliance will not be an important issue since the drug is given intravenously as a single dose. The technical requirements for administration are often (but not always) available—and when they are not, the risks of thrombolytic administration may outweigh the benefits.

Two issues remain to be resolved, both dealing with the magnitude of treatment impact. Pneumonia is an important comorbid condition, accounting for one third of deaths, at least in some charity hospitals. However, rates of cardiac death are still sufficiently high (11.1%) that the RRR we can achieve with streptokinase (28%) will result in an NNT of 32 for the overall population. For subgroups of patients, however, the NNT will range from 16 to 179, depending on the age and the size of the infarct (see Table 2B3-2). The 40-year-old man with an inferior myocardial infarction has an expected mortality of only 2% over the course of the next 30 days, suggesting an NNT of close to 200.

Should we recommend streptokinase for this patient? Although we have confirmed the applicability of the thrombolytic data on the effectiveness of streptokinase for centers with adequate blood-banking facilities, we must also consider cost. The cost of the drug is approximately $200 per treatment in United States dollars, in a country in which the average annual per capita income is $1000.[46]

Judging whether to give streptokinase will depend on who pays for the treatment (in the Philippines, usually the patients themselves must pay), patient and family values, what resources are available (resources usually are very limited in a charity hospital setting), and competing needs (for example, the need for antibiotics because of a high incidence of pneumonia, in turn a result of overcrowding in the wards).

For equally applicable treatments, our final decision may differ for a much less costly but equally effective and applicable treatment such as aspirin for the patient with myocardial infarction. When informed of the small absolute benefit in mortality reduction he would achieve with streptokinase and the small increase in risk of stroke (about 1 in 1000) with treatment, he declines the streptokinase.

# References

1. Midgette AS, O'Connor GT, Baron JA, Bell J. Effect of intravenous streptokinase on early mortality in patients with suspected acute myocardial infarction: a meta-analysis by anatomic location of infarction. *Ann Intern Med.* 1990;113: 961-968.

2. ISIS-2 Collaborative Group. Randomised trial of intravenous streptokinase, oral aspirin, both, or neither among 17,187 cases of suspected acute myocardial infarction: ISIS-2. *Lancet.* 1988;2:349-360.

3. Schmid CH, Lau J, McIntosh MW, Cappelleri JC. An empirical study of the effect of the control rate as a predictor of treatment efficacy in meta-analysis of clinical trials. *Stat Med.* 1998;17:1923-1942.

4. Gottlieb SS, McCarter RJ, Vogel RA. Effect of beta-blockade on mortality among high-risk and low-risk patients after myocardial infarction. *N Engl J Med.* 1998;339:489-497.

5. McAlister FA, Taylor L, Teo KK, et al. The treatment and prevention of coronary heart disease in Canada: do older patients receive efficacious therapies? *J Am Geriatr Soc.* 1999;47:811-818.

6. Falkner B, Kushner H. Effect of chronic sodium loading on cardiovascular response in young blacks and whites. *Hypertension.* 1990;15:36-43.

7. Wilson TW. History of salt supplies in West Africa and blood pressure today. *Lancet.* 1986;1:784-786.

8. World Health Organization. World malaria situation in 1992. Part 1. *Wkly Epidemiol Rec.* 1994;69:309-314.

9. Canlas MM, Dominguez AE, Abarquez RF. Ten year review of the clinicopathologic findings of coronary artery disease at the University of the Philippines, Philippine General Hospital (1969 - 1978). *Phil J Int Med.* 1980;18:65-74.

10. Roberts WC, Potkin BN, Solus DE, Reddy SG. Mode of death, frequency of healed and acute myocardial infarction, number of major epicardial coronary arteries severely narrowed by atherosclerotic plaque, and heart weight in fatal atherosclerotic coronary artery disease: analysis of 889 patients studied at necropsy. *J Am Coll Cardiol.* 1990;15:196-202.

11. Balgos AA, Lopez MB, delos Santos E, et al. The significance of risk factors in myocardial infarction—a 2-year retrospective study at the University of the Philippines, Philippine General Hospital. *Phil J Cardiol.* 1984;12:104-108.

12. Farmer JA, Gotto AM. Risk factors for coronary artery disease. In: Braunwald E, ed. *Heart Disease—A Textbook of Cardiovascular Medicine.* 4th ed. Philadelphia: WB Saunders Co; 1992.

13. Horai Y, Ishizaki T. Pharmacogenetics and its clinical implication: N-acetylation polymorphism. *Ration Drug Ther.* 1987;21:1-7.

14. Goodman LS, Gillman A, Rall TW, Nies AS, Taylor P. Principles of therapeutics. In: *The Pharmacologic Basis of Therapeutics.* 8th ed. New York: Pergamon Press Inc; 1991:71-73.

15. Ward J, Brenneman G, Letson GW, Heyward WL. Limited efficacy of a Haemophilus influenzae type b conjugate vaccine in Alaska Native infants. The Alaska H. influenza Vaccine Study Group. *N Engl J Med.* 1990;323: 1393-1401.

16. Martino E, Safran M, Aghini-Lombardi F, et al. Environmental iodine intake and thyroid dysfunction during chronic amiodarone therapy. *Ann Intern Med.* 1984;101:28-34.

17. Dela Paz AG, Pineda NE, Justiniani RP, et al. Thrombolysis in acute myocardial infarction. *Phil J Cardiol.* 1988;17:185-188.

18. Bulatao J. *Split-Level Christianity.* Philippines: University of St Tomas Press; 1966.

19. Raja SN, Williams S, McGee R. Multidimensional health locus of control beliefs and psychological health for a sample of mothers. *Soc Sci Med.* 1994;39:213-220.

20. Chambers BR, You RX, Donnan GA. Carotid endarterectomy for asymptomatic carotid stenosis (Cochrane Review). In: *The Cochrane Library*, Issue 4, 2000. Oxford: Update Software.

21. Barnett HJ, Eliasziw M, Meldrum HE, Taylor DW. Do the facts and figures warrant a 10 fold increase in the performance of carotid endarterectomy on asymptomatic patients? *Neurology.* 1996;46:603-608.

22. Tu JV, Hannan EL, Anderson GM, et al. The fall and rise of carotid endarterectomy in the United States and Canada. *N Engl J Med.* 1998;339:1441-1447.

23. Gersh BJ, Opie LH. Antithrombotic agents: platelet inhibitors, anticoagulants and fibrinolytics. In: Opie LH, ed. *Drugs for the Heart.* 3rd ed. Philadelphia: WB Saunders Co; 1991.

24. Glasziou PP, Irwig LM. An evidence based approach to individualising treatment. *BMJ.* 1995;311:1356-1359.

25. Sazawal S, Black RE. Meta-analysis of intervention trials on case management of pneumonia in community settings. *Lancet.* 1992;340:528-533.

26. Lupisan SP. Validity of the WHO-recommended Acute Respiratory Infection (ARI) case assessment in a malaria hyperendemic area in the Philippines (ongoing study).

27. ISIP Study Group. Acute myocardial infarction in tertiary centers in Metro Manila: in-hospital survival and physicians' practices. (Unpublished.)

28. Rothwell PM. Can overall results of clinical trials be applied to all patients? *Lancet.* 1995;345:1616-1619.

29. Bailey KR. Generalizing the results of randomized clinical trials. *Control Clinical Trials.* 1994;15:15-23.

30. The Executive Committee for the Asymptomatic Carotid Atherosclerosis Study. Endarterectomy for asymptomatic carotid artery stenosis. *JAMA.* 1995;273:1421-1428.

31. The European Carotid Surgery Trialists' Collaborative Group. Randomised trial of endarterectomy for recently symptomatic carotid stenosis: final results of the MRC European Carotid Surgery Trial. *Lancet.* 1998;351:1379-1387.

32. Sharp SJ, Thompson SG, Altman DG. The relation between treatment benefit and underlying risk in meta-analysis. *BMJ.* 1996;313:735-738.

33. Smith GD, Egger M. Who benefits from medical interventions? *BMJ.* 1994;308:72-74.

34. Oxman AD, Guyatt GH. A consumer's guide to subgroup analysis. *Ann Intern Med.* 1992;116;78-84.

35. Yusuf S, Wittes J, Probstfield J, Tyroler HA. Analysis and interpretation of treatment effects in subgroups of patients in randomized clinical trials. *JAMA.* 1991;266:93-98.

36. Ioannidis JP, Lau J. Heterogeneity of the baseline risk within patient populations of clinical trials: a proposed evaluation algorithm. *Am J Epidemiol.* 1998;148:1117-1126.

37. Grover SA, Lowensteyn I, Esrey KL, Steinert Y, Joseph L, Abrahamowicz M. Do doctors accurately assess coronary risk in their patients? Preliminary results of the coronary health assessment study. *BMJ.* 1995;310:975-978.

38. Atrial Fibrillation Investigators. Risk factors for stroke and efficacy of antithrombotic therapy in atrial fibrillation: analysis of pooled data from five randomized controlled trials. *Arch Intern Med.* 1994;154:1449-1457.

39. Elneihoum AM, Goransson M, Falke P, Janzon L. Three-year survival and recurrence after stroke in Malmo, Sweden: an analysis of stroke registry data. *Stroke.* 1998;29:2114-2117.

40. Chatellier G, Zapletal E, Lemaitre D, Menard J, Degoulet P. The number needed to treat: a clinically useful nomogram in its proper context. *BMJ.* 1996;312: 426-429.

41. Cook RJ, Sackett DL. The number needed to treat: a clinically useful measure of treatment effect. *BMJ.* 1995;310:452-454.

42. Barnett HJ, Taylor DW, Eliasziw M, et al. Benefit of carotid endarterectomy in patients with symptomatic moderate or severe stenosis. North American Symptomatic Carotid Endarterectomy Trial Collaborators. *N Engl J Med.* 1998;339:1415-1425.

43. Straus SE, McQuay HJM, Moore RA, Sackett DL. A proposed patient-centred method of delivering information about the risks and benefits of therapy: the likelihood of being helped versus harmed. *BMJ.* Submitted.

44. Keys A. *Seven Countries: A Multivariate Analysis of Death and Coronary Heart Disease.* Cambridge: Harvard University Press; 1980.

45. Tuomilehto J, Kuulasmaa K. WHO MONICA Project: assessing CHD mortality and morbidity. *Int J Epidemiol.* 1989;18:S38-45.

46. *World Development Report 2000/2001.* Washington, DC: World Bank; 2000.

# THERAPY AND APPLYING THE RESULTS

## Example Numbers Needed to Treat

Christina Lacchetti, Gordon Guyatt, and PJ Devereaux

Sharon Straus also made substantive contributions to this section

## IN THIS SECTION

# HOW CAN WE SUMMARIZE BENEFITS AND RISKS?

Evidence-based practice requires that clinicians summarize the benefits and risks of treatment for patients. Further, when called on, clinicians must incorporate patient values and benefit/risk data to judge which management strategies are in patients' best interests (see Part 2F, "Moving From Evidence to Action, Incorporating Patient Values").

These activities require clear and vivid summaries of the magnitude of treatment benefit. The relative risk reduction (RRR, the control event rate minus the treatment event rate divided by the control event rate), the absolute risk reduction (ARR, the control event rate minus the treatment event rate), and the number needed to treat (NNT) represent alternative ways of summarizing the impact of treatment (see Part 2B2, "Therapy and Understanding the Results, Measures of Association"). In this section, we provide a number of examples of the last of these, the NNT.

# THE NUMBER NEEDED TO TREAT IN WEIGHING BENEFIT AND HARM

The NNT, the number of patients the clinician must treat for a particular period of time to prevent one adverse target event, may be the most attractive single measure. Arithmetically, the NNT is the inverse of the absolute risk reduction (ARR). Clinicians could therefore simply take the ARR from a trial, calculate its inverse, and derive an NNT for their patients. Such an approach, however, can be profoundly misleading.

Consider, for instance, the Global Utilization of Streptokinase and Tissue Plasminogen Activator for Occluded Coronary Arteries (GUSTO) trial, which reported the mortality in the 30 days after hospital admission of approximately 20,000 patients who received streptokinase and approximately 10,000 who received tissue plasminogen activator (TPA).[1] In the patients receiving TPA, the risk of dying was 6.3%; in those receiving streptokinase, the risk was 7.3%. The relative risk of dying with TPA is therefore 6.3/7.3 (86%); RRR, 1.0-0.86 (14%); ARR, 7.3-6.3 (1%); and NNT, 1.0/0.01 (100). When deciding on whether an individual patient required TPA, we could assume that we might treat 100 patients to prevent a single death.

Such an approach ignores the fact that after myocardial infarction, patients have very different risks of dying. The accompanying table (Table 2B3-3) tells us that in the 6 months following myocardial infarction, 1.8% of patients without heart failure or premature ventricular beats (PVBs) will die. On the other hand, 14.4% of those with more than 10 premature ventricular beats and heart failure will die.

**TABLE 2B3-3**

## Example Number Needed to Treat

| Condition or Disorder | Intervention vs Control | Outcome | Risk Groups | RRR (CI) | % ARR | NNT |
|---|---|---|---|---|---|---|
| Persons without diagnosed cardiovascular disease[a] | Pravastatin therapy vs conventional therapy | Cardiovascular event[b] over 5 years | [c] Low=<2.5%<br>Moderate=12.5%<br>High=17.5%<br>Very High=>30% | 31%<br>(17%-43%)[4] | 0.62<br>3.88<br>5.43<br>10.85 | 161<br>26<br>18<br>9 |
| Persons without diagnosed cardiovascular disease | Aspirin vs placebo | Cardiovascular event[b] over 5 years | [c] Low=<2.5%<br>Moderate=12.5%<br>High=17.5%<br>Very High=>30% | 15%<br>(1%-27%)[2] | 0.30<br>1.88<br>2.63<br>5.25 | 333<br>53<br>38<br>19 |
| Persons without diagnosed cardiovascular disease | Aspirin vs placebo | Major bleeding episodes (fatal and nonfatal) over an average of 3.8 years | NA | RR<br>Increase=74%<br>(31%-130%)[2] | 0.62 | NNH=161 |
| Congestive heart failure | Spironolactone vs placebo | Total mortality over 1 year | [d] Low=8%<br>Medium=21%<br>High=33% | 30%<br>(18%-40%)[5] | 2.40<br>6.30<br>9.90 | 42<br>16<br>10 |
| Congestive heart failure | ACE inhibitor vs placebo | Total mortality over 1 year | [d] Low=8%<br>Medium=21%<br>High=33% | 23%<br>(12%-33%)[6] | 1.84<br>4.83<br>7.59 | 54<br>21<br>13 |
| Congestive heart failure | Beta-blocker therapy vs placebo | Total mortality over 1 year | [d] Low=8%<br>Medium=21%<br>High=33% | 32%<br>(12%-47%)[7] | 2.56<br>6.72<br>10.56 | 39<br>15<br>9 |
| Acute myocardial infarction | ACE inhibitors vs placebo | Mortality over 6 months | [e] Low=1.8%<br>Medium=2.0%<br>High=9.9%<br>Very high=14.4% | 6.3%<br>(1%-10%)[9] | 0.11<br>0.13<br>0.62<br>0.91 | 882<br>794<br>160<br>110 |
| Postmyocardial infarction | Beta-blocker therapy vs placebo | Total mortality over 6 months | [e] Low=1.8%<br>Medium=2.0%<br>High=9.9%<br>Very high=14.4% | 23%<br>(15%-31%)[10] | 0.4<br>0.5<br>2.3<br>3.3 | 242<br>217<br>44<br>30 |

| Condition or Disorder | Intervention vs Control | Outcome | Risk Groups | RRR (CI) | % ARR | NNT |
|---|---|---|---|---|---|---|
| Hypertension | Antihypertensive treatment (primarily beta blockers or diuretics) vs placebo/usual care | Cardiovascular event (includes fatal/nonfatal myocardial infarction, stroke, or coronary death) over 5 years | f Low=2% Medium=5% High=10% | 25% (14%–29%)[11, 12] | 0.5 1.25 2.5 | 200 80 40 |
| Hypertension | Antihypertensive treatment (primarily beta blockers or diuretics) vs placebo/usual care | Cardiovascular event (includes fatal/nonfatal myocardial infarction, stroke, or coronary death) over 20 years | f Low=15%; Medium=30% High=50% | 25% (14%–29%)[11, 12] | 3.75 7.5 12.5% | 27 13 8 |
| Nonvalvular atrial fibrillation | Warfarin vs placebo | Stroke over 1 year | g Very low= ≤ 1% Low=4.9% Medium=5.7% High=8.1% | 62% (48%–72%)[15] | 0.62 3.04 3.53 5.02 | 161 33 28 20 |
| Rheumatoid arthritis treated with nonsteroidal anti-inflammatory drugs | Concurrent misoprostol vs placebo | Development of serious upper gastrointestinal complications over 6 months | h Low=0.4% Medium=1.0% High=9.0% | 40% (1.8%–64%)[16] | 0.16 0.40 3.60 | 625 250 28 |
| One or more unprovoked seizure | Immediate tretment with antiepileptic drugs vs treatment only after seizure recurrence | Recurrent seizures over 2 years | i Low=27% Medium=61% High=67% | 60% (40%–70%)[17] | 16.20 36.60 40.20 | 6 3 2 |
| HIV infection | Ritonavir vs placebo | AIDS-defining illness at 6 years i | Low=2.4% Med=4.3% High=7.5% Very high=12.8% | 42% (29%–52%)[18] | 1.01 1.81 3.15% 5.38% | 99 85 32 19 |
| Breast cancer | Radiotherapy plus tamoxifen vs tamoxifen alone | Any recurrence at 10 years | k Low=43% Medium=52% High=78% | 22% (13%–29%)[19] | 9.5 11.4 17.2 | 11 9 6 |

| Condition or Disorder | Intervention vs Control | Outcome | Risk Groups | RRR (CI) | % ARR | NNT |
|---|---|---|---|---|---|---|
| Symptomatic carotid stenosis | Carotid endarterectomy vs optimal medical care, including antiplatelet therapy | Stroke over 5 years | [l]Low=18.7%<br><br>Medium= 22.2%<br><br>High=27.0% | [m]RRI=20% (range, 0-44)[20]<br><br>RRR=27% (range, 5-44)<br><br>RRR=48% (range, 27-73) | ARI=3.7%<br><br>ARR=6.0%<br><br>ARR=13.0% | NNH=27<br><br>NNT=17<br><br>NNT=8 |

[a] >90% of patients studied did not have diagnosed cardiovascular disease.

[b] *Cardiovascular event* is defined as death related to coronary artery disease, nonfatal myocardial infarction, new angina, fatal or nonfatal stroke or transient ischemic attack, the development of congestive heart failure, or peripheral vascular disease.

[c] Risk varies according to a patient's sex, diabetic status, smoking status, and age. For example, low risk=patients aged 40-49 with blood pressure between 120 and 140 mm Hg systolic or 75 and 85 mm Hg diastolic, who do not have diabetes and do not smoke; moderate risk=patients aged 50 and older with blood pressure 140-160 mm Hg systolic or 85-95 mm Hg diastolic, who may have diabetes and who do not smoke; high risk=patients aged 60 and older with blood pressure 160-180 mm Hg systolic or 95-105 mm Hg diastolic, who may have diabetes and who do not smoke; very high risk=patients aged 70 and older with blood pressure 180 mm Hg systolic or 105 mm Hg diastolic, who may have diabetes and who do not smoke. Please refer to Jackson[3] to identify the various combination of factors that determine a patient's risk category.

[d] Low risk=New York Heart Association (NYHA) functional class II; medium risk=NYHA functional class III; high risk=NYHA functional class IV.[8]

[e] Low=no premature ventricular beats (PVBs) and no clinical heart failure (CHF); medium=1-10 PVBs and no CHF; high=1-10 PVBs and CHF; very high=>10 PVBs and CHF.[13]

[f] Low=diastolic blood pressure of 90 mm Hg; medium=diastolic blood pressure of 95 mm Hg; high=diastolic blood pressure of 100 mm Hg.[14]

[g] Very low risk=<65 years old with no risk factors; low risk=<65 years old, with one or more risk factors (which includes a history of hypertension, diabetes, and prior stroke or transient ischemic attack); medium risk=65-75 years old, with one or more risk factors; high risk=>75 years old with one or more risk factors.[21]

[h] Low risk=patients with none of the following risk factors: ≥ 75 yr old; history of peptic ulcer; history of GI bleeding; or history of CV disease; medium risk=patient with any single factor; high risk=patients with all 4 factors.[16]

[i] Low risk=first seizure; medium risk=second seizure; high risk=third seizure.[22]

[j] Baseline HIV-1 RNA level (copies/mL): Low=501-3000; medium=3001-10,000; high=10,001-30,000; very high >30,000.[23]

[k] Low=no nodes affected; medium=1-3 affected nodes; high >3 affected nodes.[19]

[l] Low=<50% stenosis; medium=50-69% stenosis; high=>70%.

[m] Note: Because the effects of carotid endarterectomy vary with the degree of stenosis, three different benefits or risks of surgery are presented.

RRR indicates relative risk reduction; CI, confidence interval; ARR, absolute risk reduction; NNT, number needed to treat; NNH, number needed to harm.

Applying the relative risk reduction of TPA over streptokinase, we find that TPA will reduce the risk of death in patients without heart failure or PVBs from 1.8% to 1.548%. Thus, we must treat 397 patients in this low-risk group with TPA to prevent a death. For patients with more than 10 PVPs and heart failure, TPA reduces the risk from 14.4% to 12.4%. We must therefore treat approximately 47 high-risk patients with TPA to prevent a death. Considering that an additional two patients per 1000 who receive TPA vs streptokinase will have a stroke—and the number needed to harm (NNH) is 500—and considering the large additional cost of TPA over streptokinase, the clinician may make different decisions about which thrombolytic agent to administer to these the low- and high-risk patients.

This example tells us that when considering the NNT associated with treating a particular patient, we must consider the risk group from which that patient comes (see Part 2B3, "Therapy and Applying the Results, Applying Results to Individual Patients"). In this example, we have assumed a constant RRR across risk groups. In general, this assumption is warranted (see Part 2B2, "Therapy and Understanding the Results, Measures of Association"). In Table 2B3-3, we have applied the RRR associated with a variety of treatment to groups of patients at varying levels of risk and we have calculated the associated NNTs. In our final example, carotid endarterectomy in patients with varying degrees of stenosis, both the relative risk reduction and the absolute risk reduction vary across risk groups.

# THE NUMBER NEEDED TO TREAT IN WEIGHING BENEFIT AND HARM—OTHER EXAMPLES

The TPA/streptokinase example also illustrates the usefulness of the NNT in helping clinicians judge the degree of benefit and the degree of harm patients can expect from therapy. One of the examples in the table further illustrates this point. As a result of taking aspirin, patients with hypertension without known coronary artery disease can expect a reduction of approximately 15% in their relative risk of cardiovascular related events.[2] For an otherwise low-risk woman with hypertension and a baseline risk of cardiovascular related event of between 2.5% and 5%,[3] this translates into an NNT of approximately 200 during a 5-year period. However, as presented in the table, for every 161 patients treated with aspirin, one would experience a major hemorrhage. Thus, in 1000 patients, aspirin would be responsible for preventing five cardiovascular events, but it would also be responsible for causing approximately six serious bleeding episodes. Recommending aspirin to such low-risk patients would be questionable at best. For a patient at high risk for cardiovascular events (eg, a man with hypertension and diabetes over the age of 70 years), the NNT of approximately 20 (in 1000 patients, 50 cardiovascular events prevented by aspirin and six bleeding episodes caused by aspirin) suggests that recommending aspirin may be much more appropriate.

Finally, another example from Table 2B3-3 emphasizes the importance of considering the time frame in evaluating the NNT. During a 5-year period, the NNT for prevention of major cardiovascular events with antihypertensive treatment in low-, medium-, and high-risk patients is, respectively, 200, 80, and 40. Over a time frame of 20 years, the corresponding numbers are 27, 13, and 8. These figures help demonstrate that how one presents NNT data can determine the impact of the information on clinicians and patients.

Clinicians can use the data from the table in in making treatment decisions with patients. More important, the results illustrate the importance of considering individual patients' baseline risk and the RRR associated with treatment before advising patients about the optimal management of their health problems.

# References

1. The GUSTO Investigators. An international randomized trial comparing four thrombolytic strategies for acute myocardial infarction. *N Engl J Med.* 1993;329:673-682.

2. Hansson L, Zanchetti A, Carruthers SG, et al. Effects of intensive blood-pressure lowering and low-dose aspirin in patients with hypertension: principal results of the Hypertension Optimal Treatment (HOT) randomised trial. *Lancet.* 1998;351:1755-1762.

3. Jackson R. Updated New Zealand cardiovascular disease risk-benefit prediction guide. *BMJ.* 2000;320:709-710.

4. Shepherd J, Cobbe SM, Ford I, et al. Prevention of coronary heart disease with pravastatin in men with hypercholesterolemia. *N Engl J Med.* 1995; 333:1301-1307.

5. Pitt B, Zannad F, Remme WJ, et al. The effect of spironolactone on morbidity and mortality in patients with severe heart failure. *N Engl J Med.* 1999;341:709-717.

6. Garg R, Yusuf S. Overview of randomized trials of angiotensin-converting enzyme inhibitors on mortality and morbidity in patients with heart failure. Collaborative Group on ACE Inhibitor Trials. *JAMA.* 1995;273:1450-1456.

7. Lechat P, Packer M, Chalon S, Cucherat M, Arab T, Boissel JP. Clinical effects of beta-adrenergic blockade in chronic heart failure: a meta-analysis of double-blind, placebo-controlled, randomized trials. *Circulation.* 1998;98:1184-1191.

8. Matoba M, Matsui S, Hirakawa T, et al. Long-term prognosis of patients with congestive heart failure. *Jpn Circ J.* 1990;54:57-61.

9. ACE inhibitor Myocardial Infarction Collaborative Group. Indications for ACE inhibitors in early treatment of acute myocardial infarction: systematic overview of individual data from 100,000 patients in randomized trials. *Circulation.* 1998;97:2202-2212.

10. Freemantle N, Cleland J, Young P, Mason J, Harrison J. Beta blockade after myocardial infarction: systematic review and meta regression analysis. *BMJ.* 1999;318:1730-1737.

11. Collins R, Peto R, MacMahon S, et al. Blood pressure, stroke, and coronary heart disease. Part 2. Short-term reductions in blood pressure: overview of randomised drug trials in their epidemiological context. *Lancet.* 1990;335:827-838.

12. Gueyffier F, Boutitie F, Boissel JP, et al. Effect of antihypertensive drug treatment on cardiovascular outcomes in women and men: a meta-analysis of individual patient data from randomized, controlled trials. *Ann Intern Med.* 1997;126:761-767.

13. Maggioni AP, Zuanetti G, Franzosi MG, et al. Prevalence and prognostic significance of ventricular arrhythmias after acute myocardial infarction in the fibrinolytic era: GISSI-2 results. *Circulation.* 1993;87:312-322.

14. McAlister FA, O'Connor AM, Wells G, Grover SA, Laupacis A. When should hypertension be treated? The different perspectives of Canadian family physicians and patients. *CMAJ.* 2000;163:403-408.

15. Hart RG, Benavente O, McBride R, Pearce LA. Antithrombotic therapy to prevent stroke in patients with atrial fibrillation: a meta-analysis. *Ann Intern Med.* 1999;131:492-501.

16. Silverstein FE, Graham DY, Senior JR, et al. Misoprostol reduces serious gastrointestinal complications in patients with rheumatoid arthritis receiving nonsteroidal anti-inflammatory drugs: a randomized, double-blind, placebo-controlled trial. *Ann Intern Med.* 1995;123:241-249.

17. First Seizure Trial Group. Randomized clinical trial on the efficacy of antiepileptic drugs in reducing the risk of relapse after a first unprovoked tonic-clonic seizure. *Neurology.* 1993;43:478-483.

18. Cameron DW, Heath-Chiozzi M, Danner S, et al. Randomised placebo-controlled trial of ritonavir in advanced HIV-1 disease. The Advanced HIV Disease Ritonavir Study Group. *Lancet.* 1998;351:543-549.

19. Overgaard M, Jensen MB, Overgaard J, et al. Postoperative radiotherapy in high-risk postmenopausal breast-cancer patients given adjuvant tamoxifen: Danish Breast Cancer Cooperative Group DBCG 82c randomised trial. *Lancet.* 1999;353:1641-1648.

20. Cina CS, Clase CM, Haynes BR. Refining the indications for carotid endarterectomy in patients with symptomatic carotid stenosis: a systematic review. *J Vasc Surg.* 1999;30:606-617.

21. Atrial Fibrillation Investigators. Risk factors for stroke and efficacy of antithrombotic therapy in atrial fibrillation: analysis of pooled data from five randomized controlled trials. *Arch Intern Med.* 1994;154:1449-1457.

22. Hauser WA, Rich SS, Lee JR, Annegers JF, Anderson VE. Risk of recurrent seizures after two unprovoked seizures. *N Engl J Med.* 1998;338:429-434.

23. Mellors JW, Munoz A, Giorgi JV, et al. Plasma viral load and CD4+ lymphocytes as prognostic markers of HIV-1 infection. *Ann Intern Med.* 1997;126:946-954.

24. Barnett HJ, Taylor DW, Eliasziw M, et al. Benefit of carotid endarterectomy in patients with symptomatic moderate or severe stenosis. North American Symptomatic Carotid Endarterectomy Trial Collaborators. *N Engl J Med.* 1998;339:1415-1425.

# THERAPY AND APPLYING THE RESULTS

## Surrogate Outcomes

Heiner Bucher, Gordon Guyatt, Deborah Cook,
Anne Holbrook, and Finlay McAlister

The following EBM Working Group members also made substantive
contributions to this section: Daren Heyland and Thomas Newman

## IN THIS SECTION

## CLINICAL SCENARIO

### Should We Administer Calcitonin to a Postmenopausal Osteoporotic Woman on the Basis of Its Effect on Bone Density?

You are seeing a 68-year-old woman with postmenopausal osteoporosis. Her bone mineral density, as measured by dual-energy x-ray absorptiometry, is 2.5 standard deviations below the mean value of premenopausal women. A spinal radiograph shows an old vertebral fracture. Although she is not suffering from back pain, she is concerned that she might end up like her mother, whose osteoporotic fractures have resulted in severe, long-term back pain. She has been treated previously with calcium and alendronate, a bisphosphonate, which had to be stopped because of severe dyspepsia and endoscopically verified esophagitis. She cannot switch to risedronate, another drug for which randomized trials have shown decreases in vertebral and nonvertebral fractures, because its side effect profile is similar to that of alendronate.[1] Because the patient previously has sustained two deep vein thromboses with pulmonary embolism, you rule out treatment with raloxifene, which, though effective in preventing vertebral fractures, is associated with an increase in the risk of thromboembolic complications.[2] You are looking for a therapeutic alternative and consider whether treatment with calcitonin might be an option.

# FINDING THE EVIDENCE

You have access to the Internet and connect to the National Library of Medicine's Grateful Med site. Using the Grateful Med "Find MeSH/Meta terms" function, you construct a search strategy that includes the terms "calcitonin" and "osteoporosis, postmenopausal/drug therapy." You restrict your search by including only randomized controlled trials from the "Publication types" drop-down menu. You identify many trials; as you quickly browse through the titles and abstracts, you note that all studies report on the effect of calcitonin on bone mineral density. One particular report of a study of calcitonin attracts your attention because it is by far the largest trial and it reports on changes in bone mineral density and fracture rates.[3] Despite the study's relatively large size, however, review of the article reveals that it remains too small to provide reliable estimates of the effect of calcitonin on fracture rates. You wonder if you can substitute the findings of calcitonin effects on bone density for the unavailable data regarding fractures.

Ideally, clinicians making treatment decisions should refer to methodologically strong clinical trials examining the impact of therapy on patient-important outcomes such as health-related quality of life and morbid endpoints such as stroke, myocardial infarction, and death. Often, however, conducting these trials requires such a large sample size, or long patient follow-up, that researchers or pharmaceutical companies look for alternatives. Substituting surrogate endpoints for the target event permits researchers to conduct shorter and smaller trials, thus offering an apparent solution to the dilemma.

A *surrogate endpoint* may be defined as a laboratory or physiologic measurement used as a substitute for an endpoint that measures directly how a patient feels, functions, or survives.[4] Surrogate endpoints include physiologic variables (such as bone mineral density as a surrogate endpoint for long-bone fractures, blood pressure as a surrogate endpoint for stroke, and CD4 cell count as a surrogate endpoint for AIDS and AIDS-related mortality) or measures of subclinical disease (such as degree of atherosclerosis on coronary angiography as a surrogate endpoint for myocardial infarction or coronary death).

The use of surrogate endpoints is indispensable for drug evaluation in phase II trials and early phase III trials geared to establish or verify a drug's promise of benefit. In many countries, companies may obtain drug approval by demonstrating a positive impact on surrogate endpoints. The use of surrogate endpoints for regulatory purposes reflects drug approval decisions that regulators must make in the face of public health exigencies.

Reliance on surrogate endpoints may be beneficial or harmful. On the one hand, use of the surrogate endpoint may lead to the rapid and appropriate dissemination of new treatments. For example, the decision of the US Food and Drug Administration (FDA) to approve new antiretroviral drugs based on information from trials using surrogate endpoints recognized the enormous need for effective therapies for patients with HIV infection. Subsequently, several of these drugs have proved effective in randomized trials focusing on patient-important outcomes.[5-8]

On the other hand, reliance on surrogate endpoints may lead to excess morbidity and mortality. For example, although cardiac inotropes and vasodilators may improve short-term hemodynamic function in patients with heart failure, randomized controlled trials have demonstrated excess mortality with a number of these agents, including flosequinan, milrinone, ibopamine, vesnarinone, and xamoterol (see Part 2B1, "Therapy and Validity, Surprising Results of Randomized Controlled Trials").

How are clinicians to distinguish between these two situations? A surrogate outcome will be consistently reliable only if there is a causal connection between change in surrogate and change in the clinically important outcome. Thus, the surrogate must be in the causal pathway of the disease process, and an intervention's entire effect on the clinical outcome of interest should be fully captured by a change in the surrogate. In this section, we build on previous discussions of how one can establish a causal relationship,[9] and we present an approach to the critical appraisal of studies using surrogate endpoints and the application of their results to the management of individual patients.

As our discussion will demonstrate, the clinician needs to assess far more than a single study to make the decision about the adequacy of a surrogate. Evaluation may require a comprehensive review of observational studies of the relationship between the surrogate endpoint and the target endpoint, along with a review of some or all of the randomized trials that have evaluated treatment impact on both endpoints. Although most clinicians would hesitate to take the time to conduct such an investigation, our guidelines will allow them to evaluate experts' arguments—or those of the pharmaceutical industry—for prescribing treatments on the basis of their effect on surrogate endpoints.

# ARE THE RESULTS VALID?

When we consider the validity of a surrogate endpoint, we must address two issues. First, to be consistently reliable, the surrogate must be in the causal pathway from the intervention to the outcome. Second, in considering a particular intervention, we must be confident that there are no important effects of that intervention on the outcome of interest that are not mediated through or captured by the surrogate. Our guides for validity, as presented in Table 2B3-4, bear directly on these two issues.

**TABLE 2B3-4**

### Users' Guide for a Surrogate Endpoint Trial

**Are the Results Valid?**

- Is there a strong, independent, consistent association between the surrogate endpoint and the clinical endpoint?

- Have randomized trials of other drug classes shown that improvement in the surrogate endpoint has consistently led to improvement in the target outcome?*

- Have randomized trials of the same drug class shown that improvement in the surrogate endpoint has consistently led to improvement in the target outcome?*

**What Are the Results?**

- How large, precise, and lasting was the treatment effect?

**How Can I Apply the Results to Patient Care?**

- Are the likely treatment benefits worth the potential risks and costs?*

---

* Answers to one or all of these questions should be "yes" for a surrogate trial to be an adequate guide for clinical action.

## Is There a Strong, Independent, Consistent Association Between the Surrogate Endpoint and the Clinical Endpoint?

To function as a valid substitute for an important target outcome, the surrogate endpoint must be associated with that target. In general, researchers choose surrogate endpoints because they have found a correlation between a surrogate outcome and a target outcome in observational studies, and their understanding of biologic characteristics gives them confidence in the plausiblity that changes in the surrogate will invariably lead to changes in the important outcome. The stronger the association, the more likely is the causal link between the surrogate and the target. The strength of an association is reflected in statistical measures such as the *relative risk* (RR) or the *odds ratio* (OR) (see Part 2B2, "Therapy and Understanding the Results, Measures of Association"). Many biologically plausible surrogates are associated only weakly with clinically important outcomes. For example, measures of respiratory function in patients with chronic lung disease—or conventional exercise tests in patients with heart and lung disease—are correlated only weakly with capacity to undertake activities of daily living.[10, 11] When correlations are low, the surrogate is likely to be a poor substitute for the target outcome.

In addition to the strength of the association, one's confidence in the validity of the association depends on whether it is consistent across different studies and after adjustment for known confounding variables. For example, ecologic studies such as the Seven Countries Study[12] suggested a strong correlation between serum cholesterol levels and coronary heart disease mortality even after adjusting for other predictors such as age, smoking, and systolic blood pressure. When a surrogate is associated with an outcome after adjusting for multiple other potential prognostic factors, the association is an *independent association* (see Part 2D, "Prognosis, Regression and Correlation"). Subsequent cohort studies confirmed this association and suggested that long-term reductions in serum cholesterol of 0.6 mmol/L would lower the risk of coronary heart disease by approximately 30%.[13] Similarly, cohort studies have consistently revealed that a single measurement of plasma viral load predicts the subsequent risk of AIDS or death in patients with HIV infection.[14-19] For example, in one study the proportion of patients who progressed to AIDS after 5 years in the lowest through the highest quartiles of viral load was 8%, 26%, 49%, and 62%, respectively.[19] Moreover, this association retained its predictive power after adjustment for other potential predictors such as CD4 cell count.[14-18]

## USING THE GUIDE

Let us return to our opening clinical scenario, in which you are wondering whether you can substitute bone density for fracture as a target outcome. Consider the findings from a large cohort study investigating risk factors for hip fracture. In that study,[20] postmenopausal women with bone density in the highest tertile had a hip fracture rate of 9.4 per 1000 woman-years, while women in the middle and lowest tertile had a fracture rate per 1000 woman-years of 14.7 and 27.3, respectively. Furthermore, after considering such other risk factors for osteoporotic hip fractures as maternal history of hip fracture, previous fractures from any site, poor self-rated health, use of long-acting benzodiazepines, impaired visual function, and reduced physical activity, bone mineral density continued to predict the risk of hip fracture.[20] These findings are consistent across studies concerned with the association between bone density and fracture risk.[21, 22] Thus, bone mineral density is a moderately strong, independent predictor of fracture, and it meets the first criterion for an acceptable surrogate endpoint.

Meeting this first criterion is necessary, but it is not sufficient to support reliance on a surrogate outcome. Before offering an intervention on the basis of effects on a surrogate outcome, you should note a consistent relationship between surrogate and target outcome in randomized trials; the effect of the intervention on the surrogate must be large, precise and lasting; and the benefit/risk tradeoff must be clear.

## Have Randomized Trials of Other Drug Classes Shown That Improvement in the Surrogate Endpoint Has Consistently Led to Improvement in the Target Outcome?

Given the possibility that an association may not be causal, pathophysiologic studies, ecologic studies, and cohort studies are insufficient to definitively establish the link between surrogate and clinically important outcomes. We can confidently rely on surrogate endpoints only when long-term randomized controlled trials have consistently demonstrated that modification of the surrogate is associated with concomitant modifications in the target outcome of interest. For example, although ventricular ectopic beats are associated with adverse prognosis in patients with myocardial infarction[23] and although class I antiarrhythmic agents effectively suppress ventricular arrhythmias,[24] these drugs have proved to increase mortality when evaluated in randomized trials.[25] In this case, reliance on the surrogate endpoint of suppression of nonlethal arrhythmias led to the deaths of tens of thousands of patients.[26] This experience has led investigators evaluating antiarryhthmic drugs from other classes to realize that reduction in nonlethal arrythmias provides insufficient evidence of benefit.

The treatment of heart failure provides another instructive example. Trials of angiotensin-converting enzyme (ACE) inhibitors in patients with heart failure have demonstrated parallel increases in exercise capacity[27-30] and a decrease in mortality,[31] suggesting that clinicians may be able to rely on exercise capacity as a valid surrogate. Both milrinone[32] and epoprostol[33] have demonstrated improved exercise tolerance in patients with symptomatic heart failure. However, when these drugs were evaluated in randomized controlled trials, both showed an increase in cardiovascular mortality—which in one instance was statistically significant[34] and which in the second case led to early termination of the study.[35] Thus, exercise tolerance is inconsistent in predicting improved mortality and is therefore an invalid substitute. Other suggested surrogate endpoints in patients with heart failure have included ejection fraction, heart rate variability, and markers of autonomic function.[36] The dopaminergic agent ibopamine positively influences all three surrogate endpoints, yet a randomized trial demonstrated that the drug increases mortality in patients with heart failure.[37] In another example, the positive impact of growth hormone on a number of surrogate outcomes, including nitrogen balance and facilitating weaning from mechanical ventilation, led to high optimism about its likely effect on mortality in critically ill patients.[38,39] Yet, two randomized trials demonstrated a large increase in mortality with growth hormone.[40]

We can contrast this situation with randomized trials that have consistently shown that modification of CD4 cell count is associated with change in important outcomes. A number of trials comparing different classes of antiretroviral therapies have demonstrated that patients randomized to more potent drug regimens had higher CD4 cell counts and were less likely to progress to AIDS or death.[8,41] Even though there is no guarantee that the next trial using a different class of drugs will show the same pattern, these results greatly strengthen our inference that if therapy for HIV infection increases CD4 cell count, a reduction in AIDS-related mortality will result.

## USING THE GUIDE

Returning to our opening clinical scenario, trials of etidronate[42,43] and alendronate[44] for the prevention of osteoporotic fractures in postmenopausal women have shown parallel increases in bone mineral density and in reduced incidence of new vertebral fractures. This would suggest that clinicians might rely on bone density to evaluate new drugs in osteoporosis, assuming that if they saw increases in bone density, fracture reduction would follow.

However, another secondary prevention trial in postmenopausal women using sodium fluoride showed divergent results.[45] Although sodium fluoride increased bone mineral density at the lumbar spine by 35% over a 5-year period, more vertebral and nonvertebral fractures occurred in the intervention group than in the placebo group (163 vertebral and 72 nonvertebral fractures occurred in 101 women treated with sodium fluoride, vs 136 vertebral and 24 nonvertebral fractures in 101 women receiving placebo). In another randomized trial, sodium fluoride again showed a large increase in bone density without any change in fracture rate.[46] Inferences on the basis of unchanged bone density may also be problematic. A study of calcium carbonate malate and vitamin D in elderly patients showed virtually no change in bone density, but researchers noted a reduction in fracture risk of approximately 50%.[47] Thus, increase in bone mineral density as a surrogate endpoint has shown an inconsistent relationship to osteoporotic fractures.

## Have Randomized Trials of the Same Drug Class Shown That Improvement in the Surrogate Endpoint Has Consistently Led to Improvement in the Target Outcome?

Clinicians are in a stronger position to rely on surrogate endpoints if the new drug they are considering is from a class of drugs in which the relationship between changes in the surrogate endpoint and changes in the target outcome has been verified through randomized controlled trials. In hypertensive patients, for instance, thiazide has been shown to reduce blood pressure and patient-important outcomes such as stroke. Thus, we would be much more comfortable relying on reduction in blood pressure to justify administering a thiazide diuretic than to justify offering a novel antihypertensive agent from another drug class.[48]

For example, although in one randomized controlled trial, dihydropyridine calcium-channel blocker has been shown to reduce clinically important outcomes in hypertensive patients,[49] four other trials have shown that these agents are less efficacious than thiazides or ACE inhibitors in preventing patient-important clinical endpoints despite exerting similar degrees of blood pressure lowering.[50-53]

Several large trials of primary and secondary prevention of coronary heart disease with statins have consistently shown that these drugs reduce cardiovascular adverse outcomes.[54] We could therefore assume that a new statin with a similar LDL cholesterol-lowering potency may also reduce clinically important outcomes. However, we would be very reluctant to generalize to another class of lipid-lowering agents since trials of one such class (the fibrates) have shown that these drugs reduce the incidence of myocardial infarction but increase the risk of mortality from other causes (with no impact on overall mortality).[54-56]

These examples highlight the point we made earlier: confidence in a surrogate outcome depends on the assumption that the surrogate captures the full relationship between the treatment and the outcome.[57,58] This assumption can be violated in two ways. First, treatment may have a beneficial mechanism of effect on the outcome independent of its effect on the surrogate. For instance, while ACE inhibitors and calcium-channel blockers appear to reduce blood pressure levels and the incidence of stroke equally well, one explanation for the superior effect of ACE inhibitors vs calcium antagonists on other patient-important outcomes in hypertension such as myocardial infarction or congestive heart failure is that ACE inhibitors may have biologic effects independent of blood pressure lowering that calcium antagonists do not share.[59,60]

Second, treatment may have deleterious effects on the outcome that are not mediated through the surrogate. Mortality-increasing effects of fibrates, rather than inability to lower morbidity and mortality through cholesterol reduction, probably explain the lack of effect of fibrates on patient-important outcomes. That such additional effects are less likely across than within drug classes is what makes us more inclined to rely on within-class evidence from surrogate outcomes.

This criterion is complicated by the variable definitions of drug class. A manufacturer of a drug related to a class of agents with a consistent positive association between modification of a surrogate endpoint and modification of the target (such as a beta-blocker in patients who have sustained a myocardial infarction) will naturally argue for a broad definition of class. Manufacturers of agents that are related to drugs with known or suspected adverse effects on target events (eg, clofibrate or some calcium antagonists) are likely to argue, on the other hand, that the chemical or physiologic connection is not sufficiently close for the new drug to be relegated to the same class as the harmful agent (see Part 2B3, "Therapy and Applying the Results, Drug Class Effects").

## USING THE GUIDE

**R**eturning to the opening scenario, we have established that because of the inconsistent relationship between increase in bone mineral density and fracture reduction, we would be reluctant to offer the patient a new antiosteoporotic agent solely on the basis of evidence of its effect on the surrogate endpoint. Calcitonin, the drug we are considering, is a hormone and thus represents a different class of drugs for the prevention of osteoporotic fractures. Therefore, it is likely that its mechanisms of action will be considerably different from those of the bisphosphonates. Accordingly, the conclusion that similar reductions in loss of bone density will lead to parallel reductions in clinical fractures is questionable.

In Table 2B3-5, we apply our validity criteria to a number of controversial examples of the use of surrogate endpoints.

**TABLE 2B3-5**

### Selected Controversial Examples of Applied Validity Criteria for the Critical Evaluation of Studies Using Surrogate Endpoints

| Types of Intervention (References) | Surrogate Endpoint | Endpoint | Criterion 1 (References) | Criterion 2 (References) | Criterion 3 (References) |
|---|---|---|---|---|---|
| | | | Is there a strong, independent, consistent association between the surrogate endpoint and the clinical endpoint? | Is there evidence from randomized trials in other drug classes that improvement in the surrogate endpoint has consistently led to improvement in the target outcome? | Is there evidence from randomized trials in the same drug class that improvement in the surrogate endpoint has consistently led to improvement in the target outcome? |
| *Hormone* Calcitonin[3] | Bone mineral density | Osteoporotic fractures | yes[22-24] | no[45, 46] | no[3, 68] |

| Types of Intervention (References) | Surrogate Endpoint | Endpoint | Criterion 1 (References) | Criterion 2 (References) | Criterion 3 (References) |
|---|---|---|---|---|---|
| *Proteinase inhibitor** | HIV-1 viral plasma load | AIDS or death | | | |
| Nelfinavir[61] | | | yes[14-18] | yes[62-64] | yes[8, 41] |
| *Reverse transcriptase inhibitor* | | | | | |
| Abacavir[65] | | | yes[14-18] | yes[63, 64, 66] | yes[62, 66] |
| *Proteinase inhibitor** | CD4 cell count | AIDS or death | | | |
| Nelfinavir[71] | | | yes[14-18] | yes[62-64] | yes[8, 41] |
| *Reverse transcriptase inhibitor* | | | | | |
| Abacavir[65] | | | yes[14-18] | yes[63, 64, 66] | yes[62, 66] |
| *Antihypertensive drugs* | Blood pressure reduction | Stroke, myocardial infarction, cardiovascular mortality | | | |
| Calcium antagonist dihydropyridine | | | yes[67, 68] | yes[69] | no[50-53] |
| | | | yes[67, 68] | yes[69] | yes[69] |
| New thiazide diuretic | | | | | |
| *Antilipidemic drugs* | Cholesterol reduction or LDL-cholesterol reduction | Myocardial infarction or death from myocardial infarction | | | |
| Atorvastatin[70, 71] | | | yes[12, 72] | no[54] | yes[54] |
| Bezafibrate[73, 74] | | | yes[12, 72] | no[54] | no[54] |

\* In combination therapy with two reverse transcriptase inhibitors.

# WHAT ARE THE RESULTS?

## How Large, Precise, and Lasting Was the Treatment Effect?

When considering results, we are interested not only in whether an intervention alters a surrogate endpoint, but also in the magnitude, precision, and duration of the effect. If an intervention shows large reductions in the surrogate endpoint, the 95% confidence intervals around those large reductions are narrow, and the effect persists over a sufficiently long period of time, our confidence that the target outcome will be favorably affected increases. Positive effects that are smaller, with wider confidence intervals and shorter duration of follow-up, leave us less confident.

We have already cited evidence suggesting that CD4 counts may be an acceptable surrogate endpoint for mortality in patients with HIV infection. A randomized controlled trial of immediate vs delayed zidovudine therapy in asymptomatic patients with HIV infection reported a positive result for immediate therapy, largely on the basis of the existence of a greater proportion of treated patients with CD4 cell counts above 350/mm³ at a median follow-up of 1.7 years.[75] Subsequently, the Concorde study addressed the same question in a randomized controlled trial with a median follow-up of 3.3 years.[76] The Concorde investigators found a continuous decline in CD4 cells in both the treatment and the control groups, but the median difference of 30 cells/mm³ in favor of treated patients at study termination was statistically significant. However, the study showed no effect of zidovudine in terms of reduced progression to AIDS or death. The median CD4 cell difference was insufficient to impact on clinically important outcomes. The Concorde authors came to the following conclusion: the small but highly significant and persistent difference in CD4 count between the groups was not translated into a significant clinical benefit and it "called into question the uncritical use of CD4 cell counts as a surrogate endpoint."[76] Had the Concorde analysis that showed significantly shorter times to reach a CD4 count of 350/mm³ in the control group been regarded as fundamental, the trial might have been stopped early on the basis of a false-positive result. The message here is that even for surrogate endpoints that provide reliable information about patient-important endpoints, the effect on the surrogate must be large, robust, and of sufficient duration before inferences about patient-important effects become credible.

## USING THE GUIDE

Returning to our scenario, the dose-finding trial of calcitonin in post-menopausal women with osteoporotic fractures demonstrated that after 2 years of treatment, calcitonin-treated patients in the group receiving the highest dose (200 IU, intranasally) showed an increase in bone mineral density at the lumbar spine of 3.0% (95% confidence interval [CI], 1.8%–4.2%) compared to a slight increase in the control group of 1.0% (95% CI, 0–2.0%).[3] This difference in change over time was statistically significant ($P = .048$). As we will illustrate when we consider weighing benefits and risks, the magnitude of the effect on the surrogate endpoint may or may not help us estimate the magnitude of possible impact on the target outcome.

# How Can I Apply the Results to Patient Care?

The questions clinicians should ask themselves in applying the results are the same ones we have suggested for any issue of therapy or prevention (see Part 2B3, "Therapy and Applying the Results, Applying Results to Individual Patients"). These three questions have to do with whether the results can be applied to the care of patients in your practice, whether all important outcomes were considered, and whether the likely benefits are worth the risks of treatment.

The question, "Can the results be applied to the patient before me?" refers to the extent to which that patient is similar to those who participated in the published studies under consideration and the extent to which the therapy—along with the associated technologies for monitoring and responding to complications—is available in your setting. The question, "Were all important outcomes considered?" relates to the focus of this book, namely, was the primary outcome really the one in which patients will be interested? This second criterion also draws issues of adverse intervention effects to our attention. Applying the third criterion, judging whether the benefits are worth the treatment risks, presents particular challenges when investigators have focused on surrogate endpoints, and we will discuss this criterion in some detail.

## Are the Likely Treatment Benefits Worth the Potential Risks and Costs?

To know whether to offer a treatment to patients, clinicians must be able to estimate the magnitude of the likely benefit. When the available data are limited to the effect on a surrogate endpoint, estimating the extent to which treatment will reduce patient-important outcomes becomes a challenge.

One approach is to extrapolate from one or more randomized controlled trials assessing a related intervention in a similar patient population that provides both surrogate endpoint and target outcome data. For example, until recently there were very few long-term data on the efficacy of lovastatin in reducing patient-important outcomes in any population. However, one could extrapolate from short-term dose efficacy studies assessing the surrogate endpoint of cholesterol lowering. Thus, since treatment with 40 mg of lovastatin daily produced a degree of LDL cholesterol lowering that was similar to that of 40 mg of pravastatin (31% reduction, vs 34% reduction in the CURVES Study[77]), one could theorize that long-term benefits from lovastatin would be similar to those of pravastatin. Subsequently, the AFCAPS/TexCAPS Trial (a 5-year trial assessing the efficacy of lovastatin in the primary prevention of ischemic heart disease)[78] did confirm that this agent had a benefit profile similar to that of pravastatin (as determined by the 5-year primary prevention WOSCOPS Trial).[79] The relative risk reductions and 95% confidence intervals for myocardial infarction were 40% (17%-57%) and 31% (17%-43%), respectively. This approach is likely to be seriously flawed when one is extrapolating from trials of another class of drugs.

Consider the consequences of trying to ascertain the effect of calcitonin on fractures on the basis of bone density results. Recognizing the limitations of the approach described above, we could examine the results of randomized controlled trials of alendronate (a drug from a different class in which we have data on the same surrogate endpoint as well as clinical endpoints such as fracture reduction). Although oral alendronate treatment with 10 mg or greater appears to improve vertebral bone density by 7.5% better than controls over a 2-year period,[44] treatment with calcitonin (200 IU intranasally per day) is associated with only a 3.0% improvement over the same time frame. A systematic review of the alendronate trials[80] reported a 29% reduction in relative risk of nonvertebral fracture over a period of 2 years. Only one trial studied symptomatic vertebral fractures in women with decreased bone density and an existing vertebral fracture.[81] This study demonstrated a relative risk reduction of 55% with alendronate and suggested that for the patient we are considering, the risk over 3 years of a nonvertebral fracture would be approximately 15%; symptomatic vertebral fracture would be about 5%. Given the relative risk reductions with alendronate, over a 3-year period one would need to treat approximately 25 women to prevent a nonvertebral fracture, and 40 women would need to be treated over the same time period to prevent a symptomatic vertebral fracture.

Since the improvement in bone mineral density with calcitonin is at less than 50% of the effect of alendronate, we would anticipate a considerably lower reduction in fracture risk with calcitonin. However, 3-year interim results of a randomized controlled trial of calcitonin published in abstract form showed a 37% relative risk reduction of vertebral fractures with this therapy, despite less increase in bone mineral density than was seen with the alendronate trials.[82] These findings serve to emphasize the dangers of extrapolating results across drug classes when there is uncertainty as to whether the effects on clinically important outcomes are mediated in the same fashion by the two comparison drugs.

# CLINICAL RESOLUTION

We have found a strong, consistent, independent, and biologically plausible association between bone mineral density and vertebral and nonvertebral fractures. Randomized controlled trials, however, have failed to show a consistent association between increased bone density and reduced fracture across all drug classes.

Because the patient before us is at substantial risk of fracture over the short term, the number needed to treat to prevent both nonvertebral and vertebral fractures is moderate, as is the absolute benefit she might expect. Moreover, she is interested in longer-term fracture prevention, and her risk will grow over time. However, she is unable to tolerate the drugs that have the strongest evidence of efficacy. Ultimately, as the treating physician you must make a decision among a number of interventions with limited evidence of effectiveness in reducing fracture—calcitonin, hormone replacement therapy, or vitamin D and calcium—as well as varying costs and risks of side effects. You will ensure that your patient understands the uncertainty about the benefit on patient-important endpoints when she makes her decision regarding whether to begin a therapeutic regimen with calcitonin.

When we use surrogate endpoints to make inferences about expected benefit, we are making assumptions regarding the link between the surrogate endpoint and the target outcome. In this section, we have outlined criteria that you can use to decide when these assumptions might be appropriate. Even if a surrogate endpoint meets all of these criteria, inferences about a treatment benefit may still prove to be misleading. Thus, treatment recommendations based on surrogate outcome effects can never be as strong as if the results focused on a patient-important target outcome.

These considerations emphasize that waiting for results from randomized trials investigating the effect of the intervention on outcomes of unequivocal importance to patients is the only definitive solution to the surrogate outcome dilemma. The large number of instances in which reliance on surrogate endpoints has led—or might have led—clinicians astray argues for the wisdom of this conservative approach (see Part 2B1, "Therapy and Validity, Surprising Results of Randomized Controlled Trials"). On the other hand, when a patient's risk of serious morbidity or mortality is high, a wait-and-see strategy may pose problems for many patients and their physicians.

We encourage clinicians to critically question therapeutic interventions in which the only proof of efficacy is from surrogate endpoint data. When the surrogate endpoint meets all of our validity criteria, when the effect of the intervention on the surrogate endpoint is large, when the patient's risk of the target outcome is high, when the patient places a high value on avoiding the target outcome, and when there are no satisfactory alternative therapies, clinicians may choose to recommend therapy on the basis of randomized controlled trials evaluating only surrogate endpoints. In other situations, clinicians must carefully consider the known side effects and costs of therapy, along with the possibility of unanticipated adverse effects, before recommending an intervention solely on the basis of surrogate endpoint data.

# ADDENDUM

The publication of the Chesnut et al study,[83] unavailable at the time we constructed the opening clinical scenario, provides data regarding the impact of calcitonin on fractures—and obviates the necessity of relying on bone density findings.

# References

1. Harris ST, Watts NB, Genant HK, et al, for the Vertebral Efficacy with Risedronate Therapy (VERT) Study Group. Effects of risedronate treatment on vertebral and nonvertebral fractures in women with postmenopausal osteoporosis: a randomized controlled trial. *JAMA*. 1999;282:1344-1352.

2. Ettinger B, Black DM, Mitlak BH, et al, for the Multiple Outcomes of Raloxifene Evaluation (MORE) Investigators. Reduction of vertebral fracture risk in postmenopausal women with osteoporosis treated with raloxifene: results from a 3-year randomized clinical trial. *JAMA*. 1999;282:637-645.

3. Overgaard K, Hansen MA, Jensen SB, Christiansen C. Effect of salcatonin given intranasally on bone mass and fracture rates in established osteoporosis: a dose-response study. *BMJ*. 1992;305:556-561.

4. Temple RJ. A regulatory authority's opinion about surrogate endpoints. In: Nimmo WS, Tucker GT, eds. *Clinical Measurement in Drug Evaluation*. New York: John Wiley & Sons; 1995.

5. Hammer SM, Katzenstein DA, Hughes MD, et al, for the AIDS Clinical Trials Group Study 175 Study Team. A trial comparing nucleoside monotherapy with combination therapy in HIV-infected adults with CD4 cell counts from 200 to 500 per cubic millimeter. *N Engl J Med*. 1996;335:1081-1090.

6. Delta Coordinating Committee. Delta: a randomised double-blind controlled trial comparing combinations of zidovudine plus didanosine or zalcitabine with zidovudine alone in HIV-infected individuals. *Lancet*. 1996;348:283-291.

7. Saravolatz LD, Winslow DL, Collins G, et al, for the Investigators for the Terry Beirn Community Programs for Clinical Research on AIDS. Zidovudine alone or in combination with didanosine or zalcitabine in HIV-infected patients with the acquired immunodeficiency syndrome or fewer than 200 CD4 cells per cubic millimeter. *N Engl J Med*. 1996;335:1099-1106.

8. Hammer SM, Squires KE, Hughes MD, et al, for the AIDS Clinical Trials Group 320 Study Team. A controlled trial of two nucleoside analogues plus indinavir in persons with human immunodeficiency virus infection and CD4 cell counts of 200 per cubic millimeter or less. *N Engl J Med*. 1997;337:725-733.

9. How to read clinical journals, IV: to determine etiology or causation. *CMAJ*. 1981;124:985-990.

10. Guyatt GH, Thompson PJ, Berman LB, et al. How should we measure function in patients with chronic heart and lung disease? *J Chronic Dis*. 1985;38:517-524.

11. Mahler DA, Weinberg DH, Wells CK, Feinstein AR. The measurement of dyspnea: contents, interobserver agreement, and physiologic correlates of two new clinical indexes. *Chest*. 1984;85:751-758.

12. Verschuren WM, Jacobs DR, Bloemberg BP, et al. Serum total cholesterol and long-term coronary heart disease mortality in different cultures: twenty-five-year follow-up of the seven countries study. *JAMA*. 1995;274:131-136.

13. Law MR, Wald NJ, Thompson SG. By how much and how quickly does reduction in serum cholesterol concentration lower risk of ischaemic heart disease? *BMJ*. 1994;308:367-372.

14. Mellors JW, Rinaldo CR Jr, Gupta P, White RM, Todd JA, Kingsley LA. Prognosis in HIV-1 infection predicted by the quantity of virus in plasma. *Science*. 1996;272:1167-1170.

15. Mellors JW, Kingsley LA, Rinaldo CR Jr, et al. Quantitation of HIV-1 RNA in plasma predicts outcome after seroconversion. *Ann Intern Med*. 1995;122:573-579.

16. Ruiz L, Romeu J, Clotet B, et al. Quantitative HIV-1 RNA as a marker of clinical stability and survival in a cohort of 302 patients with a mean CD4 cell count of 300 x $10^6$/l. *AIDS*. 1996;10:F39-F44.

17. O'Brien TR, Blattner WA, Waters D, et al. Serum HIV-1 RNA levels and time to development of AIDS in the Multicenter Hemophilia Cohort Study. *JAMA*. 1996;276:105-110.

18. Yerly S, Perneger TV, Hirschel B, et al, for the Swiss HIV Cohort Study. A critical assessment of the prognostic value of HIV-1 RNA levels and CD4+ cell counts in HIV-infected patients. *Arch Intern Med*. 1998;158:247-252.

19. Ho DD. Viral counts count in HIV infection. *Science*. 1996;272:1124-1125.

20. Cummings SR, Nevitt MC, Browner WS, et al, for the Study of Osteoporotic Fractures Research Group. Risk factors for hip fracture in white women. *N Engl J Med*. 1995;332:767-773.

21. Marshall D, Johnell O, Wedel H. Meta-analysis of how well measures of bone mineral density predict occurrence of osteoporotic fractures. *BMJ*. 1996;312:1254-1259.

22. Huang C, Ross PD, Wasnich RD. Short-term and long-term fracture prediction by bone mass measurements: a prospective study. *J Bone Miner Res*. 1998;13:107-113.

23. Bigger JT Jr, Fleiss JL, Kleiger R, Miller JP, Rolnitzky LM. The relationships among ventricular arrhythmias, left ventricular dysfunction, and mortality in the 2 years after myocardial infarction. *Circulation*. 1984;69:250-258.

24. McAlister FA, Teo KK. Antiarrhythmic therapies for the prevention of sudden cardiac death. *Drugs*. 1997;54:235-252.

25. Echt DS, Liebson PR, Mitchell LB, et al, for the Cardiac Arrhythmia Suppression Trial. Mortality and morbidity in patients receiving encainide, flecainide, or placebo. *N Engl J Med*. 1991;324:781-788.

26. Moore TJ. *Deadly Medicine: Why Tens of Thousands of Heart Patients Died in America's Worst Drug Disaster*. New York: Simon & Schuster; 1995.

27. Drexler H, Banhardt U, Meinertz T, Wollschlager H, Lehmann M, Just H. Contrasting peripheral short-term and long-term effects of converting enzyme inhibition in patients with congestive heart failure: a double-blind, placebo-controlled trial. *Circulation*. 1989;79:491-502.

28. Lewis GR. Comparison of lisinopril versus placebo for congestive heart failure. *Am J Cardiol*. 1989;63:12D-16D.

29. Giles TD, Fisher MB, Rush JE. Lisinopril and captopril in the treatment of heart failure in older patients: comparison of a long- and short-acting angiotensin-converting enzyme inhibitor. *Am J Med*. 1988;85:44-47.

30. Riegger GA. Effects of quinapril on exercise tolerance in patients with mild to moderate heart failure. *Eur Heart J*. 1991;12:705-711.

31. Garg R, Yusuf S. Overview of randomized trials of angiotensin-converting enzyme inhibitors on mortality and morbidity in patients with heart failure. Collaborative Group on ACE Inhibitor Trials. *JAMA*. 1995;273:1450-1456.

32. DiBianco R, Shabetai R, Kostuk W, Moran J, Schlant RC, Wright R. A comparison of oral milrinone, digoxin, and their combination in the treatment of patients with chronic heart failure. *N Engl J Med*. 1989;320:677-683.

33. Sueta CA, Gheorghiade M, Adams KF Jr, et al, for the Epoprostenol Multicenter Research Group. Safety and efficacy of epoprostenol in patients with severe congestive heart failure. *Am J Cardiol*. 1995;75:34A-43A.

34. Packer M, Carver JR, Rodeheffer RJ, et al, for the PROMISE Study Research Group. Effect of oral milrinone on mortality in severe chronic heart failure. *N Engl J Med*. 1991;325:1468-1475.

35. Califf RM, Adams KF, McKenna WJ, et al. A randomized controlled trial of epoprostenol therapy for severe congestive heart failure: The Flolan International Randomized Survival Trial (FIRST). *Am Heart J*. 1997;134:44-54.

36. Yee KM, Struthers AD. Can drug effects on mortality in heart failure be predicted by any surrogate measure? *Eur Heart J*. 1997;18:1860-1864.

37. Hampton JR, van Veldhuisen DJ, Kleber FX, et al, for the Second Prospective Randomised Study of Ibopamine on Mortality and Efficacy (PRIME II) Investigators. Randomised study of effect of ibopamine on survival in patients with advanced severe heart failure. *Lancet*. 1997;349:971-977.

38. Jiang ZM, He GZ, Zhang SY, et al. Low-dose growth hormone and hypocaloric nutrition attenuate the protein-catabolic response after major operation. *Ann Surg*. 1989;210:513-524.

39. Knox JB, Wilmore DW, Demling RH, Sarraf P, Santos AA. Use of growth hormone for postoperative respiratory failure. *Am J Surg*. 1996;171:576-580.

40. Takala J, Ruokonen E, Webster NR, et al. Increased mortality associated with growth hormone treatment in critically ill adults. *N Engl J Med*. 1999;341:785-792.

41. Cameron DW, Heath-Chiozzi M, Danner S, et al, for the Advanced HIV Disease Ritonavir Study Group. Randomised placebo-controlled trial of ritonavir in advanced HIV-1 disease. *Lancet*. 1998;351:543-549.

42. Watts NB, Harris ST, Genant HK, et al. Intermittent cyclical etidronate treatment of postmenopausal osteoporosis. *N Engl J Med*. 1990;323:73-79.

43. Storm T, Thamsborg G, Steiniche T, Genant HK, Sorensen OH. Effect of intermittent cyclical etidronate therapy on bone mass and fracture rate in women with postmenopausal osteoporosis. *N Engl J Med*. 1990;322:1265-1271.

44. Liberman UA, Weiss SR, Broll J, et al, for the Alendronate Phase III Osteoporosis Treatment Study Group. Effect of oral alendronate on bone mineral density and the incidence of fractures in postmenopausal osteoporosis. *N Engl J Med*. 1995;333:1437-1443.

45. Riggs BL, Hodgson SF, O'Fallon WM, et al. Effect of fluoride treatment on the fracture rate in postmenopausal women with osteoporosis. *N Engl J Med*. 1990;322:802-809.

46. Meunier PJ, Sebert JL, Reginster JY, et al. Fluoride salts are no better at preventing new vertebral fractures than calcium-vitamin D in postmenopausal osteoporosis: the FAVO Study. *Osteoporos Int*. 1998;8:4-12.

47. Dawson-Hughes B, Harris SS, Krall EA, Dallal GE. Effect of calcium and vitamin D supplementation on bone density in men and women 65 years of age or older. *N Engl J Med*. 1997;337:670-676.

48. McAlister FA, Straus S, Sackett D. Randomized clinical trials of antihypertensive drugs: all that glitters is not gold. *CMAJ*. 1998;159:488-490.

49. Staessen JA, Fagard R, Thijs L, et al, for the Systolic Hypertension in Europe (Syst-Eur) Trial Investigators. Randomised double-blind comparison of placebo and active treatment for older patients with isolated systolic hypertension. *Lancet*. 1997;350:757-764.

50. Psaty BM, Siscovick DS, Weiss NS, et al. Hypertension and outcomes research: from clinical trials to clinical epidemiology. *Am J Hypertens*. 1996;9:178-183.

51. Borhani NO, Mercuri M, Borhani PA, et al. Final outcome results of the Multicenter Isradipine Diuretic Atherosclerosis Study (MIDAS): a randomized controlled trial. *JAMA*. 1996;276:785-791.

52. Tatti P, Pahor M, Byington RP, et al. Outcome results of the Fosinopril Versus Amlodipine Cardiovascular Events Randomized Trial (FACET) in patients with hypertension and NIDDM. *Diabetes Care*. 1998;21:597-603.

53. Estacio RO, Jeffers BW, Hiatt WR, Biggerstaff SL, Gifford N, Schrier RW. The effect of nisoldipine as compared with enalapril on cardiovascular outcomes in patients with non-insulin-dependent diabetes and hypertension. *N Engl J Med*. 1998;338:645-652.

54. Bucher HC, Griffith LE, Guyatt GH. Systematic review on the risk and benefit of different cholesterol-lowering interventions. *Arterioscler Thromb Vasc Biol*. 1999;19:187-195.

55. Muldoon MF, Manuck SB, Matthews KA. Lowering cholesterol concentrations and mortality: a quantitative review of primary prevention trials. *BMJ*. 1990;301:309-314.

56. Smith GD, Song F, Sheldon TA. Cholesterol lowering and mortality: the importance of considering initial level of risk. *BMJ*. 1993;306:1367-1373.

57. Prentice RL. Surrogate endpoints in clinical trials: definition and operational criteria. *Stat Med*. 1989;8:431-440.

58. Fleming TR. Surrogate markers in AIDS and cancer trials. *Stat Med*. 1994;13:1423-1435.

59. Pahor M, Psaty BM, Alderman MH, et al. Health outcomes associated with calcium antagonists compared with other first-line antihypertensive therapies: a meta-analysis of randomised controlled trials. *Lancet*. 2000;356:1949-1954.

60. Neal B, MacMahon S, Chapman N. Effects of ACE inhibitors, calcium antagonists, and other blood-pressure-lowering drugs: results of prospectively designed overviews of randomised trials. Blood Pressure Lowering Treatment Trialists' Collaboration. *Lancet*. 2000;356:1955-1964.

61. Clendeninn N, Quart B, Anderson R, Knowles M, Chang Y. Analysis of long-term virologic data from the viracept (nelfinavir) 511 protocol using 3 HIV-RNA assays. In: *Abstracts from the 5ᵗʰ Conference on Retroviruses and Opportunistic Infections.* February 3,1998; Chicago, IL. Available at: www.retroconference.org/abs/absset.htm. Accessed January 12, 2001.

62. Brun-Vezinet F, Boucher C, Loveday C, et al. HIV-1 viral load, phenotype, and resistance in a subset of drug-naive participants from the Delta trial. The national virology groups. Delta virology working group and coordinating committee. *Lancet*. 1997;350:983-990.

63. Montaner JS, Reiss P, Cooper D, et al. A randomized, double-blind trial comparing combinations of nevirapine, didanosine, and zidovudine for HIV-infected patients: the INCAS trial. Italy, the Netherlands, Canada and Australia study. *JAMA*. 1998;279:930-937.

64. CEASAR Coordinating Committee. Randomised trial of addition of lamivudine or lamivudine plus loviride to zidovudine-containing regimens for patients with HIV-1 infection: the CAESAR trial. *Lancet*. 1997;349:1413-1421.

65. Fischl M, Greenberg S, Clumeck N, et al. Safety and activity of abacavir (1592, ABC) with 3TC/ZDV in antiretroviral naive subjects [abstract]. Presented at: 12th World AIDS Conference; June 28-July 3, 1998; Geneva, Switzerland.

66. Katzenstein DA, Hammer SM, Hughes MD, et al. The relation of virologic and immunologic markers to clinical outcomes after nucleoside therapy in HIV-infected adults with 200 to 500 CD4 cells per cubic millimeter. AIDS Clinical Trials Group Study 175 Virology Study Team. *N Engl J Med*. 1996;335:1091-1098.

67. Collins R, Peto R, MacMahon S, et al. Blood pressure, stroke, and coronary heart disease. Part 2, short-term reductions in blood pressure: overview of randomised drug trials in their epidemiological context. *Lancet*. 1990;335:827-838.

68. MacMahon S, Peto R, Cutler J, et al. Blood pressure, stroke, and coronary heart disease. Part 1, prolonged differences in blood pressure: prospective observational studies corrected for the regression dilution bias. *Lancet*. 1990;335:765-774.

69. Psaty BM, Smith NL, Siscovick DS, et al. Health outcomes associated with antihypertensive therapies used as first-line agents: a systematic review and meta-analysis. *JAMA*. 1997;277:739-745.

70. Heinonen TM, Stein E, Weiss SR, et al. The lipid-lowering effects of atorvastatin, a new HMG-coA reductase inhibitor: results of a randomized, double-masked study. *Clin Ther*. 1996;18:853-863.

71. Bakker-Arkema RG, Davidson MH, Goldstein RJ, et al. Efficacy and safety of a new HMG-coA reductase inhibitor, atorvastatin, in patients with hypertriglyceridemia. *JAMA*. 1996;275:128-133.

72. Law MR, Wald NJ, Thompson SG. By how much and how quickly does reduction in serum cholesterol concentration lower risk of ischaemic heart disease? *BMJ*. 1994;308:367-372.

73. Winocour PH, Durrington PN, Bhatagnar D, et al. The effect of bezafibrate on very low density lipoprotein (VLDL), intermediate density lipoprotein (IDL), and low density lipoprotein (LDL) composition in type 1 diabetes associated with hypercholesterolaemia or combined hyperlipidaemia. *Atherosclerosis*. 1992;93:83-94.

74. Jones IR, Swai A, Taylor R, Miller M, Laker MF, Alberti KG. Lowering of plasma glucose concentrations with bezafibrate in patients with moderately controlled NIDDM. *Diabetes Care*. 1990;13:855-863.

75. Cooper DA, Gatell JM, Kroon S, et al, for the European-Australian Collaborative Group. Zidovudine in persons with asymptomatic HIV infection and CD4+ cell counts greater than 400 per cubic millimeter. *N Engl J Med*. 1993;329:297-303.

76. Concorde Coordinating Committee. Concorde: MRC/ANRS randomised double-blind controlled trial of immediate and deferred zidovudine in symptom-free HIV infection. *Lancet*. 1994;343:871-881.

77. Jones P, Kafonek S, Laurora I, Hunninghake D. Comparative dose efficacy study of atorvastatin versus simvastatin, pravastatin, lovastatin, and fluvastatin in patients with hypercholesterolemia (the CURVES Study). *Am J Cardiol*. 1998;81:582-587.

78. Downs JR, Clearfield M, Weis S, et al, for the Air Force/Texas Coronary Atherosclerosis Prevention Study. Primary prevention of acute coronary events with lovastatin in men and women with average cholesterol levels: results of AFCAPS/TexCAPS. *JAMA*. 1998;279:1615-1622.

79. Shepherd J, Cobbe SM, Ford I, et al, for the West of Scotland Coronary Prevention Study Group. Prevention of coronary heart disease with pravastatin in men with hypercholesterolemia. *N Engl J Med*. 1995;333:1301-1307.

80. Karpf DB, Shapiro DR, Seeman E, et al, for the Alendronate Osteoporosis Treatment Study Groups. Prevention of nonvertebral fractures by alendronate: a meta-analysis. *JAMA*. 1997;277:1159-1164.

81. Black DM, Cummings SR, Karpf DB, et al, for the Fracture Intervention Trial Research Group. Randomised trial of effect of alendronate on risk of fracture in women with existing vertebral fractures. *Lancet*. 1996;348:1535-1541.

82. Stock JL, Avioli IV, Baylink DJ, et al. Calcitonin-salmon nasal spray reduces the incidence of new vertebral fractures in postmenopausal women: three year interim results of the PROOF study. *J Bone Miner Res*. 1997:S149.

83. Chesnut CH, Silverman S, Andriano K, et al. A randomized trial of nasal spray salmon calcitonin in postmenopausal women with established osteoporosis: the Prevent Recurrence of Osteoporotic Fractures Study. *Am J Med*. 2000;109:267-276.

# THERAPY AND APPLYING THE RESULTS

## Drug Class Effects

Finlay McAlister, Andreas Laupacis, and George Wells

The following EBM Working Group members also made substantive contributions to this section: Gordon Guyatt, Jonathan Craig, and Jim Nishikawa

## IN THIS SECTION

## CLINICAL SCENARIO

### Which Statin Is Best—Or Is There Any Difference?

As a busy primary care physician, you care for many patients with elevated serum cholesterol levels. A speaker at a recent continuing medical education event reviewed the benefits of cholesterol-lowering therapy, particularly with hydroxymethylglutaryl-coenzyme A reductase inhibitors (statins) in the primary and secondary prevention of ischemic heart disease, but the speaker did not recommend a particular statin. You decide to consider statin therapy for patients in your practice with elevated cholesterol levels, but you are uncertain as to which of the six statins currently available is the best. You ask a local cardiologist and endocrinologist for their opinions and each suggests a different statin, citing a different rationale and different studies. You then contact local pharmaceutical representatives to provide you with the evidence that their statin is better than that of their competitors, and the representative provides another rationale and another study. Faced with a variety of competing claims, you realize that you need a framework for grading the strength of these studies.

Most classes of drugs include multiple compounds, and the interests of clinicians, manufacturers, and purchasers may conflict around questions of whether a particular drug is more effective, more safe, or more cost-effective than others in its class.[1] In this section, we review the types of evidence commonly cited to support the use of a particular drug over another of the same class, and we provide a hierarchy for grading studies that compare same-class drugs. Although there is no uniformly accepted definition of a *drug class*, and some would argue that drug class cannot be defined at all, drugs generally belong to the same class for one of three reasons: their chemical structure is similar, their mechanisms of action are similar, or their pharmacologic effects are similar (Table 2B3-6). For the purposes of this discussion, we will consider a drug class to include those drugs that share a similar chemical structure and mechanism of action. Most classes of drugs include multiple compounds; and because of their similar mechanisms of action, they are generally believed to confer similar pharmacologic effects and clinical outcomes (*class effects*). This assumption is a key medical heuristic that underlies clinical practice guidelines in which evidence from studies involving one or more drugs within a class is extrapolated to other drugs of the same class. For example, beta-blockers are recommended to survivors of myocardial infarction or angiotensin-converting enzyme (ACE) inhibitors are recommended to patients with heart failure. In this circumstance, clinicians are likely to be interested in the drug within each class with the most attractive efficacy/safety ratio; payers will pursue the most cost-effective drug from a class; and manufacturers will have a vested interest in ensuring that their drug is prescribed as much as possible.

**TABLE 2B3-6**

## Different Definitions of Drug Classes

| Definition | Example |
|---|---|
| A group of drugs with similar chemical structure | Dihydropyridine calcium channel blockers have a dihydropyridine ring. |
| A group of drugs with similar mechanism of action | Calcium channel blockers block the voltage-dependent calcium channels on the surfaces of cell membranes. |
| A group of drugs with similar pharmacologic effects | Antihypertensive agents (for example, calcium channel blockers, ACE* inhibitors, beta blockers, thiazides, and alpha blockers) lower blood pressure. |

* ACE indicates angiotensin-converting enzyme.

The *absolute treatment effect* seen with a drug, defined by the absolute risk reduction (ARR) or number needed to treat (NNT) (see Part 1B1, "Therapy"; see also Part 2B2, "Therapy and Understanding the Results, Measures of Association), is influenced by the baseline risk or control event rate (CER) of those patients in whom it is used. Thus, the absolute risk reduction (ARR) varies considerably among different groups of patients. On the other hand, the relative treatment effect of a drug, defined by the relative risk reduction (RRR), is often—but not always—similar regardless of the baseline risk of trial participants (see Part 2B3, "Therapy and Applying the Results, Applying Results to Individual Patients"). If two drugs are tested in separate placebo-controlled trials, only proportional effects such as the RRR seen with each drug can be compared (and then only under the assumption of constant RRR over different CERs). Although the point estimates of effect size vary with the play of chance, we can consider a class effect to be present when drugs with similar mechanisms of action generate RRRs or odds ratios (ORs) that are similar in direction and magnitude. For example, the Collaborative Group on ACE Inhibitor Trials[2] suggested that there is a class effect for ACE inhibitors in patients with symptomatic heart failure despite the fact that the OR point estimates for effects on total mortality ranged from 0.14 (95% CI, 0 to 7.6) for perindopril (one trial, 125 patients) to 0.78 (95% CI, 0.67-0.91) for enalapril (seven trials, 3381 patients). Our confidence in this class effect stems from the recognition that the overall OR in 32 trials involving 7105 patients was 0.77 (95% CI, 0.67-0.88), the confidence intervals for each of the ACE inhibitors overlapped, and there was no statistical heterogeneity between trials of different agents.

# The Risks of Assuming a Drug Class Effect

Although drugs of the same class typically exhibit similar pharmacologic effects and clinical outcomes, this may not always be the case. Consider, for example, the current controversy over the safety of oral d-sotalol in patients surviving myocardial infarction who develop congestive heart failure. This controversy erupted after the publication of the SWORD Trial in 1996,[3] which suggested an increase in mortality with d-sotalol in contrast to the demonstrated decrease in mortality with other beta blockers. However, in this context, it is useful to recall a previous controversy over the efficacy of beta blockers with intrinsic sympathetic activity (ISA) in patients with myocardial infarction. Although an earlier meta-analysis[4] suggested that the treatment effect was larger with non-ISA beta blockers than with ISA beta blockers, subsequent trials[5] failed to confirm this and the totality of the evidence[6] suggests that there is little difference between beta-blocker subgroups. Thus, it would seem reasonable to accept a priori that drugs within the same class exert similar effects, unless there is clear evidence of important differences.

However, this assumption can lead to two important errors in extrapolation with major clinical consequences. First, when a class of drugs (such as the thiazide diuretics) all produce similar pharmacologic effects (blood pressure lowering) and similar clinical effects (reduction in the number of strokes), a second class of drugs (for example, the calcium-channel blockers) that produce the same pharmacologic effects might be assumed to produce the same clinical benefit. In the absence of randomized controlled trials verifying that final step, this type of extrapolation may be in error. For example, certain calcium-channel blockers have unfavorable effects on total mortality.[7] In addition, even within the same class, individual drugs may have different physiologic effects other than the mechanism of action that defined them as being in the same class. To the extent that this is true, it may be inaccurate to extrapolate the clinical outcomes shown in randomized trials of one drug in a class to another drug in that class that has not been subjected to similar outcome-centered trials. For example, some authors have argued that, although all of the statins act on the HMG-coenzyme A reductase, they may have different nonlipid effects on the atherothrombotic process—which may influence their clinical efficacy.[8]

To reduce the risk of faulty extrapolation and to maximize the optimal selection of treatments within a class of drugs, it is useful to develop and apply a hierarchy of evidence when making decisions about the comparative clinical efficacy and safety of drugs within a class.

# Levels of Evidence

Table 2B3-7 presents suggested levels of evidence for comparing one drug with other drugs in the same class. This comparison should occur as part of a systematic review of all the relevant evidence on the effects of a treatment, identified and assessed by sound and transparent methods (see Part 1E, "Summarizing the

Evidence"). The key question that a meta-analysis should address with regard to class effect is whether the individual drugs explain the variability in results across trials—or within trials that directly compare different drugs (see Part 2E, "Summarizing the Evidence, Evaluating Differences in Study Results"; see also Part 2E, "Summarizing the Evidence, When to Believe a Subgroup Analysis"). Table 2B3-8 summarizes the relevant statin trials and presents details of each trial and the relevant clinically important outcomes.

**TABLE 2B3-7**

## Levels of Evidence for Comparing the Efficacy of Drugs Within the Same Class

| Level | Comparison | Study Patients | Outcomes | Threats to Validity |
|---|---|---|---|---|
| 1 | Within a RCT making a direct comparison | Drawn from the same population (by definition) | Patient-important outcomes* | • Failure to conceal randomization scheme<br>• Failure to achieve blinding<br>• Failure to achieve complete follow-up |
| 2 | Within a head-to-head RCT | Identical (by definition) | Validated surrogate outcomes† | • Those of level 1<br>• Validity of surrogate outcome for clinically important outcomes |
| 2 | Across RCTs of different drugs vs placebo | Similar or different (in disease and risk factor status) | Patient-important outcomes or validated surrogate outcomes | • Those of level 1, plus differences between trials in:<br>• Patient characteristics<br>• Methodologic quality (adequacy of blinding, allocation concealment, etc)<br>• Endpoint definitions<br>• Adherence rates |
| 3 | Across subgroup analyses from RCTs of different drugs vs placebo | Similar or different | Patient-important outcomes or surrogate outcomes | • Those of levels 1 and 2, plus<br>• Multiple comparisons, post hoc data collection<br>• Underpowered subgroups<br>• Misclassification into subgroups |
| 3 | Across RCTs of different drugs vs placebo | Similar or different | Unvalidated surrogate outcomes | • Surrogate outcomes may not capture all of the effects (beneficial or hazardous) of a therapeutic agent |
| 4 | Between nonrandomized studies (observational studies and administrative database research) | Similar or different | Patient-important outcomes | • Confounding by indication, compliance, and/or calendar time<br>• Unknown/unmeasured confounders<br>• Measurement error<br>• For outcomes research: limited databases, coding systems not suitable for research |

* *Patient-important outcomes* refer to long-term efficacy data and the particular endpoints depend on the condition being treated. For statins used to prevent or treat atherosclerotic disease, patient-important outcomes would include all-cause mortality, myocardial infarction, and stroke.

† *Surrogate outcomes* are considered validated only when the relationship between the surrogate outcome and patient-important outcomes has been firmly established in long-term RCTs.

**TABLE 2B3-8**

## Features of Randomized Controlled Trials of Statin Drugs Designed to Detect Differences in Patient-Important Outcomes

| Trial | 4S[20] | WOSCOPS[21] | CARE[22] | AFCAPS/ TexCAPS[23] | LIPID[24] |
|---|---|---|---|---|---|
| Study design | Secondary prevention; multicenter | Primary prevention; one center | Secondary prevention; multicenter | Primary prevention; multicenter | Secondary prevention; multicenter |
| Treatment (daily dose) | Simvastatin 20 mg | Pravastatin 40 mg | Pravastatin 40 mg | Lovastatin 40 mg | Pravastatin 40 mg |
| Patient inclusion criteria | 35-70 years; prior angina or acute myocardial infarction (AMI); fasting total cholesterol, 5.5-8.0 mmol/L | 45-64 years; no prior AMI; fasting LDL cholesterol, 4.0-6.0 mmol/L | 21-75 years; prior AMI; fasting LDL cholesterol, 3.0-4.5 mmol/L | 45-73 years (males) or 55-73 years (females); no prior AMI; fasting LDL cholesterol, 3.4-4.9 mmol/L | 31-75 years; prior AMI or unstable angina; fasting total cholesterol, 4-7 mmol/L |
| Cointerventions | Aspirin (37%); beta blockers (57%) | None | Aspirin (83%); beta blockers (40%) | None | Aspirin (82%); beta blockers (47%) |
| Duration of follow-up (years) | 5.4 (median) | 4.9 (mean) | 5.0 (median) | 5.2 (mean) | 6.1 (mean) |

### Patients

| | | | | | |
|---|---|---|---|---|---|
| Number | 4444 | 6595 | 4159 | 6605 | 9014 |
| Mean age (years) | 58.6 | 55.2 | 59 | 58 | 62 |
| Males (%) | 81 | 100 | 86 | 85 | 83 |
| Smokers (%) | 26 | 44 | 21 | 12 | 10 |
| With diabetes mellitus (%) | 5 | 1 | 15 | 2 | 9 |

### Baseline Serum Cholesterol Levels (mean)

| | | | | | |
|---|---|---|---|---|---|
| Total (mmol/L) | 6.8 | 7.0 | 5.4 | 5.7 | 5.6 |
| LDL (mmol/L) | 4.9 | 5.0 | 3.6 | 3.9 | 3.9 |

### Control Event Rates

| | | | | | |
|---|---|---|---|---|---|
| For death | 11.5% | 4.1% | 9.4% | 0.44% | 14.1% |
| For AMI | 22.6% | 7.9% | 10% | 0.56% | 10.3% |

| Trial | 4S[20] | WOSCOPS[21] | CARE[22] | AFCAPS/TexCAPS[23] | LIPID[24] |
|---|---|---|---|---|---|
| **Treatment Effects** **% Change in Lipids (Active Treatment vs Placebo)** | | | | | |
| Total cholesterol | -25% | -20% | -20% | -18% | -18% |
| LDL cholesterol | -35% | -26% | -28% | -25% | -25% |
| HDL cholesterol | +8% | +5% | +5% | +6% | +5% |
| Triglycerides | -10% | -12% | -14% | -15% | -11% |
| **Relative risk reductions** | | | | | |
| For death (95% CI) | 30% (15%-42%) | 22% (0-40%) | 9% (−12%- 26%) | -4% (CIs not given) | 22% (13%- 31%) |
| For AMI (95% CI) | 27% (20%-34%) | 31% (17%- 43%) | 25% (8%-39%) | 40% (17%- 57%) | 29% (18%- 38%) |
| **Number Needed to Treat*** | | | | | |
| To prevent one death[†] | 27 (5 years) | 111 (5 years) | 125 (5 years) | 5000 to harm[‡] | 32 (6 years) |
| To prevent one AMI | 10 (5 years) | 42 (5 years) | 40 (5 years) | 435 (5 years) | 34 (6 years) |

4S indicates Scandinavian Simvastatin Survival Study; WOSCOPS, West of Scotland Coronary Prevention Study; CARE, Cholesterol and Recurrent Events Trial; AFCAPS/TexCAPS, Air Force/Texas Coronary Atherosclerosis Prevention Study; LIPID, Long-term Intervention With Pravastatin in Ischaemic Disease Study; AMI, acute myocardial infarction.

\* Point estimates only

† Years in parentheses indicate number of years needed to treat that number of patients to prevent 1 event.

‡ Since all-cause mortality was nonsignificantly increased in active treatment arm, results are presented as number needed to treat to cause one death.

## Level 1 Studies

*Level 1 studies* comprise randomized trials providing direct comparisons of the drug of interest with other drugs of the same class, rather than with a placebo, for their effects on important outcomes.

Although direct comparisons from RCTs generate the strongest evidence for the decision maker, there are still issues clinicians must consider (see Table 2B3-7). First, at least one of the drugs should have been shown to have a clinically important impact vs placebo in previous trials carried out in a population that is similar to that of the current trial. Second, the choice of appropriate dose for each drug is a complicated issue, as this will affect the outcomes and safety profiles for both drugs. Finally, one must carefully consider the trial size and methods before equivalence of two drugs. Equivalence trials require much larger sample sizes than standard trials[9] (see Part 2B2, "Therapy and Understanding the Results, Confidence Intervals") and laxity in trial conduct or patient compliance will tend to mask any real differences between drugs.

The choice of important outcomes for level 1 studies depends on the target intervention. In the case of therapies designed to prevent or arrest atherosclerosis (such as statins), this implies long-term efficacy data on events such as myocardial infarction, stroke, and all-cause mortality. On the other hand, for interventions designed to treat symptomatic diseases (such as gastroesophageal reflux disease), important outcomes could include symptom scores and other quality-of-life measures.

Although there are examples of level 1 evidence in other branches of medicine (such as head-to-head trials of the selective 5-hydroxytryptamine type-3 receptor antagonists for postoperative nausea and vomiting,[10, 11]) they occur rarely in the cardiovascular literature. Our literature search failed to find any level 1 evidence for statins.

## Level 2 Studies

*Level 2 studies* comprise (1) RCTs providing direct comparisons of the drug of interest with other drugs of the same class rather than with a placebo for their effects on validated surrogate outcomes or (2) comparisons across two or more trials comparing active agents with placebos, rather than with one another, for effects on clinically important outcomes or validated surrogate outcomes.

Although ecologic studies, cohort studies, and RCTs with prestatin lipid-lowering agents supported the lipid-lowering hypothesis (ie, that lowering LDL cholesterol lowers the risk of atherosclerotic heart disease),[12] it was not until the publication of the large-scale statin trials[13-17] (see Table 2B3-8 for full description of trials and acronyms used in this section) consistently linking reductions in LDL cholesterol to reductions in morbidity and mortality that were confident accepting the surrogate endpoint of LDL-cholesterol lowering as a proxy for patient-important outcomes. Thus, to accept direct comparisons for surrogate outcomes as level 2 evidence, at least one of the drugs being compared must have demonstrated efficacy in long-term trials with patient-important outcomes.

Although a randomized trial[18] comparing four statins for their effects on LDL cholesterol, HDL cholesterol, and triglycerides over an 8-week period would be an example of level 2 evidence, it is important also to incorporate considerations of the size and duration of trials in the decision-making process (as we will discuss later in this section).

On the other hand, one can make a number of level 2 comparisons among various statins. For example, one can compare the treatment effects seen with simvastatin vs pravastatin in secondary prevention trials (such as the 4S[13] and LIPID[17] studies; see Table 2B3-8). Although consistency of effects in such comparisons would be strong evidence for the presence of a class effect, these comparisons are less useful in determining whether one drug is more efficacious than another since the advantages of randomization are lost because the comparison is essentially that is between two or more cohorts (see Part 2E, "Summarizing the Evidence, When to Believe a Subgroup Analysis"). In addition to the potential biases outlined in Table 2B3-7, there is also the possibility of confounding between a patient's risk/responsiveness and exposure to a particular treatment in those situations where patients from different trials have different risk status. In other words, drugs may be equally effective, but one may appear superior because it was tested in a population that is more responsive to the intervention. This could occur if, for example, we compared the statin used in a primary prevention trial (such as lovastatin in AFCAPS/TexCAPS[16]) with another statin tested in a secondary prevention trial (such as simvastatin in 4S[13]). For instance, the relative risk reduction may be larger in secondary prevention trials, regardless of which statin is used. If this were the case, one would risk attributing a larger effect to the drug used in the secondary prevention trial, when the difference had nothing at all to do with the drug. Comparisons such as these, across studies of patients at varying risk, would be valid only when relative risk reduction is independent of baseline risk, an assumption that some have questioned for the statins.[19-24]

It is theoretically possible to compare the efficacy of two drugs tested in separate placebo-controlled trials. As outlined by Bucher et al,[25] an indirect estimate of the association between drugs A and B can be obtained by comparing the odds ratio (OR), or relative risk, from studies of drug A vs placebo (p) and from studies comparing drug B vs placebo: $OR_{A vs B} = OR_{A vs p} / OR_{B vs p}$. However, this assumes that none of the potential biases outlined in Table 2B3-9 are operative and that an intervention's treatment effect is consistent across different patient subgroups. Furthermore, these indirect estimates may provide substantially different effect-size estimates than direct comparisons of drug A against drug B. For example, a systematic review of strategies to prevent *Pneumocystis carinii* pneumonia in HIV-positive patients documented that the indirect comparison of trimethoprim-sulfamethoxazole (T-S) vs dapsone/pyrimethamine (D/P) suggested a much larger effect size from T-S (OR, 0.37; 95% CI, 0.21-0.65) than was seen in the direct comparisons (overall OR, 0.64 in the nine trials of T-S vs D/P; 95% CI, 0.45-0.90).[25] Thus, the strength of inference from indirect comparisons is limited.

Level 3 studies and level 4 studies have numerous flaws, as outlined below, and are best viewed as exercises in hypothesis generation.

## Level 3 Studies

*Level 3 studies* comprise (1) comparisons across subgroups from different placebo-controlled trials or (2) comparisons across placebo-controlled trials in which outcomes are restricted to unvalidated surrogate markers.

In addition to the biases that affect higher-level studies, comparisons based on subgroup analyses are potentially flawed (Table 2B3-7). Both simple statistics and experience have taught us that many initial subgroup conclusions (especially when they are the result of *data-dredging*) are subsequently shown to be wrong (see Part 2E, "Summarizing the Evidence, When to Believe a Subgroup Analysis"). An example of such a comparison would be looking at the efficacy of simvastatin in the 4S subgroup with the lowest lipid levels (241 patients with total cholesterol levels ranging from 5.5 to 6.24 mmol/L)[20] vs the efficacy of pravastatin in the CARE subgroup with comparable lipid profiles (2087 patients with total cholesterol levels ranging from 5.4 to 6.21 mmol/L).[15]

Level 3 evidence may also include the use of surrogate markers that, although they may lie along a recognized pathogenetic pathway from mechanisms of action to important clinical outcomes, have not been validated in long-term randomized controlled trials. This would involve, for example, making inferences about reduction in fractures from the effects on bone density of two different bisphosphanates in two independent randomized trials.

## Level 4 Studies

*Level 4 studies* comprise comparisons involving or confined to nonrandomized evidence. Evidence yielded from level 4 studies is possible only for conditions such as hypertension or hyperlipidemia, in which there are a large number of potential treatments that are commonly used by practitioners. Nonrandomized evidence can include cohort or case-control studies, modeling studies (using risk prediction equations such as that derived from the Framingham data[26]), or outcomes research using administrative databases. Although these type of analyses can provide useful insights particularly with respect to dose-response relationships,[27] they are best viewed as exercises in hypothesis generation. In particular, outcomes research studies, originally developed to determine whether the efficacy of interventions proved in randomized trials have their anticipated impacts at a population level, have sometimes been used to pursue the primary determination of efficacy—a purpose for which they were not intended (see Part 2B, "Therapy and Harm, Outcomes of Health Services"). When used for this latter purpose, in addition to the limitations common with the other observational data listed in Table 2B3-9, they present unique problems in interpretation that restrict the validity of inferences drawn from them about the relative efficacy of medications from the same class.[28]

Advocates of pravastatin suggest that it has anti-inflammatory properties beyond those of other statins that may lead to a reduction in coronary events (including myocardial infarction and coronary death) beyond that achieved by lipid reduction. An example of level 4 evidence is a recent reanalysis of the

WOSCOPS database that explored this hypothesis. In this study, investigators compared the observed coronary event rates in pravastatin-treated patients to those predicted from the Framingham coronary event risk equation.[20] The investigators used the constellation of risk factors and mean on-treatment cholesterol levels observed in the trial to determine the expected event rate, finding a greater reduction in events than one would expect from the difference in cholesterol levels between the two groups. They inferred that pravastatin may have an efficacy exceeding that of other statins.[20]

# OTHER CONSIDERATIONS

## Amount of Efficacy Evidence

Thus far, we have focused on the validity of the evidence. However, it is important also to recognize that other factors—the number, size, and duration of studies—are essential in the decision-making process. Certainly, the superiority of one drug within a class can be definitively established only with level 1 evidence. However, although level 1 evidence would be ideal for establishing that a group of drugs exert a class effect (ie, by showing narrow confidence limits around the difference between drugs), we recognize that such evidence rarely is available. Furthermore, it is unlikely to ever be available for many classes of drugs, owing to difficulties in funding and conducting such large trials that are unlikely to appeal to researchers, manufacturers, or funding agencies. In this situation, the amount of level 2 evidence becomes important. For instance, one would be more confident in concluding the existence of a class effect if there were a number of placebo-controlled trials demonstrating that various drugs from the same class had similar treatment effects. However, our intent here is not to set a single level that must be achieved before a drug can be claimed to be superior to others in its class or before a class effect can be established. These are decisions that individual clinicians or policy makers must make, taking into account their local circumstances and individual confidence levels.

## Drug Safety

During the past decade, drugs within the same class that have often proved to have different safety profiles (for example, practolol causes sclerosing peritonitis and keratoconjunctivitis, whereas other beta blockers do not cause these conditions; ticlopidine causes more neutropenia than clopidogrel; phenylbutazone causes agranulocytosis, whereas other nonsteroidal anti-inflammatory agents do not). Although not the primary focus of this section, considerations of drug safety are part of any treatment or purchasing decision, and we therefore offer a set of levels of evidence for determining safety in Table 2B3-9. The first tests of a drug in humans (*phase I studies*) are designed to determine the maximally tolerated dose, and clinical trials (*phase II* and *phase III studies*) generally are designed to determine the efficacy of the drug. As such, the sample sizes of neither are adequate to detect uncommon adverse effects. The inverse rule of 3 tells us that to be 95% sure of seeing at least one adverse drug reaction that occurs once in every $x$ patients, you need to follow $3x$ patients.[29] Given the size and duration of most clinical trials, adverse effects that occur in fewer than one in 1000 participants or that take more than 6 months to appear generally will remain undetected.[30]

TABLE 2B3-9

## Levels of Evidence for Comparing the Safety of Drugs Within the Same Class

| Level | Properties | Advantages | Threats to Validity |
|-------|-----------|------------|---------------------|
| 1 | RCTs | Only design that will permit the detection of adverse effects when the adverse effect is similar to the event that treatment is trying to prevent | Underpowered for detecting adverse effects |
| 2 | Cohort | Prospective data collection, defined cohort | Critically depends on follow-up, classification, and measurement accuracy |
| 3 | Case-control | Inexpensive and quickly performed | Selection and recall bias; temporal relationship may not be clear |
| 4 | Postmarketing surveillance | If sufficiently large, can detect rare but important adverse effects | No (or unmatched) control group; critically depends on follow-up, classification, and measurement accuracy |
| 5 | Case series | Inexpensive and quickly performed | Small sample size; selection bias; no control group |
| 6 | Case reports | Inexpensive and quickly performed | Small sample size; selection bias; no control group |

Aside from generally being too small to detect rare side effects, randomized controlled trials have other limitations as a methodology for estimating drug toxicity. Researchers conducting RCTs tend to focus on reduction of negative target outcomes and often do not invest resources in close or comprehensive toxicity monitoring. In addition, such trials often exclude patients at high risk for drug toxicity. Because of these limitations, RCTs are at risk of underestimating drug toxicity.

Nevertheless, when investigators rigorously monitor possible toxic effects, RCTs remain the strongest design for detecting real differences in adverse effects such as the different rates of intracranial bleeding with different thrombolytic agents,[31,32] and rigorous meta-analysis of such trials can give an unbiased estimate of excess hazards. In the absence of good RCT data regarding toxicity, we believe that premarketing safety data must be considered preliminary; large *phase IV studies* (or systematic analysis of postmarketing surveillance data) are necessary to confirm the safety of new drugs.

## Convenience and Compliance

Although once-a-day medications are more convenient and usually have higher compliance rates than drugs that require multiple doses during one day, evidence on drug compliance derived from trials may translate poorly into clincal practice. For instance, although compliance with the various statins during the course of the trials described in Table 2B3-8 ranged from 90% to 94%, analyses of administrative databases in Canada and the United States[33] revealed that only 50% of statin-treated patients were still taking their medication 1 year after it was prescribed.

## Cost

Faced with a decision as to whether a new drug should be offered to eligible patients within a given population, clinicians and policymakers (including, for instance, those responsible for deciding whether a drug will be available to beneficiaries of a drug benefit plan may have different (although not mutually exclusive) perspectives. For clinicians, this decision usually hinges on the efficacy, safety, convenience, compliance, and cost of the new drug vs the old one, as well as the applicability of the trial evidence to their patient.[34] However, for policymakers these issues will form only one piece of the puzzle, and they must also evaluate drug efficiency (". . . the effects or end results achieved in relation to the effort expended in terms of money, resources, and time"),[35] affordability, and what, in terms of other health resources foregone, will be the cost if resources are allocated toward a new drug (*opportunity costs*). The efficiency of any intervention is determined by formal economic analysis (see Part 2F, "Moving From Evidence to Action, Economic Analysis"). Although *cost-minimization analysis* is the simplest and least controversial of the economic analysis techniques, it requires proof that the outcomes with both alternatives are the same. As this rarely exists, the policymaker must rely on other types of analyses (*cost-effectiveness, cost-benefit*, or *cost-utility analyses*) that involve varying degrees of assumption and guesswork. As pointed out by Naylor and colleagues,[36] economic analyses should be viewed as "promising, clearly helpful, still in need of refinement and open, like any new technology, to both wise use and well-intentioned abuse."

Further hampering the policymaker's task, the decision as to whether a new drug is efficient enough to warrant its adoption depends critically on the social, political, and economic realities of their particular health care setting. Thus, attempts to establish universal cutpoints, using cost/quality-adjusted life-year (QALY) ratios, have been largely unsuccessful.[37] Although there are occasions where there is compelling evidence for adoption or a drug (ie, the new drug is as effective or more effective than others of its class and is less costly) or rejection of a drug (ie, the new drug is less effective than others of its class and is more costly), much of the time the policymaker is operating in a cost-utility gray zone between these two extremes.[36]

## USING THE GUIDE

Let us return to the opening clinical scenario. Given the qualitative consistency of the RRR for acute myocardial infarction in patients treated with three of the statins in large trials with clinically important outcomes (Table 2B3-8) and the convincing nature of LDL-cholesterol lowering as a surrogate outcome,[12, 22, 38-40] you conclude that there is a class effect of statin drugs on the occurrence of ischemic heart disease. In the apparent absence of differences in safety or compliance profile between the various statins, you decide to pursue a cost-minimization strategy. Although the newer statin has been evaluated only for cholesterol-lowering efficacy in a short-term trial (ie, one of less than 6 months' duration), you decide to prescribe it, as it is the least expensive statin in his local setting.

## CLINICAL RESOLUTION

We cannot expect routine achievement of the ideal of evaluating every drug in each class (and, indeed, every dose and every formulation) in RCTs with active comparators from the same class for their effects on important outcomes. Advocates of newer drugs within a class must provide evidence of equivalence (or superiority) to the older agents and randomized comparative trials . . . remain the preferred evidentiary standard.[41] However, this gold standard is not always attainable, and in the case of the statins, RCTs would require very large sample sizes and long follow-up to permit the detection of significant differences in myocardial infarction or death between two different statins. Discussions about class effects will benefit from citing the levels of evidence behind the arguments and recognizing the strengths and weaknesses inherent in each study design.

# References

1. Skolnick AA. Drug firm suit fails to halt publication of Canadian Health Technology Report. *JAMA*. 1998;280:683-684.

2. Garg R, Yusuf S, for the Collaborative Group on ACE Inhibitor Trials. Overview of randomized trials of angiotensin-converting enzyme inhibitors on mortality and morbidity in patients with heart failure. *JAMA*. 1995;273:1450-1456.

3. Waldo AL, Camm AJ, deRuyter H, et al, for the SWORD Investigators. Effect of d-sotalol on mortality in patients with left ventricular dysfunction after recent and remote myocardial infarction: survival with oral d-sotalol. *Lancet*. 1996;348:7-12.

4. Yusuf S, Peto R, Lewis J, Collins R, Sleight P. Beta blockade during and after myocardial infarction: an overview of the randomized trials. *Prog Cardiovasc Dis*. 1985;27:335-371.

5. Boissel JP, Leizorovicz A, Picolet H, Peyrieux JC. Secondary prevention after high-risk acute myocardial infarction with low-dose acebutolol. *Am J Cardiol*. 1990;66:251-260.

6. McAlister FA, Teo KK. Antiarrhythmic therapies for the prevention of sudden cardiac death. *Drugs*. 1997;54:235-252.

7. Furberg CD, Psaty BM. Calcium antagonists: not appropriate as first line antihypertensive agents. *Am J Hypertens*. 1996;9:122-125.

8. Rosenson RS, Tangney CC. Antiatherothrombotic properties of statins: implications for cardiovascular event reduction. *JAMA*. 1998;279:1643-1650.

9. Donner A. Approaches to sample size estimation in the design of clinical trials—a review. *Stat Med*. 1984;3:199-214.

10. Naguib M, el Bakry AK, Khoshim MH, et al. Prophylactic antiemetic therapy with ondansetron, tropisetron, granisetron and metoclopramide in patients undergoing laparoscopic cholecystectomy: a randomized, double-blind comparison with placebo. *Can J Anaesth*. 1996;43:226-231.

11. Korttila K, Clergue F, Leeser J, et al. Intravenous dolasetron and ondansetron in prevention of postoperative nausea and vomiting: a multicenter, double-blind, placebo-controlled study. *Acta Anaesthesiol Scand*. 1997;41:914-922.

12. Law MR, Wald NJ, Thompson SG. By how much and how quickly does reduction in serum cholesterol concentration lower risk of ischaemic heart disease? *BMJ*. 1994;308:367-372.

13. Scandinavian Simvastatin Survival Study Group. Randomised trial of cholesterol lowering in 4444 patients with coronary heart disease: the Scandinavian Simvastatin Survival Study (4S). *Lancet*. 1994;344:1383-1389.

14. Shepherd J, Cobbe SM, Ford I, et al, for the West of Scotland Coronary Prevention Study Group. Prevention of coronary heart disease with pravastatin in men with hypercholesterolemia. *N Engl J Med*. 1995;333:1301-1307.

15. Sacks FM, Pfeffer MA, Moye LA, et al, for the Cholesterol and Recurrent Events Trial Investigators. The effect of pravastatin on coronary events after myocardial infarction in patients with average cholesterol levels. *N Engl J Med*. 1996;335:1001-1009.

16. Downs JR, Clearfield M, Weis S, et al, for the AFCAPS/TexCAPS Research Group. Primary prevention of acute coronary events with lovastatin in men and women with average cholesterol levels: results of AFCAPS/TexCAPS. Air Force/Texas Coronary Atherosclerosis Prevention Study. *JAMA*. 1998;279: 1615-1622.

17. The Long-term Intervention With Pravastatin in Ischaemic Disease (LIPID) Study Group. Prevention of cardiovascular events and death with pravastatin in patients with coronary heart disease and a broad range of initial cholesterol levels. *N Engl J Med*. 1998;339:1349-1357.

18. Jones P, Kafonek S, Laurora I, Hunninghake D. Comparative dose efficacy study of atorvastatin versus simvastatin, pravastatin, lovastatin, and fluvastatin in patients with hypercholesterolemia. *Am J Cardiol*. 1998;81:582-587.

19. Sacks FM, Moye LA, Davis BR, et al. Relationship between plasma LDL concentrations during treatment with pravastatin and recurrent coronary events in the cholesterol and recurrent events trial. *Circulation*. 1998;97:1446-1452.

20. Scandinavian Simvastatin Survival Study Group. Baseline serum cholesterol and treatment effect in the Scandinavian Simvastatin Survival Study (4S). *Lancet*. 1995;345:1274-1275.

21. West of Scotland Coronary Prevention Study Group. Influence of pravastatin and plasma lipids on clinical events in the West of Scotland Coronary Prevention Study (WOSCOPS). *Circulation*. 1998;97:1440-1445.

22. Fager G, Wiklund O. Cholesterol reduction and clinical benefit: are there limits to our expectations? *Arterioscler Thromb Vasc Biol*. 1997;17:3527-3533.

23. Davey Smith G, Song F, Sheldon TA. Cholesterol lowering and mortality: the importance of considering initial level of risk. *BMJ*. 1993;306:1367-1373.

24. Sacks FM, Gibson CM, Rosner B, Pasternak RC, Stone PH, for the Harvard Atherosclerosis Reversibility Project Research Group. The influence of pretreatment low density lipoprotein cholesterol concentrations on the effect of hypocholesterolemic therapy on coronary atherosclerosis in angiographic trials. *Am J Cardiol*. 1995;76:78C-85C.

25. Bucher HC, Guyatt GH, Griffith LE, Walter SD. The results of direct and indirect treatment comparisons in meta-analysis of randomized controlled trials. *J Clin Epidemiol*. 1997;50:683-691.

26. Anderson KM, Wilson PWF, Odell PM, Kannel WB. An updated coronary risk profile: a statement for health professionals. *Circulation*. 1991;83:356-362.

27. Psaty BM, Siscovick DS, Weiss NS, et al. Hypertension and outcomes research: from clinical trials to clinical epidemiology. *Am J Hypertens*. 1996;9:178-183.

28. Marshall WJS. Administrative databases: fact or fiction? *CMAJ*. 1998;158: 489-490.

29. Sackett DL, Haynes RB, Gent M, Taylor DW. Compliance. In: Inman WHW, ed. *Monitoring for Drug Safety*. Philadelphia: Lippincott; 1980.

30. McDonald CJ. Medical heuristics: the silent adjudicators of clinical practice. *Ann Intern Med*. 1996;124:56-62.

31. Third International Study of Infarct Survival Collaborative Group. ISIS-3: A randomised comparison of streptokinase vs. tissue plasminogen activator vs. anistreplase and of aspirin plus heparin vs. aspirin alone among 41 299 cases of suspected acute myocardial infarction. *Lancet*. 1992;339:753-770.

32. Gruppo Italiano per lo Studio della Sopravvivenza nell'Infarto Miocardico. GISSI-2: A factorial randomised trial of alteplase versus streptokinase and heparin versus no heparin among 12,490 patients with acute myocardial infarction. *Lancet*. 1990;336:65-71.

33. Avorn J, Monette J, Lacour A, et al. Persistence of use of lipid-lowering medications: a cross-national study. *JAMA*. 1998;279:1458-1462.

34. Dans AL, Dans LF, Guyatt GH, Richardson S, for the Evidence-Based Medicine Working Group. Users' guides to the medical literature, XIV: how to decide on the applicability of clinical trial results to your patient. *JAMA*. 1998;279:545-549.

35. Last JM. *A Dictionary of Epidemiology*. New York: Oxford University Press; 1995.

36. Naylor CD, Williams JI, Basinski A, Goel V. Technology assessment and cost-effectiveness analysis: misguided guidelines? *CMAJ*. 1993;148:921-924.

37. Laupacis A, Feeny D, Detsky AS, Tugwell PX. How attractive does a new technology have to be to warrant adoption and utilization? Tentative guidelines for using clinical and economic evaluations. *CMAJ*. 1992;146:473-481.

38. Gotto AM Jr. Cholesterol management in theory and practice. *Circulation*. 1997;96:4424-4430.

39. Grover SA, Paquet S, Levinton C, Coupal L, Zowall H. Estimating the benefits of modifying cardiovascular risk factors: a comparison of primary versus secondary prevention. *Arch Intern Med*. 1998;158:655-662.

40. Lacour A, Derderian F, Lelorier J. Comparison of efficacy and cost among lipid-lowering agents in patients with primary hypercholesterolemia. *Can J Cardiol*. 1998;14:355-361.

41. Tu JV, Naylor CD. Choosing among drugs of different price for similar indications. *Can J Cardiol*. 1998;14:349-351.

# THERAPY AND APPLYING THE RESULTS
## Qualitative Research

Mita Giacomini, Deborah Cook, and Gordon Guyatt

The following EBM Working Group members also made substantive contributions to this section: Trisha Greenhalgh, Eric Bass, Hui Lee, Lee Green, and Sharon Straus

## IN THIS SECTION

## CLINICAL SCENARIO

### How Might a Form That Records Patients' Wishes About End-of-Life Care Affect Patient-Physician Interaction?

**A**t a meeting of your hospital's Continuous Quality Improvement Committee, the last agenda item is an initiative "to enhance patient-clinician communication." The committee chair proposes that all medical charts include a form to record patient wishes about cardiopulmonary resuscitation and end-of-life care. The committee members agree in principle on the goals of enhanced communication and more accurate documentation of patient preferences. However, you raise concerns about how these forms might change the nature of end-of-life decision making and how they might even impair communication. As the meeting draws to a close, you pose a question to the group for discussion the following week: could end-of-life care preference forms unduly constrain dialogue between clinicians and patients or family members?

# FINDING THE EVIDENCE

Emerging from the meeting, you resolve to learn more about the influence of institutional record keeping on do-not-resuscitate (DNR) communication during acute illness. Back in your office, you log on to your computer and do a quick search of MEDLINE combining the search terms "resuscitation orders" (508 hits) and "patient-physician relations" (5040 hits) and "patient participation" (1680 hits)." Of 11 citations, one publication is a cultural analysis that you pick up from your hospital library en route to clinic.[1] The objectives of this study are directly relevant to your concern:

". . . to examine the use of the Limitations of Medical Care form in the context of actual hospital practice, . . . to evaluate interactive elements of the resuscitation decision, . . . [and] to explore what is said when discussing code status, how information is communicated among parties involved, and the meaning that underlies this communication."

*Quantitative research* (such as epidemiologic investigations and clinical trials) aims to test well-specified hypotheses concerning predetermined variables. These studies are essentially deductive in their approach; they begin with carefully considered hypotheses that the studies are designed to test. However, medicine is not only a quantitative science, but also is an interpretive art.[2] Interpretive research asks questions about social interactions using qualitative methods.[3] *Qualitative research* offers insight into social, emotional, and experiential phenomena in health care. Examples include inquiry about the meaning of illness to individuals and families, or about the attitudes and behavior of patients and clinicians. Qualitative research is inductive, aiming to discover important variables and to generate coherent theories and hypotheses. For example, Ventres et al[1] explored what patient-physician communication occurred during discussions about resuscitation and how the use of a standard form influenced communication between physicians and families about DNR orders. Another qualitative study probed why family members select certain processes for discontinuing life support.[4]

Just as clinicians use complementary types of information to draw clinical conclusions, complementary research methods are often useful to examine different aspects of a health problem.[5-7] Qualitative studies offer a rigorous alternative to armchair hypothesizing for areas in which insight may not be well established or for which conventional theories seem inadequate. Qualitative and quantitative studies make useful contributions to knowledge in themselves. They may also be used in tandem—qualitative investigation can be undertaken to generate theories and identify relevant variables and quantitative investigation can be undertaken to test the implied hypotheses about relationships between those variables. We refer readers elsewhere for details about how to conduct qualitative research,[8-12] as well as for further information concerning the attributes and limitations of qualitative vs quantitative research approaches.[13-19]

Our standard approach to using an article from the medical literature based on quantitative research in patient care is readily applicable to using an article based on qualitative research (Table 2B3-10). We ask: (1) Are the results of this study valid? (2) What are the results? and (3) How do the results apply to patient care?

**TABLE 2B3-10**

**Users' Guides for an Article Reporting the Results of Qualitative Research in Health Care**

**Are the Results Valid?**
- Was the choice of participants explicit and comprehensive?
- Was data collection sufficiently comprehensive and detailed?
- Were the data analyzed appropriately and the findings corroborated adequately?

**What Are the Results?**

**How Can I Apply the Results to Patient Care?**
- Does the study offer helpful theoretical conclusions?
- Does the study help me understand the context of my practice?
- Does the study help me understand my relationships with patients and their families?

# ARE THE RESULTS VALID?

The Methods section of a qualitative study should describe several aspects of the research design, including (1) the way study participants were selected, (2) the methods used to generate data, (3) the comprehensiveness of data collection, and (4) procedures for analyzing the data and validating the findings. General guidelines to help readers determine whether the findings of a qualitative study provide a valid picture of human experience and interaction are described below.

## Was the Choice of Participants Explicit and Comprehensive?

Qualitative studies discover and describe important influences and effects, particularly in terms of social dynamics and peoples' subjective realities.[3,20] Thus, the focus of a study may be the experience of individuals or the dynamic interactions of groups—or what we may learn from documents, artifacts, interactions, dialogues, or incidents.

The exploratory nature of qualitative research requires investigators not to prespecify a study population in strict terms, lest important people be overlooked. Consecutive or random selection of participants, common in quantitative research, is replaced by a conscious selection of a small number of individuals meeting particular criteria—a process called *purposive sampling*. This type of sampling usually aims to cover a range of potentially relevant social phenomena and perspectives from an appropriate array of data sources. Selection criteria often evolve over the course of analysis and investigators return repeatedly to the data to explore new cases or new angles. Purposive sampling might aim to represent any of the following: typical cases, unusual cases, critical cases, cases that reflect important political issues, or cases with connections to other cases (ie, *snowball sampling*).[21,22] Least compelling is the pursuit of merely convenient cases that are accessed most easily. Readers of qualitative studies should look for sound reasoning describing and justifying the participant selection strategies.

Having decided on a selection process, qualitative researchers need to sample a sufficient number of participants. The issue here is not one of adequate sample size in the statistical sense, but, rather, of achieving an adequate breadth of perspective to avoid presenting a misleading picture. Although careful purposive sampling can lead to considerable breadth of perspective with a small sample size, there will always be a minimal sample size that puts a study at risk of obtaining a narrow or idiosyncratic sample.

## USING THE GUIDE

Ventres et al[1] focused not on the patient but, rather, on the social interaction among several parties: patient, family members, nurses, social workers, clergy, and residents involved in resuscitation discussions about a particular patient. These researchers conducted their study over a period of 4 months, during which family practice residents identified eight hospitalized patients about whom they had discussions regarding resuscitation. The authors did not specify their criteria for choosing the two cases they ultimately summarized in detail, leaving readers unable to judge their appropriateness and how comprehensively they illustrate communication issues involving resuscitation directives in the hospital. Furthermore, examining only three cases in which resuscitation is discussed is unlikely to capture the diversity of perspectives, content, and styles found in such conversations, and it could produce a limited description. The authors themselves note that this small number of cases is a potential study limitation and that more variability may have yielded further insight into other possible structures of resuscitation discussions.

## Was Data Collection Sufficiently Comprehensive and Detailed?

Qualitative research will be valid insofar as it provides a comprehensive, detailed picture of experiences and interactions on which it focuses. Investigators must sample all relevant people and situations and use all appropriate data collection strategies. In terms of sampling all relevant people and situations, capturing the experiences of patients, families, physicians, nurses, other health care workers, and system managers may all be important.

In terms of data collection strategies, qualitative researchers have three basic strategies from which to choose (Figure 2B3-1). The first is to witness events and record them as they occur, the technical term for which is field observation. The second strategy is to question participants directly about their experience, known as the interview. Finally, researchers may review written material, known as document analysis. Clinicians should consider whether investigators have used all three sources of information—and if not, whether they could have obtained a more complete or accurate picture had they used other sources. Within each source, qualitative researchers have alternative methods from which to choose, and their choice may influence the validity of the results (Figure 2B3-1).

**FIGURE 2B3-1**

### Sources of Information in Qualitative Research

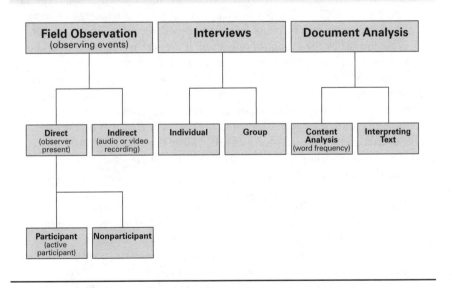

**Field Observation.** The purpose of field observation is to record social phenomena directly and prospectively. Investigators may spend time in the social milieu they are studying and record observations in the form of detailed field notes or journals, an approach called direct observation. Having chosen direct observation, they must consider how their presence might influence their findings and make further choices accordingly. In nonparticipant direct observation, the researcher stays relatively uninvolved. The crucial question for critical appraisal is whether in the particular social setting such nonparticipant observation will effectively be ignored by study participants, or might instead inadvertently influence participants' behavior. For example, a researcher in a crowded waiting room may go unnoticed and hence will be able to observe the natural unfolding of events. By contrast, in a clinic examining room she may be conspicuous—and significantly change the social interactions she is there to observe.

In nonparticipant direct observation, the researcher is acknowledged as a part of the social setting, either as a researcher per se or as a more directly involved actor (eg, social worker, ethicist, committee member, and so on). Again, the question for critical appraisal is whether the dual observer-participant role allows access to natural, candid social interactions among other participants in the setting.

The investigators may avoid the issue of their presence influencing participant behavior altogether by choosing to use video or audio recordings—indirect observation. However, this approach also has drawbacks. First, audio or video recorders can occupy a social role and be perceived by participants as partaking in surveillance, thus influencing participants' behavior. Second, recorders' observational powers are limited by their range of operation: if the action is moving around or if visual cues are missing, they may lose important information.

Regardless of the approach that investigators choose, they can never control the effect of the researcher or the researcher's equipment on the social setting (a common goal of experimental study designs). Interactions between researchers and those they study are paradoxically but necessarily regarded as both a useful source of data and a potential source of bias.[23] More than one observational technique (eg, personal observations and tape recordings of dialogue) sometimes can be used to capture more detailed data and to help analyze observer effects.

**Interviews.** A second potential source of information is the interview. The most popular interviews are semistructured in-depth individual interviews and focus groups. Structured approaches such as standardized questionnaires are usually inappropriate for qualitative research because they presuppose too much of what respondents might say and they do not allow respondents to relate experiences in their own terms. These problems limit the opportunity to gain insight into personal and social phenomena. In addition, they can impose the investigators' preconceived notions on the data.

The appropriate interview method depends on the topic. Individual interviews tend to be more useful than group interviews for evoking personal experiences and perspectives, particularly on sensitive topics. Group interviews tend to be more useful than individual interviews for capturing interpersonal dynamics, language, and culture. *Focus groups* can be appropriate for discussing emotionally sensitive topics if participants feel empowered speaking in the presence of peers; however, the public forum of a focus group can also inhibit candid disclosure.[24, 25] Critical readers should look for the rationale for choosing a particular approach and should assess its appropriateness for the topics addressed. Using more than one interview method may be helpful in capturing a wider range of information.

Document Analysis. Finally, documents such as medical charts, journals, correspondence, and other material artifacts can provide qualitative data.[26] These are especially useful in policy, historic, or organizational studies of health care. There are different approaches to the analysis of documents. One involves counting specific content elements (eg, frequencies of particular words), whereas the other involves interpreting text as one would interpret any other form of communication (eg, seeking nuances of meaning and considering context). The former approach, especially if used alone, rarely provides adequate information for a qualitative, interpretive analysis.

Regardless of the source and method investigators choose, to avoid focusing on particular, potentially misleading aspects of the data, the chosen approach must be comprehensive. Several aspects of a qualitative report indicate how extensively the investigators collected data: the number of observations, interviews, or documents; the duration of the observations; the duration of the study period; the diversity of units of analysis and data collection techniques; the number of investigators involved in collecting and analyzing data; and the degree of investigators' involvement in data collection and analysis notes.[27-30] Taping and transcribing interviews (or other dialogue) is desirable. Records of investigators' thoughts and experiences helps to isolate personal biases, as well as to use personal experiences as analytically useful information.[31] The details of the report should allow the clinician to see a clear correspondence between the empirical data and the interpreted findings.

How comprehensive and detailed was data collection in the study by Ventres et al? Both before and after the discussions, interviews were conducted with patients, family members, nurses, social workers, clergy, and physicians regarding the decision-making process. Including patients, family members, and several members of the health care team as participants in this study increased the number of perspectives from which the issue of resuscitation was considered. No key participants' perspectives seem to have been overlooked in the data collection.

In terms of data collection strategies, Ventres et al used three types: participant observation, audiotapes of discussions, and semistructured interviews. Details of the interview strategy and transcription process appear in appendixes following the article and provide additional information about the content of the interviews and techniques used to elicit responses. The investigators asked three types of questions to elicit opinions on contrasting hypothetical patient situations: *open-ended, semistructured, and contrast questions*. An observer also made written records of nonverbal interactions, which are not well captured by audiotape. Finally, the investigators recorded secondary interpretive data (ie, their personal interpretations of the discussions they observed). The use of multiple data collection methods and sources adds rigor to this study because it allows investigators to examine discussions of the limitations of medical care from several angles and to capture information with one method that may be overlooked with another method.

## Were the Data Analyzed Appropriately and the Findings Corroborated Adequately?

Qualitative researchers begin with a general exploratory question and preliminary concepts. They then collect relevant data, observe patterns in the data, organize these into a *conceptual framework*, and resume data collection to both explore and challenge this conceptual framework. This cycle may be repeated several times. The iterations among data collection, analysis, and theory development continues until a conceptual framework is well developed and further observations yield minimal or no new information to further challenge or elaborate the framework (a point variously referred to as *theoretical saturation*[32] or *informational redundancy*[33]). This analysis-stopping criterion is so basic to qualitative analysis that authors seldom declare that they have reached this point; they assume readers will understand.

In the course of analysis, key findings are also corroborated using multiple sources of information, a process called *triangulation*. Triangulation is a metaphor and does not mean literally that three or more sources are required. The appropriate number of sources will depend upon the importance of the findings, their implications for theory, and the investigators' confidence in their validity. Because no two qualitative data sources will generate exactly the same interpretation, much of the art of qualitative interpretation involves exploring why and how different information sources yield slightly different results.[34]

Readers may encounter several useful triangulation techniques for validating qualitative data and their interpretation in analysis.[35,36] *Investigator triangulation* requires more than one investigator to collect and analyze the raw data, such that the findings emerge through consensus between or among investigators. This is best accomplished by an investigative team. Use of external investigators is controversial because their involvement in the case could be too superficial to yield deep understanding.[35] If team members represent different disciplines, this helps to prevent personal or disciplinary biases of a single researcher from excessively influencing the findings. *Member checking* involves sharing draft study findings with the participants to inquire whether their viewpoints were faithfully interpreted, to determine whether there are gross errors of fact, and to ascertain whether the account makes sense to participants with different perspectives. *Theory triangulation*[37] is a process whereby emergent findings are corroborated with existing social science theories.[35] It is conventional for authors to report how their qualitative findings relate to prevailing social theory, although it is controversial whether such theories should be used to guide the research design or analysis.

Some qualitative research reports describe the use of qualitative analysis software packages. Readers should not equate the use of computers with analytic rigor. Such software is merely a data management tool offering efficient methods for storing, organizing, and retrieving qualitative data. These programs do not perform analysis. The investigators themselves conduct the analysis as they create the key words, categories, and logical relationships used to organize and interpret the electronic data. The validity of qualitative study findings depend on these investigator judgments, which cannot be programmed into software packages.

We indicated earlier that qualitative data collection must be comprehensive: adequate in its breadth and depth to yield a meaningful description. The closely related criterion for judging whether the data were analyzed appropriately is whether this comprehensiveness was determined in part by research results themselves, with the aims of challenging, elaborating, and corroborating the findings. This is most apparent when researchers state that they alternated between data collection and analysis, collected data with the purpose of elucidating the analysis-in-progress, collected data until analytic saturation or redundancy was reached, or triangulated findings using any of the methods mentioned.

Ventres et al[1] approached data coding using three broad preliminary concepts in patient-clinician communication: control, giving and withholding information, and attentiveness. Investigators commonly use sensible, broad conceptual categories such as these to help make sense of their data, but they also are commonly revised in the course of analysis. These investigators noted that data collection and analysis proceeded iteratively, reporting that "data collected and analyzed on the first members of the sample influenced the collection of information on subsequent members."[1] They used several triangulation techniques, including methodologic triangulation (using several data collection methods involving participant observation, audiotaping, and semistructured interviews), investigator triangulation (use of duplicate interpretation of audiotapes), disciplinary triangulation (interpretation from clinical, anthropologic, psychiatric, and sociologic perspectives), and member checking (assessment by both professional and lay participants in the study).

In addition, the authors report that the principal author and a sociolinguist reviewed the audiotapes blinded to "all but necessary case information." However, it is unclear which data were and were not available to these investigators prior to analysis. Readers cannot assume that blinding necessarily improved the rigor of the analysis, as limiting access to data also limits investigators' ability to make well-informed interpretations of possibly complex social interactions.

We note that the final findings of Ventres et al quite appropriately do not strictly follow their three provisional analytic categories (control, information-giving, and attentiveness), but instead reveal more specific and concrete dynamics focusing on (1) the tendency of the Limitations of Medical Care form to frame discussions in a way that excludes patient values and beliefs, (2) family-physician differences in reasoning style, and (3) consequential confusion between instrumental treatment decisions and more general goals of care.[1] This progression suggests that the conceptual findings did develop as a result of the empirical observations. The authors relate their findings back to general social, health policy, and ethical concerns about who is—and who should be—in control of limitations-of-care decision processes.

## USING THE GUIDE

**W**e conclude that the Ventres et al[1] study had marked limitations with respect to our first validity criterion, the selection and number of cases. The breadth of the sample was probably too narrow to capture the diversity of communication and decision-making styles concerning end-of-life treatment, and the basis on which the authors chose their three cases is uncertain. However, the investigators were extremely comprehensive in their exploration of the cases. Analytic rigor is evidenced by the corroboration (triangulation) of findings among different sources of data, multidisciplinary investigators, and critiques of the analysis by study participants. Thus, the study will provide some insight into the impact of a Limitations of Medical Care form on patient-clinician communication, and we can move to consider the results and how we can apply those results to the care of patients.

# WHAT ARE THE RESULTS?

The product of a qualitative study is a narrative that tries to represent faithfully and accurately the social worlds or phenomena studied.[38] A good qualitative report provides enough descriptive detail to evoke a vivid picture of the social setting or interactions studied. To do this, authors typically illustrate key findings with data excerpts from field notes, interview transcripts, or documents. These data should clearly support the main points and offer contextual detail. The use of examples and references to sources gives the reader insight into the nature of the social phenomenon under consideration as well as the sensibility of how investigators interpreted it.

In their Results section, Ventres et al[1] describe the case histories of two patients and those involved in their care. These two stories are organized chronologically (rather than conceptually), which helps draw the reader into the events and discussions as they unfold. The narratives are liberally illustrated with excerpts from interviews and taped discussions, which give readers more intimate insight into the situations studied. The excerpts also support the authors' interpretations of the structure of these life-support discussions (ie, as involving characteristic content, dyadic conversation, and ambiguity that pervades the discussion). Although the exposition is restricted to two cases and selected excerpts, the information is rich and coherently organized. In their narrative, Ventres and colleagues describe how use of the Limitation of Medical Care form, which is intended to facilitate decision making, made clinician-patient dialogue routine to meet bureaucratic needs, and narrowed rather than enhanced communication about resuscitation.

# HOW CAN I APPLY THE RESULTS TO PATIENT CARE?

## Does the Study Offer Helpful Theoretical Conclusions?

Qualitative inquiry aims to develop theoretical conclusions. Other authors have described systematic approaches to theory development.[32, 39-46] Although the most important test of a theory may be its intuitive appeal—do you find the constructs compelling?—you may gauge its usefulness by certain general characteristics.

To be useful, a theory should be adequately coherent, comprehensive, and relevant. Elder and Miller[47] suggest that coherent theory possesses the qualities of parsimony (ie, it will invoke a minimal number of assumptions), consistency (ie, it is in accordance with what is already known and inconsistencies are well explored and explained), clarity (ie, it expresses ideas evocatively and sensibly), and fertility (ie, it suggests promising directions for further investigation). On a concrete level, narrative arguments should be logical and plausible; metaphors should provide useful analogies; and illustrative frameworks such as diagrams should meaningfully label the elements and relationships depicted.

Theory consists of concepts and their relationships. Concepts are the basic building blocks of theory. Often (but not always), concepts will be organized hierarchically, including one overriding concept (perhaps a useful metaphor), a few broad categories within it, and a series of subcategories within those categories. Relationships between conceptual categories may take a form similar to quantitative relationships between variables (eg, characterized by changes in one variable causing an increase or decrease in another variable). Alternatively, categories may have qualitative effects on each other (eg, one phenomenon may frame the form that another phenomenon can take).

Authors may use one of several devices to explain how they developed theoretical conclusions. For example, a report may offer a chronological description of the experience of initial disorientation investigators felt on entering the field—and from there lead the reader through the key discovery experiences that form the key elements of the author's findings.

Conceptual frameworks are strongest when their categories or variables embrace a full range of observed empirical phenomena. Although illustrative data excerpts offer only glimpses into the analytic process, they help demonstrate how the investigators interpreted the data. If the illustrative examples do not seem to fit well with the interpretive explanation, the validity of the rest of the analysis comes into question.

Readers should look for whether the results of a qualitative research report address the way the findings relate to other theory in the field. An empirically developed theory need not agree with existing beliefs. Regardless of whether it agrees or not, authors should describe its relationship to prevailing theories and beliefs in a critical manner.[48, 49]

Ventres et al[1] offer relatively pragmatic theoretical conclusions about how an administrative form can both reflect and reinforce mechanistic objective-oriented dialogue facilitating the neglect of patient needs, values, and beliefs. In this study, the hospital's Limitation of Medical Care form was used as both the foundation for dialogue and the vehicle for expression of patient wishes. Ventres et al describe how the form—together with conventional physician communication styles—can have the adverse effect of structuring conversations to obstruct candid exchange of beliefs and feelings and obscure patient and family wishes. Ideally, the study might have developed a more comprehensive model of communication about life support or of how administrative forms express (or suppress) meaningful health directives. The report offers modest formal theory, but it does offer valid, evocative evidence of what occurred during life-support discussions.

The study's findings allow the practicing clinician to stand apart from the clinical encounter and view some common communication dynamics from a critical distance. Normally, clinicians are directly involved in their discussions with patients and families and cannot both participate actively in a conversation and analyze it objectively. Clinicians reading the Ventres et al study[1] may recognize in the scenarios something of themselves, the people they care for, and the administrative forms they use. The study highlights the potential tyranny of administrative forms when they are used to structure sensitive personal discussions. The theoretical insight that forms can play an active role in communication may help clinicians recognize this dynamic in other settings.

## Does the Study Help Me Understand the Context of My Practice?

One criterion for the generalizability of a qualitative study is whether it provides a useful road map for readers to understand and navigate in similar social settings themselves. The North American cultural value of autonomy was encoded in 1991 by the US Congress in the Patient Self-Determination Act;[16] since then, many health care systems have created documents such as advance directives and other decision tools to systematize conversations about life support.

The article by Ventres et al[1] invites us to contemplate this policy trend critically. Readers may reflect on how business metaphors have infiltrated clinical practice and how these types of resuscitation documents symbolically contractualize health care at the end of life, especially when patients are referred to as "clients" and health care workers are referred to as "providers." In this study, discussions about resuscitation were intervention specific, focusing on a series of basic and advanced life-support technologies, in part due to the task-oriented prompts of the Limitation of Medical Care form. One family member of a patient unable to speak for himself explained that "resuscitation was not appropriate in Indian culture."[1] The resident continued to describe the technical details of resuscitation even after the family had made it clear that none were desired, which made this family member feel as though the physician did not really trust the family's decision (or implicitly, their portrayal of their loved one's wishes, were he able to speak for himself).

## Does the Study Help Me Understand My Relationships With Patients and Their Families?

Interpretive research offers clinicians an understanding of roles and relationships. Many qualitative studies of interest to clinicians focus on communication among patients, families, and caregivers. Other studies describe behaviors of these groups, either in isolation or during interactions with others.

In the study by Ventres et al,[1] the acuity and severity of the patients' illness meant that dialogue typically occurred between resident physicians and family members, rather than with patients themselves. The investigators studied only a small number of patients and physicians-in-training, all in a university hospital, limiting the range of discussion styles that were identified. Some clinicians may be more likely to have prior long-term relationships with patients than the family practice residents in the setting of this study, allowing conversations about wishes regarding desired intensity of care to occur in advance—in the relative comfort of the outpatient setting, rather than during an acute illness episode. Regardless of whether you work with residents or not (or whether you are a resident yourself), a report such as this one affords an opportunity to evaluate frankly how you broach end-of-life discussions with hospitalized patients and to ask yourself whether you can relate to the communication styles described in the study—and if you can, what implications this has for your practice.

# CLINICAL RESOLUTION

Reflecting on the article by Ventres and colleagues,[1] you think back to the Continuous Quality Improvement Committee meeting you attended this morning about patient-clinician communication. Since your hospital's proposal for a Limitations of Medical Care form is similar to the one described in the article by Ventres et al, you wonder to what extent the introduction of this form might shift your own discussions with patients away from eliciting illness experiences and understanding values toward a more routine dialogue with patients or next-of-kin regarding the technologic aspects of basic and advanced life support.

You decide that at the next meeting you will share the evidence you found about the risk of making conversations between clinicians and patients mundane, should such a Limitation of Medical Care form be introduced at your hospital. You plan to precirculate the Ventres et al[1] article, and you recommend that the committee use it to help outline the potential advantages and disadvantages of introducing such a document in your hospital. Meanwhile, if this form is adopted, you plan to request that the committee evaluate its influence on end-of-life discussions, using multidisciplinary qualitative research methods.

# References

1. Ventres W, Nichter M, Reed R, Frankel R. Limitation of medical care: an ethnographic analysis. *J Clin Ethics*. 1993;4:134-145.

2. Battista RN, Hodge MJ, Vineis P. Medicine, practice, and guidelines: the uneasy juncture of science and art. *J Clin Epidemiol*. 1995;48:875-880.

3. Hughes J. The interpretive alternative. In: *The Philosophy of Social Research*. New York: Longman; 1990:89-112.

4. Tilden VP, Tolle SW, Garland MJ, Nelson CA. Decisions about life-sustaining treatment: impact of physicians' behaviors on the family. *Arch Intern Med*. 1995;155:633-638.

5. Rosenfield PL. The potential of transdisciplinary research for sustaining and extending linkages between the health and social sciences. *Soc Sci Med*. 1992;35:1343-1357.

6. Stange KC, Zyzanski SJ. Integrating qualitative and quantitative research methods. *Fam Med*. 1989;21:448-451.

7. Goering P, Streiner D. Reconcilable differences: the marriage of qualitative and quantitative methods. *Can J Psychiatry*. 1996;41:491-497.

8. Denzin NK, Lincoln YS, eds. *Handbook of Qualitative Research*. Thousand Oaks: Sage Publications; 1994.

9. Corbin J, Strauss A. Grounded theory research: procedures, canons, and evaluative criteria. *Qualitative Sociology*. 1990;13:3-23.

10. Strauss A, Corbin J. Grounded theory methodology: an overview. In: Denzin NK, Lincoln YS, eds. *Handbook of Qualitative Research*. Thousand Oaks: Sage Publications; 1994:273-285.

11. Lincoln YS, Guba EG. *Naturalistic Inquiry*. London: Sage Publications; 1985.

12. Patton MQ. *Qualitative Evaluation and Research Methods*. London: Sage Publications; 1990.

13. Poses RM, Isen AM. Qualitative research in medicine and health care: questions and controversy. *J Gen Intern Med*. 1998;13:32-38.

14. Robling MR, Owen PA, Allery LA, et al. In defense of qualitative research: responses to the Poses and Isen Perspectives article [letter to the editor]. *J Gen Intern Med*. 1998;13:64-72.

15. Guba EG, Lincoln YS. Competing paradigms in qualitative research. In: Denzin NK, Lincoln YS, eds. *Handbook of Qualitative Research*. Thousand Oaks: Sage Publications; 1994:105-117.

16. Morse J. Is qualitative research complete? *Qualitative Health Res*. 1996;6:3-5.

17. Smith JK. Quantitative versus qualitative research: an attempt to clarify the issue. *Educ Researcher*. 1983;12:6-13.

18. Neumann WL. The meanings of methodology. In: *Social Research Methods*. Boston: Allyn & Bacon; 1991:43-66.

19. Waitzkin H. On studying the discourse of medical encounters: a critique of quantitative and qualitative methods and a proposal for reasonable compromise. *Med Care*. 1990;28:473-488.

20. Lincoln YS, Guba EG. Constructed realities. In: *Naturalistic Inquiry*. London: Sage Publications; 1985:70-91.

21. Patton MQ. Designing qualitative studies. In: *Qualitative Evaluation and Research Methods*. London: Sage Publications;1990:145-198.

22. Lincoln YS, Guba EG. Doing what comes naturally. In: *Naturalistic Inquiry*. London: Sage Publications; 1985:187-220.

23. Lincoln YS, Guba EG. The disturbing and disturbed observer. In: *Naturalistic Inquiry*. London: Sage Publications; 1985:92-109.

24. Kitzinger J. Qualitative research: introducing focus groups. *BMJ*. 1995;311: 299-302.

25. Steward DW, Shamdasani PN. Group dynamics and focus group research. In: *Focus Groups: Theory and Practice*. London: Sage Publications; 1990:33-50.

26. Hodder I. The interpretation of documents and material culture. In: Denzin N, Lincoln Y. *Handbook of Qualitative Research*. London: Sage Publications; 1994:393-402.

27. Kirk J, Miller ML. *Reliability and Validity in Qualitative Research*. London: Sage Publications; 1986.

28. Schatzman L, Strauss AL. Strategy for recording. In: *Field Research: Strategies for a Natural Sociology*. Englewood Cliffs: Prentice-Hall; 1973:94-107.

29. Lincoln YS, Guba EG. Implementing the naturalistic inquiry. In: *Naturalistic Inquiry*. London: Sage Publications; 1985:250-288.

30. Patton MQ. Fieldwork strategies and observation methods. In: *Qualitative Evaluation and Research Methods*. London: Sage Publications; 1990:199-276.

31. Patton MQ. Qualitative analysis and interpretation. In: *Qualitative Evaluation and Research Methods*. London: Sage Publications; 1990:371-459.

32. Glaser B, Strauss AL. The constant comparative methods of qualitative analysis. In: *Discovery of Grounded Theory*. New York: Aldine de Gruyter; 1967: 101-116.

33. Lincoln YS, Guba EG. Designing a naturalistic inquiry. In: *Naturalistic Inquiry*. London: Sage Publications; 1985:221-249.

34. Stake R. Triangulation. In: *The Art of Case Study Research*. London: Sage Publications; 1995:107-120.

35. Lincoln YS, Guba EG. Establishing trustworthiness. In: *Naturalistic Inquiry*. London: Sage Publications; 1985:289-331.

36. Patton MQ. Enhancing the quality and credibility of qualitative analysis. In: *Qualitative Evaluation and Research Methods*. London: Sage Publications; 1990:460-506.

37. Denzin NK. *Sociological Methods*. New York: McGraw Hill; 1978.

38. Altheide DL, Johnson JM. Criteria for assessing interpretive validity in qualitative research. In: Denzin N, Lincoln Y. *Handbook of Qualitative Research*. London: Sage Publications; 1994:485-499.

39. Schatzman L, Strauss AL. Strategy for analyzing. In: *Field Research: Strategies for a Natural Sociology*. Englewood Cliffs: Prentice-Hall; 1973:108-127.

40. Strauss A, Corbin J. Process. In: *Basics of Qualitative Research: Grounded Theory Procedures and Techniques*. London: Sage Publications; 1990:143-157.

41. Strauss A, Corbin J. Techniques for enhancing theoretical sensitivity. In: *Basics of Qualitative Research: Grounded Theory Procedures and Techniques*. London: Sage Publications; 1990:75-95.

42. Strauss A, Corbin J. Open coding. In: *Basics of Qualitative Research: Grounded Theory Procedures and Techniques*. London: Sage Publications; 1990:61-74.

43. Strauss A, Corbin J. Axial coding. In: *Basics of Qualitative Research: Grounded Theory Procedures and Techniques*. London: Sage Publications; 1990:96-115.

44. Strauss A, Corbin J. Selective coding. In: *Basics of Qualitative Research: Grounded Theory Procedures and Techniques*. London: Sage Publications; 1990:116-142.

45. Strauss A, Corbin J. The conditional matrix. In: *Basics of Qualitative Research: Grounded Theory Procedures and Techniques*. London: Sage Publications; 1990:158-174.

46. Miles M, Huberman M. Tactics for generating meaning. In: *Qualitative Data Analysis*. London: Sage Publications; 1994:245-262.

47. Elder NC, Miller WL. Reading and evaluating qualitative research studies. *J Fam Pract*. 1995;41:279-85.

48. Hamberg K, Johansson E, Lindgren G, Westman G. Scientific rigour in qualitative research: examples from a study of women's health in family practice. *Fam Pract*. 1994;11:176-181.

49. Strauss A, Corbin J. The uses of literature. In: *Basics of Qualitative Research: Grounded Theory Procedures and Techniques*. London: Sage Publications; 1990:48-56.

# DIAGNOSIS
## Clinical Manifestations of Disease

W. Scott Richardson, Mark Wilson, John Williams,
Virginia Moyer, and C. David Naylor

The following EBM Working Group members also made substantive
contributions to this section: Gordon Guyatt, Peter Wyer,
Jonathan Craig, Deborah Cook, Luz Maria Letelier,
James Nishikawa, Jeroen Lijmer, and Roman Jaeschke

## IN THIS SECTION

# CLINICAL SCENARIO

## Do Normal Pulses and Equal Blood Pressure in Both Arms Rule Out Aortic Dissection in a Man With Chest Pain?

You are a general internist going about your duties in a community teaching hospital when you are suddenly summoned to the emergency department to evaluate a 58-year-old man with chest discomfort. The patient has described sudden onset of severe pain in the center of his chest radiating to his neck and mid-back. He has essential hypertension, for which he takes a diuretic. En route to examine him, you hypothesize that myocardial ischemia or myocardial infarction may be the cause of his discomfort and you consider whether you should actively exclude a diagnosis of aortic dissection.

In the emergency department, you interview and examine the patient, focusing on his thorax and cardiovascular system. You find a normal thoracic wall, clear lungs, equal pulses, a diastolic murmur of aortic regurgitation, and diastolic hypotension with blood pressure of 162/56 mm Hg. The electrocardiogram shows left ventricular hypertrophy, but no signs of ischemia or infarction. The initial set of cardiac enzymes is normal. The portable chest radiograph is difficult to interpret, but may show widening of the mediastinum. An arterial blood gas shows mild respiratory alkalosis and normal oxygenation. By now, your suspicion of acute aortic dissection has grown, so you arrange definitive testing and, after explaining the situation to the patient and family, consult with the cardiothoracic surgical team. They advise starting the patient on esmolol and a very low dose of sodium nitroprusside while they finish what they are doing in the operating room.

While you await the test results, a resident on duty in the emergency department inquires about the patient. Together, you review the clinical findings seen with aortic dissection and then discuss the findings found useful in determining whether a patient is having a myocardial infarction.[1] The resident asks whether the normal pulses and equal blood pressures in the arms can rule out dissection without further testing. You do not know the answer to this question for certain, and you wonder if there are clinical findings that are sufficiently powerful to rule out aortic dissection when they are absent. Rather than guess, you decide to look up the answer during your wait for the test results.

# FINDING THE EVIDENCE

You begin by articulating the first knowledge gap as a question: "in patients with confirmed acute aortic dissection, how frequently would a detailed and careful evaluation yield each of several clinical findings, such as pain radiation to the back, pulse asymmetry, or diastolic hypotension?" You find mention of various findings with dissection in two textbooks, but neither reports how often these findings occur. You turn to one of the department's computers. It is networked to the hospital's library, where MEDLINE is available on CD-ROM. In the MEDLINE file since 1966, you combine two MeSH terms, "aneurysm, dissecting" (5027 citations) and "aortic aneurysm, thoracic" (1699 citations), with "aortic dissection" as a text word (2330 citations) to yield a set of 6410 citations. Next, you use the floating subheadings "di" for diagnosis (applied to articles that include clinical findings from patient examination) and "co" for complications (indicates conditions that coexist or follow the specified disease process). Combining these sets yields 86 citations, which drops to 33 when you limit your search to adult patients and English-language studies. Scrolling through these titles, you find one citation by Spittell and colleagues[2] that is linked to the full-text online article in your library. The article describes the presentation in 235 patients who were ultimately diagnosed as having aortic dissection.

Table 2C-1 summarizes the guides for interpreting an article about the clinical manifestations of disease.

**TABLE 2C-1**

## Users' Guides for an Article About the Clinical Manifestations of Disease

**Are the Results Valid?**

- Did the investigators enroll the right patients? Was the patient sample representative of those with the disorder?
- Was the definitive diagnostic standard appropriate? Was the diagnosis verified using credible criteria that were independent of the clinical manifestations under study?
- Were clinical manifestations sought thoroughly, carefully, and consistently?
- Were clinical manifestations classified by when and how they occurred?

**What Are the Results?**

- How frequently did the clinical manifestations of disease occur?
- How precise were these estimates of frequency?
- When and how did these clinical manifestations occur in the course of disease?

**How Can I Apply the Results to Patient Care?**

- Are the study patients similar to those in my own practice?
- Is it unlikely that the disease manifestations have changed since this evidence was gathered?
- How can I use the results in generating a differential diagnosis?

# ARE THE RESULTS VALID?

## Did the Investigators Enroll the Right Patients? Was the Patient Sample Representative of Those With the Disorder?

Ideally, a study sample will mirror the population of persons with the target condition, so that the frequency of clinical manifestations in the sample approximates that in the underlying population. Such a patient sample is termed representative. The more representative the sample is, the more accurate are the resulting frequencies of clinical findings.[3]

To judge the representativeness of the study sample, we suggest three tactics. First, examine the setting from which study patients come. Patients seen in referral care settings might have higher proportions of unusual findings or illnesses that are harder to diagnose, yielding different frequencies of clinical manifestations than patients diagnosed in community practice.[4] Second, examine the methods the investigators used to identify and include the study patients and to exclude others. Ask yourself if they included all important demographic groups (ie, those characterized by age, gender, race, and so on) or if they excluded important subgroups. Third, examine the description of the study patients' illnesses. Are patients with mild, moderate, and severe symptoms present? If different clinical patterns of disease are known, does the sample include patients with each pattern?

Combining these three considerations, you can judge whether the spectrum of included patients is sufficiently broad and full that the study can yield valid results about clinical manifestations of this disease. For instance, in a study of the clinical findings in patients with thyrotoxic periodic paralysis, the investigators included only the 19 patients who were hospitalized during an episode of paralysis, excluding 11 patients who were diagnosed during the study period but who were not admitted.[5] To the extent that clinical manifestations differed in hospitalized patients, such a restriction might introduce bias into the study.

Investigators may deliberately choose the more limited task of describing the manifestations of a disease in a purposefully narrowed target population, whether it is demographic (eg, a study of the findings of myocardial infarction in elderly patients[6]), prognostic (eg, a study of the clinical findings before death in patients with fatal pulmonary embolism[7]), or by site of care (eg, a study of the findings in patients with ruptured abdominal aortic aneurysm who present to internists in their offices, rather than emergency departments[8]). In such situations, you can look to see whether the study sample is representative of the limited target population.

Spittell et al[2] studied patients from the Mayo Clinic, which provides both community hospital care and tertiary referral care. The study sample had patients with aortic dissection that was both acute (of shorter than 2 weeks' duration) in 158 (67%) and chronic (of longer than 2 weeks' duration) in 78 (33%). In 60 patients, the initial clinical impression was a diagnosis other than aortic dissection. The sample included patients with sudden death, including 10 out-of-hospital cardiac arrests and five that occurred in the hospital. It also included 11 patients without pain but with other symptoms, along with 33 patients without pain or other symptoms who had abnormal chest radiographs. Thus, the study sample displays a wide array of clinical presentations likely to be representative of the full spectrum of this disorder.

## Was the Definitive Diagnostic Standard Appropriate? Was the Diagnosis Verified Using Credible Criteria That Were Independent of the Clinical Manifestations Under Study?

These questions address two closely linked issues. First, how sure can the investigators be that the study patients really did have this particular disease, rather than another disease, to explain their illnesses? Although clinicians often encounter patients whose diagnoses are tentative, in a study of disease manifestations such diagnostic uncertainty could introduce bias, as the patient sample might include patients with other diseases. To minimize this threat, investigators can use a set of explicit diagnostic criteria and include in the study sample only those patients who meet these criteria. Ideally, for every disease there would be a set of published, widely accepted diagnostic criteria, including one or more well-established *reference, gold,* or *criterion standard* tests that can be reproducibly applied. Reference standards can be anatomic, physiologic, radiographic, or genetic, to name a few. To judge how the presence of disease was verified, look for which standards were used for disease verification, how they were used, and whether the standards are clinically credible.

When no reference standards exist, investigators' degree of diagnostic certainty is much lower. In these situations, known sometimes as *syndrome diagnosis,*[9] diagnostic criteria usually rely on a list of clinical features required for the diagnosis. For instance, the definition of chronic fatigue syndrome uses an explicit set of clinical features as diagnostic criteria.[10] Such explicit criteria represent an advance over an implicit, haphazard approach.

However, when investigators use these clinical manifestations to make the syndrome diagnosis, select the patient sample, and then examine the frequency of these same clinical findings in the study patients, problems arise. This creates a form of circular reasoning that can bias upward the frequencies of these findings in the study sample. For example, a study of the clinical features of 36 patients with relapsing polychondritis suffered from this *incorporation bias,* in that the investigators used diagnostic criteria that rest primarily on characteristic clinical findings.[11] Although this may be the best available method for clinical diagnosis, incorporation bias limits the inferences we can draw about the frequency of clinical manifestations. To judge the independence of verifying criteria, compare the list of these criteria with the list of clinical manifestations studied.

Spittell et al[2] studied 235 patients in whom aortic dissections were confirmed by surgical intervention (in 162), by autopsy (in 27), or by radiographic studies (in 47). They excluded patients with aortic dissection that occurred intraoperatively or during invasive catheterization procedures. Thus, the diagnoses of study patients appear to have been verified using clinically credible means that are independent of the clinical manifestations.

## Were Clinical Manifestations Sought Thoroughly, Carefully, and Consistently?

This seeking of clinical manifestations criterion addresses three closely related issues. First, were study patients evaluated thoroughly enough to detect clinical findings if they were present? Within reason, the more comprehensive the workup, the lower the chance of missing findings and drawing invalid conclusions about their frequency. Second, how did the investigators ensure that the information they gathered was correct and free of distortion? Were symptoms inquired of patients in neutral, nonjudgmental ways, or were leading questions asked that might have suggested symptoms? Were patients examined by skilled examiners? The more carefully the data were gathered, the more credible the resulting frequencies will be. Third, how consistently was the evaluation carried out? Varying assessments might yield erroneous frequencies of disease manifestations.

You may find it relatively easy to judge the thoroughness, care, and consistency of the search for manifestations when clinicians evaluated the patients prospectively using a standardized diagnostic approach. It becomes harder to judge when investigators look back on clinicians' unstandardized evaluation. For example, in a report of a retrospective analysis of disease manifestations in 68 patients with lumbar spinal stenosis, the investigators did not describe the search for clinical findings in enough detail for us to judge how well they protected against biased ascertainment.[12] Ordinarily, a prospective study of clinical manifestations of disease will provide more credible results than a retrospective study.

Spittell et al[2] retrospectively reviewed the charts of their patients after the clinical evaluations were completed. They do not explicitly describe the diagnostic evaluation. The tables of results include much detail about the clinical examination, suggesting a careful approach, but uncertainty remains about the extent of standardization during the workup.

## Were Clinical Manifestations Classified by When and How They Occurred?

Clinical manifestations of disease can range from the permanent to the fleeting. They can occur early, late, or throughout the course of the disease. Investigators would obtain the most complete information about the timing of disease manifestations if they could begin collecting data the instant the disease begins and then continue to the end of the illness. Since knowing this "zero time" with certainty is impossible for most diseases, investigators can use the next strongest approach, that of targeting all findings that occur from the onset of patients' first symptoms of this illness episode. Studies that do not start collecting at the beginning of the episode—or those that do not report the timing of evaluation relative to symptom onset—may have missed evanescent findings; and our confidence in their validity decreases. For instance, in a study of the clinical manifestations before death in 92 patients with fatal pulmonary embolism, investigators recorded findings for only the 24 hours before death, so they may have missed transient but important clues to the diagnosis that occurred before that period of time.[7]

Sometimes, studies describe qualitative findings that might be useful in clinical diagnosis, particularly when triggering initial diagnostic hypotheses. For instance, patients often describe the pain of aortic dissection as a "tearing" or "ripping" sensation that is located in the center of the torso and that reaches maximal intensity quite quickly.[13] Just as with the temporal aspects, these qualitative descriptions are more credible if clinicians have gathered them deliberately and carefully.

Spittell et al[2] describe the clinical manifestations of dissection at presentation for patients with both acute (of shorter than 2 weeks' duration) and chronic (of longer than 2 weeks' duration) illness from aortic dissection. They also describe the location of pain in relation to the site of dissection and the various clusters of pain with other findings, along with unusual findings such as hoarseness and dysphagia. Thus, despite the retrospective study design, the investigators have classified the temporal and qualitative features sufficiently accurately to provide valid results for patients with acute dissection. We may be less confident in the results for chronic dissection, since early evanescent findings might not have been detected.

# WHAT ARE THE RESULTS?

## How Frequently Did the Clinical Manifestations of Disease Occur?

Studies of clinical manifestations of disease often display the main results in a table listing the clinical findings, along with the number and percentages of patients with each of those manifestations. Since patients usually have more than one finding, these proportions are not mutually exclusive. Some studies also report the number of patients with any of the findings, either as a total or separately by particular group.

Spittell et al[2] report that 168 (74%) patients initially suffered the acute onset of severe pain, 35 (15%) were asymptomatic but had abnormal chest radiographs, and 15 (6.3%) suffered cardiac arrest or sudden death. Of the 217 of 235 (92.3%) with a record of the cardiac exam, murmurs of aortic regurgitation were detected in 22 (11%). Pulse deficits were uncommon, occurring in 14 (6%) of patients.

These results provide an example of how textbook descriptions may emphasize the presence of particular classic findings proved uncommon by systematic study. If clinicians rely on such findings, they will miss many cases. For example, experts used to describe hemoptysis as a hallmark of acute pulmonary embolism, yet of 327 patients with angiographically proved pulmonary emboli, only 30% had hemoptysis.[14] Thus, clinicians would be unwise to use the absence of hemoptysis to exclude a diagnosis of pulmonary embolism.

Systematic studies of disease manifestations may also prove some findings to be more common than is usually believed. For instance, the murmur of aortic regurgitation was detected in 40 of 124 patients with confirmed aortic dissection, suggesting that clinicians should purposefully seek this finding in suspected cases.[13]

## How Precise Were These Estimates of Frequency?

Even when valid, these frequencies of clinical manifestations are only estimates of the true frequencies. You can examine the precision of these estimates using their confidence intervals (CIs). If the authors do not provide confidence intervals for you, you can calculate them with the following formula (for 95% CI):

$$95\% \text{ CI} = P \pm 1.96 \times [P (1 - P)]/n$$

where $P$ is the proportion of patients with the finding of interest and $n$ is the number of patients in the sample. This formula becomes inaccurate when the number of cases is five or fewer, so approximations have been developed for this situation.[15, 16]

For instance, consider the clinical finding of pulse deficit, found in 14 of the 217 patients in whom it was sought by Spittell et al.[2] Using the above formula, we would start with $P = 0.06$, $(1 - P) = 0.94$, and $n = 217$. Working through the arithmetic, we find the CI to be $0.06 \pm 0.03$. Thus, although the most likely frequency of pulse deficit is 6%, it may range between 3% and 9%.

Whether you consider the confidence intervals sufficiently precise depends on how you expect to use the information. For example, for a finding that occurs in 50% of cases, you may plan to look for it on examination but not plan to use the presence or absence of this finding to exclude the diagnosis. If the confidence interval for this estimate ranged from 30% to 70%, it would not change your expected use of the information, so the result may be precise enough. On the other hand, for a finding that occurs in 97% of patients, you might hope to use its absence to help you rule out the diagnosis. If the confidence interval for this estimate ranged from 60% to 100% (the same 40-point range as before), it could mean that using this finding to exclude the diagnosis might lead you to miss up to 40% of patients with the disorder. Such a result would be too imprecise to be used to rule out the disorder of interest.

## When and How Did These Clinical Manifestations Occur in the Course of Disease?

Some studies will report the temporal sequence of symptoms in sufficient detail to characterize symptoms as presenting (ie, the symptoms prompted patients to seek care), concurring (ie, the symptoms did not prompt the seeking of care but were present initially), or eventual (ie, the symptoms were not present initially, but were found subsequently). For instance, in 100 patients with pancreatic cancer, investigators described weight loss and abdominal pain as presenting manifestations in 75 and 72 patients, respectively, whereas jaundice, commonly taught as a key presenting sign, was found in only 24 patients.[17] In addition to reporting the chronology of events, such studies can also describe the location, quality, intensity, situational context, aggravating and alleviating factors, and associated findings for the important features of the disorder.

Spittell et al[2] describe in detail the symptoms at initial assessment, both as individual findings and in clusters. The also describe the location of pain and its association with the site of dissection. They do not describe the delayed manifestations in as much detail.

# HOW CAN I APPLY THE RESULTS TO PATIENT CARE?

## Are the Study Patients Similar to Those in My Own Practice?

The closer the match between the patients in your practice and those in the study, the more confident you can be in applying the results. We suggest that you ask yourself whether the setting or the patients are so different from yours that you cannot use the results.[18] You could consider whether the patients in your practice come from a geographic, demographic, cultural, or clinical group that could be expected to differ substantively in the ways in which this particular disorder is expressed. For instance, the presenting symptoms of acute myocardial infarction were found to differ with advancing patient age. When studied in 777 elderly hospitalized patients with myocardial infarction, syncope, stroke, and acute confusion were more common and were sometimes the sole presenting symptom.[6]

Spittel et al[2] did not describe the referral filters through which their patients arrived, although we know that the Mayo Clinic provides community hospital care for Olmsted County residents along with referred care for others. Of the 235 patients, 158 (67%) were men and their mean age was very close to that of the patient in the opening scenario. The authors do not describe the patients' comorbid conditions, socioeconomic status, race, or cultural background. Thus, although some uncertainty remains, these patients are sufficiently similar to the patient in the scenario to allow application of the results.

## Is It Unlikely That the Disease Manifestations Have Changed Since This Evidence Was Gathered?

As time passes, evidence about the clinical manifestations of disease can become obsolete. New diseases can arise and old diseases can present in new ways. New disease taxonomies can be built, changing the borders between disease states. Such events can so alter the clinical manifestations of disease that previously valid studies may no longer be applicable to current practice. For example, consider how dramatically the arrival of human immunodeficiency virus disease has changed our concept of pneumonia from *Pneumocystis carinii*.[19, 20]

Similar changes can occur as the result of progress in health science or medical practice. For instance, early descriptions of *Clostridium difficile* infection emphasized severe cases of life-threatening colitis. As diagnostic testing improved and awareness of the infection became widespread, milder cases were documented and the presenting manifestations were recognized to vary widely.[21] Treatment advances can change the course of disease, so that previously common eventual clinical manifestations might occur with much less frequency. Also, new treatments bring the possibility of new iatrogenic disease, which may coexist and combine with underlying diseases in new ways.

The Spittell paper[2] was published in 1993 and reports on patients seen from 1980 to 1990. You know of no new diseases arising since then that would change the clinical features of dissection. Both diagnostic testing for suspected dissection and treatment for hypertension (a major risk factor for dissection) have changed during this period, but you expect they would not change the presenting clinical features of acute dissection.

### How Can I Use the Results in Generating a Differential Diagnosis?

For studies that prove valid and applicable to your patients, knowing the clinical manifestations of conditions that you might consider will help you generate a differential diagnosis. A few findings might occur in almost all patients with the disease. As this proportion nears 100%, the absence of these findings allows you to omit the disease from your differential diagnosis. The presence of findings that occur in the range of 10% to 90% of patients with the disease suggests that the condition should remain among those you are considering as an explanation for your patient's presentation. Some manifestations occur seldom enough—in less than 10% of patients—that their presence would not prompt consideration of the illness in your differential diagnosis.

# CLINICAL RESOLUTION

Based on the evidence from Spittell et al,[2] you and the resident agree not to use the absence of pulse asymmetry to rule out the diagnosis of aortic dissection. Given the presence of the aortic regurgitation murmur and the diastolic hypotension, along with the patient's known risk and the absence of findings for myocardial infarction, you feel even more confident in your working diagnosis of proximal aortic dissection. When completed, this patient's aortogram confirms aortic dissection of the ascending aorta and arch, complicated by aortic regurgitation. The surgical team prepares the patient for an emergency operation.

## References

1. Panju AA, Hemmelgarn BR, Guyatt GH, Simel DL. Is this patient having a myocardial infarction? *JAMA*. 1998;280:1256-1263.

2. Spittell PC, Spittell JA Jr, Joyce JW, et al. Clinical features and differential diagnosis of aortic dissection: experience with 236 cases (1980 through 1990). *Mayo Clin Proc*. 1993;68:642-651.

3. Ransohoff DF, Feinstein AR. Problems of spectrum and bias in evaluating the efficacy of diagnostic tests. *N Engl J Med*. 1978;299:926-930.

4. Fletcher RH, Fletcher SW, Wagner EH. *Clinical Epidemiology: The Essentials*. 3rd ed. Baltimore: Williams & Wilkins; 1996.

5. Manoukian MA, Foote JA, Crapo LM. Clinical and metabolic features of thyrotoxic periodic paralysis in 24 episodes. *Arch Intern Med*. 1999;159:601-606.

6. Bayer AJ, Chadha JS, Farag RR, Pathy MS. Changing presentation of myocardial infarction with increasing old age. *J Am Geriatr Soc*. 1986;34:263-266.

7. Morgenthaler TI, Ryu JH. Clinical characteristics of fatal pulmonary embolism in a referral hospital. *Mayo Clin Proc*. 1995;70:417-424.

8. Lederle FA, Parenti CM, Chute EP. Ruptured abdominal aortic aneurysm: the internist as diagnostician. *Am J Med*. 1994;96:163-167.

9. Wulff HR. *Rational Diagnosis and Treatment: An Introduction to Clinical Decision-Making*. 2nd ed. Oxford: Blackwell Scientific Publications; 1981.

10. Fukuda K, Straus SE, Hickie I, Sharpe MC, Dobins JG, Komaroff A, and the International Chroinc Fatigue Syndrom Study Group. The chronic fatigue syndrome: a comprehensive approach to its definition and study. *Ann Intern Med*. 1994;121:953-959.

11. Trentham DE, Le CH. Relapsing polychondritis. *Ann Intern Med*. 1998;129: 114-122.

12. Hall S, Bartleson JD, Onofrio BM, Baker HL Jr, Okazaki H, O'Duffy JD. Lumbar spinal stenosis: clinical features, diagnostic procedures, and results of surgical treatment in 68 patients. *Ann Intern Med*. 1985;103:271-275.

13. Slater EE, DeSanctis RW. The clinical recognition of dissecting aortic aneurysm. *Am J Med*. 1976;60:625-633.

14. Bell WR, Simon TL, DeMets DL. The clinical features of submassive and massive pulmonary emboli. *Am J Med*. 1977;62:355-360.

15. Hanley JA, Lippman-Hand A. If nothing goes wrong, is everything all right? Interpreting zero numerators. *JAMA*. 1983;249:1743-1745.

16. Newman TB. If almost nothing goes wrong, is almost everything all right? Interpreting small numerators. *JAMA*. 1995;274:1013.

17. Gudjonsson B, Livstone EM, Spiro HM. Cancer of the pancreas: diagnostic accuracy and survival statistics. *Cancer*. 1978;42:2494-2506.

18. Glasziou P, Guyatt GH, Dans LF, Straus SE, Sackett DL. Applying the results of trials and systematic reviews to patients [editorial]. *ACP Journal Club*. 1998 Nov/Dec;129:A15-A16.

19. Walzer PD, Perl DP, Krogstad DJ, Rawson PG, Schultz MG. Pneumocystis carinii pneumonia in the United States: epidemiologic, diagnostic, and clinical features. *Ann Intern Med*. 1974;80:83-93.

20. Kovacs JA, Hiemenz JW, Macher AM, et al. Pneumocystis carinii pneumonia: a comparison between patients with the acquired immunodeficiency syndrome and patients with other immunodeficiencies. *Ann Intern Med*. 1984;100:663-671.

21. Caputo GM, Weitekamp MR, Bacon AE III, Whitener C. Clostridium difficile infection: a common clinical problem for the general internist. *J Gen Intern Med*. 1994;9:528-533.

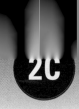

# DIAGNOSIS
## Measuring Agreement
## Beyond Chance

Thomas McGinn, Gordon Guyatt, Richard Cook,
and Maureen Meade

Roman Jaeschke also made substantive contributions to this section

## IN THIS SECTION

# CLINICIANS OFTEN DISAGREE

Clinicians often disagree in their assessment of patients. When two physicians reach different conclusions regarding the presence of a particular physical sign, either different approaches to the examination or different interpretation of the findings may be responsible for the disagreement. Similarly, disagreement between repeated applications of a diagnostic test may result from different application of the test or different interpretation of the results.

Researchers may also face difficulties in agreeing on such issues as whether patients meet the eligibility requirements for a clinical trial, whether patients in a randomized trial have experienced the outcome of interest (eg, they may disagree about whether a patient has had a transient ischemic attack or a stroke, or about whether a death should be classified as a cardiovascular death), or whether a study meets the eligibility criteria for a systematic review.

# CHANCE WILL ALWAYS BE RESPONSIBLE FOR SOME OF THE APPARENT AGREEMENT BETWEEN OBSERVERS

Any two people judging the presence or absence of an attribute will agree some of the time by chance. This means that even if the people making the assessment are doing so by guessing in a completely random way, their random guesses will agree some of the time. When investigators present agreement as raw agreement—that is, by simply counting the number of times agreement has occurred—this chance agreement gives a misleading impression.

# ALTERNATIVES FOR DEALING WITH THE PROBLEM OF AGREEMENT BY CHANCE

This section of the book describes approaches to addressing this problem of misleading results of chance agreement that statisicians have provided. So far, when we are dealing with categorical data (that is, placing patients in discrete categories such as "mild," "moderate," or "severe"; or "stage 1, 2, 3, or 4"), the most popular approach to misleading results of chance agreement is *chance-corrected agreement*. Chance-corrected agreement is quantitated as *kappa*, or *weighted kappa* (statistics used to measure nonrandom agreement between observers, investigators, or measurements).

# ONE SOLUTION TO AGREEMENT BY CHANCE: CHANCE-CORRECTED AGREEMENT, OR KAPPA

Conceptually, kappa removes the agreement by chance and informs the clinician of the extent of the possible agreement over and above chance. If the raters agree on every judgment, the total possible agreement is always 100%.

Figure 2C-1 depicts a situation in which agreement by chance is 50%, leaving possible agreement above and beyond chance of 50%. As depicted in the figure, the raters have achieved an agreement of 75%. Of this 75%, 50% was achieved by chance alone. Of the remaining possible 50% agreement, the raters have achieved half, resulting in a kappa value of 0.25/0.50, or 0.50.

**FIGURE 2C-1**

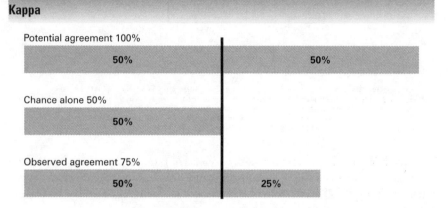

Kappa

kappa = 0.25/0.50 = 0.50 (good agreement)

# CALCULATING KAPPA

How is kappa calculated? Assume that two observers are assessing the presence of Murphy sign, which may help clinicians detect an enlarged gallbladder. However, they have no skill at detecting the presence or absence of Murphy sign and their evaluations are no better than blind guesses. Let us say they are both guessing in a ratio of 50:50; they guess that Murphy sign is present half of the time and that it is absent half of the time. On average, if both raters were evaluating the same 100 patients, they would achieve the results presented in Figure 2C-2. Referring to that figure, you observe that these results demonstrate that the two cells that tally the raw agreement, A and D, include 50% of the observations. Thus, simply by guessing (and thus by chance), the raters have achieved 50% agreement.

**FIGURE 2C-2**

## Agreement by Chance When Both Reviewers Are Guessing in a Ratio of 50% Target Positive and 50% Target Negative

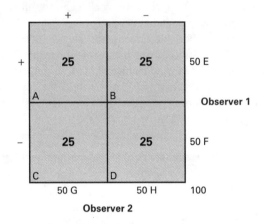

+ indicates target positive and – refers to target negative. In this case, + is Murphy sign present and – is Murphy sign absent. **A,** Patients in whom both observers find the sign present. **B,** Patients in whom observer 1 finds the sign present, and observer 2 finds the sign absent. **C,** Patients in whom observer 1 finds the sign absent, and observer 2 finds the sign present. **D,** Patients in whom both observers find the sign absent. **E,** Patients in whom observer 1 finds the sign present. **F,** Patients in whom observer 1 finds the sign absent. **G,** Patients in whom observer 2 finds the sign present. **H,** Patients in whom observer 2 finds the sign absent.

What happens if the raters repeat the exercise of rating 100 patients, but this time each guesses in a ratio of 80% positive and 20% negative? Figure 2C-3 depicts what, on average, will occur. Now, the agreement (see cells A and D) has increased to 68%.

**FIGURE 2C-3**

## Agreement by Chance When Both Reviewers Are Guessing in a Ratio of 80% Target Positive and 20% Target Negative

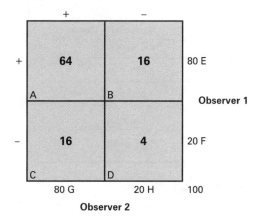

+ indicates target positive and – refers to target negative. In this case, + is Murphy sign present and – is Murphy sign absent.

What is the arithmetic involved in filling in the table to determine the level of agreement that occurs by chance? The procedure involves multiplying the marginal totals (E, F, G, and H) and dividing by the total number of patients. Alternatively, one can multiply the marginal totals, expressed as a proportion. In this example, for instance, we calculate how many observations we expect by chance to fall in cell A, we multiply E x G, and we divide by 100. Similarly, to calculate the number of observations we expect in cell D, we multiply F x H and we divide by 100.

Were we to repeat this arithmetic exercise with different marginal totals, we would find that as the proportion of observations classified as positive becomes progressively more extreme (that is, as it moves away from 50%), the agreement by chance increases. The average chance agreement changes, as shown in Table 2C-2, as two observers classify an increasing higher proportion of patients in one category or the other (such as, positive and negative; sign present or absent).

**TABLE 2C-2**

## Relationship Between the Proportion Positive and the Expected Agreement by Chance

| Proportion Positive (E/T = G/T)* | Agreement by Chance |
|---|---|
| 0.5 | 0.5 (50%) |
| 0.6 | 0.52 (52%) |
| 0.7 | 0.59 (59%) |
| 0.8 | 0.64 (64%) |
| 0.9 | 0.81 (81%) |

\* E/T and G/T refer to letters in Figures 2C-2 and 2C-3; E/T indicates the proportion of patients observer 1 finds positive; G/T refers to the proportion of patients observer 2 finds positive.

Figure 2C-4 illustrates the calculation of kappa with a hypothetical data set. First, we calculate the agreement observed: in 40 patients, the two observers agreed that Murphy sign was positive (cell A) and they further agreed that in another 40 patients it was negative (cell D). Thus, the total agreement is 40 + 40, or 80.

**FIGURE 2C-4**

## Observed and Expected Agreement

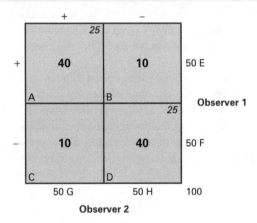

+ indicates target positive and – refers to target negative. In this case, + is Murphy sign present and – is Murphy sign absent. Expected agreement by chance appears in italics in cells A and D.

Next, we calculate the agreement by chance by multiplying the marginal totals E and G and dividing by 100, and by multiplying the marginal totals H and F and dividing by 100. The total agreement by chance is 25 + 25, or 50. We can then calculate kappa using the principle illustrated in Figure 2C-1.

$$\frac{\text{(agreement observed – agreement by chance)}}{\text{(agreement possible – agreement by chance)}}$$

or in this case:

$$\frac{80 - 50}{100 - 50} = 30/50 = 0.6.$$

# KAPPA WITH THREE OR MORE RATERS OR THREE OR MORE CATEGORIES

Using similar principles, one can calculate chance-corrected agreement when there are more than two raters.[1] Furthermore, one can calculate kappa when raters place patients into more than two categories (eg, patients with heart failure may be rated as New York Heart Association class I, II, III, or IV). In these situations, one may give partial credit for intermediate levels of agreement (eg, one observer may classify a patient as class II while another may observe the same patient as class III) by adopting a so-called weighted kappa statistic (weighted because full agreement gets full credit, and partial agreement gets partial credit).[2]

There are a number of approaches to valuing the kappa levels raters achieve. One option is the following: 0 = poor agreement; 0 to 0.2 = slight agreement; 0.2 to 0.4 = fair agreement; 0.4 to 0.6 = moderate agreement; 0.6 to 0.8 = substantial agreement; and values of 0.8 to 1.0 represent almost perfect agreement.[3]

Examples of chance-corrected agreement that investigators have calculated in clinical studies are as follows: exercise stress test cardiac T wave changes, kappa = 0.25[4]; jugular venous distention, kappa = 0.50[5]; presence or absence of a goiter, kappa = 0.82 to 0.95[6,7]; Straight Leg Raising (SLR) for diagnosis of low back pain, kappa = 0.82.[8]

# A LIMITATION OF KAPPA

Despite its intuitive appeal and widespread use, the statistical kappa has an important disadvantage: as a result of the higher level of chance agreement when distributions become more extreme, the possible agreement above chance agreement becomes small and it is very difficult to achieve even moderate values of kappa. Thus, if one uses the same raters in a variety of settings, as the proportion of positive ratings becomes extreme, kappa will decrease even if the way the raters interpret diagnostic information does not change.[4-6]

# AN ALTERNATIVE TO KAPPA: CHANCE-INDEPENDENT AGREEMENT OR PHI

One solution to this problem is chance-independent agreement using the *phi* statistic, which is a relatively new approach to assessing observer agreement.[7] One begins by estimating the odds ratio from a 2 x 2 table displaying the agreement between two observers. Figure 2C-5 contrasts the formulas for raw agreement, kappa, and phi.

**FIGURE 2C-5**

## Calculations of Agreement

$$\text{Raw agreement} = \frac{a + d}{a + b + c + d}$$

$$\text{Kappa} = \frac{\text{observed agreement} - \text{expected agreement}}{1 - \text{expected agreement}}$$

$$\text{where observed agreement} = \frac{a + d}{a + b + c + d}$$

$$\text{and expected agreement} = \frac{(a + b)(a + c)}{a + b + c + d} + \frac{(c + d)(b + d)}{a + b + c + d}$$

$$\text{Odds Ratio (OR)} = \frac{ad}{bc}$$

$$\text{Phi} = \frac{\sqrt{OR} - 1}{\sqrt{OR} + 1} = \frac{\sqrt{ab} - \sqrt{bc}}{\sqrt{ad} - \sqrt{bc}}$$

The odds ratio (OR = *ad/bc* in Figure 2C-5) provides the basis for calculating phi. The odds ratio is simply the odds of a positive classification by rater B when rater A gives a positive classification divided by the odds of a positive classification by rater B when rater A gives a negative classification (see Part 2B2, "Therapy and Understanding the Results, Measures of Association"). The odds ratio would not change if we were to reverse the rows and columns. Thus, it does not matter which observer we identify as observer A and which one we identify as observer B. The odds ratio provides a natural measure of agreement. This agreement can be made more easily interpretable by converting it into a form that takes values from –1.0 (representing extreme disagreement) to 1.0 (representing extreme agreement).

The phi statistic makes this conversion using the following formula:

$$\text{phi} = \frac{\sqrt{OR} - 1}{\sqrt{OR} + 1} = \frac{\sqrt{ad} - \sqrt{bc}}{\sqrt{ad} + \sqrt{bc}}$$

When both margins are 0.5 (that is, when both raters conclude that 50% of the patients are positive and 50% are negative for the trait of interest), phi is equal to kappa.

# ADVANTAGES OF PHI OVER OTHER APPROACHES

The use of phi has three important advantages over other approaches. First, it is independent of the level-of-chance agreement. Thus, investigators could expect to find similar levels of phi whether the distribution of results is 50% positive and 50% negative or whether it is 90% positive and 10% negative. This is not true for measures of the kappa statistic, a chance-corrected index of agreement.

Second, phi allows statistical modeling approaches that the kappa statistic does not offer. For instance, such flexibility allows investigators to take advantage of all ratings when observers assess patients on multiple occasions.[7] Third, phi allows testing of whether differences in agreement between pairings of raters are statistically significant, an option that is not available with kappa.[7] Fourth, since phi is based on the odds ratio, one can carry out exact analyses. This feature is particularly attractive when the sample is small or if there is a zero cell in the chart.[8]

Statisticians may disagree about the relative usefulness of kappa and phi. Most important from clinicians' point of view is to ensure that investigators do not mislead by presenting only raw agreement.

## References

1. Cohen J. Weighted kappa: Nominal scale agreement with provision for scaled disagreement or partial credit. *Psychol Bull*. 1968;70:213-220.

2. Landis JR, Koch GG. The measurement of observer agreement for categorical data. *Biometrics*. 1977;33:159-174.

3. Maclure M, Willett WC. Misinterpretation and misuse of the kappa statistic. *Am J Epidemiol*. 1987;126:161-169.

4. Blackburn H. The exercise electrocardiogram: differences in interpretation. *Am J Cardiol*. 1968;21:871.

5. Cook DJ. Clinical assessment of central venous pressure in the critically ill. *Am J Med Sci*. 1990;229:175-178.

6. Kilpatrick R, Milne JS, Rushbrooke M, Wilson ESB. A survey of thyroid enlargement in two general practices in Great Britain. *BMJ.* 1963;1:29-34.

7. Troffer WR, Cochrane AL, Benjamin IT, Mial WE, Exley D. A goitre survey in the Vale of Glam-organ. *Bri J Prev Soc Med.* 1962;16:16-21.

8. McComb PF, Fairbank J, Cockersole BC, Pynsent PB. 1989 Volvo Award in clinical sciences. Reproducibility of physical signs in low back pain. *Spine.* 1989;14:908-918.

9. Thompson WD, Walter SD. A reappraisal of the kappa coefficient. *J Clin Epidemiol.* 1988;41:949-958.

10. Feinstein AR, Cicchetti DV. High agreement but low kappa, I: the problems of two paradoxes. *J Clin Epidemiol.* 1990;43:543-549.

11. Cook RJ, Farewell VT. Conditional inference for subject-specific and marginal agreement: two families of agreement measures. *Can J Stat.* 1995;23:333-344.

12. Meade MO, Cook RJ, Guyatt GH, et al. Interobserver variation in interpreting chest radiographs for the diagnosis of acute respiratory distress syndrome. *Am J Respir Crit Care Med.* 2000;161:85-90.

13. Armitage P, Colton T, eds. *Encyclopedia of Biostatistics.* Chichester: John Wiley and Sons; 1998.

# DIAGNOSIS
## Clinical Prediction Rules

Thomas McGinn, Gordon Guyatt, Peter Wyer,
C. David Naylor, and Ian Stiell

## IN THIS SECTION

## CLINICAL SCENARIO

### Can a Clinical Prediction Rule Reduce Unnecessary Ankle Radiographs?

You are the medical director of a busy inner-city emergency department. Faced with a limited budget and pressure to improve efficiency, you have conducted an audit of radiologic procedures ordered for minor trauma and have found that the rate of radiographs ordered for ankle and knee trauma is high. You are aware of the Ottawa Ankle Rules,[1,2] the guidelines that identify patients for whom ankle radiographs can be omitted without adverse consequences (Figure 2C-6). In addition, you are well aware that a small number of faculty and residents currently rely on these guidelines to make quick frontline decisions in the emergency department.

You are interested in knowing the accuracy of the guidelines, whether they are applicable to the population of patients in your hospital, and whether you should be implementing them in your own practice. Further, you wonder if implementing the guidelines can change clinical behavior and reduce costs without compromising quality care. You decide to consult the original medical literature and to assess the evidence for yourself.

**FIGURE 2C-6**

## Ottawa Ankle Rules

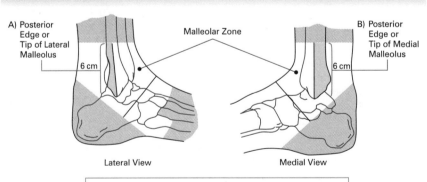

A) Posterior Edge or Tip of Lateral Malleolus

Malleolar Zone

B) Posterior Edge or Tip of Medial Malleolus

6 cm

6 cm

Lateral View

Medial View

An ankle x-ray series is required only if there is any pain in the malleolar zone and any of these findings:
1. Bone tenderness at A
   or
2. Bone tenderness at B
   or
3. Inability to bear weight both immediately and in emergency department

# FINDING THE EVIDENCE

Currently *prediction rules* or *decision rules* have no separate medical subject (MeSH) heading in the National Library of Medicine (NLM) MEDLINE database. Logging onto the Internet, you search PubMed under the MeSH heading "ankle fractures" and cross it with the text words "rules" and "decision rules." This search yields five citations, of which three deal directly with the Ottawa clinical prediction rules for ankle fractures.[1-3]

In reviewing these articles and deciding whether to implement changes in your emergency department, you require criteria for deciding on the strength of the inference you can make about the accuracy and impact of the Ottawa Ankle Rules. This section will provide you with the tools to answer those questions.

# CLINICAL PREDICTION RULES

Establishing a patient's diagnosis and prognosis are closely linked activities that are central to every physician's practice. The diagnoses we make—and our assessment of patients' prognoses—often determine the recommendations we make to patients. Clinical experience provides us with an intuitive sense of which findings on history, physical examination, and laboratory or radiologic investigation are critical in making an accurate diagnosis or an accurate assessment of a patient's prognostic fate. Although it can often be extraordinarily accurate, this intuition may sometimes be misleading. Clinical prediction rules attempt to formally test, simplify, and increase the accuracy of clinicians' diagnostic and prognostic assessments.

A *clinical prediction rule* can be defined as a clinical tool that quantifies the individual contributions that various components of the history, physical examination, and basic laboratory results make toward the diagnosis, prognosis, or likely response to treatment in an individual patient.[4] This definition is equally applicable to what have been called clinical prediction guides and clinical decision rules.

"Prediction" implies helping the clinician to better decide on a future clinical event. "Decision" implies directing the clinician to a specific course of action. As you will see, application of clinical prediction rules sometimes results in a decision and other times in a prediction, but also often in a probability or a likelihood ratio that the clinician applies to a current diagnostic problem. In this last application, the name "clinical diagnosis rule" or "clinical diagnosis guide" might be more precisely accurate. We will use the term "clinical prediction rule" regardless of whether the output of the "rule" is a suggested clinical course of action, the probability of a future event, or an increase or decrease in the likelihood of a particular diagnosis.

Whatever the clinical prediction rule is generating—a decision, a prediction, or a change in diagnostic probability—it is most likely to be useful in situations in which decision making is complex, when the clinical stakes are high, or when there are opportunities to achieve cost savings without compromising patient care.

Developing and testing a clinical prediction rule involves three steps: (1) the creation or derivation of the rule, (2) the testing or validation of the rule, and (3) the assessment of the impact of the rule on clinical behavior—the impact analysis. The validation process may require several studies to fully test the accuracy of the rule at different clinical sites (Figure 2C-7). Each step in the development of a clinical prediction rule may be published separately by different authors, or all three steps may be included in one article. Table 2C-3 presents a hierarchy of evidence that can guide clinicians in assessing the full range of evidence supporting use of a clinical prediction rule in their practice.

**FIGURE 2C-7**

## Development and Testing of a Clinical Prediction Rule

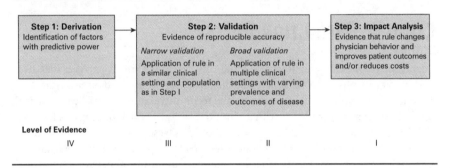

| Step 1: Derivation | Step 2: Validation | | Step 3: Impact Analysis |
|---|---|---|---|
| Identification of factors with predictive power | Evidence of reproducible accuracy | | Evidence that rule changes physician behavior and improves patient outcomes and/or reduces costs |
| | *Narrow validation* | *Broad validation* | |
| | Application of rule in a similar clinical setting and population as in Step I | Application of rule in multiple clinical settings with varying prevalence and outcomes of disease | |

Level of Evidence

| IV | III | II | I |

**TABLE 2C-3**

## Hierarchy of Evidence for Clinical Prediction Rules

**Level I:** Rules that can be used in a wide variety of settings with confidence that they can change clinician behavior and improve patient outcomes

At this level, rules must have at least one prospective validation in a different population plus one impact analysis, along with a demonstration of change in clinician behavior with beneficial consequences.

**Level II:** Rules that can be used in various settings with confidence in their accuracy

At this level, rules must have demonstrated accuracy either via one large prospective study including a broad spectrum of patients and clinicians, or via validation in several smaller settings that differ from one another.

**Level III:** Rules that clinicians may consider using with caution and only if patients in the study are similar to those in your clinical setting

These rules have been validated in only one narrow prospective sample.

**Level IV:** Rules that need further evaluation before they can be applied clinically

These rules have been derived but not validated or have been validated only in split samples, large retrospective databases, or by means of statistical techniques.

Note that this hierarchy applies only to clinical prediction rules intended for application in clinical practice. Investigators may use identical methodology to generate equations that stratify patients into different risk groups. These equations can then be used for statistical adjustment in studies involving large databases. These not-so-clinical prediction rules do not involve application by frontline practitioners and thus would require a somewhat different hierarchy of strength of evidence. We will now review the steps in the development and testing of a clinical prediction rule, relating each stage of the process to the hierarchy of evidence presented in Table 2C-3.

# DEVELOPING A CLINICAL PREDICTION RULE

Our search revealed three articles related to the Ottawa Ankle Rules, the first of which described the clinical prediction rules derivation.[1] Clinical prediction rules developers begin by constructing a list of potential predictors of the outcome of interest—in this case, ankle fractures demonstrated on ankle radiograph. The list typically includes items from the history, physical exam, and basic laboratory tests. The investigators then examine a group of patients and determine (1) whether the candidate clinical predictors are present, and (2) each patient's status on the outcome of interest—in this case, the result of the ankle radiograph. Statistical analysis reveals which predictors are most powerful and which predictors can be omitted from the rule without loss of predictive power. Typically, the statistical techniques used in this process are based on logistic regression (see Part 2D, "Prognosis, Regression and Correlation"). Other techniques that investigators sometimes use include *discriminant analysis*, which produces equations similar to regression analysis,[5] *recursive partitioning analysis*, which divides the patient population into smaller and smaller groups based upon discriminating risk factors,[6] and neural networks.[7]

Clinical prediction rules that have been derived but not validated should not be considered ready for clinical application (see Table 2C-3). Investigators interested in performing the validation of a clinical prediction rule, however, need criteria to judge whether the derivation process has been well done and, thus, whether the rule is promising enough to address certain questions before moving forward to the validation phase (see Table 2C-4).

Interested readers can find a complete discussion of the derivation process and these criteria in a paper by Laupacis et al.[4]

**TABLE 2C-4**

## Methodologic Standards for Derivation of a Clinical Decision Rule

- Were all important predictors included in the derivation process?
- Were all important predictors present in significant proportion of the study population?
- Were the outcome event and predictors clearly defined?
- Were those assessing the outcome event blinded to the presence of the predictors and were those assessing the presence of predictors blinded to the outcome event?
- Was the sample size adequate (including an adequate number of outcome events)?
- Does the rule make clinical sense?

# VALIDATION

There are three reasons why even rigorously derived clinical prediction rules are not ready for application in clinical practice without further validation. First, the prediction rules derived from one set of patients may reflect associations between given predictors and outcomes that occur primarily because of the play of chance. If that is so, a different set of predictors will emerge in a different group of patients, even if they come from the same setting. Second, predictors may be idiosyncratic to the population, to the clinicians using the rule, or to other aspects of the design of individual studies. If that is so, the rule may fail in a new setting. Finally, because of problems in the feasibility of rule application in the clinical setting, clinicians may fail to implement a rule comprehensively or accurately. The result would be that a rule succeeds in theory, but fails in practice.

Statistical methods can deal with the first of these problems. For instance, investigators may split their population into two groups, using one to develop the rule and the other to test it. Alternatively, they may use more sophisticated statistical methods built on the same logic. Conceptually, these approaches involve removing one patient from the sample, generating the rule using the remainder of the patients, and testing it on the patient who was removed from the sample. One repeats this procedure, sometimes referred to as a *bootstrap technique*, in sequence for every patient under study.

Although statistical validations within the same setting or group of patients reduce the chance that the rule reflects the play of chance rather than true associations, they fail to address the other two threats to validity. The success of the clinical prediction rule may be peculiar to the particular populations of patients and clinicians involved in the derivation study. Even if this is not so, clinicians may have difficulties using the rule in practice, difficulties that compromise its predictive power. Thus, to ascend from level IV in our hierarchy of evidence, studies must involve the use of the rule by clinicians in clinical practice.

A clinical prediction rule developed to predict serious outcomes (for example, heart failure or ventricular arrhythmia) in syncope patients highlights the importance of validation.[8] Investigators derived the rule using data from 252 patients who presented to the emergency department; subsequently, they attempted to prospectively validate it in a sample of 374 patients. The prediction rule gave individuals a score from 0 to 4 depending on the number of clinical predictors present. The probability of poor outcomes corresponding to almost every score in the derivation set was approximately twice that of the validation. For example, in the derivation set, the risk of a poor outcome in a patient with a score on the prediction rule of 3 was estimated to be 52%. By contrast, a patient with the same score in the validation set had a probability of a poor outcome of only 27%. This variation in results may have been caused by a difference in the severity of the syncope cases entered into the two studies—or by different criteria for generating a score of 3. Because of the risk that it will provide misleading information when applied in a real-world clinical setting, we situate a clinical prediction rule that has undergone development without validation as level IV in our hierarchy (see Table 2C-3).

Despite this major limitation, clinicians can still extract clinically relevant messages from an article describing the development of a clinical prediction rule. They may wish to note the most important predictors and to consider them more carefully in their own practice. They may also consider giving less importance to variables that failed to show predictive power. For instance, in developing a clinical prediction rule to predict mortality from pneumonia, investigators found that the white blood cell count had no bearing on subsequent mortality.[9] Hence, clinicians may wish to put less weight on the white blood cell count when making decisions about admitting pneumonia patients to the hospital.

To move up the hierarchy, clinical prediction rules must provide additional evidence of validity. The second article in our search described the refinement and prospective validation of the Ottawa Ankle Rules.[2] Validation of a clinical prediction rule involves demonstrating that its repeated application as part of the process of clinical care leads to the same results. Ideally, validation entails the investigators applying the rule prospectively in a new population with a prevalence and spectrum of disease that differs from that of the patients in whom the rule was derived. It is important to be sure that the clinical prediction rule performs similarly in a variety of populations in the hands of a variety of clinicians who work in a variety of institutions. Also important is to be sure that it works well when clinicians are consciously applying it as a rule, rather than as a statistical derivation from a large number of potential predictors.

If the setting in which the prediction rule was originally developed was limited and its validation has been confined to this setting, application by clinicians working in other settings is less secure. Validation in a similar setting can take a number of forms. Most simply, after developing the prediction rule, the investigators return to their population, draw a new sample of patients, and then test the rule's performance. Thus, we classify rules that have been validated in the same—or very similar—limited or narrow populations as the sample used in the development phase as level III on our hierarchy, and we recommend that clinicians use the result cautiously (see Table 2C-3).

In the derivation phase, if investigators draw patients from a sufficiently hetero-geneous population across a variety of institutions, testing the rule in the same population provides strong validation. Validation in a new population provides the clinician with strong inferences about the usefulness of the rule, corresponding to level II in our hierarchy (see Table 2C-3). The more numerous and diverse the settings in which the rule is tested and found accurate, the more likely it is that it will generalize to an untested setting.[10]

The Ottawa Ankle Rule was first derived in two large, university-based emer-gency departments in Ottawa[9] and was then prospectively validated in a large sample of patients from the same emergency departments.[2] At this stage, the rule would be classified as level II in our hierarchy because of the large number and diversity of patients and physicians involved in the study. Since that initial valida-tion, the rule has been validated in several different clinical settings with relatively consistent results.[11-14] This evidence further strengthens our inference about its predictive power.

Many clinical prediction rules are derived and then validated on a small, nar-rowly selected group of patients (level III). One such rule was derived to predict preserved left ventricular (LV) function after myocardial infarction.[15] The initial derivation and validation were performed on 314 patients who had been admitted to a tertiary care center. The prediction rule was first derived using 162 patients and then was validated using 152 patients in the same setting. The prediction rule demonstrated that of patients in whom the rule suggested LV function had been preserved, this was, in fact, true in 99%. At this stage in the rule development, the rule would be considered to be level III, only to be used in similar settings as the validation study, ie, in similar cardiac care units. The rule was further validated in two larger trials, one trial using 213 patients[16] from one site and a larger trial using 1891 patients from several different institutions.[17] In both settings, of patients in whom the rule suggested LV function had been preserved, 11% had abnormal LV function. This drop in accuracy changes the potential use and implications of the rule in clinical practice. At this point in development, the rule would be considered to fall within the category of level II, meaning that the rule can used in clinical set-tings with a high degree of confidence, but with adjusted results. The development of this rule highlights the importance of the validation of a clinical prediction rule on a diverse patient population before it can be broadly applied.

Regardless of whether investigators have conducted their validation study in a similar, narrow (level III) or broad, heterogeneous, or different (level II) popula-tion, their results allow stronger inferences if they have adhered to a number of methodologic standards (Table 2C-5). Interested readers can find a complete dis-cussion on the validation process and these criteria in a paper by Laupacis et al.[4]

**TABLE 2C-5**

## Methodologic Standards for Validation of a Clinical Prediction Rule

- Were the patients chosen in an unbiased fashion and do they represent a wide spectrum of severity of disease?
- Was there a blinded assessment of the criterion standard for all patients?
- Was there an explicit and accurate interpretation of the predictor variables and the actual rule without knowledge of the outcome?
- Was there 100% follow-up of those enrolled?

If those evaluating predictor status of study patients are aware of the outcome, or if those assessing the outcome are aware of patients' status with respect to the predictors, their assessments may be biased. For instance, in a clinical prediction rule developed to predict the presence of pneumonia in patients presenting with cough,[18] the authors make no mention of blinding during either the derivation process or the validation process. Knowledge of history or physical examination findings may have influenced the judgments of the unblinded radiologists.

The investigators testing the Ottawa Ankle Rules enrolled consecutive patients, obtained radiographs for all of them, and ensured that not only were the clinicians assessing the clinical predictors unaware of the radiologic results, but the radiologists had no knowledge of the clinical data.

# INTERPRETING THE RESULTS

Regardless of the level of evidence associated with a clinical prediction rule, its usefulness will depend on its predictive power. Investigators may report their results in a variety of ways. First, the results may dictate a specific course of action. The ankle component of the Ottawa Ankle Rules states that an ankle series is indicated only for patients with pain near the malleoli plus either inability to bear weight or localized bone tenderness at the posterior edge or tip of either malleolus (see Figure 2C-6). Underlying this decision are the sensitivity and specificity of their rule as a diagnostic test (see Part 1C2, "Diagnostic Tests"). In the development process, all patients with fracture had a positive result (sensitivity of 100%), but only 40% of those without fractures had a negative result (specificity of 40%). These results suggest that if clinicians order radiographs only for those patients with a positive result, they will not miss any fractures and will avoid the test in 40% of those without a fracture.

The validation study confirmed these results; in particular, the test maintained a sensitivity of 100%. This is particularly reassuring because the sample size was sufficiently large to result in a narrow confidence interval around the estimate of sensitivity (95% CI, 93%-100%). Thus, clinicians adopting the rule would miss very few, if any, fractures.

Another way of reporting clinical prediction rule results is in terms of probability of the target condition being present given a particular result. For example, a recent prediction rule for pulmonary embolus derived and validated by Wells and colleagues[19] accurately placed patients into low (3.4%; 95% CI, 2.2%-5%) intermediate (28%; 95% CI, 23.4%-32.2%), or high (78%; 95% CI, 69.2%-89.6%) probability categories. When investigators report prediction rule results in this fashion, they are implicitly incorporating all clinical information. In doing so, they remove any need for clinicians to consider independent information in deciding about the likelihood of the diagnosis or about a patient's prognosis.

Finally, prediction rules may also report their results as likelihood ratios, or as absolute or relative risks. For example the CAGE (Cut down, Annoyed, Guilty, Eye-opener), a prediction rule for detecting alcoholism, has been reported as likelihood ratios (for example, for CAGE scores of 0/4, LR = 0.14; for scores of 1/4, LR = 1.5; for scores of 2/4, LR = 4.5; for scores of 3/4, LR = 13; and for scores of 4/4, LR = 100). In this example, the probability of disease, alcoholism, depends on the combination of the prevalence of disease in the community and the score on the CAGE prediction rule.[20] When investigators report their results as likelihood ratios, they are implicitly suggesting that clinicians should use other, independent information to generate a pretest (or prerule) probability. Clinicians can then use the likelihood ratios generated by the rule to establish a posttest probability. (For approaches to using likelihood ratios, see Part 1C2, "Diagnostic Tests.")

# TESTING THE RULE'S IMPACT

Use of clinical prediction rules involves remembering predictor variables and often entails making calculations to determine a patient's probability of having the target outcome. Pocket cards and computer algorithms can facilitate the task of using complex clinical prediction rules. Nonetheless, they demand clinician time and energy, and their use is warranted only if they change physician behavior and if that behavior change results in improved patient outcomes or reduced costs while maintaining quality. If these conditions are not met, regardless of the accuracy of a clinical prediction rule, attempts to use it systematically will be a waste of time.

There are a number of reasons why an accurate prediction rule may not produce a change in behavior or an improvement in outcomes. First, clinicians' intuitive estimation of probabilities may be as good as, if not better than, the rule. If this is so, clinical prediction rule information will not improve their practice. Second, the calculations involved may be cumbersome and as a result, clinicians may not utilize the rule. Even worse, they may miscalculate. Third, there may be practical barriers to acting on the results of the clinical prediction rule. For instance, in the case of the Ottawa Ankle Rule, clinicians may be sufficiently concerned about protecting themselves against litigation that they may order radiographs despite a prediction rule result suggesting a negligible probability of fracture.

These are the considerations that lead us to (1) classify a clinical prediction rule with evidence of accuracy in diverse populations as level II, and (2) insist on a positive result from a study of impact before a clinical prediction rule ascends to level I.

Ideally, an impact study would randomize patients—or larger administrative units—to either apply or not apply the clinical prediction rule and follow patients for all relevant outcomes (including quality of life, morbidity, and resource utilization). Randomization of individual patients is unlikely to be appropriate because one would expect the participating clinicians to incorporate the rule into the care of all patients. A suitable alternative is to randomize institutions or practice settings and to conduct analyses appropriate to these larger units of randomization. Another potential design is to look at a single group before and after clinicians began to use the clinical prediction rule, but choice of a before/after study will substantially reduce the strength of inference.

Investigators examining the impact of the Ottawa Ankle Rule randomized six emergency departments to use or not use their prediction rule.[3] Just prior to initiating the study, one center dropped out, leaving a total of five emergency departments—two in the intervention group and three in the usual-care group. The intervention consisted of (1) introducing the prediction rule at a general meeting, (2) distributing pocket cards summarizing the rule, (3) posting the rule throughout the emergency department, and (4) applying preprinted data collection forms to each patient chart. In the control group, the only intervention was the introduction of preprinted data collection forms without the Ottawa rule attached to each chart. A total of 1911 eligible patients were entered into the study—1005 in the control group and 906 in the intervention group. There were 691 radiographs requested in the intervention group and 996 requested in the control group. In an analysis that focused on the ordering physician, the investigators found that the mean proportion of patients referred for radiography was 99.6% in the control group and 78.9% in the intervention group ($P = .03$). The investigators noted three missed fractures in the intervention group, none of which led to adverse outcomes. Thus, the investigators demonstrated a positive resource utilization impact of the Ottawa ankle rule (decreased test ordering) without increase in adverse outcomes, moving the clinical prediction rule to level I in the hierarchy (see Table 2C-3).

# CLINICAL RESOLUTION

Let us return to the opening clinical scenario. You have found level I evidence supporting the use of the Ottawa decision rule in reducing unnecessary ankle radiographs in patients presenting to the emergency department with ankle injuries. You therefore feel confident that you can productively utilize the rule in your own practice. Another recent study makes you aware that changing the behavior of your colleagues to realize the possible reductions in cost may be a challenge. Cameron and Naylor reported on an initiative in which clinicians expert in the use of the Ottawa Ankle Rule trained 16 other individuals to teach the use of the rule.[21]

These individuals returned to their emergency departments armed with slides, overheads, a 13-minute instructional video, and a mandate to train their colleagues locally and regionally in the use of the rule.

Unfortunately, this program led to no change in the use of ankle radiography. The results demonstrate that even the availability of a level I clinical prediction rule may require local implementation strategies with known effectiveness in changing provider behavior to ensure implementation.[22-24]

Clinical prediction rules inform our clinical judgment and have the potential to change clinical behavior and reduce unnecessary costs while maintaining quality of care and patient satisfaction. The challenge for clinicians is to evaluate the strength of the rule and its likely impact—and to find ways of efficiently incorporating level I rules into their daily practice.

Clinicians can access a summary of clinical prediction rules that highlights their level of evidence on the Internet (med.mssm.edu/ebm).

# References

1. Stiell IG, Greenberg GH, McKnight RD, Nair RC, McDowell I, Worthington JR. A study to develop clinical decision rules for the use of radiography in acute ankle injuries. *Ann Emerg Med*. 1992;21:384-390.

2. Stiell IG, Greenberg GH, McKnight RD, et al. Decision rules for the use of radiography in acute ankle injuries: refinement and prospective validation. *JAMA*. 1993;269:1127-1132.

3. Auleley GR, Ravaud P, Giraudeau B, et al. Implementation of the Ottawa ankle rules in France: a multicenter randomized controlled trial. *JAMA*. 1997;277:1935-1939.

4. Laupacis A, Sekar N, Stiell IG. Clinical prediction rules: a review and suggested modifications of methodological standards. *JAMA*. 1997;277:488-494.

5. Rudy TE, Kubinski JA, Boston JR. Multivariate analysis and repeated measurements: a primer. *J Crit Care*. 1992;7:30-41.

6. Cook EF, Goldman L. Empiric comparison of multivariate analytic techniques: advantages and disadvantages of recursive partitioning analysis. *J Chronic Dis*. 1984;37:721-731.

7. Baxt WG. Application of artificial neural networks to clinical medicine. *Lancet*. 1995;346:1135-1138.

8. Martin TP, Hanusa BH, Kapoor WN. Risk stratification of patients with syncope. *Ann Emerg Med*. 1997;29:459-466.

9. Fine MJ, Auble TE, Yealy DM, et al. A prediction rule to identify low-risk patients with community-acquired pneumonia. *N Engl J Med*. 1997;336:243-250.

10. Justice AC, Covinsky KE, Berlin JA. Assessing the generalizability of prognostic information. *Ann Intern Med*. 1999;130:515-524.

11. Lucchesi GM, Jackson RE, Peacock WF, Cerasani C, Swor RA. Sensitivity of the Ottawa rules. *Ann Emerg Med*. 1995;26:1-5.

12. Kelly AM, Richards D, Kerr L, et al. Failed validation of a clinical decision rule for the use of radiography in acute ankle injury. *N Z Med J*. 1994;107:294-295.

13. Stiell I, Wells G, Laupacis A, et al, for the Multicentre Ankle Rule Study Group. Multicentre trial to introduce the Ottawa ankle rules for use of radiography in acute ankle injuries. *BMJ*. 1995;311:594-597.

14. Auleley GR, Kerboull L, Durieux P, Cosquer M, Courpied JP, Ravaud P. Validation of the Ottawa ankle rules in France: a study in the surgical emergency department of a teaching hospital. *Ann Emerg Med*. 1998;32:14-18.

15. Silver MT, Rose GA, Paul SD, O'Donnell CJ, O'Gara PT, Eagle KA. A clinical rule to predict preserved left ventricular ejection fraction in patients after myocardial infarction. *Ann Intern Med*. 1994;121:750-756.

16. Tobin K, Stomel R, Harber D, Karavite D, Sievers J, Eagle K. Validation in a community hospital setting of a clinical rule to predict preserved left ventricular ejection fraction in patients after myocardial infarction. *Arch Intern Med*. 1999;159:353-357.

17. Krumholz HM, Howes CJ, Murillo JE, Vaccarino LV, Radford MJ, Ellerbeck EF. Validation of a clinical prediction rule for left ventricular ejection fraction after myocardial infarction in patients > or = 65 years old. *Am J Cardiol*. 1997;80:11-15.

18. Heckerling PS, Tape TG, Wigton RS, et al. Clinical prediction rule for pulmonary infiltrates. *Ann Intern Med*. 1990;113:664-670.

19. Wells PS, Ginsberg JS, Anderson DR, et al. Use of a clinical model for safe management of patients with suspected pulmonary embolism. *Ann Intern Med*. 1998;129:997-1005.

20. Buchsbaum DG, Buchanan RG, Centor RM, Schnoll SH, Lawton MJ. Screening for alcohol abuse using CAGE scores and likelihood ratios. *Ann Intern Med*. 1991;115:774-777.

21. Cameron C, Naylor CD. No impact from active dissemination of the Ottawa Ankle Rules: further evidence of the need for local implementation of practice guidelines. *CMAJ*. 1999;160:1165-1168.

22. Davis DA, Thomson MA, Oxman AD, Haynes RB. Changing physician performance: a systematic review of the effect of continuing medical education strategies. *JAMA*. 1995;274:700-705.

23. Cabana MD, Rand CS, Powe NR, et al. Why don't physicians follow clinical practice guidelines? A framework for improvement. *JAMA*. 1999;282:1458-1465.

24. Davis D, O'Brien MA, Freemantle N, Wolf FM, Mazmanian P, Taylor-Vaisey A. Impact of formal continuing medical education: do conferences, workshops, rounds, and other traditional continuing education activities change physician behavior or health care outcomes? *JAMA*. 1999;282:867-874.

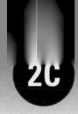

# 2C

# DIAGNOSIS
## Examples of Likelihood Ratios

### Luz Maria Letelier, Bruce Weaver, and Victor Montori

The following EBM Working Group members also made substantive contributions to this section: Gordon Guyatt and Jonathan Craig

## IN THIS SECTION

# Likelihood Ratios

In Part 1C, "The Process of Diagnosis," we introduced the concept of the likelihood ratio (LR) and explained its significance. In this section, we explore the concept in greater depth by presenting some examples of LRs along with the associated 95% confidence intervals. For each test, we describe the population to whom the test was applied and the range of prevalence (pretest probability) found for each target condition (disease). Our choice of conditions has been idiosyncratic and has represented the interests of the lead author (L.M.L.), who is a secondary care general internist. However, we did restrict ourselves to tests in current use at the time of publication of this book (and so do not offer a technical description of the tests). The lead author conducted all searches and summaries, without duplicate adjudication of eligibility or data extraction.

# Methods for Summarizing the Information on Likelihood Ratios

## Eligibility Criteria

For each test and target condition under consideration, we included studies that met each of the following criteria:

- The authors presented LRs or sufficient data to allow their calculation.

- The investigators compared the test to a gold standard that was defined in advance and that met the following criteria: (1) at the time of the study, it was in wide use and no better standard was available; (2) when the decision to apply the gold standard was unrelated to the results of the test, it was applied to at least 50% of eligible patients; and (3) when the decision to apply the gold standard may have been influenced by test results, it was applied to 90% of eligible patients—or it was blindly applied.

- The investigators enrolled patients similar to those seen in clinical practice in whom the test might be reasonably applied.

- The authors reported their results in English, Spanish, or Italian.

We excluded studies that met the following criteria:

- The study was concerned with predicting long-term outcomes.

- The study evaluated diagnostic models, including multiple tests such as decision trees, diagnostic algorithms, neural networks, or computer-based pattern recognition systems.

## Literature Search

We searched Best Evidence (1991-2000) and MEDLINE (1966-2000), and we reviewed the *JAMA* series entitled the "Rational Clinical Examination" (1992-2000) and references from a diagnostic textbook.[1] We also reviewed the citations of articles we found for additional potentially eligible studies.

For every pair of target condition and test, we searched the databases using the following search strategy template using both MeSH subject headings and text words (Figure 2C-8):

**FIGURE 2C-8**

## Search Strategy Template

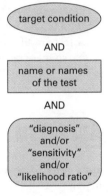

A typical search strategy example is shown in Figure 2C-9.

**FIGURE 2C-9**

## Sample Search Strategy

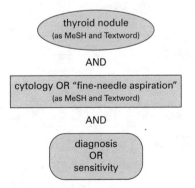

## Selection Process

When we found a good-quality systematic review,[2] we generally used it as our data source, although we sometimes reviewed the original trials to obtain the data required for our own statistical analysis. For systematic reviews done before 1997, we updated the searches using the authors' own search strategies.

## Statistical Analysis

Likelihood ratios and 95% confidence intervals for individual 2 x 2 and 2 x J (that is, two outcomes—target present and target absent—but J levels of test result) tables were computed using methods described by Simel et al.[3] We computed random-effect pooled estimates of the LRs (with delta = 0.25 added to each cell count) using the general meta-analytic method advanced by Fleiss.[4]

In calculating summary LRs, we did not take into account study quality, differences in calibration between centers, or differences in study population beyond those of our eligibility criteria, so these results are not considered to qualify as a formal meta-analysis.

# ABDOMINAL AORTIC ANEURYSM

In the following studies, investigators enrolled asymptomatic people with risk factors for abdominal aortic aneurysm (AAA). Their gold or reference standard was abdominal ultrasound. We found the results in one recent systematic review (Table 2C-6).

TABLE 2C-6

### Likelihood Ratios for Tests for Detection of Abdominal Aortic Aneurysm in Asymptomatic People

| Prevalence (Pretest Probability) | Patients Included (Number) | Test | Result | LR (95% CI) | Reference |
|---|---|---|---|---|---|
| Target condition: AAA ≥ 3 cm | | | | | |
| 1%–28% | 2955 | Abdominal palpation directed toward AAA detection | Positive | 12 (7.4–20) | 5 |
| | | | Negative | 0.72 (0.65–0.81) | |
| Target condition: AAA ≥ 4 cm | | | | | |
| 1%–28% | 2955 | Abdominal palpation directed toward AAA detection | Positive | 6 (8.6–29) | 5 |
| | | | Negative | 0.51 (0.38–0.67) | |

AAA indicates abnormal aortic aneurysm; LR, likelihood ratio; CI, confidence interval.

# ACUTE APPENDICITIS

In the following studies, investigators enrolled patients with right lower quadrant pain or acute abdominal pain (for less than 1 week), including children over 2 years of age. Their gold or reference standards for the diagnosis of appendicitis included surgery and histopathology or clinical follow-up.

Our literature search uncovered 342 potentially eligible titles or abstracts that we retrieved of which 45 appeared potentially pertinent and were reviewed in detail and 20 were included (Table 2C-7).

**TABLE 2C-7**

## Likelihood Ratios of Tests for the Diagnosis of Appendicitis

| Prevalence (Pretest Probability) | Patients Included (Number) | Test | Result | LR (95% CI) | References |
|---|---|---|---|---|---|
| 12%–26% | 2447 | History or Physical Examination | | | 6–13 |
| | | Rigidity | Present | 3.8 (3.0–4.8) | |
| | | | Absent | 0.82 (0.79–0.85) | |
| | | Psoas sign* | Present | 2.7 (1.5–4.7) | |
| | | | Absent | 0.82 (0.76–0.99) | |
| | | Pain migration from epigastrium or periumbilical area to right lower quadrant | Present | 2.4 (1.4–4.2) | |
| | | | Absent | 0.55 (0.38–0.78) | |
| | | Guarding | Present | 2.2 (1.6–3.0) | |
| | | | Absent | 0.34 (0.22–0.53) | |
| | | Pain located in right lower quadrant | Present | 2.2 (0.77–6.1) | |
| | | | Absent | 0.29 (0.11–0.77) | |
| | | Rebound sign† | Present | 1.9 (1.6–2.2) | |
| | | | Absent | 0.36 (0.25–0.52) | |
| | | Fever; vomiting; anorexia; nausea | Present | 0.5–2.0 | |

| Prevalence (Pretest Probability) | Patients Included (Number) | Test | Result | LR (95% CI) | References |
|---|---|---|---|---|---|
| | | Radiologic Findings | | | |
| 54%–64% | 200 | Abdominal and pelvic high-resolution computed tomography (CT) with intravenous and oral contrast media | Positive<br><br>Negative | 11 (4.9–25)<br><br>0.08 (0.04–0.15) | 14, 15 |
| 21%–54% | 1737 | Ultrasound by radiologist or trained surgeon with or without graded compression technique | Positive<br><br>Negative | 23 (19–44)<br><br>0.22 (0.18–0.35) | 16–19 |
| 30%–53% | 808 | Abdominal and pelvic helical CT scan, or just focused to the appendix, without IV contrast media, but with oral, colonic, or no intestinal contrast media | Positive<br><br>Negative | 26 (16–42)<br><br>0.05 (0.03–0.10) | 20–26 |

\* Psoas sign: A sign of irritation of the psoas muscle, it is elicited by having the patient extend the leg (ipsilateral to the location of abdominal pain) at the hip against resistance (by the examiner) while lying on the unaffected side. If abdominal pain appears or is exacerbated with this maneuver, the sign is considered positive. In acute appendicitis, this sign may be positive on the right side.

† Rebound sign: A sign of peritoneal inflammation, it is elicited by first palpating deeply and slowly an area of the abdomen distant from the location of abdominal pain followed by quick removal of the palpating hand. If abdominal pain appears or is exacerbated with removal of the palpating hand, the sign is considered positive.

LR indicates likelihood ratio; CI, confidence interval.

# ACUTE MYOCARDIAL INFARCTION

In the following studies of the diagnosis of acute myocardial infarction, investigators enrolled patients admitted for suspected myocardial infarction (MI) or consulting emergency departments for chest pain. Their reference standard included the results of cardiac enzyme determinations and electrocardiographic changes. We found the results in one recent systematic review (Table 2C-8).

**TABLE 2C-8**

## Likelihood Ratios for Tests for the Diagnosis of Myocardial Infarction in Patients Admitted for Suspected Myocardial Infarction or Consulting Emergency Departments for Chest Pain

| Prevalence (Pretest Probability) | Patients Included (Number) | Test | Result | LR (95% CI) | Reference |
|---|---|---|---|---|---|
| 12%–45% | 14,838 | **History** | | | 27 |
| | | Radiation of pain to left and right arm | Present | 7.1 (3.6–14.2) | |
| | | Radiation of pain to right shoulder | Present | 2.9 (1.4–6.0) | |
| | | Radiation of pain to left arm | Present | 2.3 (1.7–3.1) | |
| | | Pleuritic chest pain | Present | 0.2 (0.2–0.3) | |
| | | Sharp or stabbing chest pain | Present | 0.3 (0.2–0.5) | |
| | | Positional chest pain | Present | 0.3 (0.2–0.4) | |
| 12%–45% | 14,838 | **Physical Examination** | | | 27 |
| | | Third heart sound | Present | 3.2 (1.6–6.5) | |
| | | Pulmonary crackles | Present | 2.1 (1.4–3.1) | |
| 12%–85% | 13,940 | **Electrocardiogram** | | | 27 |
| | | New ST segment elevation | Present | 5.7–54* | |
| | | Any ST segment elevation | Present | 11 (7.1–18) | |
| | | New ST segment depression | Present | 3.0–5.2* | |
| | | Any ST segment depression | Present | 3.2 (2.5–4.1) | |
| | | New conduction defect | Present | 6.3 (2.5–16) | |
| | | Any conduction defect | Present | 2.7 (1.4–5.4) | |
| | | New Q wave | Present | 5.3–25* | |
| | | Any Q wave | Present | 3.9 (2.7–5.7) | |

| Prevalence (Pretest Probability) | Patients Included (Number) | Test | Result | LR (95% CI) | Reference |
|---|---|---|---|---|---|
| | | T wave peaking or inverted >1 mm | Present | 3.1† | |
| | | New T wave inversion | Present | 2.4–2.8* | |

\* Expressed as range due to heterogeneity of studies.

† Insufficient data to determine CI.

LR indicates likelihood ratio; CI, confidence interval.

# COMMUNITY-ACQUIRED PNEUMONIA

In the following studies of the diagnosis of community acquired pneumonia, investigators enrolled patients with fever, cough, or other respiratory symptoms— or those suspected of having pneumonia, excluding those with nosocomial infections and inmunosuppression. Their reference standard was defined as the presence of definite or suspicious new infiltrates on chest radiograph. We found the results in one recent overview and four of its selected studies (Table 2C-9).

**TABLE 2C-9**

**Likelihood Ratios for Tests for the Diagnosis of Community-Acquired Pneumonia in Symptomatic Patients Suspected of Having Pneumonia**

| Prevalence (Pretest Probability) | Patients Included (Number) | Test | Result | LR (95% CI ) | References |
|---|---|---|---|---|---|
| 3%–38% | | History | | | |
| | 1118 | Dementia* | Present | 3.4  (1.6–6.5) | 28 |
| | | | Absent | 0.94 (0.90–0.99) | |
| | 255 | Cough | Present | 1.5  (1.3–1.8) | 31 |
| | | | Absent | 0.39 (0.20–0.77) | |
| | 1118 | Past medical history of asthma | Present | 0.30 (0.16–0.54) | 32 |
| | | | Absent | 1.2  (1.2–1.3) | |
| | | Dyspnea, sputum production, chills or night sweats, myalgias, sore throat, rhinorrhea | | 2.0–0.5 | 28 |

| Prevalence (Pretest Probability) | Patients Included (Number) | Test | Result | LR (95% CI ) | References |
|---|---|---|---|---|---|
| 3%–38% | | Physical Examination | | | |
| | 483 | Asymmetric respiration | Present | 80 (1.3–5,003) | 29 |
| | | | Absent | 0.96 (0.90–1.0) | |
| | 1909 | Egophony | Present | 4.0 (2.0–8.1) | 28, 29, 32 |
| | | | Absent | 0.93 (0.88–0.99) | |
| | 1118 | Bronchial breath sounds | Present | 3.5 (2.0–5.6) | 28 |
| | | | Absent | 0.90 (0.83–0.96) | |
| | 1426 | Dullness to percussion | Present | 3.0 (1.6–5.8) | 30, 32 |
| | | | Absent | 0.86 (0.74–1.0) | |
| | 308 | Respiration rate > 30/min | Present | 2.6 (1.6–4.1) | 28 |
| | | | Absent | 0.80 (0.70–0.90) | |
| | 1426 | Decreased breath sounds | Present | 2.4 (2.0–2.9) | 30, 32 |
| | | | Absent | 0.71 (0.59–0.86) | |
| | 2164 | Temperature >37.8°C or >100°F | Present | 2.3 (1.5–3.5) | 29–32 |
| | | | Absent | 0.67 (0.58–0.77) | |
| | 1601 | Respiration rate > 25/min | Present | 2.2 (1.0–5.0) | 29, 32 |
| | | | Absent | 0.80 (0.71–0.90) | |
| | 2164 | Crackles heard on chest auscultation | Present | 2.1 (1.5–2.9) | 29–32 |
| | | | Absent | 0.77 (0.65–0.91) | |
| | 308 | Any abnormal vital sign | Present | 1.2 (1.1–1.3) | 28 |
| | | | Absent | 0.18 (0.07–0.46) | |
| | | Respiration rate > 20; heart rate > 120; rhonchi heard on chest auscultation | | 2.0–0.5 | 28 |

\* Significant cognitive impairment with ineffective airway protection mechanisms.

LR indicates likelihood ratio; CI, confidence interval.

# DEEP VENOUS THROMBOSIS

In the following studies, investigators enrolled symptomatic hospitalized or ambulatory patients suspected of having a first episode of deep venous thrombosis (DVT). Their reference standard was venography. After reviewing 15 potentially pertinent articles in detail, we determined that nine articles met inclusion criteria, including three recent systematic reviews (Table 2C-10).

**TABLE 2C-10**

## Likelihood Ratios for Tests for Diagnosis of Deep Venous Thrombosis in Symptomatic Patients

| Prevalence (Pretest Probability) | Patients Included (Number) | Test | Result | LR (95% CI) | References |
|---|---|---|---|---|---|
| Target condition: All DVT, including distal (isolated calf DVT) and proximal DVT* | | | | | |
| | 2658 | Ultrasonography | Positive | 15[†] | 35 |
| | | | Negative | 0.12[†] | |
| | 1156 | Impedance plethysmography | Abnormal | 10[†] | 35 |
| | | | Normal | 0.18[†] | |
| 25%–49% | | D-dimer (Assay) | Results (Expressed in ng/mL) | | |
| | 516 | Latex | > 200 | 5.0 (2.1–12) | 38–40 |
| | | | < 200 | 0.31 (0.22–0.45) | |
| | 56 | Latex | > 500 | 6.1[†] | 36 |
| | | | < 500 | 0.27[†] | |
| | 92 | Latex | > 1500 | 2.9[†] | 36 |
| | | | < 1500 | 0.36[†] | |
| | 111 | ELISA[‡] | > 200 | 1.7 (1.2–2.5) | 38, 39 |
| | | | < 200 | 0.03 (0–0.43) | |
| | 92 | ELISA | > 250 | 1.6[†] | 36 |
| | | | < 250 | 0.05[†] | |

| Prevalence (Pretest Probability) | Patients Included (Number) | Test | Result | LR (95% CI) | References |
|---|---|---|---|---|---|
| 92 | | Inmunofiltration (Nycomed) | > 500 | 1.26[†] | 41 |
| | | | < 500 | 0.2[†] | |
| | 214 | Blood agglutination (SimpliRed) qualitative | Positive | 3.9[†] | 37 |
| | | | Negative | 0.14[†] | |

**Target Condition: Proximal DVT (popliteal or more proximal veins)\***

| | 2658 | Ultrasonography | Positive | 49[†] | 35 |
|---|---|---|---|---|---|
| | | | Negative | 0.03[†] | |
| | 1156 | Impedance plethysmography | Abnormal | 8.4[†] | 35 |
| | | | Normal | 0.09[†] | |

\* See Figure 2C-10 for a clinical scoring model to estimate the prevalence of DVT.

† Insufficient data available to determine CI.

‡ Enzyme-Linked Immunosorbent Assay.

DVT indicates deep venous thrombosis; LR likelihood ratio; CI, confidence interval.

The chart shown in Figure 2C-10 shows a simplified clinical scoring model for patients with deep venous thrombosis. It was developed by Anand et al[33] to estimate the prevalence of this condition.

**FIGURE 2C-10**

### Clinical Scoring Model to Estimate the Prevalence of Deep Venous Thrombosis

| | |
|---|---|
| Active cancer | + 1 |
| Paralysis, paresis, or recent plaster immobilization of lower extremity | + 1 |
| Recently bedridden > 3 days of major surgery within weeks | + 1 |
| Localized tenderness along distribution of deep venous system | + 1 |
| Swelling of entire leg | + 1 |
| Calf swelling > 3 cm compared to asymptomatic leg | + 1 |
| Pitting edema (greater in symptomatic leg) | + 1 |
| Collateral superficial veins (nonvaricose) | + 1 |
| Alternative diagnosis as likely or greater than DVT | − 2 |

Score

**Results:**

| | | Prevalence (95%CI) |
|---|---|---|
| High probability | 3 or more | 75% (63%–81%) |
| Moderate probability | 1 or 2 | 17% (12%–23%) |
| Low probability | 0 or less | 3% (1.7%–5.9%) |

# HYPOVOLEMIA

In the following studies of the diagnosis of hypovolemia, investigators enrolled patients 60 years of age or older with acute conditions associated with vomiting, diarrhea, or decreased oral intake. Their reference standards included chemical measures such as serum sodium, blood urea nitrogen (BUN), the BUN-to-creatinine ratio, and osmolality. We found the results in one recent systematic review (Table 2C-11).

TABLE 2C-11

## Likelihood Ratios for Diagnosis of Hypovolemia in Patients 60 Years of Age or Older Experiencing Acute Conditions Associated With Volume Loss

| Prevalence | Patients Included (Number) | Test | Result | LR (95% CI) | References |
|---|---|---|---|---|---|
| Not available | | **Skin/Mucosal Exam** | | | |
| | 38 | Sunken eyes | Present | 3.4  (1.0–12) | 42 |
| | | | Absent | 0.50  (0.3–0.7) | |
| | 86 | Dry axilla | Present | 2.8  (1.4–5.4) | 42 |
| | | | Absent | 0.6  (0.4–1.0) | |
| | 38 | Dry tongue | Present | 2.1  (0.8–5.8) | 42 |
| | | | Absent | 0.6  (0.3–1.0) | |
| | 38 | Dry mouth and nose mucosa | Present | 2.0  (1.0–4.0) | 42 |
| | | | Absent | 0.3  (0.1–0.6) | |
| | 38 | Longitudinal furrows on tongue | Present | 2.0  (1.0–4.0) | 42 |
| | | | Absent | 0.3  (0.1–0.6) | |
| | | **Neurologic Signs** | | | |
| | 38 | Unclear speech | Present | 3.1  (0.9–11) | 42 |
| | | | Absent | 0.5  (0.4–0.8) | |
| | 38 | Weak upper or lower extremities | Present | 2.3  (0.6–8.6) | 42 |
| | | | Absent | 0.7  (0.5–1.0) | |
| | 38 | Confusion | Present | 2.1  (0.8–5.7) | 42 |
| | | | Absent | 0.6  (0.4–1.0) | |

LR indicates likelihood ratio; CI, confidence interval.

# IRON-DEFICIENCY ANEMIA

In the following studies of the diagnosis of iron deficiency anemia, investigators enrolled anemic patients with hemoglobin levels less than 11.7 g/dL and less than 13.0g/dL for women and men, respectively. Their reference standard was a bone marrow aspirate stained for iron. Our literature search identified 204 reports that seemed relevant based on their titles and abstracts. Of those, 37 appeared pertinent and were reviewed in detail, with seven fulfilling inclusion criteria (Table 2C-12).

**TABLE 2C-12**

## Likelihood Ratios for Tests for Diagnosis of Iron-Deficiency Anemia in Patients With Anemia

| Prevalence (Pretest Probability) | Patients Included (Number) | Test | Result | Likelihood Ratio (95% CI) | References |
|---|---|---|---|---|---|
| 21%–50% | 2798 | Serum ferritin ($\mu$g/L) | < 15 | 55 (35–84) | 43, 44 |
| | | | 15–25 | 9.3 (6.3–14) | |
| | | | 25–35 | 2.5 (2.1–3.0) | |
| | | | 35–45 | 1.8 (1.5–2.2) | |
| | | | 45–100 | 0.54 (0.48–0.60) | |
| | | | > 100 | 0.08 (0.06–0.11) | |
| 21%–50% | 536 | Mean cell volume ($\mu$m$^3$) | < 70 | 13 (6.1–19) | 43 |
| | | | 70–75 | 3.3 (2.0–4.7) | |
| | | | 75–85 | 1.0 (0.69–1.31) | |
| | | | 85–90 | 0.76 (0.56–0.96) | |
| | | | > 90 | 0.29 (0.21–0.37) | |
| 21%–50% | 764 | Transferrin saturation (%) | < 5 | 11 (6.4–15) | 43 |
| | | | 5–10 | 2.5 (2.0–3.1) | |
| | | | 10–20 | 0.81 (0.70–0.92) | |
| | | | 20–30 | 0.52 (0.41–0.63) | |
| | | | 30–50 | 0.43 (0.31–0.55) | |
| | | | >50 | 0.15 (0.06–0.24) | |
| 21%–50% | 278 | Red cell protoporphyrin ($\mu$g/dL) | > 350 | 8.3 (2.6–14) | 43 |
| | | | 350–250 | 6.1 (2.8–9.3) | |
| | | | 250–150 | 2.0 (1.4–2.6) | |
| | | | 150–50 | 0.56 (0.48–0.64) | |
| | | | < 50 | 0.12 (0.0–0.25) | |
| 21%–50% | 273 | Red cell volume distribution | > 21 | 2.7 (1.3–4.1) | 43 |
| | | | 21–17 | 1.8 (1.4–2.2) | |
| | | | 17–15 | 0.84 (0.63–1.1) | |
| | | | < 15 | 0.61 (0.48–0.74) | |

| Prevalence (Pretest Probability) | Patients Included (Number) | Test | Result | LR (95% CI) | References |
|---|---|---|---|---|---|
| **Patients With Anemia and Chronic Renal Failure on Hemodialysis or Peritoneal Dialysis** | | | | | |
| 9%–50% | 190 | Serum ferritin (µg / L) | < 50 | 12 (4.4–32) | 45–49 |
| | | | 50–100 | 2.3 (0.70–7.3) | |
| | | | 100–300 | 0.64 (0.32–1.2) | |
| | | | > 300 | 0.27 (0.12–0.61) | |
| **Patients With Anemia and Cirrhosis** | | | | | |
| 40% | 72 | Serum ferritin (µg/L) | < 50 | 22* | 49 |
| | | | 50–400 | 1.0–1.8 | |
| | | | 400–1000 | 0.13* | |
| | | | 1000–2200 | 0.19* | |

\* Insufficient data to determine confidence intervals.

LR indicates likelihood ratio; CI, confidence interval.

# PERIPHERAL ARTERIAL DISEASE OR PERIPHERAL VASCULAR INSUFFICIENCY

In the following studies of the diagnosis of peripheral artery disease or peripheral vascular insufficiency, investigators used the ankle to arm (brachial) systolic pressure index (AAI) as a reference standard. We found the results in one recent overview and its selected studies (Table 2C-13).

**TABLE 2C-13**

## Likelihood Ratios for Tests for Diagnosis of Peripheral Artery Disease

| Prevalence (Pretest Probability) | Number of Patient Legs Included | Test | Result | LR (95% CI) | | References |
|---|---|---|---|---|---|---|
| **Patients: Asymptomatic/Symptomatic With Risk Factors for Atherosclerosis or With Classic Peripheral Arterial Disease History** | | | | | | |
| **Target Outcome: Severe PAD = > AAI < 0.5** | | | | | | |
| If asymptomatic or symptomatic with risk factors*: 10%–12%. If symptomatic with classic PAD history: 71% | 605 | Venous filling time | > 20 seconds | 3.6 | (1.9–6.8) | 50, 51 53, 54 |
| | | | < 20 seconds | 0.8 | (0.7–1.0) | |

| Prevalence (Pretest Probability) | Number of Patient Legs Included | Test | Result | LR (95% CI) | References |
|---|---|---|---|---|---|
| " | 854 | Tibial and/or dorsalis pedis pulse | Weak/absent | 3.2 (2.7–3.9) | 50, 51 |
| | | | Present | 0.19 (0.03–1.15) | |
| " | 605 | Absent lower limb hair, atrophic skin, cool skin, blue/purple skin, capillary refilling time, > 5 sec | | 0.5–2.0 | 52 |

**Patients: Asymptomatic or Symptomatic With Risk Factors for Atherosclerosis or With Any Leg Complaint on Walking With or Without Risk Factors**

**Target Outcome: Moderate PAD (AAI < 0.9)**

| Prevalence (Pretest Probability) | Number of Patient Legs Included | Test | Result | LR (95% CI) | References |
|---|---|---|---|---|---|
| 10%–12% | 4597 | Tibial or dorsalis pedis pulse, or both | Weak or absent | 8.9 (7.1–11) | 51, 53, 54 |
| | | | Present | 0.33 (0.28–0.40) | |
| 10%–12% | 4910 | Wound or sores on foot or toes | Present | 6.9 (2.9–16) | 54 |
| | | | Absent | 0.98 (0.97–1.0) | |
| " | 5418 | Femoral pulse | Weak or absent | 6.7 (4.3–10) | 53, 54 |
| | | | Present | 0.94 (0.91–0.96) | |
| " | 4910 | Unilateral cooler skin | Present | 5.8 (4.0–8.4) | 54 |
| | | | Absent | 0.92 (0.89–0.95) | |
| " | 5,418 | Femoral bruit | Present | 5.4 (4.5–6.5) | 53, 54 |
| | | | Absent | 0.78 (0.70–0.86) | |
| " | 4,910 | Abnormal color on feet or leg | Present | 2.8 (2.4–3.2) | 54 |
| | | | Absent | 0.74 (0.69–0.80) | |

**Patients: Classic PAD History**

**Target Outcome: Moderate PAD (AAI < 0.9)**

| Prevalence (Pretest Probability) | Number of Patient Legs Included | Test | Result | LR (95% CI) | References |
|---|---|---|---|---|---|
| 71% | 4597 | Tibial or dorsalis pedis pulse, or both | Weak or absent | 8.9 (7.1–11) | 51, 53, 54 |
| | | | Present | 0.33 (0.28–0.40) | |

\* Risk factors include dyslipidemia, diabetes mellitus, smoking, hypertension, and cardiovascular disease.

PAD indicates peripheral artery disease; LR, likelihood ratio; CI, confidence interval.

# THYROID NODULE

In the following studies of the diagnosis of malignancy in thyroid nodules (primary or metastatic cancer or lymphoma), investigators enrolled patients with normal thyroid function and palpable thyroid nodules. The nodules could be solid or cystic and solitary or dominant if multiple nodules were present. Their reference standard was histopathologic examination after surgical excision or clinical follow-up. We found the results after identifying 67 reports on the basis of their titles and abstracts, of which 30 seemed pertinent and were reviewed in detail, with seven fulfilling inclusion criteria (Table 2C-14).

**TABLE 2C-14**

**Likelihood Ratios for the Diagnosis of Malignancy in Euthyroid Patients With a Single or Dominant Thyroid Nodule**

| Prevalence (Pretest Probability) | Patients Included (Number) | Test | Result | LR (95% CI) | References |
|---|---|---|---|---|---|
| 20% | 132 | Fine-needle aspiration cytology guided with ultrasound | Malignant | 226 (4.4–11,739) | 55 |
| | | | Suspicious | 1.3 (0.52–3.2) | |
| | | | Insufficient | 2.7 (0.52–15) | |
| | | | Benign | 0.24 (0.11–0.52) | |
| 7%–22% | 868 | Fine-needle aspiration cytology not guided | Malignant | 34 (15–74 ) | 56–61 |
| | | | Suspicious | 1.7 (0.94–3.0) | |
| | | | Insufficient | 0.5 (0.27–0.76) | |
| | | | Benign | 0.23 (0.13–0.42) | |

# THROMBOEMBOLISM OR ACUTE PULMONARY EMBOLISM

In the following studies of the diagnosis of acute pulmonary embolism (PE), the investigators used angiography or clinical follow-up for more than 1 year as their reference standard. Normal ventilation-perfusion scan was used to rule out PE only on trials using clinical assessment, electrocardiogram, or chest radiograph. We identified 475 reports based on their titles and abstracts, of which 112 seemed pertinent and were reviewed in detail, with 16 fulfilling inclusion criteria (Table 2C-15).

**TABLE 2C-15**

## Likelihood Ratios for Tests for the Diagnosis of Pulmonary Embolism

| Prevalence (Pretest Probability) | Patients Included (Number) | Test | Result | LR (95% CI) | References |
|---|---|---|---|---|---|
| | | | | | |
| Patients: Those Suspected of Having Acute Pulmonary Embolism (PE) Who Have Had Symptoms for the Past 24 Hours | | | | | |
| 32%–44% | | **History/Physical Examination** | | * | |
| | 78 | Blood pressure | < 100/70 | 3.1 | 62 |
| | | | >100/70 | 0.8 | |
| | 78 | Ventricular diastolic gallop | Present | 3.0 | 62 |
| | | | Absent | 0.9 | |
| | 78 | Congestive heart failure | Present | 0.3 | 62 |
| | | | Absent | 1.2 | |
| | 403 | Risk factors[†] Symptoms[†] Signs[†] | | 0.5–2.0 | 62–64 |
| 41%–44% | | **Electrocardiogram** | | * | |
| | 78 | S-I / Q-III / T-III | Present | 2.4 | 62 |
| | | | Absent | 0.88 | |
| | 78 | Inverted T waves V1→V3 | Present | 2.3 | 62 |
| | | | Absent | 0.94 | |
| | 78 | Normal | Present | 0.82 | 62 |
| | | | Absent | 2.2 | |
| | 78 | Right bundle-branch block Right ventricular hypertrophy | | 0.5–2.0 | 62 |
| 27%–44% | | **Chest Radiograph** | | | |
| | 1203 | • Normal • Pulmonary edema • Enlarged hilum or mediastinum • Prominent central artery • Atelectasis • Pleural effusion | | 0.5–2.0 | 65, 66 |

| Prevalence (Pretest Probability) | Patients Included (Number) | Test | Result | LR (95% CI) | | References |
|---|---|---|---|---|---|---|
| 31% | 98 | Latex d-dimer (ng/mL) | > 500 | 2.8 | (1.5–5.2) | 36, 67 |
| | | | < 500 | 0.61 | (0.42–0.89) | |
| | | | > 250 | 1.7 | (1.2–2.4) | |
| | | | <250 | 0.47 | (0.25–0.88) | |
| 31%–57% | | **CT scan** | | | | |
| | 60 | Contrast-enhanced electron-beam CT | Positive | 22 | (3.4–113) | 70 |
| | | | Negative | 0.36 | (0.21–0.64) | |
| | 224 | Helical CT | Positive | 13 | (6.1–26) | 68, 69 |
| | | | Negative | 0.13 | (0.03–0.51) | |
| 29% | 881 | Ventilation-perfusion scintigram (V/Q scan) | High probability | 18 | (11–31) | 71 |
| | | | Intermediate probability | 1.2 | (1.0–1.5) | |
| | | | Low probability | 0.36 | (0.26–0.49) | |
| | | | Normal | 0.10 | (0.04–0.25) | |

**Patients: Those With Suspected PE and Normal Chest Radiograph**

| | | | | | | |
|---|---|---|---|---|---|---|
| 15% | 133 | Ventilation-perfusion scintigram (V/Q scan) | High probability | 10 | | 72 |
| | | | Intermediate probability | 1.7 | | |
| | | | Low probability | 1.1 | | |
| | | | Normal | 0.2 | | |
| 15% | 110 | Dyspnea and $Pao_2$ | <70 | 2.8 | | 72 |
| | | | >70 | 0.58 | | |
| 15% | 110 | $Pao_2$ | <70 | 2.2 | | 72 |
| | | | >70 | 0.62 | | |

**Patients: Those Suspected of PE With Normal Chest Radiograph and No Prior Cardiopulmonary Disease**

| | | | | | | |
|---|---|---|---|---|---|---|
| 15% | 110 | Dyspnea and $Pao^2$ | < 60 | 6 | | 72 |
| | | | > 60 | 0.84 | | |
| | | | < 70 | 3.6 | | |
| | | | > 70 | 0.77 | | |

| Prevalence (Pretest Probability) | Patients Included (Number) | Test | Result | LR (95% CI) | References |
|---|---|---|---|---|---|
| **Patients: Those Suspected of PE Without Cardiopulmonary Disease** | | | | | |
| Not available | 70 | Hepatojugular reflux | Present | 11 | 64 |
| | | | Absent | 0.7 | |
| | 70 | Hepatomegaly | Present | 3 | 64 |
| | | | Absent | 0.89 | |
| | 70 | ECG: S-I / Q-III | Present | 3.7 | 64 |
| | | | Absent | 0.6 | |
| | 70 | ECG: inverted T waves | Present | 1.3 | 64 |
| | | | Absent | 0.88 | |
| | 70 | Chest radiograph: atelectasis | Present | 3.6 | 64 |
| | | | Absent | 0.77 | |
| | 364 | Chest radiograph: Westermark sign‡ | Present | 3.5 | 63 |
| | | | Absent | 0.95 | |
| | 364 | Chest radiograph: pulmonary edema | Present | 0.31 | 63 |
| | | | Absent | 1.1 | |

\* Insufficient data to determine 95% CI.

† Risk factors: immobilization, surgery, trauma, malignancy, previous DVT, estrogen, postpartum, stroke. Symptoms: dyspnea, hemoptysis, any type of chest pain, cough, leg pain, or swelling. Signs: fever, heart rate >100, respiratory rate >20, crackles, wheezes, third or fourth heart sounds, increased pulmonic component of second heart sound, Homan sign, actual DVT, edema, varices.

‡ Westermark sign = prominent pulmonary artery and decreased pulmonary vasculature.

LR indicates likelihood ratio; CI, confidence interval.

The following tables of likelihood ratio are a summary from the *JAMA* series on The Rational Clinical Examination, without being updated here. From this series we included only those articles that explicitly described a test or maneuver from the physical exam, the gold standard used for comparison, and the patients included in the studies assessed. In general, we present the likelihood ratio given in the articles, but for those that did not pool their results, we used the original articles to make the 2 x J tables and, using the statistical methods already described, compiled a pooled estimate of the likelihood ratio.

# ASCITES

In the following study of the diagnosis of ascites, investigators enrolled patients suspected of having liver disease or ascites using abdominal ultrasound as their reference standard[73] (Table 2C-16).

**TABLE 2C-16**

## Likelihood Ratios for Tests for Diagnosing Ascites in Patients Suspected of Having Liver Disease or Ascites

| Prevalence (Pretest Probability) | Patients Included (Number) | Test | Result | LR (95% CI) | Reference |
|---|---|---|---|---|---|
| 29%–33% | Not applicable | History | | * | 73 |
| | | Increased girth | Present | 4.6 | |
| | | | Absent | 0.17 | |
| | | Recent weight gain | Present | 3.2 | |
| | | | Absent | 0.42 | |
| | | Hepatitis | Present | 3.2 | |
| | | | Absent | 0.80 | |
| | | Ankle swelling | Present | 2.8 | |
| | | | Absent | 0.10 | |
| | | Heart failure or alcoholism or carcinoma | | 0.5–2.0 | |
| | | **Physical Examination** | | | |
| | | Fluid wave | Present | 6.0  (3.3–11) | |
| | | | Absent | 0.4  (0.3–0.6) | |
| | | Shifting dullness | Present | 2.7  (1.9–3.9) | |
| | | | Absent | 0.3  (0.2–0.6) | |
| | | Flank dullness | Present | 2.0  (1.5–2.9) | |
| | | | Absent | 0.3  (0.1–0.7) | |
| | | Bulging flanks | Present | 2.0  (1.5–2.6) | |
| | | | Absent | 0.3  (0.2–0.6) | |

* Insufficient data to determine 95% CI.

# CAROTID ARTERY STENOSIS

In the following studies of the diagnosis of carotid artery stenosis (defined as stenosis of more than 50% of the arterial lumen), investigators enrolled patients undergoing angiography for transient ischemic attacks or other neurologic conditions using the results of carotid angiography as their reference standard[74-77] (Table 2C-17).

**TABLE 2C-17**

**Likelihood Ratios for Tests for Diagnosis of Carotid Artery Stenosis (>50%) in Symptomatic Patients Undergoing Cerebral Angiography**

| Prevalence | Patients (Number) | Test | Result | Likelihood Ratio (95% CI) | References |
|---|---|---|---|---|---|
| 8.2%–38% | 2011 | Carotid bruit | Present | 4.4 (2.9–6.8) | 74–77 |
| | | | Absent | 0.62 (0.45–0.86) | |

# ALCOHOLISM

In the following studies of the diagnosis of alcohol abuse or dependence, investigators enrolled hospitalized patients from psychiatric, orthopedic, and medical wards, and ambulatory medicine patients using the *DSM-III* or *DSM III-R* criteria or multidisciplinary team diagnosis as the reference standard[78-81] (Table 2C-18).

**TABLE 2C-18**

**Likelihood Ratios for Tests for the Diagnosis of Alcohol Abuse or Dependence**

| Prevalence | Patients Included (Number) | Test | Result | Likelihood Ratio (95% CI) | References |
|---|---|---|---|---|---|
| 22%–39% | 1705 | CAGE* questionnaire | 4 | 120 (27–535) | 78–81 |
| | | | 3 | 19 (7.7–45) | |
| | | | 2 | 3.7 (1.7–7.8) | |
| | | | 1 | 1.3 (0.99–1.8) | |
| | | | 0 | 0.15 (0.12–0.18) | |

\* CAGE stands for:

    C : have you ever felt you ought to CUT down on your drinking?

    A : have people ANNOYED you by criticizing your drinking?

    G : have you ever feel bad or GUILTY about your drinking?

    E : have you ever had a drink first thing in the morning to steady your nerves or get rid of a hangover (EYE opener)?

The CAGE questionnaire score results from adding 1 point for each question answered affirmatively.

# HYPERTENSION

In the following study of the diagnosis of renovascular hypertension, investigators enrolled patients with hypertension referred to arteriography using renal arteriography as the reference standard[82] (Table 2C-19).

**TABLE 2C-19**

**Likelihood Ratios for Tests for Diagnosis of Renovascular Hypertension**

| Prevalence | Patients Included (Number) | Test | Result | Likelihood Ratio (95% CI) | Reference |
|---|---|---|---|---|---|
| 24% | 263 | Systolic and diastolic abdominal bruit | Present | 39 (9.4–160) | 82 |
| | | | Absent | 0.62 (0.51–0.75) | |
| 23% | 118 | Any epigastric or flank systolic bruit | Present | 6.4 (3.2–12.6) | 82 |
| | | | Absent | 0.42 (0.25–0.68) | |

# AIRFLOW LIMITATION

In the following study of the diagnosis of chronic or acute airflow limitation (asthma attack), investigators enrolled patients with current respiratory symptoms and used spirometry as their reference standard[78] (Table 2C-20).

**TABLE 2C-20**

**Likelihood Ratios for Tests for Diagnosis of Acute or Chronic Airflow Limitation in Symptomatic Patients**

| Prevalence | Patients Included (Number) | Test | Result | Likelihood Ratio (95% CI) | Reference |
|---|---|---|---|---|---|
| Not applicable | Not applicable | History | | * | 83 |
| | | Smoking pack-year | >70 | 8.0 | |
| | | | <70 | 0.63 | |
| | | Smoking | Ever | 1.8 | |
| | | | Never | 0.16 | |

| Prevalence | Patients Included (Number) | Test | Result | Likelihood Ratio (95% CI) | Reference |
|---|---|---|---|---|---|
| | | Sputum production (> 1/4 cup) | Present | 4.0 | |
| | | | Absent | 0.84 | |
| | | Wheezing | Present | 3.8 | |
| | | | Absent | 0.66 | |
| | | Exertional dyspnea (grade 4) | Present | 3.0 | |
| | | | Absent | 0.98 | |
| | | Exertional dyspnea (any grade) | Present | 2.2 | |
| | | | Absent | 0.83 | |
| | | Coughing or orthopnea | | 0.5–2 | |
| | | **Physical Examination** | | | |
| | | Wheezing | Present | 36 | |
| | | | Absent | 0.85 | |
| | | Decreased heart dullness | Present | 10 | |
| | | | Absent | 0.88 | |
| | | Match test[†] | Positive | 7.1 | |
| | | | Negative | 0.43 | |
| | | Chest hyperresonance on percussion | Present | 4.8 | |
| | | | Absent | 0.73 | |
| | | Subxiphoid palpation of cardiac apex impulse | Present | 4.6 | |
| | | | Absent | 0.94 | |
| | | Forced expiratory time (seconds) | > 9 | 4.8 | |
| | | | 9–6 | 2.7 | |
| | | | < 6 | 0.45 | |

\* Not enough data for 95% CI.

† Match test: inability to extinguish a lighted match held 10 cm from the mouth.

# PIGMENTED SKIN LESION

In the following study of the diagnosis of melanoma, investigators enrolled patients with pigmented skin lesions and used biopsy of the lesions as their reference standard[84] (Table 2C-21).

**TABLE 2C-21**

**Likelihood Ratios for Tests for Diagnosis of Melanoma in Patients With Pigmented Skin Lesions**

| Prevalence | Patients (Number) | Test | Result | Likelihood Ratio (95% CI) | Reference |
|---|---|---|---|---|---|
| 3% | 192 | ABCD(E) checklist* | BCD positive | 62 (19–170) | 84 |
| | | | BCD negative | 0 (0–0.5) | |

\* ABCD(E) checklist

    A: asymmetry

    B: border irregularity

    C: color variegation

    D: diameter > 6 mm

    E: elevation

# CONCLUSION

In this section we have described a series of likelihood ratios supported by high-quality evidence of historical clues, physical examination signs, and laboratory tests to aid in the diagnosis of common medical problems.

## References

1. Black E, Bordley D, Tape T, Panzer R. *Diagnostic Strategies for Common Medical Problems.* 2nd ed. Philadelphia: American College of Physicians; 1999.

2. Oxman AD, Cook DJ, Guyatt GH, Evidence-Based Medicine Working Group. Users' guides to the medical literature, VI: how to use an overview. *JAMA.* 1994;272:1367-1371.

3. Simel DL, Samsa GP, Matchar DB. Likelihood ratios with confidence: sample size estimation for diagnostic test studies. *J Clin Epidemiol.* 1991;44:763-770.

4. Fleiss JL. The statistical basis of meta-analysis. *Stat Methods Med Res*. 1993;2:121-145.

5. Lederle FA, Simel DL. Does this patient have abdominal aortic aneurysm? *JAMA*. 1999;281:77-82.

6. Nauta RJ, Magnant C. Observation versus operation for abdominal pain in the right lower quadrant: roles of the clinical examination and the leukocyte count. *Am J Surg*. 1986;151:746-748.

7. Dixon JM, Elton RA, Rainey JB, Macleod DA. Rectal examination in patients with pain in the right lower quadrant of the abdomen. *BMJ*. 1991;302:386-388.

8. Liddington MI, Thomson WH. Rebound tenderness test. *Br J Surg*. 1991;78:795-796.

9. Izbicki JR, Knoefel WT, et al. Accurate diagnosis of acute appendicitis: a retrospective and prospective analysis of 686 patients. *Eur J Surg*. 1992;158:227-231.

10. John H, Neff U, Kelemen M. Appendicitis diagnosis today: clinical and ultrasonic deductions. *World J Surg*. 1993;17:243-249.

11. Eskelinen M, Ikonen J, Lipponen P. The value of history-taking, physical examination, and computer assistance in the diagnosis of acute appendicitis in patients more than 50 years old. *Scand J Gastroenterol*. 1995;30:349-355.

12. Wagner JM, McKinney WP, Carpenter JL. Does this patient have appendicitis? *JAMA*. 1996;276:1589-1594.

13. Andersson RE, Hugander AP, Ghazi SH, et al. Diagnostic value of disease history, clinical presentation, and inflammatory parameters of appendicitis. *World J Surg*. 1999;23:133-140.

14. Balthazar EJ, Megibow AJ, Siegel SE, Birnbaum BA. Appendicitis: prospective evaluation with high-resolution CT. *Radiology*. 1991;180:21-24.

15. Balthazar EJ, Birnbaum BA, Yee J, Megibow AJ, Roshkow J, Gray C. Acute appendicitis: CT and US correlation in 100 patients. *Radiology*. 1994;190:31-35.

16. Puylaert JB, Rutgers PH, Lalisang RI, et al. A prospective study of ultrasonography in the diagnosis of appendicitis. *N Engl J Med*. 1987;317:666-669.

17. Schwerk WB, Wichtrup B, Ruschoff J, Rothmund M. Acute and perforated appendicitis: current experience with ultrasound-aided diagnosis. *World J Surg*. 1990;14:271-276.

18. Zielke A, Hasse C, Sitter H, Rothmund M. Influence of ultrasound on clinical decision making in acute appendicitis: a prospective study. *Eur J Surg*. 1998;164:201-209.

19. Rao PM, Rhea JT, Novelline RA, et al. Helical CT technique for the diagnosis of appendicitis: prospective evaluation of a focused appendix CT examination. *Radiology*. 1997;202:139-144.

20. Lane MJ, Katz DS, Ross BA, Clautice-Engle TL, Mindelzun RE, Jeffrey RB Jr. Unenhanced helical CT for suspected acute appendicitis. *Am J Roentgenol*. 1997;168:405-409.

21. Rao PM, Rhea JT, Novelline RA, Mostafavi AA, Lawrason JN, McCabe CJ. Helical CT combined with contrast material administered only through the colon for imaging of suspected appendicitis. *Am J Roentgenol*. 1997;169: 1275-1280.

22. Rao PM, Rhea JT, Novelline RA, Mostafavi AA, McCabe CJ. Effect of computed tomography of the appendix on treatment of patients and use of hospital resources. *N Engl J Med*. 1998;338:141-146.

23. Funaki B, Grosskreutz SR, Funaki CN. Using unenhanced helical CT with enteric contrast material for suspected appendicitis in patients treated at a community hospital. *Am J Roentgenol*. 1998;171:997-1001.

24. Lane MJ, Liu DM, Huynh MD, Jeffrey RB Jr, Mindelzun RE, Katz DS. Suspected acute appendicitis: nonenhanced helical CT in 300 consecutive patients. *Radiology*. 1999;213:341-346.

25. Rao PM, Feltmate CM, Rhea JT, Schulick AH, Novelline RA. Helical computed tomography in differentiating appendicitis and acute gynecologic conditions. *Obstet Gynecol*. 1999;93:417-421.

26. Panju AA, Hemmelgarn BR, Guyatt GH, Simel DL. Is this patient having a myocardial infarction? *JAMA*. 1998;280:1256-1263.

27. Metlay JP, Kapoor WN, Fine MJ. Does this patient have community-acquired pneumonia? Diagnosing pneumonia by history and physical examination. *JAMA*. 1997;278:1440-1445.

28. Diehr P, Wood RW, Bushyhead J, Krueger L, Wolcott B, Tompkins RK. Prediction of pneumonia in outpatients with acute cough—a statistical approach. *J Chronic Dis*. 1984;37:215-225.

29. Gennis P, Gallagher J, Falvo C, Baker S, Than W. Clinical criteria for the detection of pneumonia in adults: guidelines for ordering chest roentgenograms in the emergency department. *J Emerg Med*. 1989;7:263-268.

30. Singal BM, Hedges JR, Radack KL. Decision rules and clinical prediction of pneumonia: evaluation of low-yield criteria. *Ann Emerg Med*. 1989;18:13-20.

31. Heckerling PS, Tape TG, Wigton RS, et al. Clinical prediction rule for pulmonary infiltrates. *Ann Intern Med*. 1990;113:664-670.

32. Wells PS, Anderson DR, Bormanis J, et al. Value of assessment of pretest probability of deep-vein thrombosis in clinical management. *Lancet*. 1997;350:1795-1798.

33. Anand SS, Wells PS, Hunt D, Brill-Edwards P, Cook D, Ginsberg JS. Does this patient have deep vein thrombosis? *JAMA*. 1998;279:1094-1099.

34. Kearon C, Julian JA, Newman TE, Ginsberg JS. Noninvasive diagnosis of deep venous thrombosis. McMaster Diagnostic Imaging Practice Guidelines Initiative. *Ann Intern Med*. 1998;128:663-677.

35. Becker DM, Philbrick JT, Bachhuber TL, Humphries JE. D-dimer testing and acute venous thromboembolism: a shortcut to accurate diagnosis? *Arch Intern Med*. 1996;156:939-946.

36. Wells PS, Brill-Edwards P, Stevens P, et al. A novel and rapid whole-blood assay for D-dimer in patients with clinically suspected deep vein thrombosis. *Circulation*. 1995;91:2184-2187.

37. Heaton DC, Billings JD, Hickton CM. Assessment of D dimer assays for the diagnosis of deep vein thrombosis. *J Lab Clin Med*. 1987;110:588-591.

38. Bounameaux H, Schneider PA, Reber G, de Moerloose P, Krahenbuhl B. Measurement of plasma D-dimer for diagnosis of deep venous thrombosis. *Am J Clin Pathol*. 1989;91:82-85.

39. Pini M, Quintavalla R, Pattacini C, et al. Combined use of strain-gauge plethysmography and latex D-dimer test in clinically suspected deep venous thrombosis. *Fibrinolysis*. 1993;7:391-396.

40. Dale S, Gogstad GO, Brosstad F, et al. Comparison of three D-dimer assays for the diagnosis of DVT: ELISA, latex and an immunofiltration assay (NycoCard D-Dimer). *Thromb Haemost*. 1994;71:270-274.

41. McGee S, Abernethy WB III, Simel DL. Is this patient hypovolemic? *JAMA*. 1999;281:1022-1029.

42. Guyatt GH, Oxman AD, Ali M, Willan A, McIlroy W, Patterson C. Laboratory diagnosis of iron-deficiency anemia: an overview. *J Gen Intern Med*. 1992;7:145-153.

43. Punnonen K, Irjala K, Rajamaki A. Serum transferrin receptor and its ratio to serum ferritin in the diagnosis of iron deficiency. *Blood*. 1997;89:1052-1057.

44. Hussein S, Prieto J, O'Shea M, Hoffbrand AV, Baillod RA, Moorhead JF. Serum ferritin assay and iron status in chronic renal failure and haemodialysis. *BMJ*. 1975;1:546-548.

45. Milman N, Christensen TE, Pedersen NS, Visfeldt J. Serum ferritin and bone marrow iron in non-dialysis, peritoneal dialysis and hemodialysis patients with chronic renal failure. *Acta Med Scand*. 1980;207:201-205.

46. Blumberg AB, Marti HR, Graber CG. Serum ferritin and bone marrow iron in patients undergoing continuous ambulatory peritoneal dialysis. *JAMA*. 1983;250:3317-3319.

47. Kalantar-Zadeh K, Hoffken B, Wunsch H, Fink H, Kleiner M, Luft FC. Diagnosis of iron deficiency anemia in renal failure patients during the post-erythropoietin era. *Am J Kidney Dis*. 1995;26:292-299.

48. Fernandez-Rodriguez AM, Guindeo-Casasus MC, Molero-Labarta T, et al. Diagnosis of iron deficiency in chronic renal failure. *Am J Kidney Dis*. 1999;34:508-513.

49. Intragumtornchai T, Rojnukkarin P, Swasdikul D, Israsena S. The role of serum ferritin in the diagnosis of iron deficiency anaemia in patients with liver cirrhosis. *J Intern Med*. 1998;243:233-241.

50. Boyko EJ, Ahroni JH, Davignon D, Stensel V, Prigeon RL, Smith DG. Diagnostic utility of the history and physical examination for peripheral vascular disease among patients with diabetes mellitus. *J Clin Epidemiol*. 1997;50:659-668.

51. Christensen JH, Freundlich M, Jacobsen BA, Falstie-Jensen N. Clinical relevance of pedal pulse palpation in patients suspected of peripheral arterial insufficiency. *J Intern Med*. 1989;226:95-99.

52. McGee SR, Boyko EJ. Physical examination and chronic lower-extremity ischemia: a critical review. *Arch Intern Med*. 1998;158:1357-1364.

53. Criqui MH, Fronek A, Klauber MR, Barrett-Connor E, Gabriel S. The sensitivity, specificity, and predictive value of traditional clinical evaluation of peripheral arterial disease: results from noninvasive testing in a defined population. *Circulation*. 1985;71:516-522.

54. Stoffers HE, Kester AD, Kaiser V, Rinkens PE, Knottnerus JA. Diagnostic value of signs and symptoms associated with peripheral arterial occlusive disease seen in general practice: a multivariable approach. *Med Decis Making*. 1997;17:61-70.

55. Cochand-Priollet B, Guillausseau PJ, Chagnon S, et al. The diagnostic value of fine-needle aspiration biopsy under ultrasonography in nonfunctional thyroid nodules: a prospective study comparing cytologic and histologic findings. *Am J Med*. 1994;97:152-157.

56. Walfish PG, Hazani E, Strawbridge HT, Miskin M, Rosen IB. A prospective study of combined ultrasonography and needle aspiration biopsy in the assessment of the hypofunctioning thyroid nodule. *Surgery*. 1977;82:474-482.

57. Prinz RA, O'Morchoe PJ, Barbato AL, et al. Fine needle aspiration biopsy of thyroid nodules. *Ann Surg*. 1983;198:70-73.

58. Jones AJ, Aitman TJ, Edmonds CJ, Burke M, Hudson E, Tellez M. Comparison of fine needle aspiration cytology, radioisotopic and ultrasound scanning in the management of thyroid nodules. *Postgrad Med J*. 1990;66:914-917.

59. Cusick EL, MacIntosh CA, Krukowski ZH, Williams VM, Ewen SW, Matheson NA. Management of isolated thyroid swellings: a prospective six year study of fine needle aspiration cytology in diagnosis. *BMJ*. 1990;301:318-321.

60. Perez JA, Pisano R, Kinast C, Valencia V, Araneda M, Mera ME. Needle aspiration cytology in euthyroid uninodular goiter. *Rev Med Chil*. 1991;119:158-163.

61. Piromalli D, Martelli G, Del Prato I, Collini P, Pilotti S. The role of fine needle aspiration in the diagnosis of thyroid nodules: analysis of 795 consecutive cases. *J Surg Oncol*. 1992;50:247-250.

62. Hildner FJ, Ormond RS. Accuracy of the clinical diagnosis of pulmonary embolism. *JAMA*. 1967;202:567-570.

63. Stein PD, Terrin ML, Hales CA, et al. Clinical, laboratory, roentgenographic, and electrocardiographic findings in patients with acute pulmonary embolism and no pre-existing cardiac or pulmonary disease. *Chest*. 1991;100:598-603.

64. Nazeyrollas P, Metz D, Jolly D, et al. Use of transthoracic Doppler echocardiography combined with clinical and electrocardiographic data to predict acute pulmonary embolism. *Eur Heart J*. 1996;17:779-786.

65. Worsley DF, Alavi A, Aronchick JM, Chen JT, Greenspan RH, Ravin CE. Chest radiographic findings in patients with acute pulmonary embolism: observations from the PIOPED Study. *Radiology*. 1993 Oct;189:133-136.

66. Moons KG, van Es GA, Michel BC, Buller HR, Habbema JD, Grobbee DE. Redundancy of single diagnostic test evaluation. *Epidemiology*. 1999; 10:276-281.

67. Kutinsky I, Blakley S, Roche V. Normal D-dimer levels in patients with pulmonary embolism. *Arch Intern Med*. 1999;159:1569-1572.

68. Rathbun SW, Raskob GE, Whitsett TL. Sensitivity and specificity of helical computed tomography in the diagnosis of pulmonary embolism: a systematic review. *Ann Intern Med*. 2000;132:227-232.

69. Drucker EA, Rivitz SM, Shepard JA, et al. Acute pulmonary embolism: assessment of helical CT for diagnosis. *Radiology*. 1998;209:235-241.

70. Teigen CL, Maus TP, Sheedy PF II, et al. Pulmonary embolism: diagnosis with contrast-enhanced electron-beam CT and comparison with pulmonary angiography. *Radiology*. 1995;194:313-319.

71. Value of the ventilation/perfusion scan in acute pulmonary embolism. Results of the Prospective Investigation of Pulmonary Embolism Diagnosis (PIOPED). The PIOPED Investigators. *JAMA*. 1990;263:2753-2759.

72. Stein PD, Alavi A, Gottschalk A, et al. Usefulness of noninvasive diagnostic tools for diagnosis of acute pulmonary embolism in patients with a normal chest radiograph. *Am J Cardiol*. 1991;67:1117-1120.

73. Williams JW Jr, Simel DL. Does this patient have ascites? How to divine fluid in the abdomen. *JAMA*. 1992;267:2645-2648.

74. Ziegler DK, Zileli T, Dick A, Sebaugh JL. Correlation of bruits over the carotid artery with angiographically demonstrated lesions. *Neurology*. 1971;21: 860-865.

75. Ingall TJ, Homer D, Whisnant JP, Baker HL Jr, O'Fallon WM. Predictive value of carotid bruit for carotid atherosclerosis. *Arch Neurol*. 1989;46:418-422.

76. Hankey GJ, Warlow CP. Symptomatic carotid ischaemic events: safest and most cost effective way of selecting patients for angiography, before carotid endarterectomy. *BMJ*. 1990;300:1485-1491.

77. Sauve JS, Laupacis A, Ostbye T, Feagan B, Sackett DL. Does this patient have a clinically important carotid bruit? *JAMA*. 1993;270:2843-2845.

78. Mayfield D, McLeod G, Hall P. The CAGE questionnaire: validation of a new alcoholism screening instrument. *Am J Psychiatry*. 1974;131:1121-1123.

79. Bush B, Shaw S, Cleary P, Delbanco TL, Aronson MD. Screening for alcohol abuse using the CAGE questionnaire. *Am J Med*. 1987;82:231-235.

80. Buchsbaum DG, Buchanan RG, Centor RM, Schnoll SH, Lawton MJ. Screening for alcohol abuse using CAGE scores and likelihood ratios. *Ann Intern Med*. 1991;115:774-777.

81. Kitchens JM. Does this patient have an alcohol problem? *JAMA*. 1994;272:1782-1787.

82. Turnbull JM. Is listening for abdominal bruits useful in the evaluation of hypertension? *JAMA*. 1995;274:1299-1301.

83. Holleman DR Jr, Simel DL. Does the clinical examination predict airflow limitation? *JAMA*. 1995;273:313-319.

84. Whited JD, Grichnik JM. Does this patient have a mole or a melanoma? *JAMA*. 1998;279:696-701.

# PROGNOSIS

## Regression and Correlation

Gordon Guyatt, Stephen Walter, Deborah Cook,
and Roman Jaeschke

## IN THIS SECTION

Investigators are sometimes interested in the relationship between different measures, or variables. They pose questions related to the correlation of these variables. For example, they might ask: How well does the clinical impression of a patient's symptoms and well-being predict that patient's self-report? How strong is the relationship between a patient's physical and emotional function?

By contrast, other investigators are primarily interested in causal relations between biologic phenomena. For instance, they might ask: What determines the extent to which we feel dyspneic when we exercise or when we suffer from a cardiac or respiratory illness?

Clinicians may be interested in the answers to both of these sorts of questions. To the extent that the relationship between patients' and relatives' perceptions are weak, they must obtain both perspectives on a clinical situation. If physical and emotional functions are related only weakly, then clinicians must probe both areas thoroughly. If clinicians know that hypoxemia is strongly related to dyspnea, they will be more inclined to administer oxygen to patients with dyspnea. If the demonstrated hypoxemia-dyspnea relationship is weak, they will be less inclined to administer oxygen to those patients.

We refer to the magnitude of the relationship between different variables or phenomena as *correlation*. We call the statistical techniques for predicting or making a causal inference *regression*. In this section, we will provide examples to illustrate the use of correlation and regression in the medical literature.

# CORRELATION

Let us take a simple example. Traditionally, we perform laboratory measurements of exercise capacity in patients with cardiac and respiratory illnesses using a treadmill or cycle ergometer. About 25 years ago, investigators interested in respiratory disease began to use a simpler test that is related more closely to day-to-day activity.[1] In this walk test, patients are asked to cover as much ground as they can during a specified time period (typically 6 minutes), walking in an enclosed corridor. For a number of reasons, we may be interested in the strength of the relationship between the walk test and conventional laboratory measures of exercise capacity. If the tests relate strongly enough to one another, we might be able to substitute one test for the other. In addition, the strength of the relationship might inform us as to the potential of laboratory tests of exercise capacity to predictor patients' ability to undertake physically demanding activities of daily living.

What do we mean by the strength of the relationship between two variables? A relationship between two measures is strong when patients who obtain high scores on the first variable also obtain high scores on the second variable, when those in whom we find intermediate scores on the first variable also show intermediate values on the second variable, and when patients who score low on one measure score low on the other measure. If patients who score low on one measure are equally likely to score low or high on another measure, the relationship between the two variables is poor, or weak.

We can gain a sense of the strength of the correlation by examining a visual plot relating patients' scores on the two measures. Figure 2D-1 presents such a plot relating walk test results (on the x-axis) to the results of cycle ergometer exercise test (on the y-axis). The data for this plot, and those for the subsequent analyses using walk test results, come from three studies of patients with chronic airflow limitation.[2-4] Each dot in Figure 2D-1 represents an individual patient and presents two pieces of information: the patient's walk test score and cycle ergometer exercise time. Although the walk test results are truly continuous, the cycle ergometer results tend to take only certain values because patients usually stop the test at the end of a particular level, rather than part way through a level. Examining Figure 2D-1, you can see that, in general, patients who score well on the walk test also tend to score well on the cycle ergometer exercise test, and patients who score poorly on the cycle ergometer tend to score poorly on the walk test. Yet you can find patients who represent exceptions, scoring better than most other patients on one test, and not as well on the other test.

**FIGURE 2D-1**

**Relationship Between Walk Test Results and Cycle Ergometer Exercise Test Results**

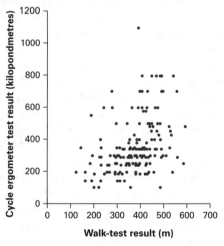

Reproduced with permission from the Canadian Medical Association.

These data therefore represent a moderate relationship between two variables, the walk test and the cycle ergometer exercise test. The strength of the relationship can be summarized in a single number, the *correlation coefficient*. The correlation coefficient, which is denoted by the letter *r*, can range from −1.0 (representing the strongest possible negative relationship, in which the person who scores the highest on one test scores the lowest on the other test) to 1.0 (representing the strongest possible positive relationship, in which the person who scores the highest on one test also scores the highest on the other test). A correlation coefficient of zero denotes no relationship between the two variables (ie, people who score high on test A have the same range of values on test B as those who score low on test A). The plot of data with a correlation of 0 looks like a starry sky.

The correlation coefficient assumes a linear relationship between the variables. There may be a relationship between the variables, but it may not take the form of a straight line when viewed visually. For example, even if scores on the variables may rise together, one may rise more slowly than the other for low values but will rise more quickly than the other for high values. If there is a strong relationship but it is not a linear one, the correlation coefficient may be misleading. In the example depicted in Figure 2D-1, the relationship does appear to approximate a straight line, and the *r* value for the correlation between the walk test and the cycle ergometer is 0.50.

Is this moderately strong correlation good or bad? It depends on how we wish to apply the information. If we were thinking of using the walk test value as a substitute for the cycle ergometer—after all, the walk test is much simpler to carry out—we would be disappointed. A correlation of 0.8 or higher would be required for us to be confident in that kind of substitution. If the correlation were any lower than 0.8, there would be too much risk that a person with a high walk test score would have mediocre or low performance on the cycle ergometer test, or that a person who did poorly on the walk test would do well on the cycle ergometer test. On the other hand, if we assume that the walk test gives a good indication of exercise capacity in daily life, the moderate correlation suggests that the cycle ergometer result tells us something (less, but still something) about day-to-day exercise capacity.

You will often see a *P* value in association with a correlation coefficient (see Part 1B1, "Therapy"). When one considers correlation coefficients, the *P* value is associated with the null hypothesis that the true correlation between the two measures is 0. Thus, the *P* value represents the probability that, if the true correlation were 0, a relationship as strong as or stronger than the one we actually observed would have occurred as a result of chance. The smaller the *P* value, the less likely it is that chance explains the apparent relationship between the two measures.

The *P* value depends not only on the strength of the relationship, but also on the sample size. In this case, we had data on both the walk test and the cycle ergometer from 179 patients; with a correlation of 0.50, the associated *P* value is $< .0001$. A relationship can be very weak, but if the sample size is sufficiently large, the *P* value may be small. For instance, with a sample size of 500, we reach the conventional threshold *P* value of .05 at a correlation of only 0.10.

In evaluating treatment effects, the size of the effect and the confidence intervals around the effect tend to be much more informative than *P* values (see Part 2B2, "Therapy and Understanding the Results, Confidence Intervals").[5] The same is true of correlations, in which the magnitude of the correlation and the confidence interval around the correlation are the key parameters. The 95% confidence interval around the correlation between the walk test and laboratory exercise tests ranges from 0.38 to 0.60.

# REGRESSION

As clinicians, we are often interested in prediction. We want to know which person will develop a disease (such as coronary artery disease) and which person will not; which patient will do well and which patient will do poorly. Regression techniques are useful in addressing this sort of question. We will once again use the walk test to illustrate the concepts involved in statistical regression.

## An Example of Regression: Predicting Walk Test Scores

Let us assume we are trying to predict patients' walk test scores using more easily measured variables: sex, height, and a measure of lung function—forced expiratory volume in 1 second ($FEV_1$). Alternatively, we can think of the investigation as examining a causal hypothesis: To what extent are patients' walk test scores determined by sex, height, and pulmonary function? Either way, we have a target or response variable that we call the *dependent variable* (in this case, the walk test) because it is influenced or determined by other variables or factors. We also have the explanatory or predictor variables, called *independent variables*: sex, height, and $FEV_1$.

Figure 2D-2, a bar graph of the walk test scores of 219 patients with chronic lung disease, demonstrates that walk test scores vary widely among patients. If we had to predict an individual's walk test score without any other information, our best guess would be the mean score of all patients (394 m). For many patients, however, this prediction would be well off the mark.

**FIGURE 2D-2**

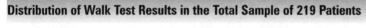

Distribution of Walk Test Results in the Total Sample of 219 Patients

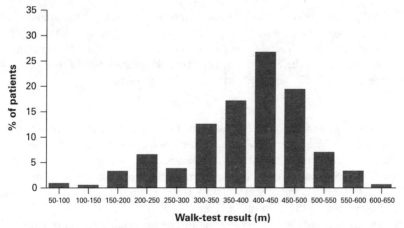

Figure 2D-3 shows the relationship between $FEV_1$ and the walk test. Note that there is a relationship between the two variables, although the relationship is not as strong as the relationship between the walk test and the exercise test depicted in Figure 2D-1. Thus, some of the differences, or variation, in walk test scores seems to be explained by, or attributable to, the patient's $FEV_1$. We can construct an equation using $FEV_1$ to predict walk test scores. Because there is only one independent variable, we call this a *univariable* or *simple regression.*[6]

**FIGURE 2D-3**

**Relationship Between $FEV_1$ and Walk Test Results in 219 Patients**

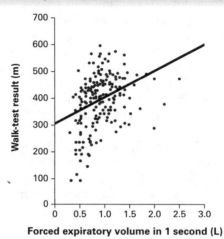

Reproduced with permission from the Canadian Medical Association.

Generally, when we construct regression equations, we refer to the predictor variable as $x$ and the target variable as $y$. The regression equation assumes a linear fit between the $FEV_1$ and the walk test data, and specifies the point at which the straight line meets the $y$-axis (the intercept) and the steepness of the line (the slope). In this case, the regression is expressed as follows:

$$y = 298 + 108x$$

where $y$ is the value of the walk test, 298 is the intercept, 108 is the slope of the line, and $x$ is the value of the $FEV_1$. In this case, the intercept of 298 has little practical meaning; it predicts the walk test distance of a patient with an $FEV_1$ of 0. The slope of 108, however, does have some meaning: it predicts that for every increase in $FEV_1$ of 1 L, the patient will walk 108 m farther. We show the regression line corresponding to this formula in Figure 2D-3.

Having constructed the regression equation, we can examine the correlation between the two variables, and we can determine whether the correlation can be explained by chance. The correlation is 0.40, suggesting that chance is a very unlikely explanation ($P = .0001$). Thus, we conclude that $FEV_1$ explains or accounts for a statistically significant proportion of the variability, or variance, in walk test scores.

We can also examine the relationship between walk test score and patients' sex (Figure 2D-4). Although there is considerable variability within the sexes, men tend to have higher scores than women. If we had to predict a man's score, we would choose the mean score of the men (410 m); to predict a woman's score, we would choose the women's mean score of 363 m.

**FIGURE 2D-4**

### Distribution of Walk Test Results in Men and in Women (Sample of 219 Patients)

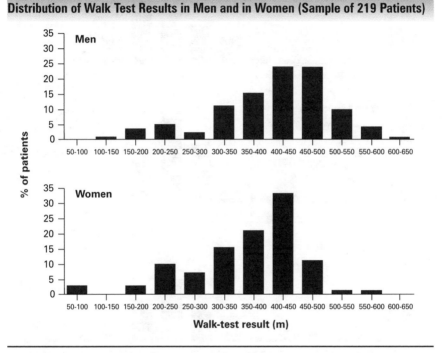

Walk-test result (m)

Reproduced with permission from the Canadian Medical Association.

We can ask the question: Does the apparent relationship between sex and walk test score result from chance? One way of answering this question is to construct another simple regression equation with walk test as the dependent variable and patient's sex as the independent variable. As it turns out, chance is an unlikely explanation of the relationship between sex and the walk test ($P = .0005$). These two examples show that the independent variable can be an either/or variable—such as sex (male or female), which we call a *dichotomous variable*—or a variable that can theoretically take any value (such as $FEV_1$), which we call a *continuous variable*.

In Figure 2D-5 we have separated the men from the women, and for each sex, we have divided them into groups with high and low $FEV_1$ results. Although there is a range of scores within each of these groups, the range is narrower than among all women or all men, and even more so than all patients; when we use the mean of any group as our best guess of the walk test score of any member of that group, we will on average be closer to the true value than if we had used the mean for all patients.

**FIGURE 2D-5**

## Distribution of Walk Test Results in Men and Women With High and Low FEV₁ (Sample of 219 Patients)

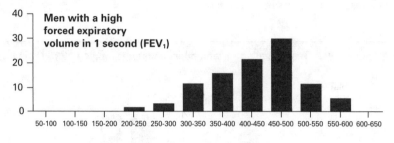

Men with a high forced expiratory volume in 1 second (FEV₁)

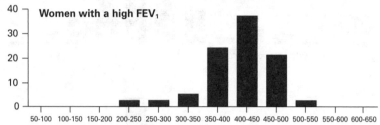

Women with a high FEV₁

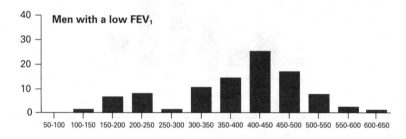

Men with a low FEV₁

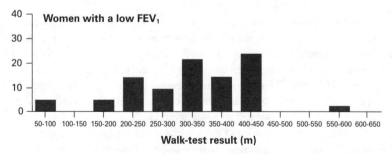

Women with a low FEV₁

Walk-test result (m)

Figure 2D-5 illustrates how we can take more than one independent variable into account at the same time in explaining or predicting the dependent variable. We can construct a mathematical model that explains or predicts the walk test score by simultaneously considering all of the independent variables and thus creating a *multivariable regression equation.*

We can learn a number of things from such an equation. First, we can determine if the variables that were associated with the dependent variable in the univariable equations each make independent contributions to explaining the variation. In the current example, we have used an approach in which the independent variable with the strongest relationship to the dependent variable is considered first, followed by the variable with the next strongest relationship. Forced expiratory volume in 1 second and sex both make independent contributions to explaining walk test results ($P < .0001$ for $FEV_1$ and $P = .03$ for sex in the multiple regression analysis), but height (which was significant at the $P = .02$ level when considered in a univariable regression) does not make a comparable contribution to the explanation.

If we had chosen both the $FEV_1$ and peak expiratory flow rates as independent variables, they would both show significant associations with walk test score. However, because $FEV_1$ and peak expiratory flow rates are associated very strongly with one another, they are unlikely to provide independent contributions to explaining the variation in walk test scores. In other words, once we take $FEV_1$ into account, peak flow rates are not likely to be of any help in predicting walk test scores—and if we first took peak flow rate into account, $FEV_1$ would not provide further explanatory power to our predictive model. Similarly, height was a significant predictor of walk test score when considered alone, but was no longer significant in the multivariable regression because of its correlation with sex and $FEV_1$.

We have emphasized how the $P$ value associated with a correlation provides little information about the strength of the relation between two values; the correlation coefficient itself is required. Similarly, knowing that sex and $FEV_1$ independently explain some of the variation in walk test scores tells us little about the power of our predictive model. Figure 2D-5 gives us some sense of the model's predictive power. Although the distributions of walk test scores in the four subgroups differ appreciably, considerable overlap remains. The regression equation can tell us the proportion of the variation in the dependent variable (that is, the differences between people in the walk test score) that is associated with each of the independent variables (sex and $FEV_1$) and, therefore, the proportion explained by the entire model. In this case, $FEV_1$ explains 15% of the variation when it is the first variable entered into the model, sex explains an additional 2% of the variation conditional on $FEV_1$ being in the model already, and the total model explains 17% of the variation. We can therefore conclude that there are many other factors that we have not measured—and, perhaps, that we cannot measure—that determine how far people with chronic lung disease can walk in 6 minutes. Other investigations using regression techniques have found that patients' experience of the intensity of their exertion, as well as the perception of the severity of their illness, may be more powerful determinants of walk test distance than is their $FEV_1$.[7]

In our example, the dependent variable—the walk test—was a continuous variable. Because the regression assumes a linear fit between the independent and dependent variables, when the dependent variable is a continuous variable and the relationship between the variables is a linear one, we refer to the regression as *linear regression*. In our next example, the dependent variable is a present/absent or dichotomous variable. Investigators sometimes use the term *logistic regression* to refer to regression models in which the target variable is dichotomous.

## Another Example of Regression: Predicting Clinically Important Bleeding

We have addressed the question of predicting which critically ill patients are at risk of clinically important gastrointestinal bleeding.[8] In this case, the dependent variable was whether or not patients had a clinically important bleeding episode. When the dependent variable is a yes/no or a dichotomous variable, we use the term *logistic* (because it uses a model that relies on logarithms) to describe the regression. The independent variables included whether patients were breathing independently or required ventilator support, and the presence or absence of coagulopathy, sepsis, hypotension, hepatic failure, or renal failure.

Table 2D-1 shows some of the results from this study, in which we followed 2252 critically ill patients and determined which of them sustained a clinically important bleeding episode. It shows that in univariable logistic regression equations, many independent variables (ie, respiratory failure, coagulopathy, hypotension, sepsis, hepatic failure, renal failure, enteral feeding, steroid administration, organ transplantation, anticoagulant therapy) were significantly associated with clinically important bleeding. For a number of variables, the odds ratio (see Part 2B2, "Therapy and Understanding the Results, Measures of Association"), which indicates the strength of the association, is quite large. However, when we constructed a multiple logistic regression equation, only two of the independent variables, ventilation and coagulopathy, were significantly and independently associated with risk of bleeding. All of the other variables that predicted bleeding in the univariate analysis were correlated either with ventilation or with coagulopathy, and therefore did not reach conventional levels of statistical significance in the multiple regression. Of those who were not ventilated, three of 1597 (0.2%) experienced a bleeding episode; of those who were ventilated, 30 of 655 (4.6%) experienced a bleeding episode. Of those with no coagulopathy, 10 of 1792 (0.6%) bled; of those with coagulopathy, 23 of 455 (5.1%) experienced a bleeding episode.

**TABLE 2D-1**

## Odds Ratios and *P* Values According to Simple (Univariable) and Multiple (Multivariable) Logistic Regression Analysis for Risk Factors for Clinically Important Gastrointestinal Bleeding in Critically Ill Patients

| | Simple Regression | | Multiple Regression | |
|---|---|---|---|---|
| Risk Factors | OR | *P* value | OR | *P* value |
| Respiratory failure | 25.5 | <.0001 | 15.6 | <.0001 |
| Coagulopathy | 9.5 | <.0001 | 4.3 | .0002 |
| Hypotension | 5.0 | .03 | 2.1 | .08 |
| Sepsis | 7.3 | <.0001 | NS | |
| Hepatic failure | 6.5 | <.0001 | NS | |
| Renal failure | 4.6 | <.0001 | NS | |
| Enteral feeding | 3.8 | .0002 | NS | |
| Steroid administration | 3.7 | .0004 | NS | |
| Organ transplant | 3.6 | .006 | NS | |
| Anticoagulant therapy | 3.3 | .004 | NS | |

OR indicates odds ratio; NS, not significant.

Our primary clinical interest was to identify a subgroup with a risk sufficiently low that bleeding prophylaxis might be withheld. Separate from the regression analysis, but suggested by its results, we divided the patients into two groups—those who were neither ventilated nor had a coagulopathy in whom the incidence of bleeding was only 2/1405 (0.14%), and those who were either ventilated or had a coagulopathy in whom 31/847 (3.7%) had a bleeding episode. Prophylaxis may reasonably be withheld in the former group.

# CONCLUSION

Correlation is a statistical tool that permits researchers to examine the strength of the relationship between two variables when neither one is necessarily considered the target variable. Regression, by contrast, examines the strength of relationship between one or more predictor variables and a target variable. Regression can be very useful in formulating predictive models that purport to assess risks, for example, the risk of myocardial infarction in a patient presenting with chest pain,[9] the risk of cardiac events in patients undergoing noncardiac surgery,[10] or the risk of bleeding in critically ill patients. Such predictive models can help us make better clinical decisions. Regardless of whether you are considering an issue of correlation or regression, you should not only consider whether the relationship between variables is statistically significant, but also the magnitude or strength of the relationship—either in terms of the proportion of variation explained or the extent to which groups with very different risks of the target event can be specified.

# References

1. McGavin CR, Gupta SP, McHardy GJ. Twelve-minute walking test for assessing disability in chronic bronchitis. *BMJ.* 1976;1:822-823.

2. Guyatt GH, Berman LB, Townsend M. Long-term outcome after respiratory rehabilitation. *CMAJ.* 1987;137:1089-1095.

3. Guyatt G, Keller J, Singer J, Halcrow S, Newhouse M. Controlled trial of respiratory muscle training in chronic airflow limitation. *Thorax.* 1992;47:598-602.

4. Goldstein RS, Gort EH, Stubbing D, Avendano MA, Guyatt GH. Randomized controlled trial of respiratory rehabilitation. *Lancet.* 1994;344:1394-1397.

5. Guyatt G, Jaeschke R, Heddle N, Cook D, Shannon H, Walter S. Basic statistics for clinicians: 2. Interpreting study results: confidence intervals. *CMAJ.* 1995;152:169-173.

6. Godfrey K. Simple linear regression. *N Engl J Med.* 1985;313:1629-1636.

7. Morgan AD, Peck DF, Buchanan DR, McHardy GJ. Effect of attitudes and beliefs on exercise tolerance in chronic bronchitis. *BMJ.* 1983;286:171-173.

8. Cook DJ, Fuller HD, Guyatt GH, et al. Risk factors for gastrointestinal bleeding in critically ill patients. *N Engl J Med.* 1994;330:377-381.

9. Pozen MW, D'Agostino RB, Selker HP, et al. A predictive instrument to improve coronary-care-unit admission practices in acute ischemic heart disease. *N Engl J Med.* 1984;310:1273-1288.

10. Detsky AS, Abrams HB, McLaughlin JR, et al. Predicting cardiac complications in patients undergoing non-cardiac surgery. *J Gen Intern Med.* 1986;1:211-219.

# SUMMARIZING THE EVIDENCE

## Publication Bias

Victor Montori and Gordon Guyatt

The following EBM Working Group members also made substantive contributions to this section: Marek Smieja, Andrew Oxman, Deborah Cook, and Trisha Greenhalgh

## IN THIS SECTION

# BIAS IN SYSTEMATIC REVIEWS

A systematic review follows a protocol describing the scope of the researcher's question, criteria for inclusion and exclusion of primary studies, a search strategy, data extraction, quality assessment procedures, and data analysis. Systematic error leading to bias can intrude at any of these steps; perhaps the most difficult type of bias for reviewers to overcome is *publication bias*. Publication bias is the selective publication of manuscripts based on the magnitude, direction, or statistical significance of the study results.

# THE MANY SOURCES OF PUBLICATION BIAS

Excluding unpublished studies from a systematic review will not bias the results of the review if the unpublished studies show, on average, the same magnitude of effect as the published reports. Unfortunately, studies that fail to reject the *null hypothesis* (those without statistically significant results), which are also called *negative studies* are less likely to be published than studies that show apparent differences between the experimental and control interventions, or *positive studies*. The magnitude and direction of a study's results may be a more important determinant of publication than study design, relevance, or quality.[1,2] Positive studies may be as much as three times more likely to be published than negative studies.[3] Journal editors' naïve belief that the peer review process guarantees the validity, quality, or representativeness of the published literature may lead them to reject systematic reviews that include unpublished data.[5] Even when they are ultimately published, negative studies face an increased delay in submission for publication.[2,4] Indeed, publication bias can intrude at virtually all stages of the planning, implementation, and dissemination of research (Table 2E-1).

**TABLE 2E-1**

### Sources of Publication Bias

| Phases of Research Publication | Actions Contributing to or Resulting in Publication Bias |
| --- | --- |
| Preliminary and pilot studies | Small studies more likely to be negative (eg, those with discarded failed hypotheses) are unpublished; some are classified as proprietary information. |
| Trial design, organization, and funding | Proposal selectively cites positive studies. |
| Institutional/ethics review board approval | No registries are kept of approved trials. |
| Study completion | Interim analysis shows that a study is likely to be negative and project is dropped. |

| Phases of Research Publication | Actions Contributing to or Resulting in Publication Bias |
| --- | --- |
| Report completion | Authors decide that reporting a negative study is worthless and uninteresting, and no time or effort is assigned. |
| Report submission | Authors decide to forgo submission of the negative study. |
| Journal selection | Authors decide to submit the report to a nonindexed, non-English, limited-circulation journal. |
| Editorial consideration | Editor decides that the negative study is not worth the peer review process and rejects manuscript. If editor decides it is worth reviewing, manuscript goes to lower-priority list. |
| Peer review | Peer reviewers conclude that the negative study does not contribute to the field and recommend rejecting the manuscript. |
| Author revision and resubmission | Author of rejected manuscript decides to forgo the revision of the negative study or to submit it to another journal (see Journal Selection above). |
| Report publication | Journal delays the publication of the negative study. |
| Lay press report | Negative study is not considered newsworthy. |
| Electronic database indexing | MEDLINE, EMBASE, Best Evidence do not scan or index articles in the journal/language of publication of the negative study. |
| Decision-maker retrieval | Health managers and policymakers do not retrieve the negative study to dictate policy. |
| Further trial evidence | New trial reports discuss their findings but do not cite the findings of the negative study. |
| Narrative review | Experts draft a review, but negative study is never cited. |
| Systematic review | Reviewer goes to extremes to identify negative reports, but misses the negative study. Industry-associated reviewer uses arbitrarily selected unpublished data "on file"; this further discredits incorporation of unpublished reports in systematic reviews. |
| Systematic review submission | Journal editors reject meta-analysis because it included unpublished reports not exposed to the rigor of peer review. Review then follows the same path described here for the negative study. |
| Practice guidelines | Evidence-based guidelines are produced based on a systematic review that missed the negative study. |
| Funding opportunities | Further funding opportunities are identified without consideration of the negative study. |

# PUBLICATION BIAS: A BIGGER DANGER IN A REVIEW WITH MANY SMALL TRIALS

Reviewers preparing a systematic review, when they fail to identify and include unpublished studies, face a risk of presenting an overly sanguine estimate of treatment effectiveness (Figure 2E-1). The risk is higher for reviews that include small studies than for those that do not include such studies.[6] Studies including large numbers of patients are less likely to remain unpublished or ignored and tend to provide more precise estimates of the treatment effect, whether positive or negative. Egger et al offer a number of examples of meta-analyses of small trials that showed a larger treatment effect than a subsequent large trial.[7] Discrepancies between results of meta-analysis and subsequent large trials may occur as often as 20% of the time,[8] and publication bias may be a major contributor to the discrepancies. Sutton et al estimated that publication bias affected 23 of 48 meta-analyses and may have changed the conclusions in four.[9]

**FIGURE 2E-1**

Treatment Effectiveness and Publication Bias

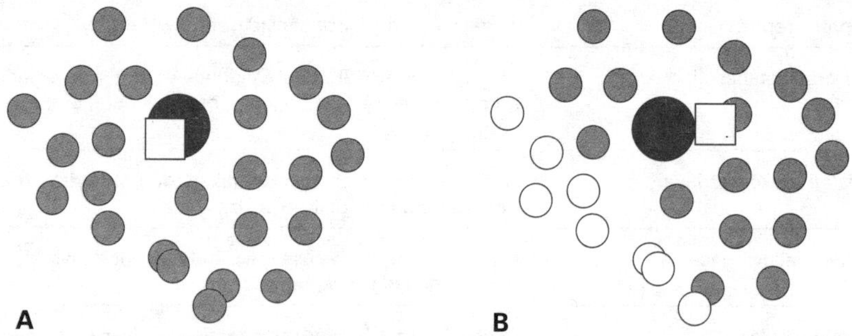

**A,** The black circle represents the underlying truth. The white square represents the pooled estimate from a systematic review of all the evidence. The small shaded circles represent the results of individual studies. **B,** The white circles represent the results of studies that the reviewers failed to identify because the studies were not published. Note the error in the pooled estimate represented by the gap between the pooled estimate (white square) and the underlying truth (black circle).

# RESEARCHERS MAY NOT SUBMIT THEIR DATA OR MAY SEND NEGATIVE STUDIES TO NON-ENGLISH LANGUAGE JOURNALS

Publication bias results more often from investigators not submitting their studies than from journals rejecting the submissions, although journal publishing policies may also play a role.[10] Researchers may fail to submit their negative studies because of lack of time or because they believe their results are uninteresting.[11] Funding sources also influence investigators' decisions regarding submission. Negative studies funded by pharmaceutical companies are less likely to get published than negative studies funded by nonprofit organizations or government agencies.[1, 12, 13] Cultural or political factors may also influence publication decisions; one report suggests that investigators from certain countries never publish a negative study.[14]

Electronic databases, including MEDLINE, limit the type and number of journals indexed. For example, 20% to 70% of randomized trials may not be identified using MEDLINE.[15] Along with journal prestige and readership, researchers deciding on submitting their work consider the likelihood of manuscript acceptance. Accordingly, they may send their positive studies to more visible sources and their negative studies to less available journals.[16] Non-English-language authors may publish their positive studies in English-language journals, and their negative—though methodologically equally strong[17]—studies in local non-English language journals that are less likely to be indexed in MEDLINE.[18] Thus, reviews that fail to seek out studies from more obscure sources may produce the same overly sanguine estimates of treatment impact as reviews that are subject to publication bias—a phenomenon known as *postpublication bias.*

Systematic reviews are less likely to suffer from postpublication bias if reviewers search a wide variety of databases, include studies published in all languages, hand-search pertinent journals, and review the reference lists of all relevant articles. Clinicians considering use of the results of a systematic review to guide their practice can be concerned less about publication bias if reviewers contact experts (in one study, 24% of references would have been missed without expert input[19]), review conference proceedings,[20] and search databases of dissertations and registries that collect studies at their inception. The Cochrane Collaboration has worked hard to achieve a rigorous search for unpublished data. In general, Cochrane reviews are more likely to conduct a comprehensive search than are average or typical reviews found elsewhere.

# STRATEGIES TO IDENTIFY LIKELY PUBLICATION BIAS

Since even such comprehensive efforts may fail to identify all unpublished studies, reviewers may conduct procedures designed to determine the likelihood that publication bias is influencing their results. In a figure that relates the precision (as measured by sample size and inverse of standard error) of studies included in a meta-analysis to the magnitude of treatment impact (as measured by effect size, relative risk reduction, and odds ratio), the resulting display should resemble an inverted funnel (Figure 2E-2). Such *funnel plots* should be symmetrical around the point estimate (dominated by the largest trials) or the results of the largest trials themselves. Asymmetry, judged by inspection, may indicate publication bias. Statistical testing[6] also may indicate publication bias, although some have questioned the statistical methods proposed.[21-23]) When asymmetry is found, the reasons may include publication bias, postpublication bias (including English-language bias), inclusion of multiple publications, poor design of small studies, fraud, and true larger effects in small studies (if, for example, compliance is higher, or the intervention is more consistently delivered).[7]

**FIGURE 2E-2A**

**Funnel Plot**

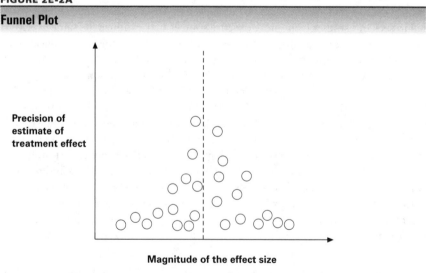

The circles represent the point estimates of the trials. The pattern of distribution resembles an inverted funnel. Larger studies tend to be closer to the pooled estimate (the dashed line). In this case, the effect sizes of the smaller studies are more or less symmetrically distributed around the pooled estimate.

## FIGURE 2E-2B

### Publication Bias

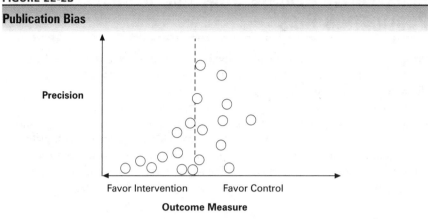

This funnel plot shows that the smaller studies are not symmetrically distributed around either the point estimate (dominated by the larger trials) or the results of the larger trials themselves. The trials expected in the bottom right quadrant are missing. This suggests publication bias—and an overestimate of the treatment effect relative to the underlying truth.

Investigators may attempt to estimate the true effect in the presence of what they believe is publication bias. They begin by removing or trimming small positive studies that do not have a negative study counterpart. This leaves a symmetric funnel plot from which the investigators calculate a putative true effect. The investigators then replace the positive studies they have removed, and hypothetical studies that mirror these positive studies are imputed or filled to create a symmetrical funnel plot that retains the new pooled effect estimate. This trim-and-fill method allows the calculation of an adjusted confidence interval and an estimate of the number of missing trials.[9]

Another method is to calculate a *fail-safe N*: this represents the number of undetected negative studies that would be needed to change the conclusions of a meta-analysis.[24] If this number is small, it suggests that the conclusion of the meta-analysis may be susceptible to publication bias. If authors have obtained the results of some unpublished studies and if published and unpublished data show different results, they have definitively established publication bias.[25,26] Perhaps the most powerful test of publication bias would come from a comparison of prospectively registered trials with published study results.[27] Because registration of trials is completed before the results are available, the results do not influence study inclusion. Indeed, prospective registration of all trials represents the ultimate solution to the problem of publication bias. Alternative suggestions include amnesty for unpublished trials, or electronic publishing of all studies[28] regardless of prior or future journal publication. These suggestions face apathy on the part of authors,[29] resistance from journal editors,[30] and the possibility of misleading presentation of data from methodologically flawed studies.[31]

# PROSPECTIVE REGISTRATION CAN REDUCE PUBLICATION BIAS

Prospective study registration with accessible results is likely to represent the best solution. Proposals exist to link prospective registration to the work of institutional review boards or ethics review boards,[32] or to the editorial process of medical journals and publishing societies.[33] Some pharmaceutical companies have made their research information available online.[34] Some journals, like *The Lancet*, have established Web sites for posting study protocols and reports of completed studies undergoing peer review.[35] Until prospective registration and complete reporting become a reality, clinicians using research reports to guide their practice must remain cognizant of the dangers of publication bias.

# A FINAL WARNING

We would add one more note of caution: readers must be alert for the potentially unscrupulous use of unpublished data. For instance, a meta-analysis based on published data showed that selective serotonin reuptake inhibitor (SSRI) antidepressant medications have the same rate of discontinuation resulting from side effects as tricyclic antidepressants (TCAs). A meta-analysis sponsored by an SSRI producer used unpublished data on file with the company to show that SSRIs are better tolerated than TCAs.[36] Two questions arise: was the choice of unpublished data selective, and what was the validity of the studies? Use of unpublished data becomes more credible if access is open to other investigators.

## References

1. Easterbrook PJ, Berlin JA, Gopalan R, Matthews DR. Publication bias in clinical research. *Lancet*. 1991;337:867-872.

2. Misakian AL, Bero LA. Publication bias and research on passive smoking: comparison of published and unpublished studies. *JAMA*. 1998;280:250-253.

3. Egger M, Smith GD. Bias in location and selection of studies. *BMJ*. 1998;316: 61-66.

4. Stern JM, Simes RJ. Publication bias: evidence of delayed publication in a cohort study of clinical research projects. *BMJ*. 1997;315:640-645.

5. Cook DJ, Guyatt GH, Ryan G, et al. Should unpublished data be included in meta-analyses? Current convictions and controversies. *JAMA*. 1993;269: 2749-2753.

6. Begg C, Berlin J. Publication bias: a problem in interpreting medical data. *J R Stat Soc A*. 1988;151:419-463.

7. Egger M, Davey Smith G, Schneider M, Minder C. Bias in meta-analysis detected by a simple, graphical test. *BMJ*. 1997;315:629-634.

8. Cappelleri JC, Ioannidis JP, Schmid CH, et al. Large trials vs meta-analysis of smaller trials: how do their results compare? *JAMA*. 1996;276:1332-1338.

9. Sutton AJ, Duval SJ, Tweedie RL, Abrams KR, Jones DR. Empirical assessment of effect of publication bias on meta-analyses. *BMJ*. 2000;320:1574-1577.

10. Callaham ML, Wears RL, Weber EJ, Barton C, Young G. Positive-outcome bias and other limitations in the outcome of research abstracts submitted to a scientific meeting. *JAMA*. 1998;280:254-257.

11. Dickersin K, Min YI. NIH clinical trials and publication bias. *Online J Curr Clin Trials*. 1993. Document No 50.

12. Dickersin K, Min YI, Meinert CL. Factors influencing publication of research results: follow-up of applications submitted to two institutional review boards. *JAMA*. 1992;267:374-378.

13. Friedberg M, Saffran B, Stinson TJ, Nelson W, Bennett CL. Evaluation of conflict of interest in economic analyses of new drugs used in oncology. *JAMA*. 1999;282:1453-1457.

14. Vickers A, Goyal N, Harland R, Rees R. Do certain countries produce only positive results? A systematic review of controlled trials. *Control Clin Trials*. 1998;19:159-166.

15. Cochrane Reviewers' Handbook 4.0 [updated June 2000]. In: Clarke M, Oxman A, eds. *Review Manager (RevMan)* [computer program]. Version 4.1. Oxford: The Cochrane Collaboration; 2000.

16. Frank E. Authors' criteria for selecting journals. *JAMA*. 1994;272:163-164.

17. Moher D, Fortin P, Jadad AR, et al. Completeness of reporting of trials published in languages other than English: implications for conduct and reporting of systematic reviews. *Lancet*. 1996;347:363-366.

18. Gregoire G, Derderian F, Le Lorier J. Selecting the language of the publications included in a meta-analysis: is there a Tower of Babel bias? *J Clin Epidemiol*. 1995;48:159-163.

19. McManus RJ, Wilson S, Delaney BC, et al. Review of the usefulness of contacting other experts when conducting a literature search for systematic reviews. *BMJ*. 1998;317:1562-1563.

20. Scherer RW, Dickersin K, Langenberg P. Full publication of results initially presented in abstracts: a meta-analysis. *JAMA*. 1994;272:158-162.

21. Irwig L, Macaskill P, Berry G, Glasziou P. Bias in meta-analysis detected by a simple, graphical test: graphical test is itself biased. *BMJ*. 1998;316:470; discussion, 470-471.

22. Stuck AE, Rubenstein LZ, Wieland D. Bias in meta-analysis detected by a simple, graphical test: asymmetry detected in funnel plot was probably due to true heterogeneity. *BMJ*. 1998;316:469; discussion, 470-471.

23. Seagroatt V, Stratton I. Bias in meta-analysis detected by a simple, graphical test: test had 10% false positive rate. *BMJ*. 1998;316:470; discussion, 470-471.

24. Gleser LJ, Olkin I. Models for estimating the number of unpublished studies. *Stat Med*. 1996;15:2493-2507.

25. Man-Son-Hing M, Wells G, Lau A. Quinine for nocturnal leg cramps: a meta-analysis including unpublished data. *J Gen Intern Med*. 1998;13:600-606.

26. Simes RJ. Confronting publication bias: a cohort design for meta-analysis. *Stat Med*. 1987;6:11-29.

27. Langhorne P. Bias in meta-analysis detected by a simple, graphical test: prospectively identified trials could be used for comparison with meta-analyses. *BMJ*. 1998;316:471.

28. Varmus H. E-Biomed: a proposal for electronic publications in the biomedical sciences [PubMed Central Web site]. 1999. Available at: www.nih.gov/welcome/director/ebiomed/ebi.htm. Accessed February 1, 2001.

29. Roberts I. An amnesty for unpublished trials: one year on, many trials are unregistered and the amnesty remains open. *BMJ*. 1998;317:763-764.

30. Relman AS. The NIH "E-biomed" proposal—a potential threat to the evaluation and orderly dissemination of new clinical studies. *N Engl J Med*. 1999;340:1828-1829.

31. Taubes G. A plan to register unpublished studies. *Science*. 1997;277:1754.

32. Boissel JP, Haugh MC. Clinical trial registries and ethics review boards: the results of a survey by the FICHTRE project. *Fundam Clin Pharmacol*. 1997;11:281-284.

33. Horton R, Smith R. Time to register randomised trials: the case is now unanswerable. *BMJ*. 1999;319:865-866.

34. Levy MD. A new register for clinical trial information. *CMAJ*. 2000;162:970-971.

35. McConnell J, Horton R. Lancet electronic research archive in international health and eprint server. *Lancet*. 1999;354:2-3.

36. Davey Smith G, Egger M. Meta-analysis: unresolved issues and future developments. *BMJ*. 1998;316:221-225.

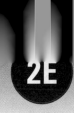

# 2E

# SUMMARIZING THE EVIDENCE

## Fixed-Effects and Random-Effects Models

Victor Montori, Gordon Guyatt, Andy Oxman, and Deborah Cook

# MODELS FOR POOLING DATA FOR META-ANALYSIS

In a meta-analysis, results from two or more primary studies are combined statistically. The meta-analyst seeking a method to pool primary study results can do so by using either a fixed-effects model or a random-effects model.[1]

The *fixed-effects model* restricts inferences to the set of studies included in the meta-analysis[2] and assumes that there is a single true value underlying all the study results. That is, the assumption is that if all studies were infinitely large, they would yield identical estimates of the effect. Thus, the observed estimates of effect differ from each other only because of random error.[3] The error term for a fixed-effects model comes only from within-study variation (study variance); the model ignores between-study variation or heterogeneity (see Part 2E, "Summarizing the Evidence, Evaluating Differences in Study Results").

By contrast, the *random-effects model* assumes that the studies included are a random sample of a population of studies addressing the question posed in the meta-analysis.[4] Each study estimates a different underlying true effect and the distribution of these effects is assumed normal around a mean value.[3] The random-effects model takes into account both within-study variability and variability in results beyond what is attributable to within-study variability.

# DIFFERENCES IN RESULTS FROM FIXED-EFFECTS AND RANDOM-EFFECTS MODELS

Compared to the fixed-effects model, the random-effects model gives smaller studies proportionally greater weight in the pooled estimate. Consequently, the direction and magnitude of the pooled estimate are influenced more by smaller studies. For the random-effects pooled estimate to be closer to the null result (ie, no treatment effect) than to the fixed-effects pooled estimate, two conditions are required. First, smaller study results must be closer to the null result than those from larger studies; second, the variability in study results must be greater than that which within-study variability can explain. If the smaller studies are farther from the null result, the random-effects model will tend to produce larger estimates of beneficial or harmful effects than will the fixed-effects model.

Thus, with one caveat, we can conclude that it is equally likely that the random-effects model will provide a more conservative, or less conservative, estimate of the treatment effect than the fixed-effects model.[5] The reservation is that the pooled estimate derived from the random-effects model will be more susceptible to publication bias, a phenomenon that primarily affects smaller studies (see Part 2E, "Summarizing the Evidence, Publication Bias").

Between-study variability beyond that which within-study variability can explain inflates the random-effects estimate of random error. An important effect of this larger error term in the analysis is that the random-effects model generally produces wider confidence intervals around the pooled estimates than the fixed-effects model. In this sense, the random effects model generally produces a more conservative assessment of the precision of the pooled estimate than the fixed-effects model.

# EXAMPLES OF DIFFERENCES IN POINT ESTIMATES AND CONFIDENCE INTERVALS FROM META-ANALYSES

Which model is preferred to conduct meta-analyses? Consider Figure 2E-3. This figure shows nine randomized controlled trials of alendronate in a dose of 5 mg to prevent fractures in sites not traditionally associated with osteoporosis. Examining the point estimates for each study, we see that three studies suggest alendronate is beneficial,[6-8] one shows no difference between treatments,[9] and five studies suggest that a control treatment is better than alendronate.[10-13] The smaller studies tend to favor the control intervention. There are large differences between the point estimates and several of the confidence intervals show little or no overlap; consider the studies by Bone et al[7] and Hosking et al[12] or the studies by Hosking et al[12] and Cummings et al.[8] Despite these appreciable differences in study results, the formal test of heterogeneity was not statistically significant ($P = .08$) (see Part 2E, "Summarizing the Evidence, Evaluating Differences in Study Results").

**FIGURE 2E-3**

## Impact of the Meta-analysis Model Chosen on the Pooled Estimate of Efficacy

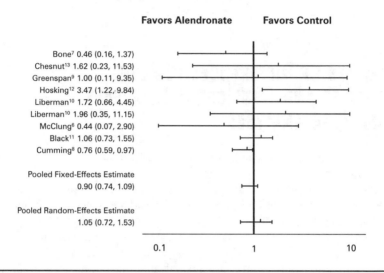

Relative Risk With 95% CI for Low-Risk Fractures After
Treatment With Alendronate

This meta-analysis includes seven small studies and two larger studies with point estimates on both sides of the line showing no difference (relative risk = 1) and some confidence intervals (in parentheses) with little or no overlap (that is, confidence intervals around estimates in different studies do not have any shared values). Using the fixed-effects model, the confidence interval is very narrow, underestimating the uncertainty about the magnitude of the effect. The random-effects model provides a more conservative estimate of the level of uncertainty about the treatment effect.

Consider the pooled estimate derived using the fixed-effects model. This pooled estimate reflects the results of the larger studies included and it favors alendronate. Because the smaller studies have a greater impact on the random-effects model results, the pooled estimate favors the control group.

Now, examine the confidence intervals around these pooled estimates. Which confidence interval better reflects the level of uncertainty we have about the true effect of the intervention? We suggest that the narrower confidence interval provided by the fixed-effects model overestimates the strength of inference we can make about the true effect of the intervention. On the other hand, the confidence interval obtained using the random-effects model provides a more realistic estimate of the range of plausible true values (see Part 2B2, "Therapy and Understanding the Results, Confidence Intervals").

Figure 2E-4 presents the results of a meta-analysis of two randomized controlled trials of raloxifene for the secondary prevention of osteoporotic vertebral fractures. The two studies had very different sample size: the trial by Ettinger et al[14] included 7705 participants, whereas the trial by Lufkin and collaborators[15] included 143 participants. The very different results of these two studies are reflected in the large difference between the point estimates and the nonoverlapping confidence intervals. In this instance, one would intuitively rely on the much larger of the two studies to suggest the magnitude and precision of our estimates of the underlying effect. We find that the extent to which the random-effects model moves the point estimate toward the smaller study and inflates the confidence interval is counterintuitive.

**FIGURE 2E-4**

**Impact of the Meta-analysis Model Chosen on the Pooled Estimate of Efficacy**

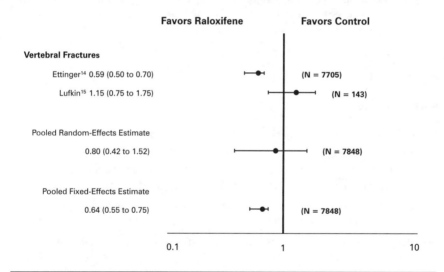

**Relative Risk With 95% Confidence Intervals for Vertebral Fractures After Treatment With Raloxifene**

| | Favors Raloxifene | Favors Control |

Vertebral Fractures

Ettinger[14] 0.59 (0.50 to 0.70)  (N = 7705)

Lufkin[15] 1.15 (0.75 to 1.75)  (N = 143)

Pooled Random-Effects Estimate

0.80 (0.42 to 1.52)  (N = 7848)

Pooled Fixed-Effects Estimate

0.64 (0.55 to 0.75)  (N = 7848)

0.1     1     10

This meta-analysis pools results from a large study and a single small study. In this case, the fixed-effects model seems to provide a sensible estimate of the uncertainty about the magnitude of the effect, while the random-effects model overestimates this uncertainty.

How should readers judge whether the appropriate model was used in a given meta-analysis? There is always some heterogeneity of results of studies included in a meta-analysis (see Part 2E, "Summarizing the Evidence, Evaluating Differences in Study Results"), and it is very unlikely that true effects are identical in varying populations of patients. Further, we are always interested in extrapolating results beyond the study sample to patients in our own practice. These considerations draw us toward the random-effects model. Furthermore, the instances in which subsequent large studies have contradicted the results of meta-analysis of small studies suggest the wisdom of a conservative estimate of confidence intervals.

On the other hand, the increased susceptibility of the random-effects model to publication bias as a result of its increased weighting of small trials is a disadvantage. It is difficult to defend use of the random-effects model in the rare instances (see Figure 2E-4) in which it generates counterintuitive results. Fortunately, these are likely to be restricted to situations in which there are very few studies, one of which is much larger than the others, and in which the point estimates differ greatly.

We do not think it appropriate to be dogmatic about choice of an analytic model. Understanding the implications associated with the choice of the model will allow clinicians to identify instances in which there may be uncertainty about the appropriateness of the model chosen for the analysis. When they identify such uncertainty, clinicians should look for results of both analytic approaches.

# References

1. Fleiss JL. The statistical basis of meta-analysis. *Stat Methods Med Res.* 1993;2:121-145.

2. Anello C, Fleiss JL. Exploratory or analytic meta-analysis: should we distinguish between them? *J Clin Epidemiol.* 1995;48:109-116.

3. Lau J, Ioannidis JP, Schmid CH. Summing up evidence: one answer is not always enough. *Lancet.* 1998;351:123-127.

4. DerSimonian R, Laird N. Meta-analysis in clinical trials. *Control Clin Trials.* 1986;7:177-188.

5. Poole C, Greenland S. Random-effects meta-analyses are not always conservative. *Am J Epidemiol.* 1999;150:469-475.

6. McClung M, Clemmesen B, Daifotis A, et al. Alendronate prevents post-menopausal bone loss in women without osteoporosis: a double-blind, randomized, controlled trial. Alendronate Osteoporosis Prevention Study Group. *Ann Intern Med.* 1998;128:253-261.

7. Bone HG, Downs RW Jr, Tucci JR, et al. Dose-response relationships for alendronate treatment in osteoporotic elderly women. Alendronate Elderly Osteoporosis Study Centers. *J Clin Endocrinol Metab.* 1997;82:265-274.

8. Cummings SR, Black DM, Thompson DE, et al. Effect of alendronate on risk of fracture in women with low bone density but without vertebral fractures: results from the Fracture Intervention Trial. *JAMA*. 1998;280:2077-2082.

9. Greenspan SL, Parker RA, Ferguson L, Rosen HN, Maitland-Ramsey L, Karpf DB. Early changes in biochemical markers of bone turnover predict the long-term response to alendronate therapy in representative elderly women: a randomized clinical trial. *J Bone Miner Res*. 1998;13:1431-1438.

10. Liberman UA, Weiss SR, Broll J, et al. Effect of oral alendronate on bone mineral density and the incidence of fractures in postmenopausal osteoporosis. The Alendronate Phase III Osteoporosis Treatment Study Group. *N Engl J Med*. 1995;333:1437-1443.

11. Black DM, Cummings SR, Karpf DB, et al. Randomised trial of effect of alendronate on risk of fracture in women with existing vertebral fractures. Fracture Intervention Trial Research Group. *Lancet*. 1996;348:1535-1541.

12. Hosking D, Chilvers CE, Christiansen C, et al. Prevention of bone loss with alendronate in postmenopausal women under 60 years of age. Early Postmenopausal Intervention Cohort Study Group. *N Engl J Med*. 1998;338:485-492.

13. Chesnut CH III, McClung MR, Ensrud KE, et al. Alendronate treatment of the postmenopausal osteoporotic woman: effect of multiple dosages on bone mass and bone remodeling. *Am J Med*. 1995;99:144-152.

14. Ettinger B, Black DM, Mitlak BH, et al. Reduction of vertebral fracture risk in postmenopausal women with osteoporosis treated with raloxifene: results from a 3-year randomized clinical trial. Multiple Outcomes of Raloxifene Evaluation (MORE) Investigators [published erratum appears in *JAMA*. 1999;282:2124]. *JAMA*. 1999;282:637-645.

15. Lufkin EG, Whitaker MD, Nickelsen T, et al. Treatment of established post-menopausal osteoporosis with raloxifene: a randomized trial. *J Bone Miner Res*. 1998;13:1747-1754.

# 2E

# SUMMARIZING THE EVIDENCE

Evaluating Differences in
Study Results

Victor Montori, Rose Hatala, and Gordon Guyatt

The following EBM Working Group members also made substantive
contributions to this section: Deborah Cook, Andrew Oxman,
and Les Irwig

## IN THIS SECTION

# Arriving at a Single Estimate of Treatment Effect

A single article may include systematic reviews of a number of discrete clinical questions. Alternatively, a single article may review a group of studies addressing a variety of related questions, the purpose being to elucidate why study results differ. However, the goal of a systematic review is often to provide a single best estimate of the effect of a treatment effect (or the power of a diagnostic test, or a patient's prognosis) that will guide clinicians in delivering care to patients. The starting assumption of a systematic review of a single, circumscribed, sensible clinical question is that across the range of patients, interventions, and outcomes included, the effect of the intervention is more or less the same (see Part 1E, "Summarizing the Evidence"). The following discussion focuses on reviews of a single issue in which the investigator's goal is to produce a quantitative summary by statistically pooling results across studies (a *meta-analysis*).

In Part 1E, "Summarizing the Evidence," we framed the dilemma that the investigator faces in conducting—and that the clinician must confront in evaluating—such a review. On the one hand, framing the question to include a broad range of patients, interventions, and ways of measuring outcome has a number of advantages. This strategy of formulating broad eligibility criteria helps avoid the bias that may occur when one focuses on a subgroup of patients (perhaps chosen because their results differ from those of other subgroups) (see Part 2E, "Summarizing the Evidence, When to Believe a Subgroup Analysis"). In addition, pooling the results of multiple studies reduces random error and increases applicability across a broad range of patients. At the same time, however, pooling the results of multiple studies risks violating the starting assumption of the analysis. The solution to this dilemma is to evaluate the extent to which results differ from study to study—that is, the *heterogeneity* of study results. This section expands on the brief discussion of how clinicians should critically appraise the assessment of study-to-study variability we presented in Part 1E, "Summarizing the Evidence."

# The Problem of Variability in Study Results: To Pool or Not to Pool?

Two studies seldom yield point estimates (the results of the study that represent the best estimate of relative risk, relative risk reduction, odds ratio, or whatever measure of effect the investigators have chosen) that are extremely close to one another, and they virtually never yield identical point estimates. Thus, in any meta-analysis that pools a number of studies, there will inevitably be some heterogeneity of results. The question is whether the heterogeneity is sufficiently great to make us uncomfortable with the investigators' decision to pool.

Consider the results of two hypothetical meta-analyses shown in Figure 2E-5 (meta-analysis A) and Figure 2E-6 (meta-analysis B). Reviewing the results of these studies, would clinicians be comfortable with pooling the results in either— or both meta-analyses? As it turns out, most clinicians will be distressed if systematic reviewers choose to pool the results of A, but will be very comfortable with the decision to pool the results in B.

**FIGURE 2E-5**

## Results of Meta-analysis A

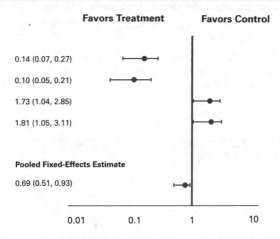

**FIGURE 2E-6**

## Results of Meta-analysis B

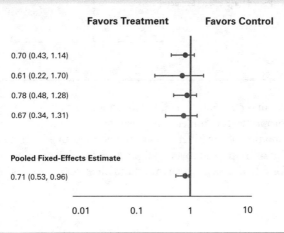

What are the implicit rules that clinicians use when they make this decision? One rule often suggested is that comfort with pooling increases when the point estimates of all studies are on the same side of the line of no effect (that is, all studies suggest benefit, or all studies suggest harm). Meta-analysis A presents the results of two studies that suggest benefit and two that suggest harm, while all studies in meta-analysis B suggest benefit. The rule apparently helps explain the intuitive assessments of the appropriateness of pooling in the two meta-analyses.

Figure 2E-7 gives us reason to question this rule. This hypothetical meta-analysis also shows point estimates on both sides of the line of no effect, but here most clinicians would be comfortable pooling the results. This leads us to reject a rule that focuses exclusively on study results suggesting benefit, or on those suggesting harm. Rather, clinicians should consider the magnitude of the differences in the point estimates of the studies. The large between-study differences in point estimates make clinicians unhappy with pooling in A; the similarity of point estimates leads to the comfort with pooling B.

**FIGURE 2E-7**

**Results of Meta-analysis C**

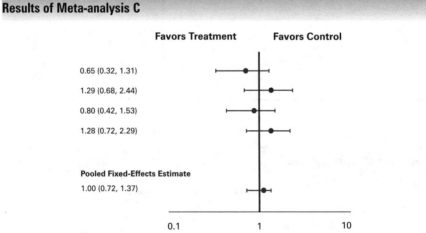

There is a second criterion that clinicians should apply when judging whether pooling is appropriate. If confidence intervals overlap widely, chance remains a plausible explanation of the differences in the point estimates. If the confidence intervals do not overlap, as in meta-analysis A, chance becomes a very unlikely explanation for differences in apparent treatment effect across studies.

# THE FORMAL STATISTICAL TEST OF HETEROGENEITY

Clinicians can also look to the results of formal statistical tests to help evaluate the validity of the pooling exercise. The null hypothesis of the *test of heterogeneity* is that the underlying effect is the same in each of the studies (eg, the relative risk in study 1 is the same as the relative risk in studies 2, 3, and 4) (see Part 2B2, "Therapy and Understanding the Results, Hypothesis Testing"). The test provides a $P$ value that represents how often one would obtain differences in study results as great or greater than those observed if the null hypothesis were true and if we repeated the studies over and over. A low $P$ value means that chance is an unlikely explanation of the differences in results from study to study. Thus, a low $P$ value in the test for heterogeneity would raise doubts about the wisdom of pooling results across studies.

We generally use our traditional cutpoint for statistical significance, which is that we have significant heterogeneity if the $P$ value is less than .05. In Figure 2E-5, we would expect this value to be very small (say, $P \leq .00001$) since it is very unlikely to see results this disparate if all studies had the same underlying effect. The $P$ values in each of Figure 2E-6 and Figure 2E-7 would be large (say, $P$ of between .8 and 1.0) since, if the null hypothesis were true, we would observe differences in effect as great as or greater than in these four studies on most repetitions of the experiments.

The test of heterogeneity is limited in that a nonsignificant result does not rule out important underlying heterogeneity of treatment effect. This test is underpowered when the meta-analysis includes a relatively small number of studies, all with small sample sizes. Under these circumstances, we might be unable to exclude chance as an explanation of differences, but we would remain suspicious that other factors (such as differences in populations, intervention, or measurement of outcome) are responsible for differences in study results (see Part 2E, "Summarizing the Evidence, When to Believe a Subgroup Analysis"). This emphasizes the need for visual inspection of differences in point estimates and in the extent to which confidence intervals overlap.

The test of heterogeneity may also provide potentially misleading results when it has a very high power. This will occur when a meta-analysis includes studies with very large sample sizes. Under these circumstances, one may see small and unimportant differences in point estimates, but because of narrow confidence intervals, a positive statistical test of heterogeneity (that is, a $P$ value that crosses the threshold—traditionally, $P < .05$).

# WHAT TO DO WHEN POOLING MAY NOT BE APPROPRIATE

What should clinicians expect of investigators when study-to-study differences in results suggest that pooling may not be appropriate? When chance becomes an unlikely explanation for differences, investigators must examine other possible explanations. In particular, differences in study participants, interventions, outcomes, and study methodology (ideally specified before the data analysis began) may explain the variation in treatment effect. (For an explanation of the principles by which clinicians should evaluate the exploration of the sources of heterogeneity, see Part 2E, "Summarizing the Evidence, When to Believe a Subgroup Analysis." For a discussion of additional issues in statistical analysis related to heterogeneity of study results, see Part 2E, "Summarizing the Evidence, Fixed-Effects and Random-Effects Models.")

What if, in the end, we are left with a large degree of unexplained between-study heterogeneity for which chance does not provide an adequate explanation? Presumably, some underlying differences in patients, interventions, outcome measurement, or methodology are responsible for these differences. Unfortunately, when unexplained heterogeneity remains, investigators have not been able to ascertain the nature of these underlying differences. Some argue that in this situation, pooling should not be conducted. Nonetheless, clinicians still need a best estimate of the treatment effect to inform their decisions. Pending further studies that may explain the differences between results, the pooled result remains the best available estimate of the treatment effect. Clinicians must nevertheless maintain extra caution in recommending treatments on the basis of pooled estimates associated with unexplained heterogeneity.

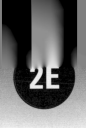

# SUMMARIZING THE EVIDENCE

## When to Believe a Subgroup Analysis

Andrew Oxman and Gordon Guyatt

The following EBM Working Group members also made substantive contributions to this section: Lee Green, Jonathan Craig, Stephen Walter, and Deborah Cook

## IN THIS SECTION

Clinicians faced with a treatment decision in a particular patient are interested in the evidence that pertains most directly to that individual. In a survey of 45 clinical trials reported in three leading medical journals, Pocock and colleagues found at least one subgroup analysis that compared the response to treatment in different categories of patients in 51% of the reports.[1] Although the investigators conducting these analyses were trying to meet clinicians' need for information specific to their individual patients, they ultimately risked misleading physicians more than enlightening them. In this section, we will present guidelines for interpreting the results of *subgroup analyses*.

Although in this section our discussion will focus on randomized controlled trials and meta-analyses of randomized controlled trials (systematic overviews), the same principles apply to any other research design. However, the assumption we start from here is that the underlying design of the studies one is examining is sound. For treatment trials, sound design involves elements of randomization, blinding, and completeness of follow-up (see Part 1B1, "Therapy"). If the study designs are not sound, the overall conclusions are suspect, let alone conclusions based on subgroup analyses.

# WHY DO INVESTIGATORS CONDUCT SUBGROUP ANALYSES?

A positive subgroup analysis suggests that there may be important difference in *treatment effect*. This difference may be across types of patients (eg, older or younger patients, or sicker or less sick ones), or across treatments (eg, low-dose or high-dose treatments, or treatment with different drugs in the same class). Although they are not ordinarily as important, differences may also occur across measurements of outcome (for example, thresholds for occurrence of stroke with important functional disability, or early or late measurement of treatment effects). When the effect is real, we say there is an interaction between class of patient, intervention, or outcome, and the magnitude of the treatment effect. When the magnitude of the difference between subgroups is both real and sufficiently large, it may influence patient management.

Determining which subgroup analyses should be undertaken, and which should be believed, remains controversial. Critics of subgroup analysis decry fishing expeditions and data-dredging exercises[2-5] that result in spurious inferences concerning subgroup effects. Advocates of subgroup analysis are alarmed at the risks of missing important differences in effect,[6,7] particularly with cavalier pooling of results[8]—which can result in meaningless conclusions about "average" effects[9] and/or failure to detect important treatment effects as a result of overly heterogeneous study populations.[10]

Even though the debate between these two camps can lead to some useful insights, clinicians need practical advice for when to believe an analysis that shows apparent difference in treatment effects across subgroups. In considering this issue, clinicians need to bear in mind the different possible measures of effect, and how the choice of measure of effect can influence inferences about subgroup differences.

# Measures of Effect and Subgroup Analyses

Consider a 40-year-old nonsmoking woman without diabetes and without a family history of heart disease, a blood pressure of 110/70 mm Hg, and an elevated serum cholesterol level with a total cholesterol-to-HDL ratio of 6. Her risk of cardiovascular death in the next decade is 2% or less. Contrast this woman with a 70-year-old male smoker with diabetes who has a positive family history of heart disease, a blood pressure of 140/85 mm Hg, and an identical serum cholesterol level and cholesterol-to-HDL ratio. His risk of a cardiovascular death in the next decade is 30% or more.

These two individuals represent extremes of high- and low-risk subgroups of candidates for lipid-lowering therapy. If one considers the absolute risk reduction these patients may achieve by taking a statin for the next decade, a subgroup effect is almost certain. The greatest absolute benefit the young woman could expect would be a risk reduction in the order of 1% (from 2% to 1%), whereas the older man might have his risk reduced by 10% or more (from 30% to 20%). We would thus conclude there is an interaction between risk stratum and the magnitude of treatment effect (ie, the biggest effects are seen in the higher-risk group).

On the other hand, the relative risk reduction (in meta-analyses of statin drugs, on the order of 30%[11]) may well be very similar in high- and low-risk patients. Indeed, meta-analyses of randomized trials of statins suggest that relative risk reductions vary little across higher- and lower-risk groups. In general, considering a wide variety of interventions, relative risk reductions tend to be relatively similar across risk groups, whereas absolute risk reductions show greater variability (see Part 2B2, "Therapy and Understanding the Results, Measures of Association"). In our discussion of subgroup analyses, we will be referring to relative risk reductions unless we state otherwise.

It is implausible that the underlying true treatment effect is identical in any two subgroups. What we are concerned about are important differences. We consider a difference important if it results in a change in a treatment decision. We cannot offer a rule for when a difference in relative risk reduction will become important, for it will depend on the patient's baseline risk, the outcome being prevented, and the side effects of therapy. We would suggest, however, that differences in relative risk reduction of less than 10% (from 20% to either 10% or 30%, for instance) will seldom be important.

In formulating guides for whether to believe a subgroup analysis, we will build on criteria that have been suggested by other authors.[12-15] Table 2E-2 summarizes the approach that we will describe in detail below. Because we believe that more serious errors tend to be committed when investigators present spurious subgroup analyses as real, we will focus on the dangers of misleading analyses that suggest different treatment effects across subgroups. We do, however, acknowledge that when sample sizes are low and the power of analyses is limited, false-negative subgroup analyses also occur.

**TABLE 2E-2**

## Guidelines for Deciding Whether Apparent Differences in Subgroup Response Are Real

- Is the subgroup difference suggested by comparisons within rather than between studies?
- Did the hypothesis precede rather than follow the analysis?
- Was the subgroup effect one of a small number of hypothesized effects tested?
- Is the magnitude of the effect large?
- Was the effect statistically significant?
- Is the effect consistent across studies?
- Is there indirect evidence that supports the hypothesized subgroup effect?

# GUIDELINES FOR INTERPRETING SUBGROUP ANALYSES

## Is the Effect Suggested by Comparisons Within Rather Than Between Studies?

Making inferences about different effect sizes in different groups on the basis of between-study differences entails a high risk in comparison with inferences made on the basis of within-study differences. For instance, one would be reluctant to conclude that treatment with propranolol results in a different magnitude of risk reduction for death after myocardial infarction than does administration of metoprolol on the basis of data from two studies—one comparing propranolol with placebo and the other comparing metoprolol with placebo. Drawing inferences about these two drugs from two different placebo-controlled studies would be making an indirect comparison of their effect. A direct comparison would involve, in a single study, patients being randomized to receive either placebo, propranolol, or metoprolol. If, in such a direct comparison in a single high-quality study, investigators demonstrated clinically important and statistically significant differences in magnitude of effect between the two active treatments, the inference would be quite strong.

In a meta-analysis examining the effectiveness of prophylaxis for gastrointestinal bleeding in critically ill patients,[16] histamine-2-receptor (H2) antagonists and antacids, when individually compared to placebo, had comparable effects in reducing overt bleeding (common odds ratios of 0.58 and 0.66, respectively). By contrast, direct comparison from studies in which patients were randomized to receive H2 antagonists or antacids demonstrated a statistically significantly greater reduction in bleeding with the H2 antagonists (common odds ratio, 0.56).

The reason that inference on the basis of between-study differences is potentially so misleading is that the apparent differentiating factor between studies will always be only one of many differences. For instance, aside from differences in the specific drugs used, different populations (eg, varying in risk of adverse outcomes), varying degrees of cointervention, or varying criteria for gastrointestinal bleeding all could explain the results. Explanations for these differences would not be plausible if the inference were based on within-study differences from randomized trials in which populations studied, control of cointervention, and outcome criteria were all identical. In this latter situation, there are only two possible explanations of the difference in effect across subgroups: either it is true or it is a chance phenomenon. The fact that chance has so often led clinicians astray means that, even for within-trial comparisons, the clinician requires other evidence for deciding when to believe a subgroup analysis.

### Did the Hypothesis Precede Rather Than Follow the Analysis?

Embedded within any large data set are a certain number of apparent, but in fact spurious, interactions. As a result, the credibility of any apparent interaction that arises out of post hoc exploration of a data set is questionable.

An example of this was the apparent finding that aspirin had a beneficial effect in the prevention of stroke in men with cerebrovascular disease, but lacked the same effect in women.[17] For a considerable period of time, the finding led many physicians to withhold aspirin for women with cerebrovascular disease. This interaction, which was "discovered"—that is, the investigators stumbled across the finding in exploring the data, rather than suspecting the interaction beforehand— in the first large trial of aspirin in patients with transient ischemic attacks, was subsequently found, in other studies and in a meta-analysis summarizing these studies,[18] to be untrue.

Whether a hypothesis preceded analysis of a data set is not necessarily a clearly distinguishable issue. At one extreme, unexpected results might be clearly responsible for generating a new hypothesis—the results are discovered by a post hoc analysis. At the other extreme, a subgroup analysis might be clearly planned for—a priori—in a study protocol to test a hypothesis suggested by prior research. In between these two extremes is a range of possibilities, and the extent to which a hypothesis arose before, during, or after the data were collected and analyzed is frequently not clear. Nevertheless, if a hypothesis has been clearly and unequivocally suggested by a different data set, one has moved from a hypothesis-generating framework to a hypothesis-testing framework.

### Was the Subgroup Effect One of a Small Number of Hypothesized Effects Tested?

Post hoc hypotheses based on subgroup analysis often arise from exploration of a data set in which many such hypotheses are considered. The greater the number of hypotheses tested, the greater the number of interactions one will discover by chance. Even if investigators have clearly specified their hypotheses in advance, the strength of inference associated with the apparent confirmation of any single hypothesis will decrease if it is one of a large number that have been tested.

Clinicians and investigators tend to underestimate the impact of chance on the results of experiments. In an imaginative investigation entitled "The Miracle of DICE Therapy for Acute Stroke," Counsell and colleagues directed participants in a practical class in statistics to roll different-colored dice numerous times to simulate 44 clinical trials of fictitious therapies.[19] Participants received the dice in pairs and were told that one die in each pair was an ordinary die representing control patients, while the other die was loaded to roll either more or fewer sixes than the control. Rolling a six represented a patient death, and all other numbers represented a survival. Some pairs of dice were red, some white, and some green, each color representing a different medication used in administering "DICE therapy." The investigators simulated trials of different size (various numbers of rolls of the paired dice) and methodologic rigor, along with the peer review and publication process.

Subgroup analysis suggested that "red" DICE therapy had a nonsignificant trend toward excess mortality; when the inferior "red" drug was excluded, along with methodologically inferior and unpublished trials and data from inexperienced centers, DICE therapy offered an impressive 39% relative risk reduction for mortality in acute stroke.

The participants, however, had been deliberately misled: the dice were not loaded. The effects observed, which closely mimicked the patterns reported in actual medical literature, resulted entirely from chance. The impressive, statistically significant effect of "properly administered" DICE therapy resulted entirely from selective subgroup analyses and exclusions.

The DICE therapy demonstration suggests that clinicians should exercise great caution in interpreting apparent subgroup effects when investigators have conducted many such analyses. For instance, in a regression analysis concerned with predictors of the impact of digoxin on heart failure patients in sinus rhythm, Lee et al tested 16 variables.[20] This relatively large number increases the level of skepticism with which clinicians should regard their finding that the presence of a third heart sound is an important predictor of digoxin response. The skepticism would be even greater if the investigators had examined each variable separately, rather than in a regression analysis that considers all 16 variables simultaneously (see Part 2D, "Prognosis, Regression and Correlation").

In another example, the Beta-Blocker Heart Attack Trial (BHAT) investigators conducted 146 subgroup comparisons.[21] Although the estimated effects of the treatment, propranolol, clustered around the overall effect, the effect in some small subgroups appeared to be either much more effective or ineffective. However, the overall pattern was completely consistent with the observed difference in effect among the various subgroups because of sampling error rather than true interactions.

Unfortunately, clinicians may not always be sure about the number of possible interactions that the investigators tested. If the investigators choose to withhold this information, reporting only those that were significant, the reader is likely to be misled.

## Is the Magnitude of the Effect Large?

As a rule, the larger the difference between the effect in a particular subgroup (or with a particular drug or dosage of drug) and the overall effect, the more plausible it is that the difference is real. At the same time, as the difference in effect size between the anomalous subgroup and the remainder of the patients becomes larger, the clinical importance of the difference increases. When sample sizes are small, however, one will see large differences in apparent effect simply by the play of chance. Were one to conclude that an interaction is real just because it is large, one would be wrong more often than right. For instance, a meta-analysis of 24 randomized trials compared the impact of sucralfate vs histamine receptor antagonists and/or antacids on the incidence of nosocomial pneumonia in criti-cally ill patients.[22] The pooled estimate showed a relative risk of 0.86 (95% CI, 0.75-0.97), suggesting a possible reduction of pneumonia with sucralfate.[22] The results of the individual studies varied, however, between a relative risk of 0.33 (a reduction of pneumonia with sucralfate of two thirds) to 1.84 (an 80% increase in the incidence of pneumonia). These differences occurred despite the fact that the results were entirely consistent with a single underlying magnitude of treatment effect for all these studies (heterogeneity $P$ value, .33) (see Part 1E, "Summarizing the Evidence"; see also Part 2E, "Summarizing the Evidence, Evaluating Differences in Study Results"). Focusing on the results of the individual studies, and on possi-ble subgroup effects, could easily have led the investigators to make spurious infer-ences about subgroup effects, capitalizing on the play of chance.

## Was the Effect Statistically Significant?

A key question that investigators must address when examining apparent subgroup differences is: if the true underlying effect were the same in all patients, how likely is it that the differences between subgroups that we observed would have occurred by chance (see Part 2B2, "Therapy and Understanding the Results, Hypothesis Testing")? For instance, in the GUSTO trial that found a 1% absolute reduction in mortality in patients with acute myocardial infarction treated with tPA rather than streptokinase, the mortality difference was 1.2% in the United States and 0.7% else-where (see Part 2F, "Moving From Evidence to Action, Economic Analysis").[23] Observers noted that patients underwent invasive revascularization with percuta-neous transluminal angioplasty or coronary artery bypass surgery more frequently in the United States. They therefore wondered whether the benefits of tPA might be greater in the context of this more aggressive approach—that is, whether there was a subgroup effect such that tPA impact was greater in the context of greater use of angioplasty and surgical therapy.

How would one go about determining whether the difference between the mag-nitude of the apparent effects in the United States and elsewhere was a real phe-nomenon, or whether it was an artifact of the play of chance? The wrong way would be to test whether the effect was significant in the United States and then, separately, to test whether the effect was significant in other countries. Figure 2E-8 illustrates just how misleading such an analysis could be.

**FIGURE 2E-8**

## Two Subgroups With an Underlying Identical Treatment Effect

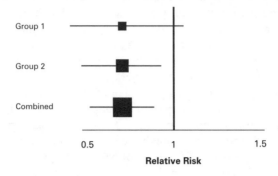

Figure 2E-8 depicts a treatment effect in two hypothetical subgroups, plus a pooled estimate combining the subgroups. The dashed line represents a relative risk of 1.0, indicating neither a beneficial nor a harmful treatment effect. The underlying truth, reflected in the results, is that the treatment effect is identical in the two subgroups. If one looks only at subgroup 2, the effect is statistically significant. In subgroup 1, because of a smaller sample size, the effect does not reach statistical significance (reflected in the confidence interval, which overlaps the line representing a treatment effect of zero). It would clearly be a mistake to conclude that treatment works in subgroup 2, but not in subgroup 1.

How should one handle this situation? Rather than asking separately: "Is the treatment effective in subgroup 1?" or "Is it effective in subgroup 2?" one should ask: "Is the effect different in subgroup 1 vs in subgroup 2?" In Figure 2E-8, the answer to that question is a resounding: "No!"

Putting the correct question into the formal framework of hypothesis testing, one asks: "how often, if there were no difference between the true underlying treatment effect in the two subgroups, would one observe differences in apparent effect as large as or larger than those we have observed?" (See Part 2B2, "Therapy, Hypothesis Testing") Returning to the example of the trial of thrombolytic therapy, the question would be: "how often, if there was no true underlying gradient of effect, would investigators find differences as large as or larger than the difference between the 1.2% and 0.7% estimates?" The $P$ value for this test was .3. That is, if the true mortality gradient between tPA and streptokinase were identical (say, 1.0%) in the US and other countries, differences as large as or larger than those observed among the US and other-country subgroups would occur 30% of the time. Thus, the data provide little support for the hypothesis that the effect of tPA differs across these settings.

Contrast this with a meta-analysis examining the impact of alendronate on nonvertebral fractures.[24] The investigators used regression methods to discover that a model in which they pooled all doses of alendronate was less powerful than a model that separated doses of less than 10 mg and 10 mg or more in explaining differences in results across studies ($P = .002$). The investigators therefore gained confidence that the apparently greater effect of doses of greater than 10 mg (RRR, 0.49) than that of lower doses (RRR, 0.13) was a real, rather than chance, phenomenon.

Investigators can use a variety of statistical techniques to explore whether chance can explain apparent subgroup differences.[9, 12, 25-28] What readers should look for are the results of a statistical test that addresses the possibility that the apparent difference in magnitude of effect between subgroups is a chance finding.

We would add two notes of caution. First, if investigators have examined a large number of subgroup hypotheses, they run the risk of generating low $P$ values in some of their analyses simply by chance. For example, investigators conducted a study of platelet-activating factor receptor antagonist (PAFra) in sepsis patients.[29] The result for all 262 patients showed a weak, nonsignificant trend in favor of active therapy.[29] A subgroup analysis of 110 patients with gram-negative bacterial infection showed a large, statistically significant advantage for PAFra. A subsequent larger study of 444 patients with gram-negative bacterial infection showed a small, nonsignificant trend in favor of PAFra almost identical to that of the prior trial analysis, which included all randomized patients.[30] The disappointed investigators might have been less surprised at the result of the second trial had they fully appreciated the limitations of their first subgroup analysis: the possible differential effect of PAFra in gram-negative bacterial infection was one of 15 subgroup hypotheses they tested.[31]

Second, if a hypothesis about an interaction has arisen out of exploration of a data set from a study, then one could make an argument for excluding that study from a meta-analysis in which the hypothesis is tested. Certainly, if the hypothesis is confirmed in a meta-analysis that excludes data from the study that originally suggested the interaction, the inference rests on stronger ground. If the statistical significance of the interaction disappears or is substantially weakened when data from the original study are excluded, the strength of inference is reduced.

## Is the Interaction Consistent Across Studies?

A hypothesis concerning differential response in a subgroup of patients may be generated by examination of data from a single study. The interaction becomes more credible if it is also found in other studies. The extent to which a rigorous systematic review of the relevant literature finds an interaction to be consistently present is probably the best single index of its credibility.

The hypothesis concerning a third heart sound as a predictor of response to digoxin in heart failure patients in sinus rhythm was tested in a second crossover randomized trial.[32] The presence of a third heart sound proved to be a weaker predictor than in the initial study, although its association with response to digoxin did reach conventional levels of statistical significance. However, a number of factors that, like a third heart sound, reflect greater severity of heart failure were associated with response to digoxin. Thus, support for a more general hypothesis—that response is related to severity of heart failure—was provided by the second study.

Other studies that have examined the efficacy of digoxin in heart failure patients in sinus rhythm have been summarized in a meta-analysis.[33] Unfortunately, none of these studies have conducted subgroup analyses addressing the issue of differential response according to differing severity of heart failure. Had these analyses been undertaken in the other available studies, the hypothesis would likely have been confirmed or refuted with substantially greater confidence. As it is, we would be inclined to view the conclusion as tentative (ie, the strength of inference is only moderate).

### Is There Indirect Evidence That Supports the Hypothesized Interaction?

We are generally more ready to believe a hypothesized interaction if there is indirect evidence (such as from animal studies or analogous situations in human biology) that make the interaction more plausible. That is, to the extent that a hypothesis is consistent with our current understanding of the biologic mechanisms of disease, we are more likely to believe it. Such understanding comes from three types of indirect evidence: studies of different populations (including animal studies); observations of interactions for similar interventions; and results of studies of other related outcomes particularly (intermediary outcomes).

The extent to which indirect evidence strengthens an inference about a hypothesized interaction varies substantially. In general, evidence from intermediary outcomes is the strongest type of indirect evidence, eg, evidence of differences in immune response that support a conclusion that there is an important difference in the clinical effectiveness of a vaccine depending on age.[34] Conversely, indirect evidence from related interventions is generally the weakest type of indirect evidence, eg, evidence of a similar interaction with other vaccines.

The human mind is sufficiently fertile that there is no shortage of biologically plausible explanations, or indirect evidence, in support of almost any observation. One quite ironic example of biologic evidence supporting a possible interaction mentioned earlier in this section comes from an early trial suggesting that aspirin reduced stroke in men, but not in women.[20] This finding stimulated animal research, which provided a biologic basis for the interaction.[35] Ultimately, however, it turned out that aspirin for stroke reduction was as effective in women as in men.[21]

# Conclusion

Criteria suggested for determining whether to believe hypotheses concerning causation have proved helpful in understanding controversial causal claims.[2,36] The criteria suggested here should be useful in deciding when to believe an analysis that suggests a differential response to treatment in a definable subgroup of patients, or with a particular drug or drug dose. At the one extreme are relatively small, marginally significant interactions based on between-study differences or generated for the first time by post hoc exploration of a single data set. At the other extreme are large, important interactions, originally suggested by both indirect evidence and direct evidence, and independently tested either in a new trial or in a meta-analysis in which the possibility of the interaction resulting from the play of chance is very low. The former should be viewed with great skepticism; the latter can form the basis of clinical decision making. The strength of inference can range from one end of this spectrum to the other. In instances when criteria are partially satisfied, further information, in the form of either new primary studies or meta-analysis, will often be desirable to strengthen the inference one way or the other, to the point where it can be confidently applied as clinical policy.

Decisions regarding how much effort to put into accumulating more evidence, and what clinical action to take, will depend on the potential benefits, risks, and costs involved. Decision thresholds, both for undertaking further research and for taking a clinical action, vary greatly. For problems with large potential benefits and small risks and costs, we are generally willing to accept lower standards of evidence than for problems with smaller potential benefits or larger risks or costs.

Deciding whether to base clinical practice on the average estimate of effect from an overall analysis (one that is more robust) or on a subgroup analysis (one that more closely reflects the specific clinical situation at hand) hinges on the criteria described above. It is tempting to take one extreme or the other, ie, always to base decisions on the overall estimate of effect or always to base decisions on the most applicable subgroup analysis. However, a thoughtful approach based on these criteria is more likely to result in the most benefit and the least harm for patients.

# References

1.  Pocock SJ, Hughes MD, Lee RJ. Statistical problems in the reporting of clinical trials: a survey of three medical journals. *N Engl J Med*. 1987;317:426-432.

2.  Fletcher RH, Fletcher SW, Wagner EH. *Clinical Epidemiology: The Essentials*. 2nd ed. Baltimore, MD: Williams & Wilkins; 1988:185-186.

3.  Feinstein AR. *Clinical Epidemiology: The Architecture of Clinical Research*. Philadelphia, PA: WB Saunders Co; 1985:306-307, 516-517.

4.  Senn S, Harrell F. On wisdom after the event. *J Clin Epidemiol*. 1997;50: 749-751.

5.  Altman DG. Within trial variation—a false trail? *J Clin Epidemiol*. 1998;51: 301-303.

6.  Horwitz RI, Singer BH, Makuch RW, Viscoli CM. On reaching the tunnel at the end of the light. *J Clin Epidemiol*. 1997;50:753-755.

7.  Feinstein AR. The problem of cogent subgroups: a clinicostatistical tragedy. *J Clin Epidemiol*. 1998;51:297-299.

8.  Goldman L, Feinstein AR. Anticoagulants and myocardial infarction: the problems of pooling, drowning, and floating. *Ann Intern Med*. 1979;90:92-94.

9.  Furberg CD, Morgan TM. Lessons from overviews of cardiovascular trials. *Stat Med*. 1987;6:295-306.

10. Horwitz RI. Complexity and contradiction in clinical trial research. *Am J Med*. 1987;82:498-510.

11. Bucher HC, Griffith LE, Guyatt GH. Systematic review on the risk and benefit of different cholesterol-lowering interventions. *Arterioscler Thromb Vasc Biol*. 1999;19:187-195.

12. Buyse ME. Analysis of clinical trial outcomes: some comments on subgroup analyses. *Control Clin Trials*. 1989;10(suppl 4):187S-194S.

13. Bulpitt CJ. Subgroup analysis. *Lancet*. 1988;2:31-34.

14. Byar DP. Assessing apparent treatment—covariate interactions in randomized clinical trials. *Stat Med*. 1985;4:255-263.

15. Shuster J, van Eys J. Interaction between prognostic factors and treatment. *Control Clin Trials*. 1983;4:209-214.

16. Cook DJ, Witt LG, Cook RJ, Guyatt GH. Stress ulcer prophylaxis in the critically ill: a meta-analysis. *Am J Med*. 1991;91:519-527.

17. The Canadian Cooperative Study Group. A randomized trial of aspirin and sulfinpyrazone in threatened stroke. *N Engl J Med*. 1978;299:53-59.

18. Antiplatelet Trialists' Collaboration. Secondary prevention of vascular disease by prolonged antiplatelet treatment. *Br Med J Clin Res Ed*. 1988;296:320-331.

19. Counsell CE, Clarke MJ, Slattery J, Sandercock PA. The miracle of DICE therapy for acute stroke: fact or fictional product of subgroup analysis? *BMJ*. 1994;309:1677-1681.

20. Lee DC, Johnson RA, Bingham JB, et al. Heart failure in outpatients: a randomized trial of digoxin versus placebo. *N Engl J Med*. 1982;306:699-705.

21. Furberg CD, Byington RP, for the Beta-Blocker Heart Attack Trial experience. What do subgroup analyses reveal about differential response to beta-blocker therapy? *Circulation*. 1983;67(6 pt 2):I98-I101.

22. Cook DJ, Reeve BK, Guyatt GH, et al. Stress ulcer prophylaxis in critically ill patients: resolving discordant meta-analyses. *JAMA*. 1996;275:308-314.

23. The GUSTO investigators. An international randomized trial comparing four thrombolytic strategies for acute myocardial infarction. *N Engl J Med*. 1993;329:673-682.

24. Cranney A, Guyatt G, Willan A, Griffith L, Krolicki N, Welch V, et al. A meta-analysis of alendronate for the treatment of osteoporosis in postmenopausal women. *JAMA*. Submitted.

25. Schneider B. Analysis of clinical trial outcomes: alternative approaches to subgroup analysis. *Control Clin Trials*. 1989;10(suppl 4):176S-186S.

26. Breslow NE, Day NE. *Statistical Methods in Cancer Research. Vol 1. The Analysis of Case-Control Studies*. Lyon: International Agency for Research on Cancer; 1980:122-159.

27. Breslow NE, Day NE. *Statistical Methods in Cancer Research. Vol 1. The Analysis of Case-Control Studies*. Lyon: International Agency for Research on Cancer; 1980:192-246.

28. Beach ML, Meier P. Choosing covariates in the analysis of clinical trials. *Control Clin Trials*. 1989;10(suppl 4):161S-175S.

29. Dhainaut JF, Tenaillon A, Le Tulzo Y, et al, for the BN 52021 Sepsis Study Group. Platelet-activating factor receptor antagonist BN 52021 in the treatment of severe sepsis: a randomized, double-blind, placebo-controlled, multicenter clinical trial. *Crit Care Med*. 1994;22:1720-1728.

30. Dhainaut JF, Tenaillon A, Hemmer M, et al, for the BN 52021 Sepsis Investigator Group. Confirmatory platelet-activating factor receptor antagonist trial in patients with severe gram-negative bacterial sepsis: a phase III, randomized, double-blind, placebo-controlled, multicenter trial. *Crit Care Med*. 1998;26:1963-1971.

31. Natanson C, Esposito CJ, Banks SM. The sirens' songs of confirmatory sepsis trials: selection bias and sampling error. *Crit Care Med*. 1998;26:1927-1931.

32. Guyatt GH, Sullivan MJ, Fallen EL, et al. A controlled trial of digoxin in congestive heart failure. *Am J Cardiol*. 1988;61:371-375.

33. Jaeschke R, Oxman AD, Guyatt GH. To what extent do congestive heart failure patients in sinus rhythm benefit from digoxin therapy? A systematic overview and meta-analysis. *Am J Med*. 1990;88:279-286.

34. Stieb DM, Frayha HH, Oxman AD, Shannon HS, Hutchison BG, Crombie FS. Effectiveness of Haemophilus influenzae type b vaccines. *CMAJ*. 1990;142:719-733.

35. Kelton JG, Hirsh J, Carter CJ, Buchanan MR. Sex differences in the antithrombotic effects of aspirin. *Blood*. 1978;52:1073-1076.

36. Hill AB. *Principles of Medical Statistics*. 9th ed. New York: Oxford University Press; 1971:312-320.

# MOVING FROM EVIDENCE TO ACTION

## Incorporating Patient Values

Gordon Guyatt, Sharon Straus, Finlay McAlister,
Brian Haynes, Jack Sinclair, PJ Devereaux,
and Christina Lacchetti

## IN THIS SECTION

## CLINICAL SCENARIO

### Would This Patient With Atrial Fibrillation Choose Aspirin or Anticoagulants?

**A** 70-year-old man who has smoked a pack of cigarettes daily for many years was well until 3 months ago, when he presented with heart palpitations. An electrocardiogram showed atrial fibrillation with a rate of 110 bpm, but was otherwise normal. Review of the patient's history, physical examination, and laboratory values showed no prior or current hypertension, a current blood pressure of 130/80 mm Hg, a normal serum cholesterol level, and no clinical or electrocardiographic findings suggesting coronary artery disease. An echocardiogram showed an enlarged atrium but normal ventricular size and function, and no wall motion abnormalities. Over the next 4 weeks, you treated the patient with metoprolol, which controlled his heart rate, plus warfarin to obtain an international normalized ratio (INR) of between 2.0 and 3.0. Attempted electrical cardioversion and a trial of amiodarone failed to convert the patient to a state of sinus rhythm.

You must now deal with the patient's persistent atrial fibrillation and consequent increased risk of an embolic stroke. You are aware that options for prophylaxis include no treatment, treatment with aspirin, or treatment with warfarin. You realize that to help the patient make a rational decision about the best treatment, you need to be able to estimate his risk of serious bleeding and stroke while receiving each of these therapeutic options.

# FINDING THE EVIDENCE

To conduct your search, you initially identify your patient population as older patients with otherwise uncomplicated nonvalvular atrial fibrillation (NVAF), but subsequently you realize that, because no studies have restricted themselves to this subgroup, you will likely have to be content with a wider population of patients with NVAF. With respect to bleeding, ideally you would like to find a randomized trial—or a meta-analysis of a set of such trials—that made direct head-to-head comparisons between treatment with placebo and with the two active agents. Once again, because of a paucity of studies making head-to-head comparisons between the three agents, you may have to compromise by relying on trials whose investigators considered warfarin and placebo separately, and aspirin and placebo separately. In addition, you are concerned that researchers conducting randomized controlled trials may select highly compliant patient populations and achieve more rigorous control of anticoagulant intensity than is possible in routine clinical practice, leading to underestimates of bleeding complications in warfarin-treated patients. Therefore, for this outcome, you are prepared to extend your search beyond randomized controlled trials to observational studies in which investigators follow patients prescribed these regimens in usual clinical settings. You are interested in rates of both bleeding and stroke.

Finally, you need to establish the baseline risk of stroke for the patient before you, information that you may extrapolate from the placebo or untreated groups in randomized trials, or from the results of observational studies. As you think about the matter further, you realize its complexity and conclude that a *decision analysis* may also be helpful.

You know that the most efficient approach to collecting high-quality evidence on a topic is to begin with the electronic evidence-based medicine resource, Best Evidence. You log on to the current version, Best Evidence 4, starting a search of the selected topic group, therapeutics, for the effectiveness of aspirin and warfarin in treatment of patients with stroke by combining the search terms "atrial fibrillation and stroke." This strategy yields 16 citations, of which two are systematic reviews that are potentially relevant to your problem.[1,2] However, both reviews address atrial fibrillation as only one of a number of risk factors for stroke, and you wonder if you can find a more specific review.

Searching for systematic reviews that focus on atrial fibrillation, you switch to the PubMed system of searching MEDLINE. You enter the terms "atrial fibrillation and stroke," then, using the Limit function, limit your results to the publication type "meta-analysis." This search strategy yields 14 meta-analyses, of which three are additional papers whose authors studied all three treatment groups and estimated the risk of both stroke and bleeding.[3-5]

Next, to get a good estimate of bleeding complications in warfarin-treated patients, you search PubMed using the terms "warfarin and atrial fibrillation and bleeding," limiting the search to English-language studies with a publication date no older than 1998. This search identifies 50 articles, one of which appears particularly relevant.[6] This study provides a current estimate of the risk of bleeding secondary to warfarin therapy in patients with atrial fibrillation from an observational study conducted in the community.

Finally, you conduct your search for a formal decision analysis using the combined search terms "atrial fibrillation and anticoagulant therapy and decision analysis." Of the citations generated, the study by Thomson et al looks most appropriate.[7]

Three of the five meta-analyses that focus on atrial fibrillation meet most validity criteria for a systematic review (see Part 1E, "Summarizing the Evidence")[2,4,5] and were published since 1999. One of these three, a meta-analysis by Hart and colleagues,[4] was more explicit in its inclusion criteria and those investigators appear to have conducted a more comprehensive search than the other two. Authors of one of the two less recent meta-analyses did not conduct a comprehensive search, but the investigators had at their disposal individual patient data that allowed them to formulate patient risk groups, which allows you to estimate your patient's risk at baseline.[3] You therefore decide to formulate estimates of baseline risk from Laupacis et al[3], but use Hart and colleagues' results[4] as the best estimate of treatment effectiveness.

In reviewing the data, you conclude that if the patient before you remains untreated, the best estimate of stroke risk (ie, both ischemic and hemorrhagic stroke) during the next year is 4.3%, and, further, that aspirin is likely to decrease this risk by approximately 22% and warfarin is likely to decrease the risk by 62%, corresponding to absolute risk reductions (ARR) of 0.95% and 2.6%, respectively, over a 1-year period. This translates into a number needed to treat (NNT) for 1 year to prevent a stroke of approximately 106 for treatment with aspirin and 39 for treatment with warfarin (see Part 2B2, "Therapy and Understanding the Results, Measures of Association"). These results are quite consistent with the relative risk reduction from direct comparisons of warfarin and aspirin of 36%. Assuming the patient starts with a 3.35% risk while taking aspirin (derived from the baseline risk of 4.3% and aspirin's 22% relative risk reduction), this corresponds to an NNT of 83, close to the NNT of 67 we would get by subtracting the NNT for warfarin from the NNT for aspirin.

Examining the likelihood of serious extracranial hemorrhage (of which gastrointestinal bleeding predominates), the meta-analysis suggests a risk of 0.6% for control patients in the warfarin trials, with a risk of 0.9% in warfarin-treated patients, yielding an absolute increase in risk of 0.3%. However, the observational study suggests a risk of 1.7% (including intracerebral bleeding risk) per year for low-risk patients.[6] You conclude that the most plausible explanation of differences between estimates from the randomized trials and the observational studies is success in avoiding excessive anticoagulation. Assuming a risk of major bleeding of approximately 0.6% in untreated patients, the data from the community study suggest that the increase in risk of serious bleeding in community patients is approximately 1% per year.

In light of your knowledge that the patient before you is intelligent, conscientious, and very concerned about his health, you anticipate a high rate of adherence; in addition, you anticipate that the bleeding risk rate of 1% represents a conservative estimate of his increased risk of serious gastrointestinal bleeding while receiving warfarin. The systematic review failed to detect any increase in the incidence of gastrointestinal bleeding with aspirin; bleeding rates were approximately 0.8% in both treated and control patients.[4]

Considering these numbers, you are aware that the treatment decision may depend on the relative value the patient places on avoiding a stroke, avoiding a gastrointestinal bleeding episode, and avoiding the inconvenience associated with anticoagulation. The decision analysis confirms your impression that the patient's values are likely to be crucial in making the decision.[7] You are now faced with the problem of how to best incorporate the patient's values into the decision.

# THE GUIDE

## Two Fundamental Strategies for Incorporating Patient Values

We have proposed in other sections of this book (see Part 1B1, "Therapy"; Part 1F, "Moving From Evidence to Action"; Part 1A, "Introduction: The Philosophy of Evidence-Based Medicine"; and Part 2B3, "Therapy and Applying the Results,

Applying Results to Individual Patients") that clinical decision making should begin by using the best evidence to estimate the benefits, risks, and costs associated with alternative courses of action. We have pointed out that since there are always advantages and disadvantages to an intervention, evidence alone cannot determine the best course of action. Most would agree that the values and preferences that the clinician must use to balance risks and benefits should be those of the patient. Findings that patients vary greatly in the value they place on different outcomes will come as no surprise.[8] Given this variability in patient's values, clinicians should proceed with great care; it is easy to assume that the patient's values are similar to one's own, yet this may well be incorrect.[9] The challenge, then, is to integrate the evidence with the patient's values.

For many—perhaps most—of our clinical decisions, the tradeoff is sufficiently clear that clinicians need not concern themselves with variability in patient values. Previously healthy patients will all want antibiotics to treat their pneumonia or their urinary tract infection, anticoagulation to treat their pulmonary embolus, or aspirin to treat their myocardial infarction. Under such circumstances, a brief explanation of the rationale for treatment and the expected benefits and side effects will suffice.

When benefits and risks are balanced more precariously and the best choice may differ across patients, clinicians must attend to the variability in patients' values. One fundamental strategy for integrating evidence with preferences involves communicating the benefits and risks to patients, thus permitting them to incorporate their own values and preferences in the decision. One advantage of this approach is that it avoids the vexing problem of measuring patients' values. Unfortunately, the problem of communicating the evidence to patients in a way that allows patients to clearly and unequivocally understand their choices is almost as vexing as the direct measurement of patient values.

A second basic strategy is to ask patients to place a relative value on the key outcomes associated with the management options. In our opening clinical scenario, for instance, the key choice is the relative value one places on avoiding a stroke vs avoiding a gastrointestinal bleeding episode.[10] One can then consider the likely outcomes of alternative courses of action and use the patient's values as the basis of trading off benefits and risks. When done in a fully quantitative way, this approach becomes a decision analysis using individual patient preferences (see Part 1F, "Moving From Evidence to Action").

Patients often have preferences not only about the outcomes, but about the decision-making process itself. These preferences can vary, and the patient's desired level of involvement should determine which approach the clinician takes.[11-13] Ethicists have characterized the alternative strategies.[14] At one end of the spectrum, the physician acts as a technician, providing the patient with information and taking no active part in the decision-making process. This corresponds to the first strategy for incorporating patient values, presenting patients with the likely benefits, risks, inconvenience, and cost and then letting patients decide. At the opposite extreme, corresponding to the second strategy, ascertaining the patient's values and then making a recommendation in light of the likely advantages and disadvantages of alternative management approaches, the clinician takes a "paternalistic" approach and decides what is best for the patient in light of that patient's preferences.

However, intermediate approaches of shared decision making are generally more popular than those at either extreme. Shared decision making uses both of the two fundamental approaches to decision making presented above: The physician typically shares the evidence, in some form, with the patient, while simultaneously attempting to understand the patient's values. Evidence that more active patient involvement in the process of health care delivery can improve outcomes and reported quality of life—and, possibly, reduce health care expenditures[15-19]—provides empirical evidence in support of secular trends toward patient autonomy and away from parental approaches.

Clinicians should temper their enthusiasm for active patient involvement in decision making with an awareness that many patients prefer parental approaches. Consider, for instance, the results of a survey of 2472 patients suffering from chronic disease (hypertension, diabetes, heart failure, myocardial infarction, or depression) completed between 1986 and 1990.[20] In response to the statement: "I prefer to leave decisions about my medical care up to my doctor," 17.1% strongly agreed, 45.5% agreed, 11.1% were uncertain, 22.5% disagreed, and only 4.8% strongly disagreed. Although it is likely that, more than a decade after this survey was conducted, patients are more enthusiastic about active involvement in decision making, these results suggest that many patients still prefer the physician to assume a primary role.

The results of this survey also emphasize the extent to which preferred decision-making styles differ. Gauging the degree to which an individual patient wants to actively participate can therefore present a challenge.[21-23] However, patients who prefer a parental approach tend to quickly chasten clinicians who try to communicate the benefits and risks with admonitions such as, "You're the doctor." Furthermore, clinicians who take a parental approach with a patient who prefers to make the decision herself risk the possibility of future legal action from that patient. Although patients are often flexible and may seek guidance not only in the ultimate decision, but in how that decision is made, sensitive clinicians will elicit the patient's preferred decision-making formula.

Regardless of the decision-making approach chosen by the patient and clinician, evidence-based medicine injects challenges into the process by insisting that clinicians consider quantitative estimates of benefits and risks, rather than just whether a treatment works or whether toxicity occurs. If clinicians leave the decisions to patients, they must effectively communicate the probabilities associated with the alternative outcomes to them. If they opt for taking responsibility for combining patient values with the evidence, they must quantify those values. A vague sense of the patient's preferences cannot fully satisfy the rigor of the optimal evidence-based medicine approach.

We will now describe some of the specific strategies associated with two decision-making models: one in which the clinician presents the patient with the likely consequences of alternative management strategies and leaves the choice to the patient, and the other in which the clinician ascertains the patient's values and provides a recommendation.

## Patient as Decision Maker: Decision Aids

If the patient wishes to play the primary role in decision making, clinicians may use intuitive approaches to communicating concepts of risk and risk reduction that they have developed through clinical experience. They will answer the patient's questions and ultimately act on the patient's decision. Alternatively, if available for a particular decision, clinicians can use a *decision aid* that presents descriptive and probabilistic information about the disease, treatment options, and potential outcomes in a patient-friendly manner.[24, 25]

A well-constructed decision aid has two advantages. One is that someone has reviewed the literature and produced a rigorous summary of the probabilities. Clinicians who doubt that the summary of probabilities is rigorous can go back to the original literature on which those probabilities are based and, using the principles of this book, determine their accuracy. A second advantage of a well-constructed decision aid is that it will offer a pretested and effective way of communicating the information to patients who may have little background in quantitative decision making. Most commonly, decision aids use visual props to present the outcome data in terms of the percentage of people with a certain condition who do well without intervention, compared to the percentage who do well with intervention. Decision aids will summarize the data regarding all outcomes of importance to patients.

Theoretically, decision aids present an attractive strategy for ensuring that patient values guide clinical decision making. What impact do decision aids actually have on clinical practice? O'Connor and colleagues conducted a systematic review, finding 17 randomized trials that used 11 different decision aids.[26] Of these 17 trials, decision aid impact on knowledge was evaluated in four. All four found greater knowledge in the decision aid group, with a pooled difference of 19 on a 100-point scale (95% CI, 14-25). Decision aids reduced decisional conflict in three of four trials in which investigators addressed this issue (mean effect, 0.3; 95% CI, 0.1-0.4 on a 5-point scale). Three studies failed to show a difference in satisfaction with the decision made, although one of these three showed increased satisfaction with the decision-making process.

The effect on the final decision has been inconsistent. For example, patients offered decision aids have proved less likely to choose coronary revascularization or mastectomy, yet more likely to accept hepatitis B vaccine.[26] Decision aids have had no impact on the proportion of parents choosing circumcision for their newborn boys, women choosing to undergo amniocentesis, or women electing to begin hormone replacement therapy.[26]

In summary, decision aids markedly increase patient knowledge and decrease discomfort with decision making as reflected in decisional conflict scores. The importance of the reduction in decisional conflict remains uncertain. Simple decision aids that clinicians can integrate into regular patient care could increase the extent to which patient values truly determine health care decisions.

## Patient as Provider of Values

The second set of approaches all begin with, at minimum, establishing the relative value the patient places on the target outcomes. Doing so requires that the patient understand the nature of those outcomes. How, for instance, would the patient imagine living with a stroke, or the experience of having a gastrointestinal bleeding episode? Patients may find a written description of the health states (such as the description of a mild and a severe stroke and a gastrointestinal bleeding episode in Table 2F-1) useful in the process of describing their preferences.

**TABLE 2F-1**

### Sample Descriptions of Mild Stroke, Severe Stroke, and Gastrointestinal Bleeding

**Mild Stroke**

Having a mild stroke causes you to slur your words. After a mild stroke, you are able to fully understand what is being said to you. Your thoughts remain clear and you can carry out a conversation without much trouble, but sometimes you cannot find the right word to use. Your thinking ability is otherwise normal. There is some weakness and numbness in your right arm and your face has a slight droop. You are able to feed, dress, and bathe yourself. However, you cannot grip objects as tightly as you could before the stroke, objects sometimes fall from your hands, and you have difficulty writing. Your condition will not get better in the future.

**Severe Stroke**

After having a severe stroke, your speech is impaired to the extent that others cannot understand your words. You can understand simple communication, but have great difficulty with more complex communication. You are not confused, but your thinking is impaired to the point that you are unable to attend to your financial matters and you cannot work. You can feed and dress yourself, but you need assistance to bathe. Your right arm and right leg are weak. You can walk with the aid of a cane. Your condition will not get better in the future.

**Gastrointestinal Bleeding**

You are vomiting bright-red blood and there is blood in your stool, which is black. You experience dizziness and are feeling unwell enough to go to the emergency department. You feel like you are going to die. You are admitted to the hospital, where the doctors insert a tube into your stomach. You require an urgent operation, followed by several blood transfusions. You are hospitalized for 10 days. You will need to take medication the next 6 months to prevent further bleeding and to raise your blood count after the bleeding. Your blood will be checked monthly. You feel extremely tired to the point of exhaustion. Your energy will gradually improve until, at 4 months after discharge from hospital, you will be back to normal.

Having made their best effort to ensure that patients understand the outcomes, clinicians can choose from among a number of ways of obtaining their values for those outcomes. They can gain a qualitative sense of their patients' preferences from a discussion without a formal structure. Alternatively, a direct comparison between outcomes may prove useful. For instance, with only two outcomes, the patient can make a direct comparative rating. The question may be: "How much worse would it be to have a stroke vs a gastrointestinal bleeding episode? Would it be equally bad? Twice as bad to have a stroke? Three times as bad?"

Using a somewhat more complex strategy, the clinician can ask the patient to place a mark on a *visual analogue scale* or "feeling thermometer" (Figure 2F-1), in which the extremes are anchored at death and full health, to represent how the patient feels about the health states in question. When, as in the case of a gastrointestinal bleeding episode and a stroke, some health states are temporary and others are permanent, the clinician must ensure that patients incorporate the duration of the health state in their rating.

**FIGURE 2F-1**

## Visual Analogue Scale as a "Feeling Thermometer"

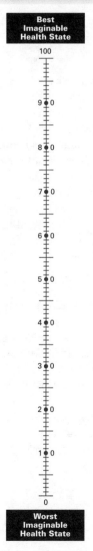

More sophisticated approaches include the time tradeoff and the standard gamble.[27] In completing the time tradeoff, patients choose between a longer period in a state of impaired health (such as recovery from severe stroke) and a shorter period in a state of full health. With the standard gamble, by contrast, patients are asked to choose between living in a state of impaired health vs taking a gamble in which they may return to full health or die immediately (see Part 2B2, "Therapy and Understanding the Results, Quality of Life"). These latter approaches—and particularly the standard gamble—come much closer to meeting assumptions that health economists argue are necessary for accurate ratings of the relative value of health states in the context of choice with uncertain outcomes.

# DECISION ANALYSIS

Regardless of the strategy clinicians use to obtain patient values, they must somehow integrate these values with the likely outcomes of the alternative management strategies. Formal decision analysis provides the most rigorous method for making this integration (see Part 1F, "Moving From Evidence to Action"). Practical software for plugging in the patient's values and conducting a patient-specific decision analysis for common clinical problems is not yet available, although it may be available in the near future. Indeed, investigators have shown that, when patients' values are used in individualized decision analyses, their decisions about anticoagulation in atrial fibrillation differ from those suggested by existing guidelines.[28] Whether the decisions would have differed had the patients been provided with the probabilities and asked to choose their preferred management strategy—as with a decision aid—remains unknown.

Even if the tools for individual decision analysis were widely available, application of the approach would depend on the availability of health care workers—probably nurses—who could devote time to eliciting patient values. Such a process may be resource intensive, and issues of how much we gain from the investment, or the intervention's cost-effectiveness (see Part 2F, "Moving From Evidence to Action, Economic Analysis"), may become very important. Exactly the same considerations apply to the use of decision aids, in which the improvement of knowledge is clear but the impact on anxiety, or on the choices patients actually make, is not as obvious.

While waiting for the software for individualized decision analysis to become available, a published decision analysis may be helpful. To apply a decision analysis to an individual patient, the values used in the analysis must approximate those of the patient, or the decision analysis must provide information about the impact of variation in patient values.

# THE LIKELIHOOD OF BEING HELPED VS HARMED

Another method of expressing information to patients that incorporates their values is the likelihood of being helped vs harmed.[29] Clinicians can apply the likelihood of being helped vs harmed to any clinical decision, and preliminary evidence suggests the approach may be useful on busy clinical services. The clinician begins by calculating the NNT and NNH for the average patients in the study or studies from which the data about treatment effectiveness and harm come (see Part 2B2, "Therapy and Understanding the Results, Measures of Association"). The clinician then adjusts the average NNT and NNH for the individual patient according to that patient's likelihood of suffering the target event that treatment is intended to prevent, and the risks it may precipitate, relative to the average patient. Having established the relative likelihood of help vs harm, the clinician explores the patient's values about the severity of adverse events that might be caused by the treatment relative to the severity of the target event that treatment helps prevent. The final adjustment of the likelihood of being helped vs harmed incorporates the patient's values.

# CLINICAL RESOLUTION

The patient in our opening clinical scenario places a very high value on avoiding a stroke (or, to put it another way, places a low value on life as a disabled person following a stroke). He places a considerably lower value on avoiding a gastrointestinal bleeding episode than on avoiding a stroke, and is minimally troubled by the inconvenience of regular monitoring of anticoagulant therapy. We will now see how the resolution of the scenario would play out given different choices about how to incorporate the patient's values.

## Semistructured Conversation

You describe to the patient the consequences of a stroke, the experience and consequences of having a serious gastrointestinal bleeding episode, and what is involved with long-term monitoring of anticoagulation. Talking with the patient, you discover his aversion to life after a stroke, his less intense aversion to a gastrointestinal bleeding episode, and his equanimity when reflecting on the need for anticoagulant monitoring. You explain his risk of stroke and his risk of bleeding should he decide to continue on anticoagulant therapy. Together, you decide that continuing with warfarin treatment ultimately is in his best interest.

In a variation of this way of resolving the problem, to help ensure the patient's understanding, you present him with a written description of what it is like to have a stroke and a gastrointestinal bleeding episode (Table 2F-1). Again, you decide together to continue warfarin.

## Decision Aids

You are aware of a decision aid for atrial fibrillation[30] that you obtain from the authors.[31] The material includes a written text and an audiotape that describes background information about atrial fibrillation, depicts mild and severe strokes, explains what the patient can expect taking either aspirin or warfarin, and provides some case studies to make the decision more vivid. Working through the audiotape and text takes the patient 30 to 45 minutes. The material is based on a single trial and is designed for patients with hypertension, both of which limit its applicability to the patient before you. However, the risks presented in the tape are close to your best estimates for him, and you decide to present the tape to the patient and discuss his interpretation.

The patient finds the tape and booklet extremely helpful. Reviewing what he has learned, you realize that he has achieved a good understanding of his options. You are pleased when he informs you he would choose anticoagulation, the option that you believe is in his best interests.

## Decision Analysis

Reviewing the published decision analysis you have found,[7] you note that the analysts have used median values from a patient survey to establish patient preferences. These turn out to be 0.88 for gastrointestinal bleeding, 0.675 for a minor stroke, and zero for a major stroke (all on a 0-1.0 scale where zero represents death and 1.0 represents full health) (see Part 2B2, "Therapy and Understanding the Results, Quality of Life"). You conclude that these values are sufficiently close to those of the presenting patient that you can use the decision analysis to guide your approach to this patient. In the decision analysis, you find a table that provides recommendations that vary according to patient age, risk factors for stroke, and blood pressure. You locate your patient's situation in these tables and, somewhat to your surprise, discover that the analysis has concluded "no clear benefit" from warfarin therapy for patients like yours. Reading more closely, you note that the authors found their model to be very sensitive to the patient's feelings about anticoagulant monitoring. In particular, they state that for patients with no disutility associated with the inconvenience of therapy (the value of life with anticoagulant monitoring and no other problems is 1.0), warfarin therapy is preferred for virtually all patients. You review these findings with the patient, who agrees to continue taking anticoagulants.

## Likelihood of Help vs Harm

During your discussion with the patient about the consequences of a stroke, gastrointestinal bleeding, and regular monitoring of anticoagulant use, you asked him to use the "feeling thermometer" (see Figure 2F-1) to estimate how he feels about each of these events. He is not concerned at all about the required laboratory monitoring, but places a value of living with a stroke at 0.2 and of living with a gastrointestinal bleed at 0.8. You use these to calculate his likelihood of being helped or harmed (LHH) from warfarin therapy vs aspirin therapy.

Using the NNTs calculated in the scenario, the LHH from warfarin vs aspirin becomes:

$$LHH = \frac{(1/NNT)}{(1/NNH)}$$

$$LHH = (1/NNT) : (1/NNH)$$

(Note: we could also use [1/absolute risk reduction] : [1/absolute risk increase] but this uses decimal fractions and may increase the likelihood of arithmetic errors.)

$$LHH = (1/83) : (1/125)$$

$$= 2 : 1$$

Therefore, you can tell the patient that warfarin is approximately twice as likely to help him as to harm him, when compared with aspirin.

Incorporating his values that you elicited, the LHH becomes:

$$LHH = (1/NNT) \times (1 - Uevent) : (1/NNH) \times (1 - Utoxicity)$$

$$= (1/83) \times (1 - 0.2) : (1/125) \times (1 - 0.8)$$

$$= 8 : 1$$

And you can now inform the patient that warfarin is approximately eight times as likely to help him as to harm him.

Alternatively, a quicker way of incorporating the patient's values is to ask the patient to rate one event against another. For example, is the adverse effect about as severe as the event the treatment prevents—or 10 times as bad or only half as severe? This rating ("s") can then be used to adjust the LHH as:

$$LHH = (1/NNT) \times s : (1/NNH).$$

# CONCLUSION

Clinicians may find a rigorous approach to clinical decision making intimidating. Finding the best evidence can be difficult, and success in this endeavor may leave uncertainties. In considering atrial fibrillation for anticoagulation, for example, should clinicians accept the very low bleeding rates patients experienced while taking warfarin in the randomized trials, or should they pay attention to the higher rates from some observational studies?

Having ascertained the likely outcomes of the alternate courses of action, the clinician must either present patients with the options and outcomes and leave it for them to choose, try to discover the patient's values and having done so suggest a course of action to the patient (the paternalistic approach), or choose the middle course of shared decision making. The patient's preferred decision-making style will guide the clinician in this regard. However, communicating the nature of the outcomes and their probabilities in a way the patient will understand, or accurately ascertaining the patient's values regarding the outcomes, remains problematic.

The results of a survey of the 45 clinician members of the Evidence-Based Medicine Working Group suggest the preliminary nature of the formal approaches to incorporating patient values in clinical decision making. All of the clinician members report that they conduct only unstructured discussions to ascertain their patient's preferences. Fifteen (33%) sometimes obtain a quantitative rating of the patient's preferences, and eight (18%) sometimes use written scenarios to enhance the patient's understanding. Six (13%) sometimes use a rating scale or other formal method for obtaining relative values of different outcomes, and 11 (24%) sometimes use clinical decision aids.

The challenges of optimal clinical decision making should not obscure the realization that clinicians face these challenges in helping patients with every management decision. For each choice, clinicians guide patients with their best estimate of the likely outcomes. They then help patients balance these outcomes in making their ultimate decision. Finding better strategies to carry out these tasks remains a frontier for evidence-based medicine.

# References

1. Hankey GJ. Anticoagulants and antiaggregants prevent strokes in high-risk patients. *ACP Journal Club.* 1994;121:60. Comment on: American College of Physicians. Guidelines for medical treatment of stroke. *Ann Intern Med.* 1994;121:54-55; and Matchar DB, McCrory DC, Barnett HJ, Feussner JR. Medical treatment for stroke prevention. *Ann Intern Med.* 1994;121:41-53. [Revised: October 1999]

2. Gubitz G. Review: 6 clinical conditions can be modified to reduce risk for a first stroke. *ACP Journal Club.* 1999;131:30-31. Comment on: Gorelick PB, Sacco RL, Smith DB, et al. Prevention of a first stroke: a review of guidelines and a multidisciplinary consensus statement from the National Stroke Association. *JAMA.* 1999;281:1112-1120.

3. Laupacis A, Boysen G, Connolly S, et al. Risk factors for stroke and efficacy of antithrombotic therapy in atrial fibrillation: analysis of pooled data from five randomized controlled trials [published erratum appears in *Arch Intern Med.* 1994;154:2254]. *Arch Intern Med.* 1994;154:1449-1457.

4. Hart RG, Benavente O, McBride R, Pearce LA. Antithrombotic therapy to prevent stroke in patients with atrial fibrillation: a meta-analysis. *Ann Intern Med.* 1999;131:492-501.

5. Segal JB, McNamara RL, Miller MR, et al. Prevention of thromboembolism in atrial fibrillation: a meta-analysis of trials of anticoagulants and antiplatelet drugs. *J Gen Intern Med.* 2000;15:56-67.

6. Kalra L, Yu G, Perez I, Lakhani A, Donalson N. Prospective cohort study to determine if trial efficacy of anticoagulation for stroke prevention in atrial fibrillation translates into clinical effectiveness. *BMJ.* 2000;320:1236-1239.

7. Thomson R, Parkin D, Eccles M, Sudlow M, Robinson A. Decision analysis and guidelines for anticoagulant therapy to prevent stroke in patients with atrial fibrillation. *Lancet.* 2000;355:956-962.

8. Samsa GP, Matchar DB, Goldstein L, et al. Utilities for major stroke: results from a survey of preferences among persons at increased risk for stroke. *Am Heart J.* 1998;136:703-713.

9. Gordon K, MacSween J, Dooley J, Camfield C, Camfield P, Smith B. Families are content to discontinue antiepileptic drugs at different risks than their physicians. *Epilepsia.* 1996;37:557-562.

10. Man-Son-Hing M, Laupacis A, O'Connor A, et al. Warfarin for atrial fibrillation: the patient's perspective. *Arch Intern Med.* 1996;156:1841-1848.

11. Strull WM, Lo B, Charles G. Do patients want to participate in medical decision making? *JAMA.* 1984;252:2990-2994.

12. Degner LF, Kristjanson LJ, Bowman D, et al. Information needs and decisional preferences in women with breast cancer. *JAMA.* 1997;277:1485-1492.

13. Stiggelbout AM, Kiebert GM. A role for the sick role: patient preferences regarding information and participation in clinical decision-making. *CMAJ.* 1997;157:383-389.

14. Emanuel EJ, Emanuel LL. Four models of the physician-patient relationship. *JAMA.* 1992;267:2221-2226.

15. Szabo E, Moody H, Hamilton T, Ang C, Kovithavongs C, Kjellstrand C. Choice of treatment improves quality of life: a study of patients undergoing dialysis. *Arch Intern Med.* 1997;157:1352-1356.

16. Greenfield S, Kaplan SH, Ware JE Jr, Yano EM, Frank HJL. Patients' participation in medical care: effects on blood sugar control and quality of life in diabetes. *J Gen Intern Med.* 1988;3:448-457.

17. Kaplan SH, Greenfield S, Ware JE Jr. Assessing the effects of physician-patient interactions on the outcomes of chronic disease. *Med Care.* 1989;27:S110-S127.

18. Schulman BA. Active patient orientation and outcomes in hypertension treatment: application of a socio-organizational perspective. *Med Care.* 1979;17:267-280.

19. Stewart MA. Effective physician-patient communication and health outcomes: a review. *CMAJ.* 1995;152:1423-1433.

20. Arora NK, McHorney CA. Patient preferences for medical decision making: who really wants to participate? *Med Care.* 2000;38:335-341.

21. Rothenbacher D, Lutz MP, Porzsolt F. Treatment decisions in palliative cancer care: patients' preferences for involvement and doctors' knowledge about it. *Eur J Cancer.* 1997;33:1184-1189.

22. Mazur DJ, Hickam DH. Patients' preferences for risk disclosure and role in decision making for invasive medical procedures. *J Gen Intern Med.* 1997;12:114-117.

23. Margalith I, Shapiro A. Anxiety and patient participation in clinical decision-making: the case of patients with ureteral calculi. *Soc Sci Med.* 1997;45:419-427.

24. Levine MN, Gafni A, Markham B, MacFarlane D. A bedside decision instrument to elicit a patient's preference concerning adjuvant chemotherapy for breast cancer. *Ann Intern Med.* 1992;117:53-58.

25. O'Connor AM. Consumer/patient decision support in the new millennium: where should our research take us? *Can J Nurs Res.* 1997;29:7-19.

26. O'Connor AM, Rostom A, Fiset V, et al. Decision aids for patients facing health treatment or screening decisions: systematic review. *BMJ.* 1999;319:731-734.

27. Torrance GW. Measurement of health state utilities for economic appraisal: a review. *J Health Econ.* 1986;5:1-30.

28. Protheroe J, Fahey T, Montgomery AA, Peters TJ. The impact of patients' preferences on the treatment of atrial fibrillation: observational study of patient based decision analysis. *BMJ.* 2000;320:1380-1384.

29. Straus SE, McQuay HJM, Moore RA, Sackett DL. A proposed patient-centered method of delivering information about the risks and benefits of therapy: the likelihood of being helped versus harmed. *Evaluation and the Health Professions*. Submitted.

30. Man-Son-Hing M, Laupacis A, O'Connor AM, et al. A patient decision aid regarding antithrombotic therapy for stroke prevention in atrial fibrillation. *JAMA.* 1999;282:737-743.

31. Laupacis A, Man-Son-Hing M, O'Connor A, et al. *Presenting the Results of SPAF III: Implications for Participating Patients* [audiocassette]. Ottawa, ON: Loeb Health Research Institute; 1996.

# Moving From Evidence to Action

## Recommendations About Screening

Alexandra Barratt, Les Irwig, Paul Glasziou, Robert Cumming,
Angela Raffle, Nicholas Hicks, JA Muir Gray,
and Gordon Guyatt

Jeroen Lijmer also made substantive contributions to this section

## IN THIS SECTION

## CLINICAL SCENARIO

### Should a 47-Year-Old Couple Undergo Colon Cancer Screening?

**Y**ou are a primary care physician seeing a 47-year-old woman and her husband of the same age. They are concerned because a friend of theirs recently was told she had colon cancer and has urged them both to undergo screening with fecal occult blood tests (FOBT) because, she says, prevention is much better than the cure she is now undergoing.

Both of these patients have no family history of colon cancer and no change in bowel habit. They ask whether you agree that they should be screened. You know that trials of FOBT screening have demonstrated that screening can reduce mortality from colorectal cancer but you also recall that FOBTs can have a high false-positive rate, which then necessitates investigation by colonoscopy. You are unsure whether screening these relatively young, asymptomatic people at average risk of colon cancer is likely to do more good than harm. You decide to check the literature to see if there are any guidelines or recommendations about screening for colorectal cancer that might help you respond to their question.

# FINDING THE EVIDENCE

Since you know that there is more than one randomized trial related to the topic, you look first for a systematic review. You log on and use PubMed to search MEDLINE using the terms "colorectal neoplasms AND mass screening AND systematic review." Your search produces a systematic review by Towler et al in the *BMJ*.[1] However, since there may be ancillary evidence that would influence your decision about whether to recommend screening to the patients before you (such as the false-positive rate of the test, the side effects of subsequent investigation and treatment, and the associated costs), you also check for a clinical practice guideline. You find the American Gastroenterological Association (AGA) guideline, "Colorectal Cancer Screening: Clinical Guidelines and Rationale,"[2] which is based on the same trials as the systematic review and also provides the additional information you were hoping to find. The full text is provided, so you print a copy to take home and read tonight.

# THE CONSEQUENCES OF SCREENING

The best way to think about screening is as a therapeutic intervention. This clarifies the methodology required to support a policy of screening: randomized trials examining the effect of screening on patient-important outcomes.[3-6] In this section, we probe specific issues introduced earlier (see Part 1F, "Moving From Evidence to Action"), focusing on those that are specific to screening and placing them in the context of the framework developed in Part 1F, "Moving From Evidence to Action."

**TABLE 2F-2**

## Users' Guides for an Article About Screening

**Are the Recommendations Valid?**

- Is there randomized trial evidence that earlier intervention works?
- Were the data identified, selected, and combined in an unbiased fashion?

**What Are the Recommendations and Will They Help You in Caring for Patients?**

- What are the benefits?
- What are the risks?
- How do benefits and risks compare in different people and with different screening strategies?
- What is the impact of individuals' values and preferences?
- What is the impact of uncertainty associated with the evidence?
- What is the cost-effectiveness?

---

Table 2F-3 presents the possible consequences of screening. Some people will have true-positive results (a) with clinically significant disease ($a^0$); a proportion of this group will benefit according to the effectiveness of treatment and the severity of the detected disease. Taking an example from a specific screening program, children found to have phenylketonuria (PKU) will experience large, long-lasting benefits. Other people will have true-positive results with inconsequential disease ($a^1$): They may experience the consequences of labeling, investigation, and treatment for a disease or risk factor that otherwise never would have affected their lives. Consider, for instance, a man in whom screening reveals low-grade prostate cancer. This person will most likely die from a coronary artery disease before his prostate cancer becomes clinically manifest. Thus, he may be advised to undergo unnecessary treatment and may experience associated adverse effects.

People with false-positive results (b) may be adversely affected by the risks associated with investigation of the screen-detected abnormality. People with false-negative results of clinically important disease ($c^0$) may experience harm if false reassurance results in delayed presentation or investigation of symptoms; some also may be angry when they discover they have disease despite having negative screening test results. By contrast, patients with false-negative results with inconsequential disease (c¹) are not harmed by their "disease" being missed because it was never destined to affect them. Patients with true-negative results (d) may experience benefit associated with an accurate reassurance of being disease free, but they may also experience inconvenience, cost, and anxiety.

**TABLE 2F-3**

**Summary of Benefits and Risks of Screening by Underlying Disease State**

| | Reference Standard Results | | |
| --- | --- | --- | --- |
| | Disease or Risk Factor Present | | Disease or Risk Factor Absent |
| Screening test positive | $a^0$ true positives (significant disease) | $a^1$ true positives (inconsequential disease) | b false positives |
| Screening test negative | $c^0$ false negatives (significant disease) | $c^1$ false negatives (inconsequential disease) | d true negatives |

**Key:**

$a^0$  Disease or risk factor that will cause symptoms in the future (significant disease)

$a^1$  Disease or risk factor asymptomatic until death (inconsequential disease)

b   False-positive results

$c^0$  Missed disease that will be significant in the future

$c^1$  Missed disease that will be inconsequential in the future

d   True-negative results

Note: sensitivity = a/a+c and specificity = d/b+d.

The longer the gap between possible detection and clinically important consequences, the greater the number of people in the inconsequential disease category ($a^1$). When screening for risk factors, very large numbers of people need to be screened and treated to prevent one adverse event years later.[7] Thus, most people found to have a risk factor at screening will be treated for inconsequential disease.

# ARE THE RECOMMENDATIONS VALID?

## Is There Randomized Trial Evidence That Earlier Intervention Works?

Guidelines recommending screening are on strong ground if they are based on randomized controlled trials in which screening is compared to conventional care. In the past, many screening programs, some of them effective (such as cervical cancer screening and screening for PKU), have been implemented on the strength of observational data. When the benefits are enormous and the downsides are minimal, there is no need for randomized trials. More often, the benefits and risks from screening are balanced more evenly. In these situations, observational studies of screening may be misleading. Survival, as measured from the time of diagnosis, may be increased not because patients live longer, but because screening lengthens the time that they know they have disease (*lead-time bias*). Patients whose disease is discovered by screening also may appear to live longer because screening tends to detect slowly progressing disease, yet tends to miss rapidly progressive disease that becomes symptomatic between screening rounds (*length-time bias*). Therefore, unless the evidence of benefit is overwhelming, randomized trial assessment is required.

Investigators may choose one of two study designs to test the impact of a screening process. The trial may assess the entire screening process (early detection and early intervention; see Figure 2F-2A), in which case people are randomized either to be screened and treated if early abnormality is detected, or not screened (and treated only if symptomatic disease occurs). Trials of mammographic screening have utilized this design.[8-10]

**FIGURE 2F-2**

## Designs for Randomized Controlled Trials of Screening

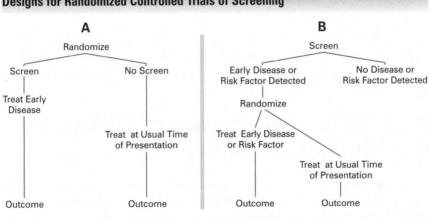

Alternatively, all participants may participate in screening and those with positive results are randomized to be treated or not treated (Figure 2F-2B). If those who receive treatment do better, then one can conclude that early treatment has provided some benefit. Investigators usually use this study design when screening detects not the disease itself, but factors that increase the risk of disease. Tests of screening programs for hypertension and high cholesterol have utilized this design.[11,12] The principles outlined in this section apply to both of the study designs (Figures 2F-2A and 2F-2B) used in addressing screening issues.

Regardless of which design is used (Figure 2F-2A or 2F-2B), a successful outcome of screening depends on optimal, or at least appropriate, application of testing and treatment that follows a positive screening test. One way investigators may deal with this issue is to include protocols for the investigative tests and therapies to be delivered if the target condition is detected. The limitation of this approach is that it may not simulate usual clinical practice, and thus may limit the applicability of the results. An alternative is to allow clinicians to manage patients as they ordinarily would, and to document the investigative tests and therapies they use. Without such monitoring, there is a risk that the clinical community will be unaware that the reason screening failed to improve outcome was because of suboptimal management of patients who had positive screening results.

### Were the Data Identified, Selected, and Combined in an Unbiased Fashion?

As is true for all guidelines, developers must specify the inclusion and exclusion criteria for the studies they choose to consider, conduct a comprehensive search, and assess the methodologic quality of the studies they include. The review by Towler et al[1] searched for published and unpublished trials and assessed their quality using criteria recommended by the Cochrane Collaboration.[13] The investigators extracted data from the trials and combined them in a meta-analysis on an intention-to-screen basis.

The AGA guideline[2] on colorectal screening used explicit inclusion and exclusion criteria and a comprehensive search to identify all the randomized trials of FOBT screening. The authors include a critical appraisal of the trials and conclude that they provide strong evidence of effectiveness, although their appraisal is limited in that they do not consider the effect of screening on health-related quality of life.

# What Are the Recommendations and Will They Help You in Caring for Patients?

A good guideline about a screening program should summarize the trial evidence about benefits and present data about the risks, for example, in a balance sheet.[14] The guideline should then provide information about how these benefits and risks can vary in subgroups of the population and under different screening strategies.

### What Are the Benefits?

What outcomes need to be measured to estimate the benefits of a screening program? Some of those who test positive will experience a reduction in mortality or an increase in quality of life. The benefit can be estimated as an absolute risk reduction (ARR) or a relative risk reduction (RRR) in adverse outcomes (see Part 2B2, "Therapy and Understanding the Results, Measures of Association"). Briefly, the ARR depends on the baseline risk of disease and thus presents a more realistic estimate of the size of the mortality benefit. By contrast, the RRR is independent of baseline risk and can lead to a misleading impression of benefit (see Table 2F-4). The number of people needed to screen to prevent an adverse outcome (NNS) provides another way of presenting benefit (see Part 2B2, "Therapy and Understanding the Results, Measures of Association").

**TABLE 2F-4**

## Comparison of Data Presented as Relative and Absolute Risk Reductions and Number Needed to Screen With Varying Baseline Risks of Disease and Constant Relative Risk

| Baseline Risk (Risk in Unscreened Group) | Risk in Screened Group | Relative Risk Reduction | Absolute Risk Reduction | Number Needed to Screen |
|---|---|---|---|---|
| 4% | 2% | 50% | 2% | 50 |
| 2% | 1% | 50% | 1% | 100 |
| 1% | 0.5% | 50% | 0.5% | 200 |
| 0.1% | 0.05% | 50% | 0.05% | 2000 |

When the benefit is a reduction in mortality, we would like to see a reduction in both disease-specific mortality and total mortality. However, because the target condition is typically only one of many causes of death, even important reductions in disease-specific mortality are unlikely to result in statistically significantly reductions in total mortality (that is, mortality due to any and all possible causes). In some conditions for which mortality is very high, it may be reasonable to expect a reduction in total mortality as well as in disease-specific mortality. An example is screening and treatment for high cholesterol among people who already have symptomatic heart disease. In this instance, the risk of death from heart disease is high and is by far the most likely cause of death; meta-analyses have shown significant effects on both disease-specific and total mortality.[15] For the most part, however, we will have to be satisfied with demonstrated reductions in disease-specific mortality only, although it is reassuring if data showing at least no increase in total mortality also are presented.

In addition to prevention of adverse outcomes, people may also regard knowledge of the presence of an abnormality as a benefit, as in antenatal screening for Down syndrome. Another potential benefit of screening comes from the reassurance afforded by a negative test, if a person is experiencing anxiety because a family member or friend has developed the target condition, or from discussion in the popular media. However, a person's self-perception as being "at risk" can be enhanced rather than reduced by being given a test. In instances in which anxiety is a result of the publicity surrounding the screening program itself, we would not view anxiety reduction as a benefit.

The AGA guideline[2] reports that the relative risk reductions from three trials of FOBT screening are, respectively, 33% (for annual screening) and 15% and 18%

(for biennial screening). An estimate of the uncertainty associated with these estimates (as one would get from the 95% confidence interval around a pooled relative risk reduction) would help the reader appreciate the range within which the true relative risk reduction plausibly lies. Based on a computer simulation, the AGA guideline for annual screening with FOBT estimates an absolute risk reduction of 1330 deaths prevented per 100,000 (13.3 per 1000) people ranging in age from 50 to 85 years of age, assuming 100% participation (Table 2F-5).

**TABLE 2F-5**

**Clinical Consequences for 1000 People Entering a Program of Annual FOBT Screening for CRC at Age 50 Years and Remaining in it Until Age 85 or Death***

| Adverse Consequences | Number of Events in 1000 People |
| --- | --- |
| Screening tests | 27,030 |
| Diagnostic evaluations (by colonoscopy) | 2263 |
| False-positive screening tests | 2158 |
| Deaths from colonoscopy complications | 0.5 |
| Bowel perforations from colonoscopy | 3.0 |
| Major bleeding episodes from colonoscopy | 7.4 |
| Minor complications from colonoscopy | 7.7 |
| **Benefits** | |
| Deaths averted | 13.3 |
| Years of life saved | 123.3 |
| Years of life gained per person whose cancer death was prevented | 9.3 |

\* Adapted from AGA guideline 1997.

## What Are the Risks?

Among those who test positive, adverse consequences may include:

- Complications arising from investigation
- Side effects of treatment
- Unnecessary treatment of persons having true-positive results with inconsequential disease
- Adverse effects of labeling or early diagnosis
- Anxiety generated by the investigations and treatment
- Costs and inconvenience incurred during investigations and treatment

The AGA guideline[2] reports that of the patients who do not have colorectal cancer, 8% to 10% will have false-positive test results (specificity, 90%-92% using rehydrated slides). In the trials, only 2% to 6% of those who tested positive actually had colon cancer (positive predictive value of 2%-6%). Thus, of every 100 screening participants with a positive test, only two to six will have cancer, but all 100 will be exposed to colonoscopy and its attendant risks (Table 2F-5). Although the colonoscopies will reveal few cancers, they will show many polyps (25% of people aged 50 years or older have polyps, some of which will be judged to need removal, depending on the size of the polyp). Part of the benefit of screening will come from removal of the small proportion of polyps that would have progressed to invasive cancer. Part of the risk of screening will come from regular colono-scopies that are recommended for people who have had a benign or inconsequen-tial polyp removed.

Among those who test negative, adverse consequences may include:

- Anxiety generated by the screening test (waiting for result)

- False reassurance (and delayed presentation of symptomatic disease later)

- Costs and inconvenience incurred during the screening test

Of those who have cancer, FOBT screening using rehydrated slides will cor-rectly identify 90% and will miss the other 10% (sensitivity of 90%), according to the AGA guideline.[2] Those who present with symptoms after a false-negative result may experience a sense of anger and betrayal that they would not suffer in the absence of a screening program.

Using computer simulation, the AGA guideline presents data on the frequency of some of these risks. Table 2F-5 summarizes data for 1000 people from 50 to 85 years of age participating in annual screening by FOBT. The model assumes those who test positive undergo colonoscopy.

We now know the magnitude of both benefits and risks (as presented in Table 2F-5). This balance sheet tells us that screening 1000 people annually with FOBT from age 50 years will prevent 13.3 deaths from colorectal cancer but will cause 0.5 death from the complications of investigation and surgery. There will also be 10.4 major complications (perforations and major bleeding episodes) and 7.7 minor complications. The authors provide no data on anxiety, but we could assume that some people will feel anxious prior to colonoscopy. Figure 2F-3 presents these data as a flow diagram.

**FIGURE 2F-3**

## Clinical Consequences for 1000 People in a Program of Annual Fecal Occult Blood Tests Screening for Colorectal Cancer

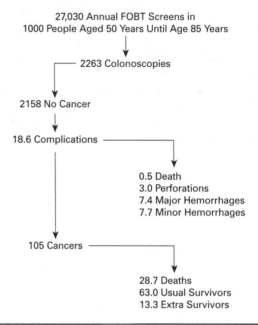

FOBT indicates fecal occult blood tests; CRC indicates colorectal cancer.

Adapted and reproduced with permission from the WB Saunders Company.

These data assume that the screening programs will deliver the same magnitude of benefit and risks as found in randomized controlled trials; this will be true only if the program is delivered to the same standard of quality as that in the trials. Otherwise, benefits will be smaller and the risks will be greater.

## How Do Benefits and Risks Compare in Different People and With Different Screening Strategies?

The AGA guideline[2] recommends that people at average risk and over 50 years of age be offered screening for colorectal cancer. The guideline discusses several screening strategies (FOBT, flexible sigmoidoscopy, barium enema, and colonoscopy) and, in relation to FOBT, recommends offering annual screening. The magnitude of benefits and adverse consequences will vary in different patients and with different screening strategies, as the following discussion reveals.

### Risk of Disease

Assuming that the relative risk reduction is constant over a broad range of risk of disease, benefits will be greater for people at higher risk of disease. For example, mortality from colorectal cancer rises with age and the mortality benefit achieved by screening rises accordingly (Figure 2F-4A). But the life-years lost to colorectal cancer are related to both the age at which mortality is highest and the length of life still available. Thus, the number of life-years that can be saved by colorectal cancer screening increases with age to about 75 years and then decreases again as life expectancy declines (Figure 2F-4B). The number of deaths averted by screening over 10 years for those aged 40, 50, and 60 years at first screening (0.2, 1.0, and 2.4 per 1000 people, respectively[1]) reflects these differences. Because of a greater benefit, it may be rational for a person aged 60 years to decide screening is worthwhile, whereas a person aged 40 years (or 80 years) with smaller potential benefit might decide it is not worthwhile.

**FIGURE 2F-4**

## Mortality and Years of Life Lost According to Age

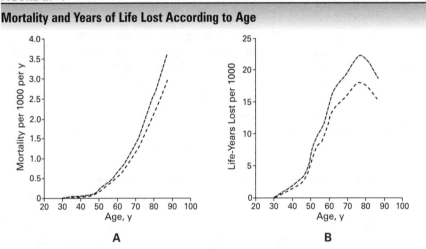

**A**, Mortality in populations participating (with) and not participating (without) in colorectal cancer screening. **B**, Years of life lost in populations participating (with) and not participating (without) in colorectal cancer screening.

Reproduced with permission from the BMJ Publishing Group.

Risk of disease—and, therefore benefits from screening—may be increased by such other factors as a family history. The AGA guideline[2] reports that people with one or more first-degree relatives (parent, sibling, child) with colorectal cancer, but without one of the specific genetic syndromes, have approximately twice the risk of developing colorectal cancer as average-risk individuals without a family history. This means that for people aged 40 years who have a first-degree relative with colorectal cancer, the incidence of colorectal cancer is comparable to that for people aged 50 years without a family history. The guideline also notes that within each age group, the risk is greatest in those whose relatives developed cancer at a younger age.

### Screening Interval
As the screening interval is shortened, the effectiveness of a screening program will tend to improve, although there is a limit to the amount of improvement that is possible. For example, screening twice as often could theoretically double the

relative mortality reduction obtainable by screening, but in practice the effect is usually much less. Cervical cancer screening, for instance, may reduce the incidence of invasive cervical cancer by 64%, 84%, and 94% if screening is conducted at 10-year, 5-year, and 1-year intervals, respectively.[16]

The frequency of risks also will increase with more frequent screening, potentially directly in proportion to the frequency of screening. Thus, we will see diminishing marginal return as the screening interval is shortened. Ultimately, the marginal risks will outweigh the marginal benefit of further reductions in the screening interval.

### Test Characteristics

If the sensitivity of a new test is greater than the test used in the trials and if it is detecting significant disease earlier, the benefit of screening will increase. But it may be that the new, apparently more sensitive, test is detecting more cases of inconsequential disease (eg, by detecting more low-grade prostate cancers or more low-grade cervical epithelial abnormalities[17]), which will increase the potential for risk. On the other hand, if specificity is improved and testing produces fewer false-positive results, net benefit will increase and the test may now be useful in groups in which the old test was not as useful.

Ideally, clinicians would look to randomized trials of the new test compared to the old test. However, new tests often appear in profusion, and randomized trials are expensive and often are interpretable only after long follow-up. Being pragmatic, we will usually need to accept that if the trials have shown that earlier detection reduces the risk of adverse effects, then a comparison of a new vs an old test only needs to examine test characteristics.

Returning to colorectal cancer screening, since we have randomized trial data of mortality reduction after early detection by FOBT, we may assume that early detection works in principle. It therefore seems reasonable to assume that early detection using other methods, such as flexible sigmoidoscopy, will also reduce mortality from colorectal cancer even though there are no published reports of randomized trials of screening with flexible sigmoidoscopy. This theoretical approach is supported by the available observational data, which do indicate benefit from other methods of screening for colorectal cancer.[2]

## What Is the Impact of Values and Preferences?

The way and extent to which people value the benefits and risk of screening can vary. For example, pregnant women who are considering fetal screening for Down syndrome may make different choices depending on the value they place on having a child with Down syndrome vs the risk of iatrogenic abortion from amniocentesis.[18]

Perception plays a large role. Individuals who choose to participate in screening programs are benefiting (in their view) from screening and other individuals are benefiting (in their view) from not participating. Individuals can make the right choice for themselves only if they have access to high-quality information about the benefits and risks of screening and if they are able to weigh that information. This probably will require much better educational materials and decision-support materials than traditionally have been provided; some examples are already available.[19, 20]

## What Is the Impact of Uncertainty Associated With the Evidence?

There is always uncertainty about the benefits and risks of screening. The 95% confidence interval around the magnitude of each benefit and adverse consequence provides an indication of the amount of uncertainty in each estimate. When sample size is limited, the confidence intervals will be wide and clinicians should alert potential screening participants that the magnitude of the benefit or risk could be considerably smaller or greater than the point estimate.

## What Is the Cost-effectiveness?

Although clinicians will be most interested in the balance of benefits and risks for individual patients, policymakers must consider issues of cost-effectiveness and local resources in their decisions (see Part 2F, "Moving From Evidence to Action, Economic Analysis").

The AGA guideline[2] reports the estimated cost-effectiveness of FOBT screening is approximately $10,000 per life-year gained among people over 50 years of age (although, like the absolute size of the benefit, it will vary with risk of disease). The AGA guideline also notes that all CRC screening strategies examined (FOBT, flexible sigmoidoscopy, barium enema, and colonoscopy) cost less than $20,000 per life-year saved.

These cost-effectiveness ratios are within the range of what is currently paid in some countries for the benefits of other screening programs such as mammographic screening for women aged 50 to 69 years (estimated at $21,400 per life year saved[21]), ultrasound screening for patients with carotid stenosis (incremental cost per quality-adjusted life-year [QALY] gained is estimated at $39,495[22]), and ultrasound screening for abdominal aortic aneurysm in men aged 60 to 80 years (estimated $41,550 per life-year gained[23]).

# CLINICAL RESOLUTION

A clinical practice guideline that addresses a question of screening should quantify the benefit of screening according to age so that you can inform patients as accurately as possible about the benefits of screening for them. The AGA guideline does not provide age-specific mortality reductions attributable to screening; therefore, you cannot easily quantify the benefit for patients in your practice. From the AGA guideline, all you can say with confidence is that screening a group of 1000 people with FOBT beginning at age 50 and continuing annually to age 85 will avert about 13 deaths from CRC. However, we know from the Towler et al systematic review[1] that the mortality benefit for people between 40 and 50 years of age is about 0.2 to1.0 deaths averted over 10 years per 1000 people screened. Next, you could outline the potential risks of screening. As noted earlier, adverse consequences are related primarily to colonoscopy. According to the AGA guideline, the risks of colonoscopy are about 0.1 to 0.3 per 1000 for death and one to three per 1000 for perforation and hemorrhage. In addition, there would also be issues of cost, inconvenience, and anxiety.

Returning to our opening clinical scenario, it is up to the patients before you to weigh whether the benefit of reduced risk of death from colorectal cancer is worth the potential adverse consequences including the inconvenience of colonoscopy and the complications arising from colonoscopy, the adverse effects of early treatment for colon cancer, side effects of treatment, and the anxiety generated by the investigations and treatment.

If they feel that they are unable to do this, then you could consider helping them to clarify their values about the possible outcomes. For example, if they are not bothered by the prospect of a colonoscopy, they would probably choose to be screened. But if either of them places a high value on avoiding colonoscopy now, he or she may prefer to reconsider screening in a few years, when the benefits will be greater than they are now.

# References

1. Towler B, Irwig L, Glasziou P, Kewenter J, Weller D, Silagy C. A systematic review of the effects of screening for colorectal cancer using the faecal occult blood test, hemoccult. *BMJ.* 1998;317:559-565.

2. Winawer SJ, Fletcher RH, Miller L, et al. Colorectal cancer screening: clinical guidelines and rationale. *Gastroenterology.* 1997;112:594-642.

3. Wilson JMG, Jungner G. *Principles and Practice of Screening for Disease.* Geneva: World Health Organization; 1968.

4. Gray JA. *Evidence-Based Healthcare.* London: Churchill Livingstone; 1997.

5. Sackett DL, Haynes RB, Tugwell P. *Clinical Epidemiology: A Basic Science for Clinical Medicine.* 2nd ed. Boston: Little, Brown; 1991.

6. Welch HG, Black WC. Evaluating randomized trials of screening. *J Gen Intern Med.* 1997;12:118-124.

7. Khaw KT, Rose G. Cholesterol screening programmes: how much potential benefit? *BMJ.* 1989;299:606-607.

8. Andersson I, Aspegren K, Janzon L, et al. Mammographic screening and mortality from breast cancer: the Malmo mammographic screening trial. *BMJ.* 1988;297:943-948.

9. Tabar L, Fagerberg G, Duffy SW, Day NE. The Swedish two county trial of mammographic screening for breast cancer: recent results and calculation of benefit. *J Epidemiol Community Health*. 1989;43:107-114.

10. Roberts MM, Alexander FE, Anderson TJ, et al. Edinburgh trial of screening for breast cancer: mortality at seven years. *Lancet*. 1990;335:241-246.

11. Multiple Risk Factor Intervention Trial Research Group. Multiple risk factor intervention trial: risk factor changes and mortality results. *JAMA*. 1982;248:1465-1477.

12. Frick MH, Elo O, Haapa K, et al. Helsinki Heart Study: primary-prevention trial with gemfibrozil in middle-aged men with dyslipidemia. Safety of treatment, changes in risk factors, and incidence of coronary heart disease. *N Engl J Med*. 1987;317:1237-1245.

13. Mulrow CD, Oxman AD, eds. Critical Appraisal of Studies. Cochrane Collaboration Handbook (updated September 1997); section 4. In: *The Cochrane Library* (database on disk and CD-ROM). The Cochrane Collaboration. Oxford: Update Software; 1997, issue 4.

14. Eddy DM. Comparing benefits and harms: the balance sheet. *JAMA*. 1990;263:2493, 2498, 2501, 2505.

15. Barratt A, Irwig L. Is cholesterol testing/treatment really beneficial? *Med J Aust*. 1993;159:644-647.

16. IARC Working Group on Evaluation of Cervical Cancer Screening Programmes. Screening for squamous cervical cancer: duration of low risk after negative results of cervical cytology and its implication for screening policies. *Br Med J Clin Res Ed*. 1986;293:659-664.

17. Raffle AE. New tests in cervical screening. *Lancet*. 1998;351:297.

18. Fletcher J, Hicks NR, Kay JD, Boyd PA. Using decision analysis to compare policies for antenatal screening for Down's syndrome. *BMJ*. 1995;311:351-356.

19. Wolf AM, Nasser JF, Wolf AM, Schorling JB. The impact of informed consent on patient interest in prostate-specific antigen screening. *Arch Intern Med*. 1996;156:1333-1336.

20. Flood AB, Wennberg JE, Nease RF Jr, Fowler FJ Jr, Ding J, Hynes LM, for the Prostate Patient Outcomes Research Team. The importance of patient preference in the decision to screen for prostate cancer. *J Gen Intern Med*. 1996;11:342-349.

21. Salzmann P, Kerlikowske K, Phillips K. Cost-effectiveness of extending screening mammography guidelines to include women 40 to 49 years of age. *Ann Intern Med*. 1997;127:955-965.

22. Yin D, Carpenter JP. Cost-effectiveness of screening for asymptomatic carotid stenosis. *J Vasc Surg*. 1998;27:245-255.

23. Frame PS, Fryback DG, Patterson C. Screening for abdominal aortic aneurysm in men ages 60 to 80 years: a cost-effectiveness analysis. *Ann Intern Med*. 1993;119:411-416.

# MOVING FROM EVIDENCE TO ACTION

Grading Recommendations—
A Qualitative Approach

Gordon Guyatt, Jack Sinclair, Deborah Cook,
Roman Jaeschke, Holger Schünemann, and Stephen Pauker

Hui Lee also made substantive contributions to this section

## IN THIS SECTION

Treatment decisions involve a trade-off between likely benefits on the one hand, and risks and costs on the other hand. To integrate these recommendations with their own clinical judgment, clinicians need to understand the basis for the clinical recommendations that experts offer them. A systematic approach to grading the strength of treatment recommendations can minimize bias and aid interpretation.

The formulation we use for establishing grades of recommendation focuses on two aspects of recommendations (Table 2F-6). The first is the degree of uncertainty in the balance between benefits of a treatment on the one hand, and risks, harms, or costs on the other. If benefits outweigh risks, negative consequences, and costs, experts will recommend that clinicians offer a treatment to typical patients. The uncertainty associated with the trade-off between benefits and risks will determine the strength of recommendations. If experts are very certain that benefits do—or do not—outweigh risks, they will make a strong recommendation (in our formulation, grade 1). If they are less certain of the magnitude of the benefits and risks and, thus, of their relative impact, they must make a weaker (grade 2) recommendation.

A second factor in grading recommendations is the methodologic quality of the underlying evidence. Randomized trials with consistent results provide unbiased, grade A recommendations. Randomized trials with inconsistent results or with major methodologic weaknesses warrant grade B recommendations. Grade C recommendations come from observational studies and from generalizations from randomized trials in one group of patients to a different group of patients. When experts find the generalization from randomized trials secure or the data from observational studies overwhelmingly compelling, they choose a C+ grade. In other instances, they choose grade C.

The remainder of this section describes the basis of the grading system in more detail. We begin by describing how methodologically strong studies can yield stronger or weaker recommendations depending on the trade-off between risks and benefits.

# HOW METHODOLOGIC QUALITY AND RISK/BENEFIT CONTRIBUTE TO GRADES OF RECOMMENDATIONS

Magnitude of benefit from treatment will have a major impact on treatment recommendations. For instance, consistent results from high-quality randomized trials suggest that both aspirin and thrombolytic agents reduce the relative risk of death after myocardial infarction by approximately 25%. Depending on their age and factors such as the presence of heart failure, typical patients with myocardial infarction face risks of death in the first 30 days after infarction of between 2% and 40%.[1] We can therefore expect a 0.5% absolute reduction in risk (from 2% to 1.5%) in the lowest-risk patients and a 10% reduction (from 40% to 30%) in the highest-risk ones. Aspirin has minimal side effects and very low cost. Thrombolytic agents seldom result in catastrophic bleeding, and streptokinase is

**TABLE 2F-6**

## Current Approach to Grades of Recommendations

| Grade of Recommendation | Clarity of Risk/Benefit | Methodologic Strength of Supporting Evidence | Implications |
|---|---|---|---|
| 1 A | Clear | Randomized trials without important limitations | Strong recommendation; can apply to most patients in most circumstances without reservation |
| 1 B | Clear | Randomized trials with important limitations (inconsistent results, nonfatal methodologic flaws) | Strong recommendation; likely to apply to most patients |
| 1 C+ | Clear | No randomized trials for this specific patient or patient population, but results from randomized trial(s) including different patients can be unequivocally extrapolated to the patient under current consideration; or overwhelming evidence from observational studies is available | Strong recommendation; can apply to most patients in most circumstances |
| 1 C | Clear | Observational studies | Intermediate-strength recommendation; may change when stronger evidence is available |
| 2 A | Unclear | Randomized trials without important limitations | Intermediate-strength recommendation; best action may differ depending on circumstances or patients' or societal values |
| 2 B | Unclear | Randomized trials with important limitations (inconsistent results, methodologic flaws) | Weak recommendation; alternative approaches likely to be better for some patients under some circumstances |
| 2 C | Unclear | Observational studies | Very weak recommendation; other alternatives may be equally reasonable |

only moderately costly. Because, even in the lowest-risk subgroups, the benefits clearly outweigh the risks, adverse consequences, and costs, administration of both aspirin and a thrombolytic agent are strongly endorsed and widely practiced. In our system of grading recommendations (Table 2F-6), both recommendations would fall within the category of grade 1A (1 because the benefits clearly outweigh the risks, A because the estimate of benefit comes from high-quality, randomized trials that yielded consistent results).

Consider two other treatment choices: whether to administer streptokinase or tissue plasminogen activator (tPA) for thrombolysis in myocardial infarction (MI); and whether to offer clopidogrel or aspirin to patients with recent ischemic stroke. Again, evidence regarding both decisions comes from high-quality RCTs and, with respect to methodologic rigor of the evidence, any recommendations will be strong. The magnitude of the relative risk reduction in mortality with tPA over streptokinase is approximately 12%.[2] (The baseline risk is 25% lower because the comparison is with patients already receiving thrombolytic therapy, corresponding to absolute risk reductions of approximately 0.4% and 3.6% in low- and high-risk patients, respectively.) However, tPA is associated with a greater risk of hemorrhagic stroke than is streptokinase, along with a substantially greater cost. Here, because it is less clear that benefits outweigh risks, adverse consequences, and costs, the recommendation cannot be as strong. The result is differing recommendations and variable practice; in general, tPA is preferred over streptokinase in the United States, whereas European physicians administer streptokinase more frequently than tPA. Recommendations regarding tPA vs streptokinase therefore would fall within the category of grade 2A.

Our best estimate, from a large and rigorous randomized trial, is that clopidogrel reduces the relative risk of subsequent stroke in patients with recent ischemic stroke by approximately 9% relative to aspirin.[3] In a patient with a 10% risk of stroke during the next year, this 9% relative risk reduction corresponds to an absolute risk reduction of approximately 1%. However, clopidogrel is far more costly than aspirin and, in contrast to thrombolytic agents, must be administered over a long period of time. Thus, despite the reduction in stroke with clopidogrel, most clinicians continue to offer aspirin as the initial treatment of patients at high risk of ischemic cerebrovascular events. Any recommendation, whether for clopidogrel or aspirin, would be associated with a grade of 2A (grade 2 because the balance between risks and benefits is not clear, A because the estimate of benefit comes from a rigorous randomized controlled trial).

Situations may even arise in which randomized trials demonstrate that treatment is beneficial but, at least in some subgroups of patients, experts may adduce strong recommendations not to treat. For instance, histamine-2-receptor antagonists, as demonstrated in a systematic review of randomized trials, reduce the relative risk of serious bleeding in critically ill patients by approximately 58%.[4] However, a spontaneously breathing patient without a coagulopathy has a risk of serious bleeding of only 0.14% without treatment.[5] This baseline risk is so low that most clinicians would not consider it worth treating to lower the relative risk by another 58% (to 0.06%)—a number needed to treat (NNT) of 1250 (see Part 2B2,

"Therapy and Understanding the Results, Measures of Association"). Depending on one's values, the recommendation not to treat could be considered to fall within the category of either grade 1A or grade 2A.

These examples illustrate how our treatment decisions depend not only on the strength of the methods, but also on the balance between benefits and downsides of treatment, including risks and costs—and on our confidence in that balance.[6,7] Depending on the balance between benefits and risks, methodologically strong studies suggesting a benefit of one agent over a placebo or another agent may lead to varying recommendations. When side effects are minimal or the patient's risk of the target event that that treatment will prevent is very high, investigators may make a strong recommendation to administer the more effective agent. When benefits and risks are closely balanced, we may see conflicting recommendations and practice. When risk reductions are small and toxicity is high, investigators may even recommend the less effective agent, or recommend not to treat at all. As the magnitude of the benefit and the magnitude of the risk become more closely balanced, decisions about administration of effective therapy also become more cost sensitive.

# THE GRADES OF RECOMMENDATIONS

## Validity, Consistency, and Generalization of Results

Investigators making treatment recommendations must consider the best estimate of the treatment effect. A rigorous systematic review will yield the strongest evidence, and a meta-analysis pooling data across trials is often appropriate for arriving at the best single estimate of the treatment effect (see Part 1E, "Summarizing the Evidence").

The decision to pool data is never completely straightforward and occasionally is fraught with controversy. For instance, on the basis of a meta-analysis of three randomized trials comparing the thrombolytic agents streptokinase and tPA, Collins and colleagues[8] have concluded that streptokinase and tPA are virtually identical in efficacy. On the other hand, tPA proponents point out that tPA administration may have been suboptimal in two of the three trials. The tPA proponents thus choose to focus on the results from GUSTO 1[2] that suggested the 12% relative risk reduction that we have noted above. Regardless of the decision regarding the best estimate, it should flow from a careful consideration of all data obtained from a systematic review of available results.

Investigators will make their strongest recommendations when their systematic review reveals one or more RCTs yielding consistent results (grade A evidence, as described in Table 2F-6). When several RCTs yield widely differing estimates of treatment effect for which there is no explanation (we label this situation "heterogeneity present"), the strength of recommendations from even rigorous RCTs is weaker (grade B evidence, as described in Table 2F-6). For example, studies examining serum ferritin as a diagnostic test for iron deficiency have shown conflicting results that so far defy definitive explanation.[9] Randomized trials of nitrate administration after myocardial infarction have shown similar variability in results.[10] In both of these examples, we must acknowledge the heterogeneity of results across studies. In doing so, any recommendation would descend from grade A to grade B.

Our confidence in recommendations also decreases if the available studies are flawed by major methodologic deficiencies that are likely to result in a biased assessment of the treatment effect. These severe methodologic limitations, which include a very large loss to follow-up, or an unblinded study with subjective outcomes highly susceptible to bias, lead us to classify studies as grade B.

Recommendations based on observational studies are weaker than those from RCTs, regardless of whether or not heterogeneity is present (grade C, as described in Table 2F-6). Grade C recommendations also include those in which we extrapolate from randomized trials involving one group of patients to a different group of patients, or to similar patients under different circumstances. For example, a recommendation for the use of spironolactone in patients with mild heart failure, when the only randomized trial has shown a mortality reduction in severe heart failure patients, might be considered a grade C recommendation (see Part 1B1, "Therapy").

Our grading scheme also includes a provision for situations in which experts are extremely confident about generalization from RCTs, or situations in which an extremely large treatment effect is shown from observational studies in which there is no apparent source of bias. For example, oral anticoagulation in patients with mechanical heart valves has not been compared to placebo in a randomized controlled trial. However, evidence from observational studies suggests that the risk of suffering thromboembolic events without anticoagulation is 12.3% annually in bileaflet aortic valves and higher for other valve types,[11] and that the pooled estimate of the relative risk reduction with oral anticoagulation is 80% (95% CI, 63%-90%). Although the observational studies are likely to overestimate the true effect, study design is very unlikely to explain the entire benefit. Thus, experts might reasonably offer a grade 1C+ recommendation for the use of oral anticoagulation in patients with mechanical heart valves (see Table 2F-6).

Similarly, investigators have not conducted randomized trials in patients with atrial fibrillation and mitral valve disease. However, RCTs show a very large (68%) and precise (95% confidence interval, 50%-79%) reduction in relative risk with warfarin in patients with nonvalvular atrial fibrillation.[12] Furthermore, the risk of embolism in mitral stenosis and atrial fibrillation is high, and the biologic mechanisms of action of embolism and of warfarin in mitral stenosis are very similar in patients with atrial fibrillation with and without mitral stenosis. Therefore, experts should classify a recommendation for use of warfarin therapy in patients with mitral stenosis and atrial fibrillation as grade 1C+.

## Evaluating the Trade-Off Between Benefits and Risks— A Qualitative Approach

When randomized trials provide precise estimates suggesting large treatment effects, and when risks and costs of therapy are small, we can confidently recommend treatment for average patients with compatible values and preferences. We have noted the examples of aspirin and thrombolysis for myocardial infarction. Another example is the prophylaxis of deep venous thrombosis after hip fracture surgery, in which heparin or low-intensity oral anticoagulation reduces the risk of deep venous thrombosis by approximately 50%.[7] Here, because sample sizes of the studies are relatively large and confidence intervals are narrow, and because prophylaxis is associated with low costs and complications, benefits clearly outweigh the downsides of therapy and the recommendation is strong (grade 1, as described in Table 2F-6).

If the balance between benefits and risks is uncertain, we may have methodologically rigorous studies providing grade A evidence and recommendations may still be weak (grade 2). Uncertainty may come from less precise estimates of benefit, harm, or costs, or from small effect sizes. We have cited examples of the use of tPA vs streptokinase in patients after myocardial infarction and the use of clopidogrel in comparison to aspirin in patients with recent ischemic stroke. Grade B or C evidence is unlikely to provide accurate, precise estimates of the balance between benefits and risks. Therefore, the recommendation in these two categories will often be grade 2.

Use of heparin after myocardial infarction in patients receiving thrombolytic and aspirin therapy provides another example. A systematic review of randomized trials suggests that in 1000 patients with infarction treated with heparin, five fewer will die, three fewer will have reinfarction, and one fewer will have a pulmonary embolus, while three more will have major bleeding episodes.[13] Further, these estimates are not precise, and beneficial effects may not persist for as long as 6 months. The small and possibly transient benefits, with relatively imprecise estimate, leave us less confident about any recommendation. Hence, the recommendation is likely to be grade 2A.

In situations in which there is doubt about the value of the trade-off, any recommendation will be weaker, moving from grade 1 to grade 2 (see Table 2F-6).

We will be able to make grade 1 recommendations only when we have precise estimates of both benefit and harm, and when the balance between the two clearly favors recommending—or not recommending—the intervention for the average patient with compatible values and preferences. Table 2F-7 summarizes how a number of factors can reduce the strength of a recommendation, moving it from grade 1 to grade 2.

Uncertainty about a recommendation to treat may be introduced if the target event we are preventing is less important (for example, we are more likely to be confident of recommendations to prevent death or stroke than asymptomatic deep venous thrombosis); if the magnitude of risk reduction in the overall group is small; if the risk is low in a particular subgroup of patients; if the estimate of the treatment effect, reflected in a wide confidence interval around the effect, is imprecise; if there is substantial potential harm associated with therapy; or if we expect a wide divergence in values even among average or typical patients. Higher costs would also lead to weaker recommendations to treat.

**TABLE 2F-7**

## Factors That May Weaken a Recommendation to Treat, Changing From Grade 1 to Grade 2

| Issue | Example |
|---|---|
| Less serious outcome | Preventing postphlebitic syndrome with thrombolytic therapy in DVT is less compelling than preventing death from pulmonary embolism |
| Smaller treatment effect | Clopidogrel vs aspirin leads to a smaller stroke reduction in TIA (8.7% RRR) than anticoagulation vs placebo in AF (68% RRR) |
| Imprecise estimate of treatment effect | Aspirin vs placebo in patients with atrial fibrillation has a wider confidence interval than aspirin for stroke prevention in patients with TIA |
| Lower risk of target event | Some surgical patients are at very low risk of postoperative DVT and pulmonary embolism, while other surgical patients have considerably higher rates of DVT and pulmonary embolism |
| Higher risk of therapy | Warfarin has a much higher risk of serious hemorrhage than aspirin |
| Higher costs | TPA has much higher cost than streptokinase in acute myocardial infarction |
| Varying values | Most young, healthy people will put a high value on prolonging their lives (and thus incur suffering to do so); the elderly and infirm are likely to vary in the value they place on prolonging their lives (and may vary in the suffering they are ready to experience to do so) |

DVT indicates deep vein thrombosis; TIA, transient ischemic attack; RRR, relative risk reduction; AF, atrial fibrillation; TPA, tissue plasminogen activator.

The more balanced the trade-off between benefits and risks, the greater is the influence of individual patient values in decision making. If they understand the benefits and risks, virtually all patients will take aspirin after myocardial infarction—or comply with prophylaxis to reduce thromboembolism after hip replacement. Thus, one way of thinking about a grade 1 recommendation is that variability in patient values or individual physician values is unlikely to influence treatment choice in average or typical patients.

When the trade-off between benefits and risks is less clear, clinicians will want to take special time and effort in ensuring that individual patient values bear strongly on the final decision (see Part 2F, "Moving From Evidence to Action, Incorporating Patient Values"). For example, patients who place a very high value on avoiding a disabling stroke might be more likely to choose streptokinase over tPA than those who do not have that priority. In considering the duration of anticoagulation after an episode of idiopathic deep venous thrombosis, patients may make different choices depending on the relative value they place on avoiding a fatal pulmonary embolus, on avoiding bleeding, and on the inconvenience and worry associated with repeated testing to determine the intensity of anticoagulation. Grade 2 recommendations are those in which variation in patient values or individual physician values will often mandate different treatment choices, even among average or typical patients.

# References

1. Stevenson R, Ranjadayalan K, Wilkinson P, Roberts R, Timmis AD. Short and long term prognosis of acute myocardial infarction since introduction of thrombolysis. *BMJ.* 1993;307:349-353.

2. The GUSTO Investigators. An international randomized trial comparing four thrombolytic strategies for acute myocardial infarction. *N Engl J Med.* 1993;329:673-682.

3. CAPRIE Steering Committee. A randomised, blinded, trial of clopidogrel versus aspirin in patients at risk of ischaemic events (CAPRIE). *Lancet.* 1996;348: 1329-1339.

4. Cook DJ, Reeve BK, Guyatt GH, et al. Stress ulcer prophylaxis in critically ill patients: resolving discordant meta-analyses. *JAMA.* 1996;275:308-314.

5. Cook DJ, Fuller HD, Guyatt GH, et al, for the Canadian Critical Care Trials Group. Risk factors for gastrointestinal bleeding in critically ill patients. *N Engl J Med.* 1994;330:377-381.

6. Guyatt GH, Sackett DL, Sinclair JC, Hayward R, Cook DJ, Cook RJ, for the Evidence-Based Medicine Working Group. Users' guides to the medical literature, IX: a method for grading health care recommendations. *JAMA.* 1995;274:1800-1804.

7. Guyatt GH, Sinclair J, Cook DJ, Glasziou P, for the Evidence-Based Medicine Working Group and the Cochrane Applicability Methods Working Group. Users' guides to the medical literature, XVI: how to use a treatment recommendation. *JAMA.* 1999;281:1836-1843.

8. Collins R, Peto R, Baigent C, Sleight P. Aspirin, heparin, and fibrinolytic therapy in suspected acute myocardial infarction. *N Engl J Med.* 1997;336:847-860.

9. Guyatt GH, Oxman AD, Ali M, Willan A, McIlroy W, Patterson C. Laboratory diagnosis of iron-deficiency anemia: an overview. *J Gen Intern Med.* 1992;7:145-153.

10. Cairns JA, Kennedy JW, Fuster V. Coronary thrombolysis. *Chest.* 1998;114(suppl 5):634S-657S.

11. Stein PD, Alpert JS, Dalen JE, Horstkotte D, Turpie AG. Antithrombotic therapy in patients with mechanical and biological prosthetic heart valves. *Chest.* 1998;114(suppl 5):602S-610S.

12. Risk factors for stroke and efficacy of antithrombotic therapy in atrial fibrillation: analysis of pooled data from five randomized controlled trials. *Arch Intern Med*. 1994;154:1449-1457.

13. Collins R, MacMahon S, Flather M, et al. Clinical effects of anticoagulant therapy in suspected acute myocardial infarction: systematic overview of randomised trials. *BMJ*. 1996;313:652-659.

# MOVING FROM EVIDENCE TO ACTION

## Grading Recommendations— A Quantitative Approach

Gordon Guyatt, Jack Sinclair, Deborah Cook,
Roman Jaeschke, and Holger Schünemann

## IN THIS SECTION

In Part 2F, "Moving From Evidence to Action, Grading Recommendations—A Qualitative Approach," we introduced a system of grading recommendations that separated two components: (1) the clarity of the tradeoff between benefits and risks of the interventions and (2) the methodologic quality of the evidence on which the recommendation rests. In this section—of potential interest to clinicians formulating recommendations for others, or to those with a methodologic or quantitative bent—we show how the tradeoff between benefits and risks can be made more explicit. We direct clinicians interested in an even more detailed and more mathematical exposition to an article by Sinclair and colleagues.[1]

# THE THRESHOLD NUMBER NEEDED TO TREAT

The decision about whether a recommendation should suggest a treatment be administered or withheld, and whether the recommendation should be grade 1 or grade 2, depends on two elements. First is the magnitude of intervention effect at which benefit exceeds the risks of therapy, including both adverse effects and costs. Second is the relationships between the estimate of the magnitude of the intervention effect, the precision of that estimate, and the threshold. We will deal with these components in turn.

In describing results of studies, we will consider the effect of the intervention on the clinical event that it is designed to prevent (the *target event*). We will focus on the relative risk (RR), which is the ratio of the risk of target events in treated patients to the risk of target events in the untreated patients, and the relative risk reduction (RRR), or 1.0 − relative risk; on the absolute risk reduction (ARR), which is the difference in the absolute risk of the target event between treatment and control groups; and on the number needed to treat (NNT), which is the number of patients one needs to treat to prevent one target event (arithmetically, the inverse of the absolute risk reduction) (see Part 2B2, "Therapy and Understanding the Results, Measures of Association").

For any treatment for any condition, it is useful to think of a threshold effect above which one would treat, and below which one would not treat (see Part 2B2, "Therapy and Understanding the Results, Confidence Intervals"). Moreover, it is informative to think of the number of patients one would need to treat to prevent a single adverse event.[2,3] Consider, for instance, the prevention of gastrointestinal bleeding in critically ill patients. Envision a group of critically ill patients who are ventilated or who have a coagulopathy and whose risk of bleeding is therefore increased to 3.7%.[4,5] Treating such patients with histamine-2-receptor antagonists reduces their relative risk by 58%, to 1.55%. In absolute terms, their risk has fallen 2.15% (Table 2F-8). The reciprocal of this absolute risk reduction is the number needed to treat (NNT). In this case, 45 patients must receive prophylaxis to prevent an episode of serious bleeding.

TABLE 2F-8

## The Decision to Administer Prophylaxis in Critically Ill Patients at High and Low Risk of Gastrointestinal Bleeding From Stress Ulceration

| | Bleeding Risk if Untreated U | Relative Risk Reduction (U – T)/U | Bleeding Risk if Treated T | Absolute Risk Reduction U – T | Number Needed to Treat 1/(U – T) to Prevent Bleeding |
|---|---|---|---|---|---|
| Critically ill patient ventilated and/or coagulopathy | 0.037 | 58% | 0.0155 | 0.0215 | 45 |
| Critically ill patient breathing spontaneously without coagulopathy | 0.0014 | 58% | 0.0006 | 0.0008 | 1250 |

Consider another group of critically ill patients whom we have already mentioned, those who are breathing spontaneously and who do not have a coagulopathy. Their risk of bleeding without treatment (the *baseline risk*) is 0.14%, their risk with treatment is 0.06%, and one must treat 1250 such patients to prevent serious bleeding (see Table 2F-8).

Should we treat either, or both, of these patients? This decision involves generating a threshold NNT. If the patients' risk without treatment is high enough and the NNT is below the threshold, we administer treatment. If the patient's risk without treatment is low enough and the NNT is therefore above the threshold, we would not treat.

Generating the threshold NNT (which we can designate as $NNT_T$) involves three steps. In the first step, we identify two sorts of undesirable events. One is the target event and the other is the adverse effects attributable to treatment. To generate the $NNT_T$, we need to specify the relative value we place on avoiding the target event in relation to the adverse consequences of treatment. If we are to include costs in our deliberations, we must also specify the costs we incur when we treat patients, the costs we save when we prevent the occurrence of the target event, the costs that we might incur as a result of preventing the target event, and the costs we incur when we look after patients who suffer adverse events associated with treatment.

In considering the decision whether to administer prophylaxis for gastrointestinal bleeding, some of the costs we specify below are based on an economic analysis from a hospital's point of view,[6] whereas others are much more approximate estimates. In this case, the cost of administering the histamine-2-receptor antagonist ranitidine during a patient's 10-day stay in the intensive care unit (calculated, as are all our costs, based on Canadian data) is approximately $65 dollars (including drug costs and costs of administering the treatment) and the cost of treating a gastrointestinal bleeding episode is $12,000.[6] Adverse effects of ranitidine include hepatitis with hepatic failure (an incidence of 0.06%,[7] with a treatment cost of $10,000 per episode) and central nervous system toxicity (an incidence of 1.5%,[8] with a cost of $500 per episode).

The second step in generating the $NNT_T$ is assigning relative values to the outcomes and relating them to dollar costs. These values may come from health workers, from administrators, from patients, or from a large random sample of the general public; one of a number of approaches (such as individual interviews or a group consensus process) might be used to assess utility (see Part 2F, "Moving From Evidence to Action, Incorporating Patient Values"). Although there is no consensus about either who should be deciding values or the best method of establishing that group's values, we would recommend individual interviews either with patients or with the general public. Whatever population and approach to eliciting values one chooses, the process would involve (in the present case) determining the degree of satisfaction, distress, or desirability that people associate with having an episode of gastrointestinal bleeding relative to an episode of liver toxicity or central nervous system toxicity. The process then involves deciding how much money should be allocated to prevent a single episode of gastrointestinal bleeding, which in turn determines the amount of money we would be willing to spend to avoid the adverse events attributable to treatment.[9]

For purposes of the present discussion, we have not actually obtained values from a random sample of the population, but have guessed at what the population might say. In this case, we would be willing to spend $3000 to prevent one episode of gastrointestinal bleeding. We have equated one episode of liver toxicity and 10 episodes of central nervous system toxicity to a serious gastrointestinal bleeding episode. Thus, we would be willing to spend $3000 to avoid one episode of liver toxicity and $300 to avoid one episode of central nervous system toxicity. We explain the algebra involved in calculating the $NNT_T$ in the Appendix; as it turns out, the figures above generate a $NNT_T$ of approximately 150.

Figure 2F-5 presents the relation between the treatment NNT, the $NNT_T$, and the risk of bleeding without treatment for critically ill patients. In constructing Figure 2F-5, we have used the relative risk reduction we can expect with administration of histamine-2-receptor antagonists (58%) and the $NNT_T$ of 150 that we have generated. The horizontal line at an NNT of 150 represents this $NNT_T$. The decreasing curve represents the NNT for any given risk of bleeding without treatment; we will call this the treatment NNT line. Points on this line include the groups of patients from Table 2F-8: patients with a risk of serious bleeding without treatment of 3.7%, for whom the NNT is 45; and patients with a risk of serious bleeding without treatment of 0.14%, for whom the NNT is 1250. The NNT line crosses the $NNT_T$ at a risk without treatment of 1.15%. Therefore, our judgment is that treatment is warranted in patients whose risk of serious bleeding without treatment is greater than 1.15%, and it is not warranted for those whose risk is less than 1.15%.

**FIGURE 2F-5**

## Relationship Between Baseline Risk and the NNT

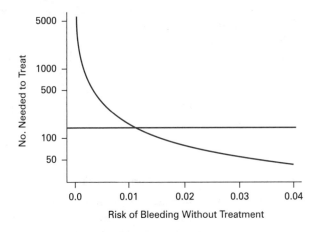

The curved line represents the number needed to treat (NNT) associated with treatment, and the horizontal line represents the threshold NNT. The NNT increases as the risk of bleeding without treatment for critically ill patients (the baseline risk) drops.

The NNT$_T$ will vary, depending on the values the clinician and patient place on its components. Some clinicians may be uncomfortable including costs as a consideration in the decision to treat. The strength of the threshold approach is that in generating an NNT$_T$, those recommending policy can make explicit the values they place on avoiding clinical events, adverse effects, and costs incurred or avoided— or they can omit costs from the consideration. In the Appendix to this book, we provide a method of calculating the NNT$_T$ without considering costs. Clinicians can examine the basis for the decision regarding the NNT$_T$, and the implications of differences in values and the lower or higher threshold generated, as a result of different values.

# COMPARING THE THRESHOLD NUMBER NEEDED TO TREAT TO THE NUMBER NEEDED TO TREAT FOR SPECIFIC GROUPS OF PATIENTS

A *meta-analysis* is a quantitative review that yields the best estimate of the treatment effect by pooling results from different trials (see Part 1E, "Summarizing the Evidence"). This estimate is called a point estimate to remind us that, although the true value lies somewhere in its neighborhood, it is unlikely to be exactly correct. Confidence intervals tell us the range within which the true treatment effect likely lies (see Part 2B2, "Therapy and Understanding the Results, Confidence Intervals").

We usually (though arbitrarily) use the 95% confidence interval, which can be interpreted as defining the range that would include the true treatment effect 95% of the time on repetition of the experiment.

Given a specified risk of a clinical event without treatment, we can use the reduction in relative risk of clinical events with treatment, and the confidence interval around that reduction in relative risk, to calculate not only the NNT, but also the confidence interval around the NNT. The relation between that confidence interval and the threshold NNT will have a profound effect on the strength of any recommendation to treat or not to treat. There are four possible relations between the threshold NNT, the point estimate of the treatment effect, and the confidence interval around the point estimate. We will examine each of these four in turn.

### Critically Ill Ventilated Patients With a Coagulopathy

First, consider critically ill patients who are being ventilated and have a coagulopathy. We have already decided that since their NNT lies below the threshold, they should be treated with histamine-2-receptor antagonists or some equivalent treatment (see Table 2F-8 and Figure 2F-5). We must remember, however, the upper boundary of the confidence interval around the NNT. This boundary represents the smallest reduction in risk, and thus the largest NNT, that is likely to be consistent with the data. In this case, the 95% confidence interval around the relative risk reduction of 58% ranges from 79% to 21%, and the corresponding confidence interval around the NNT, given the risk without treatment of 3.7%, ranges from 34 to 129. Here, the boundary of the confidence interval that represents the highest NNT consistent with the data is still less than the threshold NNT of 150. We can be confident that the treatment, for patients whose risk of bleeding is 3.7%, does more good than harm, on average, given the relative values and costs we have specified.

### Critically Ill Unventilated Patients Without Coagulopathy

Next, consider critically ill patients who neither are ventilated nor have a coagulopathy, and whose risk of bleeding is therefore 0.14%. Given the 58% relative risk reduction, we must treat 1250 such patients to prevent a bleeding episode (see Table 2F-8). The 95% confidence interval around this NNT ranges from 904 to 3401. The boundary of the confidence interval that represents the largest plausible treatment effect and, thus, the smallest NNT (904) is greater than the threshold NNT of 150. We can therefore be confident that the risks and costs of treatment outweigh the benefits.

## Critically Ill Unventilated Patients With a Coagulopathy

Now consider patients with an intermediate risk of bleeding without treatment, when the recommendation is less clear. Take, for instance, a critically ill patient with a bleeding risk of 2%. Given a relative risk reduction of 58%, we must treat 86 such patients to prevent a bleeding episode. Given the range of the 95% confidence interval around the relative risk reduction (79% to 21%), the true NNT may lie between 63 and 238. The boundary of the 95% confidence interval that represents the smallest plausible treatment effect, and thus the greatest NNT (238), is greater than the threshold NNT. Although the overall recommendation will still be to treat patients with this level of risk of bleeding, our strength of inferences will be weaker.

## Critically Ill Ventilated Patients Without Coagulopathy

Similarly, if one considers a patient with a risk of serious bleeding without treatment of 0.9%, the most likely NNT is 192, but the 95% confidence interval ranges from 141 to 529. Since the most likely NNT is above the threshold, the recommendation will be to withhold treatment, but because the 95% confidence interval overlaps the threshold NNT of 150, the strength of inference is relatively weak.

We present results from all four levels of baseline risk (0.14%, 0.9%, 2%, and 3.7%, respectively), together with the threshold NNT, in Figure 2F-6.

**FIGURE 2F-6**

### Levels of Baseline Risk and Threshold Number Needed to Treat (NNT)

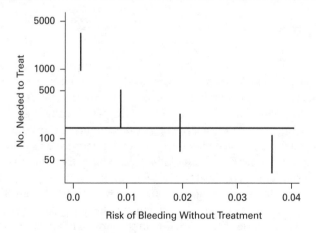

Vertical lines represent the 95% confidence intervals around treatment number needed to treat (NNT) at baseline risks of 0.14%, 0.9%, 2%, and 3.7%. The horizontal line represents the threshold NNT, 150.

# CONSIDERATIONS IN APPLYING THE QUANTITATIVE APPROACH TO GRADING RECOMMENDATIONS

There are many issues in arriving at recommendations that remain to be fully explored. The 0.05 threshold for deciding whether or not heterogeneity is statistically significant, the proposed criteria for deciding whether heterogeneity is clinically important, and the choice of 95% for the confidence interval around the treatment NNT are all arbitrary. Our choice of 95% is based on tradition. Less stringent values would lead to narrower confidence intervals (and, thus, more grade 1 recommendations) and ultimately may be judged more appropriate.

The decision about the $NNT_T$ may vary in different practice settings and from patient to patient. We suggest that those making recommendations for clinical practice be explicit about how they arrive at their $NNT_T$. They must consider all major toxicity, annoyance, or inconvenience for the patient, the administrative burden on the health care system, and the cost of treatment, and describe how they have valued each component. Limitations in the data will emphasize the need to conduct additional rigorous studies. Those making recommendations should acknowledge any limitations in their data set. If clinicians disagree with the values underlying a particular $NNT_T$ or if they work in a setting in which a particular $NNT_T$ does not apply, they can generate a new $NNT_T$ consistent with their values or practice setting. They could still use the overview evidence and the $NNT_T$ and quickly generate recommendations.

# CONCLUSION

Whether or not they use our approach to grading recommendations, those who take the responsibility for generating recommendations should clearly separate two components: the design and heterogeneity of the primary studies, on the one hand, and the magnitude and precision of the estimates of the treatment effects on the other hand. Implicitly or explicitly, grades of recommendations should estimate the uncertainty associated with the estimate of treatment effect and should note the relationship between a threshold for treatment to that uncertainty. Clinicians determining the optimal course of action for an individual patient must traverse the same path, considering, in the light of the patient's circumstances, the likely outcomes of alternative courses of action and the uncertainty associated with the estimates. Because of the similarity in the process of recommendations and individual decision making, our discussion may help clinicians label the elements of their decisions and understand the underlying uncertainty.

# Calculations: Threshold Number Needed to Treat

This appendix presents a brief outline of how we go about calculating the threshold number needed to treat, a fuller description of which can be found in a recent publication.[1] In describing how to calculate a threshold NNT, we will use the following notation:

- $NNT_T$: the threshold number needed to treat

- $Cost_{treatment}$: the cost of treating one patient

- $Cost_{target}$: the cost of treating one target event

- $Cost_{AE}$: the cost of treating one adverse event, with a further subscript 1 or 2 denoting the first and second adverse events

- $Rate_{AE}$: the proportion of treated patients who suffer an adverse event (again subscripts 1 and 2 denoting the two adverse events)

- $Value_{target}$: the dollar value we assign to preventing one target event

- $Value_{AE}$: the dollar value we assign to preventing one adverse event (again subscripts 1 and 2 denoting the two adverse events)

The general approach for generating the threshold NNT is based on the concept that at this threshold, the value of treatment inputs equals the value of treatment outputs: that is, the net cost of treating the number of patients one needs to treat to prevent one patient having the target event equals the net value of the adverse events prevented or caused by treating that number of patients.

**Treatment Input.** The value of the treatment inputs includes:

the cost of treating the number of patients that will comprise the threshold NNT:

$$(Cost_{treatment}) \ (NNT_T)$$

plus

the cost of treating the adverse events attributable to treatment in the number of patients that will comprise the threshold NNT:

$$(Cost_{AE})(Rate_{AE})(NNT_T)$$

minus

the cost of treating one target event:

$$Cost_{target}$$

**Treatment Output.** The value of the outputs includes:

the dollar value assigned to the one target event prevented:

$$\text{Value}_{target}$$

minus

the dollar value assigned to adverse events attributable to treatment:

$$(\text{Value}_{AE})(\text{Rate}_{AE})(\text{NNT}_T)$$

Thus we have:

$$[(\text{Cost}_{treatment})(\text{NNT}_T)] + [(\text{Cost}_{AE})(\text{Rate}_{AE})(\text{NNT}_T)] - \text{Cost}_{target} = \text{Value}_{target} - [(\text{Value}_{AE})(\text{Rate}_{AE})(\text{NNT}_T)]$$

Rearranging the above equation gives:

$$\text{NNT}_T [\text{Cost}_{treatment} + (\text{Cost}_{AE})(\text{Rate}_{AE})] - \text{Cost}_{target} = \text{Value}_{target} - \text{NNT}_T [(\text{Value}_{AE})(\text{Rate}_{AE})]$$

And solving for threshold NNT

$$\text{NNT}_T = \frac{\text{Cost}_{target} + \text{Value}_{target}}{\text{Cost}_{treatment} + (\text{Cost}_{AE})(\text{Rate}_{AE}) + (\text{Value}_{AE})(\text{Rate}_{AE})}$$

In the example we have used in the body of the article concerning the prevention of gastrointestinal bleeding, there are two adverse effects attributable to treatment that we must consider. The equation therefore becomes:

$$\text{NNT}_T = \frac{\text{Cost}_{target} + \text{Value}_{target}}{\text{Cost}_{treatment} + [(\text{Cost}_{AE1})(\text{Rate}_{AE1}) + (\text{Cost}_{AE2})(\text{Rate}_{AE2})] + [(\text{Value}_{AE1}(\text{Rate}_{AE1}) + (\text{Value}_{AE2})(\text{Rate}_{AE2})]}$$

Or, for multiple adverse events

$$\text{NNT}_T = \frac{\text{Cost}_{target} + \text{Value}_{target}}{\text{Cost}_{treatment} + \Sigma(\text{Cost}_{AE})(\text{Rate}_{AE}) + \Sigma(\text{Value}_{AE})(\text{Rate}_{AE})}$$

Substituting the figures from the body of the article:

$$\text{NNT}_T = \frac{12,000 + 3000}{65 + [(10,000)(0.006) + (500)(0.015)] + [(3000)(0.0006) + (300)(0.015)]}$$

$$\text{NNT}_T = \frac{15,000}{65 + 6 + 7.5 + 18 + 4.5}$$

$$\text{NNT}_T = \frac{15,000}{101}$$

$$\text{NNT}_T = 148.5$$

# References

1. Sinclair JC, Cook R, Guyatt GH, Pauker SG, Cook DJ. When should an effective treatment be used? Derivation of the threshold number needed to treat and the minimum event rate for treatment. *J Clin Epidemiol*. 2001;54: In press.

2. Laupacis A, Sackett DL, Roberts RS. An assessment of clinically useful measures of the consequences of treatment. *N Engl J Med*. 1988;318:1728-1733.

3. Guyatt GH, Sackett DL, Cook DJ, for the Evidence-Based Medicine Working Group. Users' guides to the medical literature, II: how to use an article about therapy or prevention. B. What were the results and will they help me in caring for my patients? *JAMA*. 1994;271:59-63.

4. Cook DJ, Reeve BK, Guyatt GH, et al. Stress ulcer prophylaxis in critically ill patients: resolving discordant meta-analyses. *JAMA*. 1996;275:308-314.

5. Cook DJ, Fuller HD, Guyatt GH, et al. Risk factors for gastrointestinal bleeding in critically ill patients. Canadian Critical Care Trials Group. *N Engl J Med.* 1994;330:377-381.

6. Heyland DK, Gafni A, Griffith L, et al. The clinical and economic consequence of clinically important gastrointestinal bleeding in critically ill patients. *Clin Intens Care.* 1996;7:121-125.

7. Dobbs JH, Muir JG, Smith RN. H2-antagonists and hepatitis. *Ann Intern Med*. 1986;105:803.

8. Vial T, Goubier C, Bergeret A, Cabrera F, Evreux JC, Descotes J. Side effects of ranitidine. *Drug Saf*. 1991;6:94-117.

9. Torrance GW. Measurement of health state utilities for economic appraisal. *J Health Econ*. 1986;5:1-30.

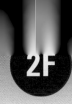

# MOVING FROM EVIDENCE TO ACTION

## Economic Analysis

Bernie O'Brien, Michael Drummond, W. Scott Richardson, Mitchell Levine, Daren Heyland, and Gordon Guyatt

The following EBM Working Group members also made substantive contributions to this section: Trisha Greenhalgh and Christina Lacchetti

## CLINICAL SCENARIO

### Are the Benefits of tPA Over Streptokinase Worth the Costs?

**Y**ou are a general internist on the staff of a large community hospital. Your chief of medicine knows of your interest in evidence-based medicine, and she asks you to help her solve a problem. The hospital's Pharmacy and Therapeutics Committee has been trying to decide on formulary guidelines for the use of streptokinase or tissue plasminogen activator (tPA) in the treatment of acute myocardial infarction. Members of the committee have been arguing for weeks about the GUSTO trial[1] and whether the added expense of tPA is worth it. The committee has reached an impasse and has asked the chief of medicine for some outside help to reach a decision. Knowing that the hospital faces pressure to keep costs down, the chief wants good information about this question to bring to the next committee meeting later this week. She asks you to help her find out if anyone has published a formal economic analysis that compares thrombolytic agents for acute MI and then help her present it to the committee.

## FINDING THE EVIDENCE

From your office computer, you enter the hospital library's current Best Evidence database using Ovid search software. Your search of thrombolytic agents for myocardial infarction yields four hits when the search term "thrombolytic therapy" is limited to economics. Of these, one looks relevant and you put it aside for further review.[2] You then switch databases and connect to the Cochrane Database, where you combine the three search terms "myocardial infarction " AND "thrombolytic therapy" AND "cost-benefit analysis," a search that yields nothing worthwhile. Next, you examine the "Abstracts of Economic Evaluations of Health Care Interventions" with the search term "thrombolytic therapy"; of the 39 hits, three appear potentially relevant.[3-5]

One of the articles is an economic analysis based directly on data from the GUSTO study.[2] Of the other three articles, all of which use modeling approaches to economic analysis, you decide to focus on the one paper that both takes a long-term (rather than a 1-year) perspective and is readily available in your local library.[3]

## COST: JUST ANOTHER OUTCOME?

In the course of their work, clinicians make many decisions about the care of individual patients. Clinicians also participate in decisions for large groups of patients, whether to set clinical policy for an institution (addressing such questions as, "Should streptokinase or tPA be recommended routinely for patients with an acute myocardial infarction who present to our hospital?") or to set health policy at a more "macro" level (addressing such questions as, "Which thrombolytic agents should our national or local health authority choose to purchase and provide for our citizens with acute myocardial infarction?"). When making decisions for such patient groups, clinicians need not only weigh the benefits and risks, but also consider whether these benefits will be worth the health care resources consumed. Resources used to provide health care are vast, but not limitless. Thus, more and more, clinicians have to convince colleagues and health policymakers that the benefits of their interventions justify the costs.

To inform these decisions, clinicians can use economic analyses of clinical practices. *Economic analysis* is a set of formal, quantitative methods used to compare two or more treatments, programs, or strategies with respect to their resource use and their expected outcomes.[6,7] If two strategies are analyzed but only costs are compared, this comparison would inform only the resource-use half of the decision and is termed a *cost analysis*. Comparing two or more strategies only by their consequences (such as in a randomized trial) informs only the outcomes portion of the decision. A full economic comparison requires that both the costs and consequences be analyzed for each of the strategies being compared.

Economic evaluations seek to inform resource allocation decisions, rather than to make them. Economic analyses, widely applied in the health care field, have informed decisions at different levels, including managing major institutions like hospitals and determining regional or national policy.[8,9]

In one sense, like physiologic function, quality of life, morbid events such as stroke and myocardial infarction, and death, cost is simply another outcome for clinicians to consider when assessing the effects of therapy. As for other outcomes, there are two fundamental strategies for discovering the impact of alternative management strategies on resource consumption. One is to conduct a single study, ideally a randomized trial, comparing two or more interventions. Such an approach asks, "*What does happen?*" (on average, and limited by the precision of the estimate) when clinicians choose management strategy A vs strategy B. The second approach is to construct a *decision tree* of events that flow from a clinical decision, using all the available evidence to estimate the probabilities of all possible outcomes—including the costs generated. This second approach asks, "*What might happen?*" if clinicians choose management strategy A vs strategy B.

Although there are fundamental similarities between cost and other outcomes, there are also important differences that we will now describe.

## Costs Are More Variable Than Other Outcomes

Whether clinicians administer tPA or streptokinase to a particular patient with myocardial infarction in Toronto or Chicago, or even in Bangkok, the relative impact on mortality is likely to be the same. Indeed, treatment effects on conventional outcomes of quality of life, morbidity, and mortality have proved on most occasions to be similar not only across geographic location, but across patient groups and ways of administering the intervention as well (see Part 2E, "Summarizing the Evidence, When to Believe a Subgroup Analysis").

In contrast to clinical endpoints, costs vary hugely across jurisdictions, not only in absolute terms but in the relative costs of different components of care, including physicians, other health workers, drugs, services, and technologic devices. For example, outpatient treatment of deep venous thrombosis (DVT) with low-molecular-weight heparin (LMWH) compared to inpatient treatment with unfractionated heparin is more cost-effective in the United States than Canada, even though LMWH is more than double the price in the United States. The reason is that the price of reduced hospital days relative to the price of LMWH is much greater in the United States than in Canada.[10]

One need not move across international—or even national, or regional, or state boundaries—to see large cost differences. Adjacent hospitals may have different success in negotiating a contract with a drug company to purchase a large volume of a drug at a low price. Drug prices in adjacent hospitals may therefore vary by a factor of 2 or more, and the resource implications of use of alternative agents may therefore differ substantially in the two institutions.

Costs also depend on how care is organized, and organization of care varies widely across jurisdictions. The same service may be delivered by a physician or a nurse practitioner, in the outpatient setting or in the hospital, and with or without administrative costs related to adjudication of patient eligibility to receive the service. If it is delivered by a physician, in the hospital, with maximal administrative costs—as our example of inpatient DVT treatment in the United States suggests—the expense will be greater than if the service is delivered on an outpatient basis, or in an institution with lower administrative costs.

The substantial dependence of resource consumption on local costs and local organization of health care delivery means that most cost data are specific to a particular jurisdiction and have limited transferability. An additional problem with randomized controlled trials is that their conduct may alter practice patterns in a way that further limits generalizability to other settings—or even to their own setting, outside of the RCT context. For example, in an economic evaluation of misoprostol, a drug for prophylaxis against gastric ulcer in patients receiving high doses of nonsteroidal anti-inflammatory drugs (NSAIDs) over long periods of time, Hillman and Bloom[11] used clinical data from a trial undertaken by Graham et al.[12] This blinded randomized trial of 3 months' duration compared misoprostol (400 mg and 800 mg daily) with placebo. An important issue for economic analysis was that prevention of ulcers by misoprostol may generate savings in health care expenditure, savings that could balance the cost of adding the drug. However, in this study, endoscopy was performed monthly. In regular clinical practice, endoscopy would be undertaken in response to symptoms. An analysis of the results from this trial would have told clinicians of the cost implications of misoprostol administration when patients undergo routine monthly endoscopy—information that would be useless, given how different such circumstances are from regular clinical practice.

The what-might-happen modeling approach of decision analysis allows investigators to deal with such problems. Hillman and Bloom,[11] for instance, adjusted observed ulcer rates to reflect the fact that 40% of endoscopically determined lesions did not produce any symptoms. Noting that compliance of patients in the trial was greater than one might expect in clinical practice, they also adjusted for lower compliance by using the ulcer rates in the evaluable cohort and by assuming that only 60% of this efficacy would be achieved in practice.

The modeling approaches of decision analysis allow investigators to deal with other problems such as inadequate length of follow-up by using available data to estimate what will happen over the long term. Decision analysts can also examine a variety of cost assumptions and ways of organizing care, and can calculate the sensitivity of their results to these alternate assumptions (see Part 1F, "Moving From Evidence to Action").

The key limitation of the decision analytic approach is that if its assumptions are flawed, it will not give us an accurate picture. For instance, Schulman et al[13] concluded that early use of zidovudine therapy in asymptomatic individuals with HIV infection was cost-effective based on projections of disease progression from a clinical trial with 1-year follow-up. However, a subsequent study with 3-year follow-up showed that the advantages of therapy in the first year were eroded in subsequent years.[14] In one review of 326 pharmacoeconomic analyses submitted to the Australian Department of Health by the pharmaceutical industry, 218 (67%) included significant problems, many of which required a detailed review to detect.[15]

The ideal, then, may be a melding of the two approaches in which the analysis rests on data from randomized trials, with adjunctive analytic decision-based modeling to adapt the results to the real-life situations in which they will be applied.[16] However, even the melding approach must use average patient values, and these averages may be very different from values or preferences of the individual patient (see Part 2F, "Moving From Evidence to Action, Incorporating Patient Values"). Furthermore, these differences may affect the optimal management strategy (see Part 1F, "Moving From Evidence to Action"). The extent to which the authors make their assumptions transparent will add to the credibility of any economic analysis.

## The Role of Costs in Clinical Decision Making Remains Controversial

Although few would deny the importance of cost considerations in setting health care policy, the relevance of costs in individual patient decision making remains controversial. Some would argue—taking an extreme of what can be called a deontological approach to distributive justice (see Part 1A, "Introduction: The Philosophy of Evidence-Based Medicine")—that the clinician's only responsibility should be to best meet the needs of the individual under her care. An alternate view—philosophically consequentialist or utilitarian—would contend that even in individual decision making, the clinician should take a broader social view. In this broader view, the effect on others of allocating resources to a particular patient's care would bear on the decision.

As health care technologies proliferate, their potential benefits and their costs increase, but their marginal benefits over less resource-intensive approaches are often small. In such a world, the arguments for bedside rationing become more compelling.[17] Our own belief is that while individual clinicians should attend primarily to the needs of the patients under their care, they should not neglect the resource implications of the advice they offer their patients. Neglect of resource issues in one patient, after all, may affect resource availability for other patients under their care. For those who disagree, this section remains relevant for consideration of health policy decisions.

## Using Cost Information to Inform Decisions Poses Special Challenges

Typically, effective treatments make patients feel better, or they reduce risk of major morbid or mortal events in the future. Moving from evidence to action then involves trading off these benefits against common immediate side effects, long-term toxicity, and the inconvenience attendant on complying with the therapeutic regimen. Individual patient values, ideally, will inform this trade-off (Part 1F, "Moving From Evidence to Action"; Part 2F, "Moving From Evidence to Action, Incorporating Patient Values").

In health care policy decisions, we must use cost information to allocate scarce resources efficiently. Let us assume that two treatments both cost, in comparison to conventional treatment and after consideration of all their consequences, $1,000,000 for each 100 patients treated for 1 year. For treatment A, the benefits achieved by this expenditure is the prevention of an average of two severe attacks of migraine headache per patient, or 200 migraine headaches. For treatment B, the benefit is avoiding a single myocardial infarction. If, in a resource-constrained environment, one had to choose between A and B, what would be the better choice?

If the choice makes you feel uncomfortable, you are in good company. Choosing between competing beneficial treatments presents daunting logistic, ethical, and political challenges. The example demonstrates how, in economic analysis, we must trade off costs against benefits, and how we must deal with very different outcomes that accrue to very different people—in this case, migraine headaches to one patient group and myocardial infarction to another—in deciding on allocation of resources.

Economic analysis must deal with the problem of the relative value of different outcomes, and the trade-off of dollar values against health. Typically, health economists turn to one of three strategies. One is to report patient-important outcomes in physical or natural units such as "life-years gained" or "migraine headaches prevented" or"myocardial infarctions prevented" (*cost-effectiveness analysis*). In a second approach, the different types of outcomes are weighted to produce a composite index of outcome, such as the quality-adjusted life-year (QALY), or healthy years equivalent[18] (we call this *cost-utility analysis*—sometimes classified as a subcategory of cost-effectiveness analysis). Quality adjustment involves placing a lower value on time spent with impaired physical and emotional function than time spent in full health. On a scale where 0 represents death and 1.0 represents full health, the greater the impairment, the lower the value of a particular health state (see Part 2B2, "Therapy and Understanding the Results, Quality of Life"). Finally, investigators may put a dollar value on additional life gained, migraine headaches prevented, or myocardial infarctions prevented. In these *cost-benefit analyses*, health care consumers consider what they would be willing to pay for programs or products that achieve particular outcomes—such as prolonging life or preventing adverse events.

In the studies from our scenario, Mark et al[2] chose cost-effectiveness as their primary analysis using the outcome "years of life saved." They considered QALYs in a secondary analysis. Kalish et al[3] chose cost-utility analysis using QALYs as their primary approach. In both cases, the value of states of health was obtained by the time trade-off approach, that is, by asking patients how many years in their current state of health they would be willing to give up to live their remaining years in excellent health. Mark et al[2] obtained these values from patients in the GUSTO trial 1 year after treatment. Kalish et al[3] obtained them from a subset of patients in the GISSI-2 trial.

Having outlined some of the challenges of economic analysis, we offer our usual structure for guides to the medical literature: Are the results valid? What are the results? How can I apply results to patient care? The issues we present in Table 2F-9 are those specific to economic analysis and are presented within the structure of our guides for practice guidelines and decision analyses (see Part 1F, "Moving From Evidence to Action").

**TABLE 2F-9**

## Users' Guides for an Article About Economic Analyses

**Are the Results Valid?**

*Did the recommendations consider all relevant patient groups, management options, and possible outcomes?*

- Did investigators adopt a sufficiently broad viewpoint?
- Are results reported separately for patients whose baseline risk differs?

*Is there a systematic review and summary of evidence linking options to outcomes for each relevant question?*

- Were costs measured accurately?
- Did investigators consider the timing of costs and consequences?

**What Are the Results?**

- What were the incremental costs and effects of each strategy?
- Do incremental costs and effects differ between subgroups?
- How much does allowance for uncertainty change the results?

**How Can I Apply the Results to Patient Care?**

- Are the treatment benefits worth the risks and costs?
- Can I expect similar costs in my setting?

# ARE THE RESULTS VALID?

## Did Investigators Adopt a Sufficiently Broad Viewpoint?

Investigators can evaluate costs and consequences from a number of viewpoints: the patient, the hospital, the third-party payer (or national or local government in some countries), or society at large. Each viewpoint may be relevant depending on the question being asked, but broader viewpoints are most relevant to those allocating health care resources. For example, an evaluation adopting the viewpoint of the hospital will be useful in estimating the budgetary impact of alternative therapies for that institution. However, economic evaluation is usually directed at informing policy from a broader societal perspective.

For example, in an evaluation of an early-discharge program, it is not sufficient to report only hospital costs, since patients discharged early may consume substantial community resources. These costs may not be borne by the hospital, but are likely to have an impact on the third-party payer or the patient in some way or another. This was a limitation of a study by Topol et al,[19] which assessed the feasibility and cost savings of hospital discharge 3 days after acute myocardial infarction, considering only hospital and professional charges. We have no knowledge of other community services consumed and whether these differed between early- and conventional-discharge patients.

One of the main reasons for considering narrower viewpoints in conducting an economic analysis is to assess the impact of change on the main budget holders, since budgets may need to be adjusted before a new therapy can be adopted—often termed the silo effect. Weisbrod et al[20] pointed out that, although a community-oriented mental illness program was worthwhile from the perspective of society as a whole, it would be more costly to the organization responsible for providing the care. Even within the same institution, narrow budgetary viewpoints can prevail. In our example comparing streptokinase with tPA, it would be wrong to focus exclusively on the relative costs of the drugs, which fall on the pharmacy budget, if there are also impacts on other hospital resource use. In the DVT example we used earlier, use of outpatient LMWH will decrease hospital cost, but whoever pays the drug budget will find their costs rising.

The patient's perspective may also merit specific consideration, if costs (eg, travel-related ones) reduce access to care. Also, some patients may not be able to participate in community care programs if these impose major costs in terms of informal nursing support in the home. However, in general, the analysis integrates the patient's perspective by measuring the consequences of therapy, such as impact on quality of life.

From a societal viewpoint, determination of costs should include the therapy's impact on the patients' ability to work and hence their contribution to the nation's productivity. The issue of inclusion or exclusion of productivity changes (known as indirect costs and benefits) remains a frequent topic of debate. On one hand, indirect costs represent resource-use changes just like those occurring in the health care system. On the other hand, production may not actually be lost if a worker is absent for a short period. Also, for longer periods of absence, employers may hire a previously unemployed worker. Furthermore, inclusion of productivity changes biases evaluations in favor of programs for individuals who are in full-time employment. Therefore, clinicians should be skeptical about any economic analysis that includes indirect costs without clearly presenting the implications.

Table 2F-10 presents the way in which the articles by Mark et al[2] and Kalish et al[3] handle these and other key methodologic issues. The first major point to note about these studies is that most of the data from Mark et al come from a single clinical trial, whereas Kalish et al used data from multiple sources to construct a decision analysis. Both studies, however, used observational databases to extrapolate survival data beyond the 1-year survival observed in the trial. This reaffirms the point that, even when investigators have good-quality clinical data available, modeling is often necessary to conduct an economic evaluation.

**TABLE 2F-10**

## Key Methodologic Features of Two Studies

|  | Mark et al[2] | Kalish et al[3] |
|---|---|---|
| Overall study design | Randomized controlled trial | Decision analysis |
| Viewpoint for analysis | Societal stated; health care payer is used | Not stated |
| Alternatives compared | tPA or streptokinase for patients with acute myocardial infarction | tPA or streptokinase for patients with acute myocardial infarction |
| Benefit measure(s) | Life-years saved and quality-adjusted life-years saved | Quality-adjusted life-years saved |
| Source(s) of effectiveness data | GUSTO trial (1 year survival) and Duke Cardiovascular Disease Database (long-term survival) | GUSTO trial (1 year survival) and Worcester Heart Attack Study (long-term survival) |
| Source(s) of quality of life (utility) weights | Sample of 2600 US patients enrolled in the GUSTO trial | GISSI-2 trial |
| Estimates of resource use | 23,105 US patients enrolled in the GUSTO trial (for initial hospitalization). Sample of 2600 US patients (for resource use up to 1 year) | Brigham and Women's Hospital and the literature |
| Source(s) of cost data | Duke cost accounting system and Medicare DRG rates | Brigham and Women's Hospital and the literature |
| Discounting | 5% per annum | 5% per annum |
| Sensitivity analysis | Varied estimates of survival and cost. Also, varied discount rate and considered importance of disabling strokes | Varied estimates of survival cost and stroke rate. Also, varied discount rate. |

tPA indicates tissue plasminogen activator; GUSTO, Global Utilization of Streptokinase and Tissue Plasminogen for Occluded Coronary Arteries; GISSI, Gruppo Italiano per lo Studio della Sopravvivenza nell'Infarto Miocardio; DRG, diagnosis related group.

Mark et al[2] point out the importance of considering a broad, societal viewpoint, whereas Kalish et al[3] do not discuss the issue. In practice, both analyses concentrate on the identification and quantification of direct medical care costs, both inside and outside the hospital. The authors do not tell us their reasons for exclusion of other cost items, such as patients' costs, but they may relate to the practical problems of data collection. Neither study considered productivity costs, but their inclusion would be unlikely to substantially influence the comparison between streptokinase and tPA.

### Are Results Reported Separately for Patients Whose Baseline Risks Differ?

The costs and consequences of treatment are likely to be related to the baseline risk in the population. For example, the cost-effectiveness of drug therapy for elevated cholesterol, compared with no treatment, will depend on age, gender, pretreatment, cholesterol level, and other risk factors; the greater the patients' risk, the lower the cost per unit of benefit.[21] Thus, secondary prevention is generally more cost-efficient than primary prevention.

Division of patients into risk categories is common in clinical practice. In a study of the cost-effectiveness of beta-blockers after acute myocardial infarction, Goldman et al[22] found that the cost per life-year gained was $2400 for those patients at high risk, compared with $13,000 for those at low risk. The differences in the cost-effectiveness ratios were driven primarily by the patient's ability to benefit from therapy (ie, if you are likely to do well without treatment, you have a limited capacity to benefit), rather than treatment cost.

Both the Mark et al[2] and Kalish et al[3] articles investigate the impact of patient age on cost-effectiveness, as older patients have a higher mortality risk and fewer years of life left to live. In addition, Mark et al[2] investigate the impact of infarction location on the cost-effectiveness estimates.

### Were Costs Measured Accurately?

Although the viewpoint determines the relevant range of costs and consequences to be included in an economic evaluation, there are many issues relating to their measurement and evaluation. First, clinicians should look for the physical quantities of resources consumed or released by the treatments, separately from their prices or unit costs. Not only does this allow them to scrutinize the method of assigning monetary values to resources, it also helps to extrapolate the results of a study from one setting to another, as prices will vary by location.

Second, there are different approaches to valuing costs or cost savings. One approach is to use published charges. However, charges may differ from real costs, depending on the sophistication of accounting systems and the relative bargaining power of health care institutions and third-party payers.[23] Where there is a systematic deviation between costs and charges, the analyst may adjust the latter by a cost-to-charge ratio. However, the relationship between charges and costs can vary markedly by institution, so simple adjustments may not suffice. From the third-party payer's perspective, charges will bear some relation to the amounts actually paid, although in some settings payments vary by payer. From a societal perspective we would like the real costs, since these reflect what society is forgoing, in benefits elsewhere, to provide a given treatment.

For example, Cohen et al[24] compared costs and charges for conventional angioplasty, directional atherectomy, stenting, and bypass surgery. Previous studies had suggested that total hospital charges for directional coronary atherectomy or intracoronary stenting are significantly higher than those for conventional angioplasty. However, when the investigators examined costs by adjusting itemized patient accounts by department-specific cost/charge ratios, the investigators found that the in-hospital costs of angioplasty and directional coronary atherectomy were similar. Also, although the cost of coronary stenting was approximately $2500 higher than that of conventional angioplasty, the magnitude of this difference was smaller than the $6300 increment previously suggested on the basis of analysis of hospital charges. Thus, clinicians may have been dissuaded from using coronary atherectomy or stenting because of the high "cost," when the apparent cost difference may have been an artifact of hospital accounting systems or bargaining power, rather than a reflection of the real value to society of the resources consumed by those procedures.

Mark et al[2] used costs from the Duke Transition One cost-accounting system, Medicare diagnosis related group (DRG) reimbursement rates, and Medicare physicians' fees in their estimations. Since the costs of the thrombolytic agents are an important component of the analysis, they calculated drug costs in two ways: from the *Drug Topics Red Book* average of 1993 wholesale prices, and from the average costs of the drugs in 16 randomly selected GUSTO hospitals. They examine the impact on cost-effectiveness of the different estimation methods. Kalish et al[3] use medication costs and Medicare DRG reimbursement rates for one hospital. They took costs of treating serious hemorrhage—and those of managing coronary artery disease and stroke—from the literature.

## Did Investigators Consider the Timing of Costs and Consequences?

A final issue in the measurement and valuation of costs and consequences relates to the adjustment for differences in their timing. Generally, people prefer benefits sooner and prefer to postpone costs because of uncertainty about the future and because resources, if invested, usually yield a positive return. The accepted way of allowing for this in economic evaluations is to discount costs and consequences occurring in the future to present values by assigning a lower weight to future costs and benefits. Following a foundational paper by Weinstein and Stason in 1977[25], cost-effectiveness analysis has usually used a 5% per annum discount rate. More recently, the US Panel on Cost Effectiveness in Health and Medicine[26] has proposed a 3% discount rate based on the inflation-adjusted rate of return on US government bonds. There are also debates about whether health outcomes should be discounted at the same rate as costs.[27, 28]

In the studies considered here, both sets of authors discount costs and benefits occurring in the future at a rate of 5% per annum. Mark et al[2] also report results for discount rates of 0% and 10%, whereas Kalish et al[3] report results for rates of 1% and 10%.

# WHAT ARE THE RESULTS?

## What Were the Incremental Costs and Effects of Each Strategy?

Let us start with the incremental costs. Look in the text and tables for the listings of all the costs considered for each treatment option, remembering that costs are the product of the quantity of a resource used and its unit price. These should include the costs incurred to produce the treatment such as the physician's time, nurse's time, materials, and so forth, which we might term the up-front costs, as well as the downstream costs due to resources consumed in the future and associated with clinical events that are attributable to the therapy. For instance, in the Mark et al paper, Table 2 lists all the resource use the authors considered, including the initial hospitalization and follow-up from 6 months to 1 year, while their Table 1 provides the unit price for specific resources. The Kalish et al article inludes a section on "costs" in their methods, with an associated Table 2 that summarizes the costs they attributed to a variety of patient events.

The study by Mark et al[2] quantifies resources used by treatment group in three periods of time over 1 year: initial hospitalization, discharge to 6 months, and 6 months to 1 year. Both treatment groups were very similar in their use of hospital resources over the year; both experienced a mean length of stay of 8 days, 3.5 of which were in the intensive care unit. In addition, both groups had the same rate of coronary artery bypass grafting (13%) and percutaneous transluminal angioplasty (31%) on initial hospitalization. As summarized in Table 2F-11, the 1-year health care costs, excluding the thrombolytic agent, were $24,990 per tPA-treated patient and $24,575 per streptokinase-treated patient. As is clear from Table 2F-11, the main cost difference between the two groups is the cost of the thrombolytic drugs themselves—$2750 for tPA and $320 for streptokinase. The overall difference in cost between tPA-treated and streptokinase-treated patients is, therefore, our incremental cost at $2845 during the first year. This is discounted at 5% per annum, for a final figure of $2710. The authors argue that there is no cost difference between the two groups after 1 year. These data for incremental costs from tPA are very similar to those estimated by Kalish et al,[3] who found a difference of $2535 in the use of tPA in preference to streptokinase to manage patients with myocardial infarction.

TABLE 2F-11

## Costs, Effects, and Cost-Effectiveness Summary for Tissue-Type Plasminogen Activator (t-PA) vs Streptokinase*

| | Treatment Group | | Difference (tPA-Streptokinase) | Discounted at 5% per Year |
|---|---|---|---|---|
| | tPA | Streptokinase | | |
| Health care costs (in US dollars) for 1 year (excluding thrombolytic drug cost)† | 24,990 | 24,575 | 415 | ... |
| Thrombolytic drug cost | 2750 | 320 | 2430 | ... |
| Total 1-year cost | 27,740 | 24,895 | 2845 | 2709.6 (=ΔC)‡ |
| Effects life expectancy, years | 15.41 | 15.27 | 0.14 | 0.0829 (=ΔE)‡ |
| Incremental cost-effectiveness of tPA | ... | ... | ... | ΔC/ΔE=$32,678 per life-year gained |

\* Data from Mark et al.[2]

† Treatment groups assumed to have no cost differences beyond 1 year.

‡ These discounted differences were not reported in the article, but have been imputed. ΔC indicates incremental cost, and ΔE, incremental effect.

tPA indicates tissue plasminogen activator.

The measure of effectiveness chosen in the Mark et al[2] study is the gain in life expectancy associated with tPA. The available follow-up experience was to 1 year, with 89.9% surviving in the streptokinase group vs 91.1% in the tPA group ($P < .001$). To translate these observations into life expectancy gains, the authors project survival curves for another 30 years or more using first a 14-year MI survivorship database from Duke University and then an assumption that survivorship will follow a statistical distribution. Having projected two survival curves, the authors calculate the area under each curve, which represents the expected value of survival time or life expectancy. For tPA patients, life expectancy was 15.41 years and for streptokinase patients it was 15.27 years. As summarized in Table 2F-11, the difference in life expectancy is 0.14 year per patient; phrased another way, for every 100 patients treated with tPA in preference to streptokinase, we would expect to gain 14 years of life.

In other situations, quantifying incremental effectiveness may be more difficult. Not all treatments change survival, and those that do not may affect different dimensions of health in many ways. For example, drug treatment of asymptomatic hypertension may result in short-term health reductions from drug side effects, in exchange for long-term expected health improvements such as reduced risk of strokes. Note that in our tPA example, the outcome is not unambiguously restricted to survival benefit because there is a small but statistically significant increased risk of nonfatal hemorrhagic stroke associated with tPA.[1] The existence of trade-offs between different aspects of health, or between length of life vs quality of life, means that to arrive at a summary measure of net effectiveness, we must implicitly or explicitly weight the desirability of different outcomes relative to each other.

There is a large and growing body of literature on quantitative approaches for combining multiple health outcomes into a single metric using patient preferences.[29] One of the most popular is the construction of quality-adjusted life-years (QALYs) as a measure that captures the impact of therapies in the two broad domains of survival and quality of life (see Part 1F, "Moving From Evidence to Action"; see also Part 2B2, "Therapy and Understanding the Results, Quality of Life"). Alternative approaches include the healthy year equivalent method.[30]

Our second thrombolytic study by Kalish et al[3] used QALYs as its primary measure of effectiveness. First, they took the same 1-year survival probabilities from the GUSTO study and projected them forward to estimate life expectancy using data from a different longitudinal study, the Worcester Heart Attack Study. Similar to Mark et al,[2] they estimated that the average life span after myocardial infarction is 14.6 years and then used GUSTO risk reductions to estimate life expectancy difference for tPA and streptokinase patients.

To derive QALYs, they applied utility weights (from death = 0 to healthy = 1) to patients surviving the MI but sustaining morbid events over time such as nonfatal stroke (utility of 0.79) or reinfarction (utility of 0.93). These utility weights were taken from the literature, based on preference measurements undertaken in the GISSI-2 trial.[31] However, given the small differences between treatment groups in risk of morbid events that receive quality adjustment in survival, although the total number of future QALYs is fewer than unadjusted life-years at 8.842 for streptokinase and 8.926 for tPA, the difference in QALYs (0.084), using 30-day GUSTO survival data, is almost identical to the effect calculated by Mark et al[2] using unadjusted life expectancy.

In summary, both studies use the efficacy data from the GUSTO trial as their starting point to conclude that tPA treatment is more costly than that with streptokinase—but that it provides an increase in survival (quality-adjusted or otherwise). Table 2F-11, using the data from Mark et al,[2] illustrates the next calculation in both studies that determines the incremental cost-effectiveness ratio for tPA. After discounting future costs and effects at 5% per year to reflect time preference (for rationale, see our first paper[32]), the difference (ie, tPA minus streptokinase) in cost per patient over the year (and, by extension, into the future because they assume no cost differences beyond 1 year) is $2710, which is divided by the difference in life expectancy per patient (0.0829) to yield a ratio of $32,678 per year of life gained.

A simple interpretation of this ratio is that it is the price at which we are buying additional years of life by using tPA in preference to streptokinase; the lower this price, the more attractive is the use of tPA. The Kalish et al study[3] reaches a similar incremental cost-effectiveness ratio (with their adjusted denominator of QALYs and using the 30-day risk reduction GUSTO data) of $30,300 per QALY. These are the main results of the studies; we will discuss their interpretation later in this section.

## Do Incremental Costs and Effects Differ Between Subgroups?

In an editorial accompanying the GUSTO economic analysis, Lee[33] stresses that the cost-effectiveness of tPA depends on how the drug is administered and to whom it is given." The first point relates mainly to the fact that the GUSTO trial had a protocol for accelerated administration of tPA; slower regimens of administration of the same drug had previously shown no clinical advantage.[34] The second point is that because some patients (eg, the elderly) have a greater prior risk of mortality, the tPA treatment effect will likely yield a higher absolute risk reduction in mortality.[1]

This second point has important implications for cost-effectiveness, as can be seen in Table 2F-12, which presents cost per life-year estimates among eight subgroups on the basis of infarction site and patient age. Because the baseline risk of mortality in MI varies by age and infarction site, the mortality benefit from treatment with tPA also varies, and it is clear from Table 2F-12 that tPA is more cost-effective in older patients with anterior infarcts. To take two extreme cases, the cost per life-year gained in a person aged 40 years or less with an inferior infarct is $203,071, compared to a person aged 75 years or more with an anterior infarct at only $13,410 per life-year gained.

**TABLE 2F-12**

### Incremental Cost-Effectiveness of Tissue-Type Plasminogen Activator vs Streptokinase in Patient Subgroups*

| | Cost (in US Dollars) Per Life-Year Gained by Age Subgroup (Years) | | | |
| --- | --- | --- | --- | --- |
| | ≤ 40 | 41–60 | 61–75 | >75 |
| Inferior myocardial infarction | 203,071 | 74,816 | 27,873 | 16,246 |
| Anterior myocardial infarction | 123,609 | 49,877 | 20,601 | 13,410 |

\* Data from the GUSTO Investigators.[1]
Data from reference 2.

## How Much Does Allowance for Uncertainty Change the Results?

Uncertainty in economic evaluation can arise either from lack of precision in estimation or from methodologic controversy. The conventional way of allowing for uncertainty in economic analyses is to undertake a *sensitivity analysis,* where the estimates for key variables are altered to assess what impact they have on study results (see Part 1F, "Moving From Evidence to Action").

In addition, conducting economic evaluations concurrently with clinical trials provides the opportunity to apply conventional tests of statistical significance to the resource quantities or costs.[35] Also, where measurements from a clinical trial inform us of the distribution of cost variables, it is possible to set the range of estimates for sensitivity analysis in relation to the statistical properties of the distribution (eg, two standard deviations from the mean). This raises a number of important issues, such as the size of the "economically important difference" when comparing the cost or cost-effectiveness of two alternatives, and the appropriateness of and methods for statistical tests on cost-effectiveness ratios.

Because economic evaluation methods are in their infancy compared with those for randomized trials, investigators still debate many issues.[36] These include the appropriateness of alternative methods for valuing outcomes, the appropriateness of considering some types of consequences (eg, the costs of lost production if individuals are away from work because of illness), and the choice of discount rate.

A useful starting point for a sensitivity analysis is to examine the impact of variation in the effectiveness measure on the cost-effectiveness estimated. For instance, investigators may assume the smallest possible estimate of a treatment effect. Ideally, such an estimate would come from the lower boundary of the confidence interval generated in a meta-analysis of available randomized trials (see Part 2B2, "Therapy and Understanding the Results, Confidence Intervals"). Investigators then examine the impact on cost-effectiveness of assuming an appreciably and plausibly smaller treatment effect.

For instance, Mark et al[2] note that, although the point estimate of the tPA treatment effect was a 1.1% increase in 1-year survival, the 95% confidence interval ranged from 0.46% to 1.74%. Applying this variation to the denominator of the incremental cost-effectiveness ratio, Mark et al[2] report a range of $71,039 per life-year gained to $18,781 around their baseline estimate of $32,678, with smaller benefit yielding a higher ratio. Both studies conclude that their estimates of cost-effectiveness are most sensitive to uncertainty in the magnitude of mortality benefit. In other words, society will have to pay more for the mortality reduction if the effect is smaller.

This particular analysis, however, only partially captures the uncertainty in the cost-effectiveness ratio because it assumes the numerator (eg, the cost) does not vary. Investigators are currently developing more formal procedures for estimating confidence intervals for cost-effectiveness ratios that permit both the numerator and the denominator to vary.[30] Both the Mark et al[2] and Kalish et al[3] papers report extensive additional sensitivity analyses, many of which relate to different methodologic choices (eg, the source of cost estimates) rather than to observed variability in the data.

# HOW CAN I APPLY THE RESULTS TO PATIENT CARE?

Having established the results of the two economic studies and the precision of the estimates, we now turn to two important issues of interpretation. The first is how incremental cost-effectiveness ratios can be interpreted to help in decision making; the second is the extent to which the cost and/or effects from the study can be applied to your practice setting.

## Are the Treatment Benefits Worth the Risks and Costs?

In Figure 2F-7 we present a framework for categorizing economic study results. This 3 x 3 matrix contains nine cells categorizing studies depending on whether the new treatment is more costly than, less costly than, or of equivalent cost to that of the control, and whether it is more effective, less effective, or equally effective.

**FIGURE 2F-7**

### Categorizing Economic Study Results

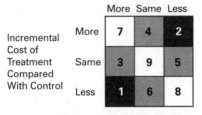

Incremental Effectiveness of
Treatment Compared With Control

|  | More | Same | Less |
|---|---|---|---|
| Incremental Cost of Treatment Compared With Control — More | 7 | 4 | 2 |
| Same | 3 | 9 | 5 |
| Less | 1 | 6 | 8 |

■ Strong Dominance for Decision
  1 = Accept Treatment
  2 = Reject Treatment

▨ Weak Dominance for Decision
  3 = Accept Treatment
  4 = Reject Treatment
  5 = Reject Treatment
  6 = Accept Treatment

☐ Nondominance; No Obvious Decisions
  7 = Is Added Effect Worth Added Cost to Adopt Treatment?
  8 = Is Reduced Effect Acceptable Given Reduced Cost to Accept Treatment?
  9 = Neutral on Cost and Effects—Other Reasons to Accept Treatment?

Nine possible outcomes arising in the comparison of treatment control in terms of incremental cost and incremental effectiveness.

In category 1, the new treatment is both less costly and more effective than control, so the new treatment is said to be strongly dominant. For example, treatment to eradicate *Helicobacter pylori* for duodenal ulcer is strongly dominant over acid suppression with a histamine-2-receptor antagonist because it both is less costly and results in fewer recurrences of ulcer over a 1-year period.[37] Category 2 represents strong dominance to reject a new therapy where the costs are higher and the effectiveness is worse than that seen with control. Four cases of so-called weak dominance follow, where either costs or effectiveness are equivalent between the two therapies: category 3, indicating weak dominance to accept the treatment (equivalent cost but better effectiveness), and category 4, indicating weak dominance to reject the treatment (greater cost with equivalent effectiveness). Similarly, categories 5 and 6 indicate weak dominance to reject and accept, respectively.

All of the shaded cells in Figure 2F-7 indicate comparative cost and effectiveness combinations that provide evidence of strong or weak dominance. To inform decision making, no further analysis, such as calculation of cost-effectiveness ratios, is required for these shaded cells. However, further analysis is needed if results fall into the nondominance, unshaded cells of 7, 8, or 9. First, it may be that the treatment is associated with no statistically significant or clinically important difference in either effectiveness or cost, although it should be noted that the process of implementation and change of programs will generate costs not captured in the analysis. The most common nondominance circumstance is category 7 (or its mirror image in category 8), where the new therapy offers additional effectiveness but at an increased cost. Both tPA studies fall within category 7, requiring calculation of the incremental cost-effectiveness ratios of the new therapy, as discussed above and as illustrated in Table 2F-11.

Having estimated the incremental cost-effectiveness of tPA over streptokinase, and assuming for the moment that these data apply to your practice setting, how do you decide whether approximately $33,000 is an acceptable price to pay for saving 1 additional year of life? The first important point to note is that this question involves a value judgment and cannot be resolved using only the study data. As noted in the conclusion of the GUSTO economic analysis, the study data can inform the decision but cannot make the choice. Some appeal must be made to external criteria to ascertain whether a jurisdiction or society is willing to pay this price for this improvement in outcome.

There are a number of approaches to the interpretation of incremental cost-effectiveness ratios. In an ideal world of complete information, we would have data indicating the health (or other) outcomes we would be forgoing from other interventions and programs, within and outside health care, not funded as a consequence of using tPA (the *opportunity cost* of tPA administration). Since data to accomplish this task are very limited, investigators have promulgated a variety of second-best interpretive strategies. One approach assumes that previous decisions to adopt new medical therapies of known cost-effectiveness reveal an underlying set of values with which to judge the acceptability of the current treatment candidate. Both of our two tPA cost-effectiveness studies use this interpretive strategy to assess their $30,000 per life-year estimates; both cite the cost-effectiveness of two to three other interventions, some noncardiac, that are currently funded; and both conclude that an acceptable cost-effectiveness threshold would be $50,000 per QALY gained (for Kalish et al[3]) and per life-year gained (for Mark et al[2]).

Investigators have debated the validity of such interpretive strategies for incremental cost-effectiveness ratios at both a theoretical[38,39] and a practical[40] level. For example, although Johannesson and Weinstein[38] maintain that prioritizing resource allocations based on rank orderings of interventions by incremental cost-effectiveness does lead to an efficient allocation of resources, not all health economists agree.[34] Most would agree that there are practical problems of comparisons between cost-effectiveness studies that may have used very different methods, data, and assumptions.[35]

In summary, we should exercise caution when drawing conclusions from incremental cost-effectiveness ratios. The ultimate criterion is one of local opportunity cost: If the money for a new program will result in decreased ability to deliver other health care interventions, what are the health benefits you will no longer realize in order to have tPA available for all? The practical difficulty in applying this criterion is that many existing programs or services currently provided may not have been evaluated. Therefore, the opportunity cost of reducing or removing them is unknown or speculative.

## Can I Expect Similar Costs in My Setting?

If costs or consequences differ in your setting, the cost-effectiveness/utility/benefit ratios from the study will not apply. We deal with issues of whether you can antici- pate the same consequences of treatment in detail in Part 2B3, "Therapy and Applying the Results, Applying Results to Individual Patients" and will focus here on costs. Applying those criteria here to the analyses of tPA vs streptokinase, we note that both economic studies used data from the large, simple, GUSTO trial,[1] in which the inclusion and exclusion criteria were sufficiently broad that patients likely reflect the mix of those suffering an acute MI in many settings. There are, however, some concerns with applicability.

Kalish et al[3] note doubt as to whether "the results achieved in the GUSTO trial are possible in actual practice, largely due to the small time delay between symp- tom onset and treatment in this trial."[29,41] The benefit of tPA in the GUSTO trial was seen primarily among patients treated within 4 hours of symptom onset,[1] and the majority of patients who have acute MI in the United States are not treated within 4 hours.[42] Another issue is whether the GUSTO efficacy data are applicable to centers outside of the US. The GUSTO trial enrolled patients from 15 different countries; the majority of these patients (56%) were recruited from the United States. United States patients were managed differently from non-US patients in a number of ways, including greater use of invasive revascularization such as PTCA and CABG, and greater use of nonprotocol medications such as antiarrhythmic agents and calcium antagonists.[43] Although mortality reduction with accelerated tPA vs streptokinase was greater in the United States (1.2% absolute decrease vs 0.7% elsewhere), this difference proved easily attributable to the play of chance ($P = .30$). In other words, if the truth were that there was no difference between the United States and other countries, differences as or greater than 1.2% vs 0.7% would be found in 30% of similar trials (see Part 2B2, "Therapy and Understanding the Results, Hypothesis Testing"). Thus, the results provide little support for the hypothesis of a different effect across countries (see Part 2E, "Summarizing the Evidence, When to Believe a Subgroup Analysis").

In considering the transferability of cost estimates between jurisdictions (such as countries, states, regions, or even, sometimes, cities), remember that the cost of a treatment is the summation of the product of physical resources consumed (eg, drugs and tests) and their unit prices. We have noted earlier how cost data may not transfer well between jurisdictions because of differing organization of practice and because of differing local prices. To address these points, a good economic evaluation should report resource use and prices separately so that a reader can ascertain whether practice patterns and prices apply to their jurisdiction. The eco- nomic analysis by Mark et al[2] gives detailed reporting of resources and prices so the reader can judge whether, for example, the 73% rate of cardiac catheterization, 31% rate of PTCA, and the 13% rate of CABG are applicable to their institution.

The GUSTO economic analysis was undertaken only on the US patients from the multinational trial and, as we have noted, the intensity of resource use was lower in other countries. Such resource use differences reflect a number of factors, including availability of resources and financial incentives to health care physicians and hospitals. For example, the length of hospital stay was significantly lower in US hospitals than in non-US hospitals (8 vs 10 days; $P < .001$), despite a greater incidence of complications among US patients. This difference likely reflects downward pressure exerted on length of stay in the United States by the prospective payment system to hospitals based on diagnosis-related groups. The greater use of invasive revascularization and medications in the United States, and the shorter hospital stay, will result in different total costs than those of other countries. On the other hand, it is possible that, if differences are applied equally to both groups, the intercountry resource use differences may have a limited impact on differences in incremental costs.

The results of the GUSTO economic analysis[2] are clearly dependent upon the relative prices of tPA and streptokinase; furthermore, we know that these relative drug prices vary among countries. For example, if the drug costs were those typical in Europe (approximately $1000 for 100 mg of tPA and $200 for 1.5 million units of streptokinase), the cost-effectiveness ratio would be $13,943 per year of life saved.

Finally, countries (or social, cultural, or political groups within countries) may differ with respect to the value they place on health benefits vs other commodities. There is no reason why $50,000 per life-year as an acceptable cost-effectiveness threshold for the United States is applicable to, say, a less-industrialized country where the opportunity cost of such resources will be much higher. The governments of various countries vary in their willingness to pay for health and health care.

# CLINICAL RESOLUTION

Returning to our opening clinical scenario and referring to the framework in Figure 2F-7, both tPA cost-effectiveness studies indicate that tPA is not dominant over streptokinase but falls within category 7, implying that a trade-off between increased effectiveness at increased cost needs to be resolved. Since the effectiveness, resource use, and price data are applicable to your hospital, you inform the committee that the analyses you have reviewed can help inform their decision but that they must make the choice and decide which cost-effectiveness threshold is acceptable. You help frame this choice as one of local opportunity cost: By diverting resources to tPA, what health benefits will be forgone from other treatments or programs no longer funded?

The committee decides that universal use of tPA in all MI cases will divert resources from other health-producing programs in the hospital (although the benefits of these programs have not been as clearly documented as the new program). The committees decides that tPA should be used selectively based on the cost-effectiveness evidence in Table 2F-12 and should involve adoption of the cutpoint of $50,000 per life year suggested by Mark et al.[2] The committee determines that the preferred clinical strategy in their hospital is streptokinase in patients aged less than 60 years with an inferior infarct and patients aged 40 years or less with an anterior infarct; all other patients would receive tPA. In making this recommendation, however, the committee recognizes that the optimal choice may differ in individual patients. For instance, among higher-risk patients in whom tPA would generally be preferred, clinicians may best serve patients who view life after a severe stroke as worse than death by administering streptokinase.[44]

# References

1. The GUSTO Investigators. An international randomized trial comparing four thrombolytic strategies for acute myocardial infarction. *N Engl J Med*. 1993;329:673-682.

2. Mark DB, Hlatky MA, Califf RM, et al. Cost effectiveness of thrombolytic therapy with tissue plasminogen activator as compared with streptokinase for acute myocardial infarction. *N Engl J Med*. 1995;332:1418-1424.

3. Kalish SC, Gurwitz JH, Krumholz HM, Avorn J. A cost-effectiveness model of thrombolytic therapy for acute myocardial infarction. *J Gen Intern Med*. 1995;10:321-330.

4. Castillo PA, Palmer CS, Halpern MT, Hatziandreu EJ, Gersh BJ. Cost-effectiveness of thrombolytic therapy for acute myocardial infarction. *Ann Pharmacother*. 1997;31:596-603.

5. Kellett J. Cost-effectiveness of accelerated tissue plasminogen activator for acute myocardial infarction. *Br J Med Econ*. 1996;10:341-359.

6. Eisenberg JM. Clinical economics: a guide to the economic analysis of clinical practices. *JAMA*. 1989;262:2879-2886.

7. Detsky AS, Naglie IG. A clinician's guide to cost-effectiveness analysis. *Ann Intern Med*. 1990;113:147-154.

8. Elixhauser A, Luce BR, Taylor WR, Reblando J. Health care CBA/CEA: an update on the growth and composition of the literature. *Med Care*. 1993;31:JS1-11, JS18-149.

9. Backhouse ME, Backhouse RJ, Edey SA. Economic evaluation bibliography. *Health Econ*. 1992;1:1-236.

10. O'Brien B, Levine M, Willan A, et al. Economic evaluation of outpatient treatment with low-molecular-weight heparin for proximal vein thrombosis. *Arch Intern Med*. 1999;159:2298-2304.

11. Hillman AL, Bloom BS. Economic effects of prophylactic use of misoprostol to prevent gastric ulcer in patients taking nonsteroidal anti-inflammatory drugs. *Arch Intern Med*. 1989;149:2061-2065.

12. Graham DY, Agrawal NM, Roth SH. Prevention of NSAID-induced gastric ulcer with misoprostol: multicentre, double-blind, placebo-controlled trial. *Lancet*. 1988;2:1277-1280.

13. Schulman KA, Lynn LA, Glick HA, Eisenberg JM. Cost effectiveness of low-dose zidovudine therapy for asymptomatic patients with human immunodeficiency virus (HIV) infection. *Ann Intern Med*. 1991;114:798-802.

14. Concorde Coordinating Committee. Concorde: MRC/ANRS randomised double-blind controlled trial of immediate and deferred zidovudine in symptom-free HIV infection. *Lancet*. 1994;343:871-881.

15. Hill SR, Mitchell AS, Henry DA. Problems with the interpretation of pharmaco-economic analyses: a review of submissions to the Australian Pharmaceutical Benefits Scheme. *JAMA*. 2000;283:2116-2121.

16. O'Brien B. Economic evaluation of pharmaceuticals: Frankenstein's monster or vampire of trials? *Med Care*. 1996;34:DS99-DS108.

17. Ubel PA. The unbearable rightness of bedside rationing. In: *Pricing Life: Why It's Time for Health Care Rationing*. Cambridge, MA: MIT Press; 2000.

18. Mehrez A, Gafni A. Quality-adjusted life years, utility theory, and healthy-years equivalents. *Med Decis Making*. 1989;9:142-149.

19. Topol EJ, Burek K, O'Neill WW, et al. A randomized controlled trial of hospital discharge three days after myocardial infarction in the era of reperfusion. *N Engl J Med*. 1988;318:1083-1088.

20. Weisbrod BA, Test MA, Stein LI. Alternative to mental hospital treatment, II: economic benefit-cost analysis. *Arch Gen Psychiatry*. 1980;37:400-405.

21. Oster G, Epstein AM. Cost-effectiveness of antihyperlipemic therapy in the prevention of coronary heart disease: the case of cholestyramine. *JAMA*. 1987;258:2381-2387.

22. Goldman L, Sia ST, Cook EF, Rutherford JD, Weinstein MC. Costs and effectiveness of routine therapy with long-term beta-adrenergic antagonists after acute myocardial infarction. *N Engl J Med*. 1988;319:152-157.

23. Finkler SA. The distinction between cost and charges. *Ann Intern Med*. 1982;96:102-109.

24. Cohen DJ, Breall JA, Ho KK, et al. Economics of elective coronary revascularization: comparison of costs and charges for conventional angioplasty, directional atherectomy, stenting and bypass surgery. *J Am Coll Cardiol*. 1993;22:1052-1059.

25. Weinstein MC, Stason WB. Foundations of cost-effectiveness analysis for health and medical practices. *N Engl J Med*. 1977;296:716-721.

26. Gold MR, Siegel JE, Russell LB, Weinstein MC, eds. *Cost-Effectiveness in Health and Medicine*. Oxford: Oxford University Press; 1966.

27. Parsonage M, Neuburger H. Discounting and health benefits. *Health Econ*. 1992;1:71-76.

28. Cairns J. Discounting and health benefits: another perspective. *Health Econ*. 1992;1:76-79.

29. Torrance GW, Feeny D. Utilities and quality-adjusted life years. *Int J Technol Assess Health Care*. 1989;5:559-575.

30. Mehrez A, Gafni A. The healthy-years equivalents: how to measure them using the standard gamble approach. *Med Decis Making*. 1991;11:140-146.

31. Glasziou PP, Bromwich S, Simes RJ. Quality of life six months after myocardial infarction treated with thrombolytic therapy. AUS-TASK Group. Australian arm of International tPA/SK Mortality Trial. *Med J Aust*. 1994;161:532-536.

32. Drummond MF, Richardson WS, O'Brien BJ, Levine M, Heyland D. Users' guides to the medical literature, XIII: how to use an article on economic analysis of clinical practice. A. Are the results of the study valid? Evidence-Based Medicine Working Group. *JAMA*. 1997;277:1552-1557.

33. Lee TH. Cost effectiveness of tissue plasminogen activator. *N Engl J Med*. 1995;332:1443-1444.

34. Ridker PM, O'Donnell C, Marder VJ, Hennekens CH. Large-scale trials of thrombolytic therapy for acute myocardial infarction: GISSI-2, ISIS-3, and GUSTO-1. *Ann Intern Med*. 1993;119:530-532.

35. O'Brien BJ, Drummond MF, Labelle RJ, Willan A. In search of power and significance: issues in the design and analysis of stochastic cost-effectiveness studies in health care. *Med Care*. 1994;32:150-163.

36. Udvarhelyi IS, Colditz GA, Rai A, Epstein AM. Cost-effectiveness and cost-benefit analyses in the medical literature: are the methods being used correctly? *Ann Intern Med*. 1992;116:238-244.

37. O'Brien B, Goeree R, Mohamed AH, Hunt R. Cost-effectiveness of *Helicobacter pylori* eradication for the long-term management of duodenal ulcer in Canada. *Arch Intern Med*. 1995;155:1958-1964.

38. Johannesson M, Weinstein MC. On the decision rules of cost-effectiveness analysis. *J Health Econ*. 1993;12:459-467.

39. Birch S, Gafni A. Changing the problem to fit the solution: Johannesson and Weinstein's (mis) application of economics to real world problems. *J Health Econ*. 1993;12:469-476.

40. Drummond M, Torrance G, Mason J. Cost-effectiveness league tables: more harm than good? *Soc Sci Med*. 1993;37:33-40.

41. Ridker PM, O'Donnell C, Marder V, Hennekens CH. A response to "Holding GUSTO up to the light." *Ann Intern Med*. 1994;120:882-885.

42. Ridker PM, Manson JE, Goldhaber SZ, Hennekens CH, Buring JE. Comparison of delay times to hospital presentation for physicians and nonphysicians with acute myocardial infarction. *Am J Cardiol*. 1992;70:10-13.

43. Van de Werf F, Topol EJ, Lee KL, et al. Variations in patient management and outcomes for acute myocardial infarction in the United States and other countries. Results from the GUSTO trial. Global Utilization of Streptokinase and Tissue Plasminogen Activator for Occluded Coronary Arteries. *JAMA.* 1995;273:1586-1591.

44. Heyland DK, Gafni A, Levine MA. Do potential patients prefer tissue plasminogen activator (TPA) over streptokinase (SK)? An evaluation of the risks and benefits of TPA from the patient's perspective. *J Clin Epidemiol.* 2000;53:888-894.

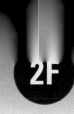

# MOVING FROM EVIDENCE TO ACTION

## Clinical Utilization Review

C. David Naylor and Gordon Guyatt

## IN THIS SECTION

# CLINICAL SCENARIO

## Are Cardiologists Performing Unnecessary PTCAs?

It is February 1996 and you are a general internist attending a medical advisory committee meeting as the newly appointed chief of staff in a large community hospital affiliated with a major health maintenance organization. A junior administrator presents data showing that the hospital's use of percutaneous transluminal coronary angioplasty (PTCA) is high, relative to similarly sized centers with a comparable number of invasive cardiologists. He insinuates that cardiologists are performing unnecessary PTCAs. The cardiologists present are infuriated, and the meeting degenerates into a shouting match. After the hospital chief executive officer brings the meeting back to order, you and the chief of cardiology agree to research the matter independently and report back in 1 week.

# FINDING THE EVIDENCE

Raw utilization data are insufficient to assess whether cardiologists at your hospital are using PTCA inappropriately. You must review their practice in light of criteria for deciding whether each application of PTCA was likely, given a balance of risks and benefits, to be in the patient's best interest. Using MEDLINE on CD-ROM, you search from 1991 to November 1995. The MeSH subject heading, "Angioplasty, Transluminal, Percutaneous Coronary," yields 2052 citations even after the search is limited to "human" and "English language" with an abstract on file. You then try "Guideline" or "practice guideline" as key words. The relevant guideline references look useful for informing a practitioner's decisions, but you cannot readily see how to translate them into criteria for auditing individual charts.

Finally, you combine PTCA with "utilization review" as a MeSH heading, and two references turn up. The abstract of one article looks directly relevant. Carried out by researchers with the RAND Corporation, the study used explicit criteria to assess the appropriateness of PTCA for 1306 randomly selected patients in 15 randomly selected New York State hospitals.[1] The investigators performed a retrospective medical record audit—similar to what you envisage may be necessary for your hospital. However, you also note that the records were drawn from 1990, raising a concern that the criteria may be outdated. Auditors rated 58% of PTCAs appropriate; 38%, uncertain; and 4%, inappropriate. The inappropriate rate varied by hospital from 1% to 9% ($P = .12$), while the uncertain rate ranged from 26% to 50% ($P = .02$). Judging from this article, your hospital would have a defensible profile if its rate of apparently inappropriate PTCA was less than 10%. But are the criteria developed by the RAND investigators valid or easily applied?

# APPROACHES TO REVIEWING A UTILIZATION REVIEW

Investigators often publish evidence about clinical management strategies in meta-analyses (see Part 1E, "Summarizing the Evidence") and recommendations for action follow in decision analyses or practice guidelines (see Part 1F, "Moving From Evidence to Action"). Meta-analyses synthesize multiple research studies, and decision analyses and practice guidelines suggest what a practitioner ought to do. However, actual practice sometimes differs from what the evidence appears to mandate, raising concerns about quality of care. Quality concerns, together with the omnipresent focus on cost containment, have led a growing cadre of researchers, insurers, administrators, and policymakers to examine what clinicians do. Their examinations may focus on outcomes, but it is not easy to determine whether an adverse outcome was due to some aspect of the care provided or attributable to the patient's clinical situation (see Part 2B, "Therapy and Harm, Outcomes of Health Services"). Indeed, even exemplary care may be associated with bad outcomes if the patient's prognosis is inherently poor. Thus, it is often more straightforward and valid to assess processes of care—the topic of this article.

In assessing clinical processes—that is, conducting a clinical utilization review—researchers and managers seek to determine whether the right service is provided to the right type of patient for the right reasons at the right time and place. The assessment may rely on expert opinion offered without explicit criteria—what one might call implicit reviews—trusting the individualized judgments of expert clinicians. Practitioners can then be assured that someone who understands the clinical world and its exigencies is appraising their work.

Unfortunately, lack of standardization renders implicit reviews unreliable.[2,3] Explicit criteria, which form the basis for most clinical utilization reviews in the literature, have the advantages of standardization and consistency, as well as transparency. Where necessary, trained staff can apply the criteria retrospectively to medical records without a major time commitment from clinicians. Such criteria may nonetheless have a weak basis in evidence, be applied in a biased or imprecise fashion, or be impractical for use in a particular practice setting. In this section we will assist clinicians in either one of two related goals: to critique a paper purporting to measure the quality of care delivered in a particular setting, and to decide whether, in conducting a utilization review, they should emulate the methods or borrow the tools used in a published study.

In the following discussion, we use the American term, *utilization review*, and the British term, *clinical audit*, interchangeably to describe this type of process-of-care assessment. We refer to *panelists* as members of the group of clinical experts that helps establish the explicit review criteria, and *auditors* as those who review patient charts or interview patients and/or physicians to obtain the information needed to apply the criteria.

We modified the basic questions used in earlier Users' Guides to consider three issues: are the criteria valid? were the criteria applied appropriately? can you use the criteria in your own practice? (See Table 2F-13.)

**TABLE 2F-13**

## Users' Guides for Appraising and Applying the Results of a Utilization Review

**Are the Criteria Valid?**

- Is there a systematic review and summary of evidence linking options to outcomes for each relevant question?
- If necessary, was an explicit, systematic, and reliable process used to tap expert opinion?
- Is there an explicit, systematic specification of values or preferences?
- If the quality of the evidence used in originally framing the criteria was weak, have the criteria themselves been correlated with patient outcomes?

**Were the Criteria Applied Appropriately?**

- Was the process of applying the criteria reliable, unbiased, and likely to yield robust conclusions?
- What is the impact of uncertainty associated with evidence and values on the criteria-based ratings of process of care?

**How Can I Apply the Criteria to Patient Care?**

- Are the criteria relevant to your practice setting?
- Have the criteria been field-tested for feasibility of use in diverse settings, including settings similar to yours?

# ARE THE CRITERIA VALID?

For process-of-care criteria to be valid, the criteria must have a direct link either to improving health or to lowering resource use without compromising health outcomes. Rather than presenting guidelines to help practitioners make clinical decisions, process-of-care criteria constitute guidelines for others to use in assessing whether a practitioner made the right decision. Despite this different focus, the questions for appraising the validity of criteria for a utilization review are similar to those one should use to assess a practice guideline or decision analysis (see Part 1F, "Moving From Evidence to Action").

## Is There a Systematic Review and Summary of Evidence Linking Options to Outcomes for Each Relevant Question?

Criteria elsewhere in this book (see Part 1E, "Summarizing the Evidence") provide guides for deciding whether the authors used explicit and rigorous methods to identify, select, and combine available evidence. How does the PTCA audit mentioned in the opening scenario of this section measure up? Reading the full article, you see at once that the authors describe some of the methods in a companion article on coronary artery bypass graft (CABG) surgery.[4] The investigators undertook a systematic literature review, with a comprehensive search and analysis of risks and benefits of PTCA in various patient subgroups.[1,4] The full literature review on PTCA is a separate background document, with explicit inclusion and exclusion criteria.[5] Like an iceberg, guidelines and clinical audit criteria often represent a visible tip that is supported by a large literature review that most journals do not wish to publish, and which most clinicians will not want to read. Thus, as is the case here, you will sometimes have to rely on a description of how the literature was assembled and distilled.

Any decision about whether a clinician has delivered quality care is only as strong as the evidentiary basis of the criteria, which may vary from blinded randomized trials with complete follow-up to weak observational studies. Are the key indications for the service covered by trial evidence, or must observational evidence, inference, and expert opinion provide support for review criteria? The need to fall back on the latter, weaker evidence reduces the validity of audit criteria.

The PTCA example is germane here. The RAND group highlights that at the time they conducted their work no randomized-trial evidence of PTCA vs alternative therapies existed for stable angina.[1] However, their literature review runs only to 1990.[1,5] Investigators have conducted many trials of PTCA vs CABG since then, and a literature search produces citations to articles reporting on one randomized trial of PTCA vs medical therapy in stable single-vessel disease,[6] and four of PTCA vs CABG published in 1993 and 1994.[7-10] This newer evidence highlights that any audit criteria must be up-to-date, as what is optimal practice at one time may be malpractice a short time later. Investigators could now create stronger criteria based on the higher-quality evidence available from these randomized trials.

### If Necessary, Was an Explicit, Systematic, and Reliable Process Used to Elicit Expert Opinion?

When investigators rely on expert opinion to help frame criteria, they should use an explicit process for selecting panelists, and a sensible, systematic method for collating the judgments of the experts. The RAND group uses an original[11] and widely emulated multispecialty panel process that the PTCA report and companion paper on CABG clearly outline.[1,4] Specifically, nominations of recognized experts by national specialty societies provided the basis for choosing a group of nine panelists on PTCA from different geographic areas of the United States, academic and private practice, and different specialties (eg, cardiac surgeons, interventional and noninterventional cardiologists, and internists).[4] Each panelist independently rates hundreds of different case scenarios on a risk-benefit scale, and each of these scenarios describes a potential indication for the procedure or clinical service in question. After the panelists review patterns of interpanelist agreement presented anonymously, the panelists rerate the scenarios at a panel meeting. The final set of panelists' ratings then determines whether a given indication is deemed potentially appropriate, uncertain, or inappropriate. Given the limited evidence from randomized trials, it seems reasonable that the panelists graded the appropriateness of PTCA as "uncertain" for 38% of the patients whose records they audited.[1]

A weakness of this method is that for any given clinical indication, the researchers never make clear whether the appropriateness ratings rested primarily on research evidence or inference, extrapolation, and opinion. On the other hand, the RAND methods compare favorably with those used to create other utilization review tools. For example, health care managers often apply various sets of diagnosis- and procedure-independent criteria to hospital records to determine whether initial or continued stay in an acute care setting is necessary. These criteria usually come, in the first instance, from implicit judgments of clinicians and utilization managers. One study found physician panels rejected from 28% to 74% of the verdicts reached by utilization review nurses using three of these instruments.[12] Nonetheless, with the diffusion of managed care, criteria such as these have an enormous and continuing impact on the lives of patients, families, and health professionals.

## Is There an Explicit, Appropriate Specification of Values or Preferences Associated With Outcomes?

The confusion of evidenced-based facts and values—by which we mean preferences exercised in trading off benefits and risks—in expert judgments is a recurrent issue in these exercises. Most treatment decisions involve trade-offs. The randomized trials of CABG vs PTCA highlight this issue. For example, PTCA has a slightly lower early mortality, along with lower initial costs and more rapid recovery from the procedure. Longer-term mortality data are similar, but patients who underwent CABG appear to achieve better symptom relief, have decreased use of medication, and require fewer subsequent procedures.[7-10] Panelists' ratings in the RAND study[1] presumably reflected these types of trade-offs, but we cannot be sure that patients themselves would make the same choices. This issue is especially important for uncertain indications, where patients' preferences must be given special weight. However, chart audits and concurrent reviews using explicit criteria do not lend themselves to capturing patients' preferences and values.

Indeed, studies of expert panels show that surgeons' ratings of surgical options are more favorable than physicians', and that medical generalists are more negative in procedural appropriateness ratings than medical specialists who do the procedure.[13-16] This again emphasizes that you should look for a clear description of how the panel was assembled along with the members' specialties and any organizations they are representing. Even when panels have similar practitioner profiles, the nationality of the panel markedly affects the criteria and the results of applying them to actual cases.[16,17] Perceptions of the values of different outcomes will continue to vary, but researchers should try to elucidate these issues whenever possible.

## If the Quality of the Evidence Used in Originally Framing the Criteria Was Weak, Have the Criteria Themselves Been Correlated With Patient Outcomes?

When audit criteria follow directly from evidence from randomized trials, clinicians can be confident of the link to outcomes. For example, systematic reviews of randomized trials of aspirin and beta-blocker use by patients following myocardial infarction have demonstrated mortality reduction.[18] Furthermore, these drugs are inexpensive and have few serious side effects. Therefore, an audit of prescribing practices after myocardial infarction that showed that patients without contraindications were not prescribed these medications would strongly suggest substandard practice.

When weaker evidence and expert opinion form the basis for criteria, investigators (and users) can strengthen the criteria by determining how outcomes correlate with adherence to the criteria. Are outcomes improved, or similar despite decreased costs? These studies are tantamount to assessing a therapeutic intervention and could be critically appraised using criteria we suggested in prior Users' Guides (see Part 1B1, "Therapy").[19, 20] For example, researchers might randomly allocate practices or practitioners to usual care vs a program of concurrent audit, focusing on the service(s) of interest.

Although the design is much weaker, the impact of utilization review criteria can also be assessed using so-called historical controls. Here one would compare patient experience before and after a program of audit or prospective case management is implemented. Yet another option is to determine whether patients meeting the criteria who do not undergo a procedure have poorer outcomes than those who receive the procedure as indicated.

For example, the RAND group assembled a cohort of 671 patients undergoing coronary angiography in six Los Angeles hospitals and followed them for a median of 2 years.[21] The investigators examined patients meeting panel criteria for revascularization. Those patients who did not undergo revascularization had significantly worse outcomes than those who received either PTCA or CABG.[21] In general, we suggest that clinicians should seek outcomes-based evidence to support the safety and/or effectiveness of various utilization review tools and managed care programs.

# WERE THE CRITERIA APPLIED APPROPRIATELY?

Audit criteria based on sound evidence can be poorly applied. This section may help clinicians to critique the published results of a utilization review undertaken for research purposes, or to apply audit criteria to their own practice setting.

### Was the Process of Applying the Criteria Reliable, Unbiased, and Likely to Yield Robust Conclusions?

Application of explicit process-of-care criteria often rests on data derived from retrospective chart reviews by professional auditors. Evidence of the reliability of these ratings (eg, if two or more auditors generate the same data from the same patients' records or if the findings agree with those of a reference auditor with proven expertise) should increase confidence in their findings (see Part 2C, "Diagnosis,

Measuring Agreement Beyond Chance"). Such reproducibility demands explicit definitions of the clinical variables incorporated into the criteria, eg, if PTCA is deemed appropriate for refractory unstable angina with one-vessel coronary disease, then there should be a clear definition of refractory unstable angina.

In the RAND study of PTCA in New York State hospitals,[1,4] the authors do not mention either the interauditor reliability of the chart review process or agreement with a criterion-standard abstractor. However, the process they used is well established, with good interabstractor reliability for other services.[22] A particular strength of the RAND process is a series of checks, wherein a nurse-specialist reviews the auditors' work, and trained physicians interpret information on key clinical details copied verbatim from the medical record.[1,4]

Standardization of explicit audit criteria and the drive for reliable work by abstractors exists in tension with a potential lack of responsiveness to mitigating clinical factors. Most utilization reviews, including the RAND PTCA study,[1,4] apply audit criteria as a screening test. To preclude false positives, experienced clinicians review cases in which the explicit review shows potential problems with the appropriateness of a service. However, this introduces more subjectivity into the audit, and raises the question as to why a sample of supposedly appropriate charts is not also reviewed for false negatives. There is no easy resolution of this tension.

As to potential biases in practice audits, these are more of a concern when implicit (nonsystematic) reviews are used in the audit. In such cases, auditors should be blinded to institutional or practitioner identity and to patient outcomes, as they are more likely to rate identical cases and care processes as inappropriate when there are severe adverse outcomes.[23] In this respect, it is unfortunate that some licensing and discipline bodies respond to complaints with unblinded implicit audits of the alleged problem practice without comparison samples from other practices. However, in explicit criteria-based audits, skewed sampling of practioners, hospitals, and patients can also introduce bias. The RAND investigators appropriately selected a random sample of both hospitals and patients for their PTCA study.

Last, it is crucial that investigators review enough cases to draw robust conclusions. In the PTCA study, auditors reviewed about 1500 charts.[1] Institutions had from 1% to 9% inappropriate procedures, but the investigators could not exclude chance as an explanation for the differences. Differences of this magnitude, if real, would be important to patients, payers, and policymakers. Thus, this sample size may have been insufficient for the investigators to detect important differences in quality among hospitals.

## What Is the Impact of Uncertainty Associated With Evidence and Values on the Criteria-Based Ratings of Process of Care?

Limitations of evidence and uncertainty about values may suggest different criteria for appropriateness, and investigators should examine the impact of these different criteria. This may be done in a number of ways. If panelists have disagreed, investigators might present alternative results based on ratings from both the harsher and more lenient raters. Alternatively, one could look at the implications of assuming that ratings of "uncertain" represent adequate, or inadequate, care. This examination of alternative ratings is a form of sensitivity analysis (see Part 1F, "Moving From Evidence to Action"). The RAND report on PTCA in New York[1] offers extensive sensitivity analyses including an exploration of how cases were placed in the uncertain category (eg, by explicit ratings of uncertain risk-benefit ratio; by being rated appropriate for revascularization rather than medical therapy, but with CABG preferred to PTCA; and by panelist disagreement).

# HOW CAN I APPLY THE CRITERIA TO PATIENT CARE?

Even if the criteria are adequate in terms of their validity, and clinicians are satisfied with their understanding of how they should ideally apply the criteria, it may not be reasonable or feasible to apply the criteria in a particular practice setting.

### Are the Criteria Relevant to Your Practice Setting and Culture?

Medical practice is always shaped by an amalgam of evidence, values, and circumstances. We noted earlier in this section that expert panels generate rather different sets of audit criteria in different countries. Although the task is difficult, clinicians should consider intangibles such as their local medical culture and practice circumstances before importing a particular set of audit criteria that may not be relevant. The stronger the evidence on which the criteria are based, the less clinicians need to consider local factors. For example, few medical cultures would reject a practical intervention that was definitively proven in a randomized trial to yield major reductions in all-cause mortality with relatively low toxicity and costs. With weaker evidence, however, the judgments are less straightforward. For example, it is unlikely that US patterns of PTCA utilization could be readily transplanted to the United Kingdom, with its tradition of comparative restraint in adopting invasive cardiovascular procedures.[16]

### Have the Criteria Been Field-Tested for Feasibility of Use in Diverse Settings, Including Settings Similar to Yours?

Even if criteria are sufficiently valid and relevant, feasibility issues may challenge implementation. For example, investigators applied the RAND criteria-based assessments of PTCA successfully in diverse hospital settings in New York,[1] but a highly skilled team of researchers and auditors did the work. Clinicians and managers will want to know how long it takes to train staff to use the criteria and the costs of available training programs. Costs per case for the audit must include training and labor charges, as well as any purchase charges for special audit forms. Clinicians must also decide whether or not to apply the criteria for concurrent case management. Errors associated with use of the criteria will have immediate consequences for individual patients and physicians in a managed care program, and the logistics of concurrent review can be daunting. Nonetheless, many busy hospitals already apply a wide range of concurrent utilization review criteria, as most practitioners, to their occasional frustration, know.

# CLINICAL RESOLUTION

This section provides an approach to critically appraising quality-of-care studies that focus on the process of delivering a service. We focused on methods that involve a blend of evidence and expert opinion or judgment, as these are widely applied in deriving utilization review criteria. However, on occasion, more straightforward approaches will be possible. As noted previously, one can draw on systematic reviews of randomized trials when the balance of benefits and risks is clear—what we elsewhere refer to as 1A recommendations to derive a set of strong criteria (see Part 1F, "Moving From Evidence to Action" and Part 2F, "Moving From Evidence to Action, Grading Recommendations—A Qualitative Approach"). One can then set aside other indications as resting in the gray zone of uncertainty where reasonable persons can disagree.[17] While this approach is simpler and less controversial, there are two problems with streamlined criteria. The first problem is that randomized trial evidence is often limited and may never become available for some procedures and clinical situations.[17,24] A commitment to evidence-based practice cannot preclude the reasonable use of clinical judgment, inference, and extrapolation.[17] The second problem is that trials are better at helping us decide what to do than what not to do. Expert panels, with all their limitations, do permit detailed assessments of inappropriate and uncertain indications.

At present, however, the proliferation of quality-of-care assessments has greatly outstripped the credible research in the field.[2,3] Despite the eager embrace of managed care, the measurement of quality of care remains difficult. Reliability of implicit assessments is low, while the available evidence for derivation of explicit criteria is often limited. Furthermore, the overall impact of these criteria on clinical behaviors, system costs, and patients' health outcomes is difficult to determine as they are seldom evaluated in formal prospective studies, and are often coupled with changes in practice organization and/or reimbursement that in themselves may change behavior.

The resolution of the scenario presented at the beginning of this section has you revisiting the library to obtain copies of articles describing the randomized studies of PTCA vs medical therapy and PTCA vs CABG that have appeared since 1990. You digest these articles with lunch at your desk in the following few days. At the next medical advisory committee meeting, you are prepared to discuss the RAND study on PTCA, as well as the new randomized trials.

However, the chief of cardiology speaks first. She informs the committee that she has been to the health records department and has visited colleagues at two area hospitals with different utilization statistics. She presents data showing that the discrepant utilization profile is almost completely attributable to urgent use of PTCA for acute myocardial infarction, which your hospital's cardiologists offer as an alternative to thrombolysis for patients presenting early after the onset of symptoms. Her literature search shows four relevant randomized trials.[25-28] The chief of cardiology rightly claims: "the trial evidence supports direct PTCA as a safe and effective alternative to intravenous thrombolysis when patients present early and are suitable candidates for emergency angioplasty."

The meeting briefly degenerates into a squabble over whether the administrator should apologize to the hospital's cardiologists, but the hospital CEO rescues his junior colleague by questioning whether the hospital can be cost-competitive if it relies more on PTCA than its neighboring institutions. Amid grumbles about the eternal bottom line from the other physicians present, you and the chief of cardiology volunteer each other to research the comparative costs of PTCA and thrombolysis for acute myocardial infarction.

# References

1. Hilborne LH, Leape LL, Bernstein SJ, et al. The appropriateness of use of percutaneous transluminal coronary angioplasty in New York State. *JAMA*. 1993;269:761-765.

2. Health Services Research Group. Quality of care, 1: what is quality and how can it be measured? *CMAJ*. 1992;146:2153-2158.

3. Health Services Research Group. Quality of care, 2: quality of care studies and their consequences. *CMAJ*. 1992;147:163-167.

4. Leape LL, Hilborne LH, Park RE, et al. The appropriateness of use of coronary artery bypass graft surgery in New York State. *JAMA*. 1993;269:753-760.

5. Hilborne LH, Leape LL, Kahan JP, Park RE, Kamberg CJ, Brook RH. *Percutaneous Transluminal Coronary Angioplasty: A Literature Review and Ratings of Appropriateness and Necessity.* Santa Monica, CA: RAND; 1991.

6. Parisi AF, Folland ED, Hartigan P, for the Veterans Affairs ACME Investigators. A comparison of angioplasty with medical therapy in the treatment of single-vessel coronary artery disease. *N Engl J Med*. 1992;326:10-16.

7. Hamm CW, Reimers J, Ischinger T, Rupprecht HJ, Berger J, Bleifeld W, for the German Angioplasty Bypass Surgery Investigation. A randomized study of coronary angioplasty compared with bypass surgery in patients with symptomatic multivessel coronary disease. *N Engl J Med*. 1994;331:1037-1043.

8. King SB III, Lembo NJ, Weintraub WS, et al, for the Emory Angioplasty versus Surgery Trial. A randomized trial comparing coronary angioplasty with coronary bypass surgery. *N Engl J Med*. 1994;331:1044-1050.

9. Coronary angioplasty versus coronary artery bypass surgery: the Randomized Intervention Treatment of Angina (RITA) trial. *Lancet*. 1993;341:573-580.

10. Rodriguez A, Boullon F, Perez-Balino N, Paviotti C, Liprandi MI, Palacios IF, for the ERACI Group. Argentine randomized trial of percutaneous transluminal coronary angioplasty versus coronary artery bypass surgery in multivessel disease (ERACI): in-hospital results and 1-year follow-up. *J Am Coll Cardiol*. 1993;22:1060-1067.

11. Brook RH, Chassin MR, Fink A, Solomon DH, Kosecoff J, Park RE. A method for the detailed assessment of the appropriateness of medical technologies. *Int J Technol Assess Health Care*. 1986;2:53-63.

12. Strumwasser I, Paranjpe NV, Ronis DL, Share D, Sell LJ. Reliability and validity of utilization review criteria. Appropriateness Evaluation Protocol, Standardized Medreview Instrument, and Intensity-Severity-Discharge criteria. *Med Care*. 1990;28:95-111.

13. Leape LL, Park RE, Kahan JP, Brook RH. Group judgments of appropriateness: the effect of panel composition. *Qual Assur Health Care*. 1992;4:151-159.

14. Fraser GM, Pilpel D, Hollis S, Kosecoff J, Brook RH. Indications for cholecystectomy: the results of a consensus panel approach. *Qual Assur Health Care*. 1993;5:75-80.

15. Kahn KL, Park RE, Brook RH, et al. The effect of comorbidity on appropriateness ratings for two gastrointestinal procedures. *J Clin Epidemiol*. 1988;41:115-122.

16. Brook RH, Kosecoff JB, Park RE, Chassin MR, Winslow CM, Hampton JR. Diagnosis and treatment of coronary disease: comparison of doctors' attitudes in the USA and the UK. *Lancet*. 1988;1:750-753.

17. Naylor CD. Grey zones of clinical practice: some limits to evidence-based medicine. *Lancet*. 1995;345:840-842.

18. Yusuf S, Wittes J, Friedman L. Overview of results of randomized clinical trials in heart disease, I: treatments following myocardial infarction. *JAMA*. 1988;260:2088-2093.

19. Guyatt GH, Sackett DL, Cook DJ, for the Evidence-Based Medicine Working Group. Users' guides to the medical literature, II: how to use an article about therapy or prevention. A: Are the results of the study valid? *JAMA*. 1993;270:2598-2601.

20. Guyatt GH, Sackett DL, Cook DJ, for the Evidence-Based Medicine Working Group. Users' guides to the medical literature, II: how to use an article about therapy or prevention. B: What were the results and will they help me in caring for my patients? *JAMA*. 1994;271:59-63.

21. Kravitz RL, Laouri M, Kahan JP, et al. Validity of criteria used for detecting underuse of coronary revascularization. *JAMA*. 1995;274:632-638.

22. Kahn KL, Kosecoff J, Chassin MR, et al. Measuring the clinical appropriateness of the use of a procedure. Can we do it? *Med Care*. 1988;26:415-422.

23. Caplan RA, Posner KL, Cheney FW. Effect of outcome on physician judgments of appropriateness of care. *JAMA*. 1991;265:1957-1960.

24. Fink A, Brook RH, Kosecoff J, Chassin MR, Solomon DH. Sufficiency of clinical literature on the appropriate uses of six medical and surgical procedures. *West J Med*. 1987;147:609-614.

25. Grines CL, Browne KF, Marco J, et al, for the Primary Angioplasty in Myocardial Infarction Study Group. A comparison of immediate angioplasty with thrombolytic therapy for acute myocardial infarction. *N Engl J Med*. 1993;328:673-679.

26. Zijlstra F, de Boer MJ, Hoorntje JC, Reiffers S, Reiber JH, Suryapranata H. A comparison of immediate coronary angioplasty with intravenous streptokinase in acute myocardial infarction. *N Engl J Med*. 1993;328:680-684.

27. Gibbons RJ, Holmes DR, Reeder GS, Bailey KR, Hopfenspirger MR, Gersh BJ, for the Mayo Coronary Care Unit and Catheterization Laboratory Groups. Immediate angioplasty compared with the administration of a thrombolytic agent followed by conservative treatment for myocardial infarction. *N Engl J Med*. 1993;328:685-691.

28. Ribeiro EE, Silva LA, Carneiro R, et al. Randomized trial of direct coronary angioplasty versus intravenous streptokinase in acute myocardial infarction. *J Am Coll Cardiol*. 1993;22:376-380.

# APPENDIX

## Calculations

Raymond Leung

## IN THIS SECTION

# TREATMENT AND HARM

(see *Part 1B1, "Therapy"; Part 1B2, "Harm"; Part 2B2, "Therapy and Understanding the Results, Measures of Association"*)

|  |  | Outcome | |
|---|---|---|---|
|  |  | **Present** | **Absent** |
| **Exposure/Treatment** | Present | a | b |
|  | Absent | c | d |

$$\text{Controlled Event Rate (CER)} \; = \; \frac{c}{(c + d)}$$

$$\text{Experimental Event Rate (EER)} \; = \; \frac{a}{(a + b)}$$

$$\text{Relative Risk (RR)} \; = \; \frac{a/(a + b)}{c/(c + d)}$$

$$\text{Relative Risk Reduction (RRR)} \; = \; 1 - RR$$

$$= \; \frac{c/(c + d) - a/(a + b)}{c/(c + d)}$$

$$\text{Absolute Risk Reduction (ARR)} \; = \; \frac{c}{c + d} - \frac{a}{a + b}$$

$$\text{Number Needed to Treat (NNT)} \; = \; \frac{1}{ARR}$$

$$\text{Odds Ratio (OR)} \; = \; \frac{a/b}{c/d} = \frac{ad}{cb}$$

Deriving number needed to treat from controlled event rate and odds ratio

$$NNT \; = \; \frac{1 - CER(1 - OR)}{CER(1 - CER)(1 - OR)}$$

Deriving number needed to harm from controlled event rate and odds ratio

$$NNH \; = \; \frac{1 + CER(1 - OR)}{CER(1 - CER)(1 - OR)}$$

# DIAGNOSIS

(see *Part 1C2, "Diagnostic Tests"*)

|  | | Reference Standard | |
|---|---|---|---|
|  | | **Positive** | **Negative** |
| **Test Result** | Positive | $a$ | $b$ |
|  | Negative | $c$ | $d$ |

$$\text{True Positive} = a$$

$$\text{True Negative} = d$$

$$\text{False Positive} = b$$

$$\text{False Negative} = c$$

$$\text{Sensitivity} = \frac{a}{a+c}$$

$$\text{Specificity} = \frac{d}{b+d}$$

$$\text{Likelihood Ratio for Positive Test (LR+)} = \frac{a/(a+c)}{b/(b+d)}$$

$$\text{Likelihood Ratio for Negative Test (LR--)} = \frac{c/(a+c)}{d/(b+d)}$$

$$\text{Positive Predictive Value (PPV)} = \frac{a}{a+b}$$

$$\text{Negative Predictive Value (NPV)} = \frac{d}{c+d}$$

$$\text{Diagnostic Accuracy} = \frac{a+d}{a+b+c+d}$$

$$\text{Pretest Probability (prevalence)} = \frac{a+c}{a+b+c+d}$$

$$\text{Pretest Odds} = \frac{prevalence}{1-prevalence} = \frac{a+c}{b+d}$$

$$\text{Posttest Odds} = \text{pretest odds} \times \text{likelihood ratio}$$

$$\text{Posttest Probability} = \text{posttest odds} / (1 + \text{posttest odds})$$

# CHANCE-CORRECTED AGREEMENT: KAPPA

(see *Part 2C, "Diagnosis, Measuring Agreement Beyond Chance"*)

|  |  | Rater B's Observation | |
|---|---|---|---|
|  |  | **Present** | **Absent** |
| **Rater A's Observation** | Present | a | b |
|  | Absent | c | d |

$$\text{Raw agreement} = \frac{a + d}{a + b + c + d}$$

$$\text{Kappa } (\kappa) = \frac{observed\ agreement - expected\ agreement}{1 - expected\ agreement}$$

$$\text{where observed agreement} = \frac{a + d}{a + b + c + d}$$

$$\text{and expected agreement} = \frac{(a + b)(a + c)}{a + b + c + d} + \frac{(c + d)(b + d)}{a + b + c + d}$$

$$\text{Odds Ratio (OR)} = \frac{ad}{bc}$$

$$\text{Phi } (\Phi) = \frac{\sqrt{OR} - 1}{\sqrt{OR} + 1} + \frac{\sqrt{ab} - \sqrt{bc}}{\sqrt{ad} + \sqrt{bc}}$$

# THRESHOLD NUMBER NEEDED TO TREAT (NNT)

(see *Part 2F, "Moving From Evidence to Action, Grading Recommendations—A Quantitative Approach"*)

$$NNT_T = \frac{Cost_{target} + value_{target}}{Cost_{treatment} + \Sigma(Cost_{AE})(Rate_{AE}) + \Sigma(Value_{AE})(Rate_{AE})}$$

Where

$NNT_T$      = the threshold number needed to treat

$Cost_{treatment}$    = the cost of treating one patient

$Cost_{target}$      = the cost of treating one target event

$Cost_{AE}$      = the cost of treating one adverse event

$Rate_{AE}$      = the proportion of treated patients who suffer an adverse event

$Value_{target}$     = the dollar value we assign to preventing one target event

$Value_{AE}$      = the dollar value we assign to preventing one adverse event

# CONFIDENCE INTERVALS

(see *Part 2B2, "Therapy and Understanding the Results, Confidence Intervals"*)

For the 2 x 2 sample set:

|       | Column 1 | Column 2 | Total |
|-------|----------|----------|-------|
| Row 1 | $a$      | $b$      | $c$   |
| Row 2 | $c$      | $d$      | $m$   |

the following confidence intervals can be calculated[1]:

| | Point Estimate | Confidence Intervals | Examples |
|---|---|---|---|
| Binomial proportion | $\dfrac{a}{n}$ | $\dfrac{a}{n} \pm z\sqrt{\dfrac{a(n-a)}{n^3}}$ | CER, EER, Sensitivity, Specificity, PPV, NPV |
| Difference between 2 proportions | $\dfrac{a}{n} - \dfrac{c}{m}$ | $\left(\dfrac{a}{n} - \dfrac{c}{m}\right) \pm z\sqrt{\dfrac{a(n-a)}{n^3} + \dfrac{c(m-c)}{m^3}}$ | ARR |
| Ratio between 2 proportions | $\dfrac{a/n}{c/m}$ | $\dfrac{a/n}{c/m} e^{\pm z\sqrt{\frac{1}{a} - \frac{1}{n} + \frac{1}{c} - \frac{1}{m}}}$ | RR, LR+, LR– |
| Ratio between 2 ratios | $\dfrac{a/b}{c/d}$ | $\dfrac{a/b}{c/d} e^{\pm z\sqrt{\frac{1}{a} + \frac{1}{b} + \frac{1}{c} + \frac{1}{d}}}$ | OR |

where $z = 1.96$ for 95% confidence intervals.

# Reference

1. SAS Institute Inc. SAS OnlineDoc, Version 8. Cary, NC: SAS Institute Inc; 1999. Availiable at: http://v8doc.sas.com/sashtml/. Accessed February 21, 2001.

# GLOSSARY

| Term | Definition | See Also |
|---|---|---|
| **Absolute Risk Increase (ARI)** | Difference in the absolute risk (percentage or proportion of patients with an outcome) in the exposed vs the unexposed. Typically used with a harmful exposure. | Absolute Risk Reduction (ARR); Number Needed to Harm (NNH) |
| **Absolute Risk Reduction (ARR)** | Difference in the absolute risk (percentage or proportion of patients with an outcome) in the exposed (experimental event rate [EER]) vs the unexposed (control event rate [CER]). Use restricted to a beneficial exposure or intervention. | Absolute Risk Increase (ARI); Number Needed to Treat (NNT); Risk |
| **Active Alternatives** | See *Differential Diagnosis* | |
| **Adjusted Analysis** | An adjusted analysis takes into account differences in prognostic factors between groups that may influence the outcome. For instance, in comparison between an experimental treatment and control, if the experimental group is on average older, and thus at higher risk of an adverse outcome, than the control group, the adjusted analysis will show a larger treatment effect than the unadjusted analysis. | Cox Regression Model |
| **Alerting Systems** | Alerting systems monitor a continuous signal or stream of data and generate a message (an alert) in response to items or patterns that might require action on the part of the clinician. | Reminder Systems |
| **Algorithm** | An explicit description of an ordered sequence of steps to be taken in patient care under specified circumstances. | |

| Term | Definition | See Also |
|------|-----------|----------|
| **Allocation Concealment** | Randomization is concealed if the person who is making the decision about enrolling a patient is unaware of whether the next patient enrolled will be entered in the treatment or control group. If randomization was not concealed, patients with better prognoses may tend to be preferentially enrolled in the active treatment arm resulting in exaggeration of the apparent benefit of therapy (or even falsely concluding that treatment is efficacious).<br><br>Used for *Concealment* | Blind |
| **Alpha Level** | The probability of erroneously concluding there is a difference between two treatments when there is in fact no difference. Typically, investigators decide on the chance of a false positive result they are willing to accept when they plan the sample size for a study. | |
| **Autocorrelation** | Autocorrelation occurs when the likelihood of an observation is not independent of its relationship with other observations. For example, autocorrelation occurs when a "good day" for a patient with chronic disease is more likely to follow a "good day" than a "bad day." | |
| **Baseline Risk** | The risk of an adverse outcome in the control group of an experiment. Synonymous with control event rate (CER). | |
| **Bayesian Analysis** | An analysis that starts with a particular probability of an event (the prior probability) and incorporates new information to generate a revised probability (a posterior probability). | |
| **Before-After Trial** | Investigation of an intervention in which the investigators compare the status of patients before and after the intervention. | Crossover Trial |
| **Bias** | A sytematic tendency to produce an outcome that differs from the underlying truth<br><br>a) **Channeling effect or Channeling bias:** The tendency of clinicians to prescribe treatment based on a patient's prognosis. As a result of the behavior, comparisons between treated and untreated patients will yield a biased estimate of treatment effect. | |

| Term | Definition | See Also |
|---|---|---|
| **Bias** (continued) | b) **Data completeness bias:** Using the information system to log episodes in the treatment group and using a manual system in the non-CDSS (computer decision support system) group can create a data completeness bias. | |
| | c) **Detection bias:** The tendency to look more carefully for an outcome in one of two groups being compared. | |
| | d) **Incorporation bias:** When investigators study a diagnostic test that incorporates features of the target outcome. | |
| | e) **Interviewer bias:** Greater probing by an interviewer in one of two groups being compared. | |
| | f) **Publication bias:** Publication bias occurs when the publication of research depends on the direction of the study results and whether they are statistically significant. | |
| | g) **Recall bias:** Recall bias occurs when patients who experience an adverse outcome have a different likelihood of recalling an exposure than the patients who do not have an adverse outcome, independent of the true extent of exposure. | |
| | h) **Surveillance bias:** Synonymous with detection bias; the tendency to look more carefully for an outcome in one of two groups being compared. | |
| | i) **Verification Bias:** Results of a diagnostic test influence whether patients are assigned to a treatment group. | |
| | Used for *Work-up Bias* | |
| **Blind** (or **Blinded** or **Masked**) | The participant of interest is unaware of whether patients have been assigned to the experimental or control group. Patients, clinicians, those monitoring outcomes, judicial assessors of outcomes, data analysts, and those writing the paper can all be blinded or masked. To avoid confusion the term *masked* is preferred in studies in which vision loss of patients is an outcome of interest. | Allocation Concealment |
| **Bootstrap Technique** | A statistical technique for estimating parameters such as standard errors and confidence intervals based on resampling from an observed data set with replacement. | |

| Term | Definition | See Also |
|------|-----------|----------|
| Case Reports | Descriptions of individual patients. | |
| Case Series | A study reporting on a consecutive collection of patients treated in a similar manner, without a control group. For example, a surgeon might describe the characteristics of an outcome for 100 consecutive patients with cerebral ischemia who received a revascularization procedure. | Consecutive Sample |
| Case-Control Study | A study designed to determine the association between an exposure and outcome in which patients are sampled by outcome (that is, some patients with the outcome of interest are selected and compared to a group of patients who have not had the outcome), and the investigator examines the proportion of patients with the exposure in the two groups. | |
| Chance-Corrected Agreement | Of the possible agreement beyond what one would expect by chance alone, the proportion achieved. | |
| Channeling Effect (or Channeling Bias) | See *Bias* | |
| Checklist Effect | The effect on clinicians' behavior of having them record information, or their orders, using a structured data collection form. | |
| Chi-square Test | A statistical test that examines the distribution of categorical outcomes in two groups, the null hypothesis of which is that the underlying distributions are identical. | |
| Clinical Prediction Rules (or Clinical Decision Rules) | A clinical prediction rule is generated by initially examining, and ultimately combining, a number of variables to predict the likelihood of a current diagnosis or a future event. Sometimes, if the likelihood is sufficiently high or low, the rule generates a suggested course of action. | |
| Cointerventions | Interventions other than treatment under study that may be differentially applied to experimental and control groups and, thus potentially bias the results of a study. | |
| Comorbidity | Disease(s) that coexist(s) in a study participant in addition to the index condition that is the subject of the study. | |

| Term | Definition | See Also |
|------|-----------|----------|
| Cohort | A group of persons with a common characteristic or set of characteristics. Typically, the group is followed for a specified period of time to determine the incidence of a disorder or complications of an established disorder (prognosis). | Cohort Study |
| Cohort Study (or Cohort Analytic Study) | Prospective investigation of the factors that might cause a disorder in which a cohort of individuals who do not have evidence of an outcome of interest but who are exposed to the putative cause are compared with a concurrent cohort who are also free of the outcome but not exposed to the putative cause. Both cohorts are then followed to compare the incidence of the outcome of interest. Used for *Prospective Study* | Cohort; Inception Cohort |
| Complete Follow-up | See *Follow-up* | |
| Computer Decision Support Systems (CDSS) | Computer software designed to aid directly in clinical decision-making about individual patients. | |
| Concealment | See *Allocation Concealment* | |
| Concepts | Concepts are the basic building blocks of theory. | |
| Conceptual Framework | An organization of ideas that provides a system of relationships between those ideas. | |
| Conditional Probabilities | The probability of a particular state, given another state. That is, the probability of A, given B – $P(A/B)$. | |
| Confidence Interval (CI) | Range of two values within which it is probable that the true value lies for the whole population of patients from whom the study patients were selected. | |
| Confounder | A factor that distorts the true relationship of the study variable of interest by virtue of also being related to the outcome of interest. Confounders are often unequally distributed among the groups being compared. Randomized studies are less likely to have their results distorted by confounders than are observational studies. Used for *Confounding Variable* | |
| Confounding Variable | See *Confounder* | |
| Consecutive Sample | A sample in which all potentially eligible patients seen over a period of time are enrolled. Used for *Sequential Sample* Case Series | |

| Term | Definition | See Also |
|------|-----------|----------|
| Consequentialist (or Utilitarian) | A consequentialist or utilitarian view of distributive justice would contend that even in individual decision-making, the clinician should take a broad social view in which the action that would provide the greatest good to the greatest number is favored. In this broader view, the effect on others of allocating resources to a particular patient's care would bear on the decision. An alternative to the deontological view. | |
| Construct Validity | A construct is a theoretically derived notion of the domain(s) we wish to measure. An understanding of the construct will lead to expectations about how an instrument should behave if it is valid. Construct validity therefore involves comparisons between measures, and examination of the logical relationships, which should exist between a measure and characteristics of patients and patient groups. | |
| Contamination | Contamination occurs when participants in either the experimental or control group receive the intervention intended for the other arm of the study. | |
| Continuous Variables | A variable that can theoretically take any value and in practice can take a large number of values with small differences between them. | |
| Control Event Rate (CER) | See *Event Rate, Baseline Risk* | |
| Control Group | A group that does not receive the experimental intervention. In many studies, the control group receives either the standard of care currently delivered in the community or the best care that is available on the basis of the current evidence. | |
| Controlled Trial | See *Randomized Controlled Trial* | |
| Convenience Sample | Individuals or groups selected at the convenience of the investigator or primarily because they were available at a convenient time or place. | |
| Corollary Orders | Orders that are needed to detect or ameliorate adverse reactions (also called response orders). | |
| Correlation | The magnitude of the relationship between different variables or phenomena. | |

| Term | Definition | See Also |
|------|-----------|----------|
| Correlation Coefficient | A numerical expression of the strength of the relationship between two variables, which can take values from –1.0 to 1.0 | |
| Cost Analysis | If two strategies are analyzed but only costs are compared, this comparison would inform only the resource-use half of the decision (the other half being the expected outcomes) and is termed a cost analysis. | |
| Cost Benefit Analysis | A form of economic analysis in which both the costs and the consequences (including increases in the length and quality of life) are expressed in monetary terms. | |
| Cost-Effectiveness Analysis | An economic analysis in which the consequences are expressed in natural units. Some examples would include cost per life saved or cost per unit of blood pressure lowered. | |
| Cost Minimization Analysis | An economic analysis conducted in situations where the consequences of the alternatives are identical, and so the only issue is their relative costs. | |
| Cost-to-Charge Ratio | Where there is a systematic deviation between costs and charges, an economic analysis may adjust charges using a cost-to-charge ratio. The goal is to approximate real costs. | |
| Cost-Utility Analysis | A type of cost-effectiveness analysis in which the consequences are expressed in terms of life-years adjusted by peoples' preferences. Typically, one considers the incremental cost per incremental gain in quality adjusted life-years (QALYs). | Quality-Adjusted Life-Year (QALY) |
| Cox Regression Model | A regression technique that allows adjustment for known differences in baseline characteristics between experimental and control groups applied to survival data. | Adjusted Analysis |
| Criterion Standard | A method having established or widely accepted accuracy for determining a diagnosis, providing a standard to which a new screening or diagnostic test can be compared. The method need not be a single or simple procedure but could include follow-up of patients to observe the evolution of their conditions or the consensus of an expert panel of clinicians, as is frequently used in the study of psychiatric conditions.<br><br>Used for *Gold Standard, Reference Standard* | |

| Term | Definition | See Also |
|------|------------|----------|
| Critiquing | When the computer evaluates a clinician's decision and generates an appropriateness rating or an alternative suggestion, the decision support approach is called critiquing. | |
| Crossover Trial | A study design in which all patients receive both experimental and control treatments in sequence. | Before-After Trial |
| Cross-Sectional Survey | The observation of a defined population at a single point in time or during a specific time interval. Exposure and outcome are determined simultaneously. | |
| Data Completeness Bias | See *Bias* | |
| Data-dredging | Searching a data set for differences between groups on particular outcomes, or in subgroups of patients, without explicit a priori hypotheses. | |
| Decision Aid | A tool that endeavors to present patients with the benefits and risks of alternative courses of action in a manner that is quantitative, comprehensive, and understandable. | |
| Decision Analysis | A systematic approach to decision making under conditions of uncertainty. It involves identifying all available alternatives and estimating the probabilities of potential outcomes associated with each alternative, valuing each outcome, and, on the basis of the probabilities and values, arriving at a quantitative estimate of the relative merit of the alternatives. | |
| Decision Tree | Most clinical decision analyses are built as decision trees. Articles about clinical decision analyses usually will include one or more diagrams showing the structure of the decision tree used for the analysis. | |
| Degrees of Freedom | A technical term in a statistical analysis that has to do with the power of the analysis. The more degrees of freedom, the more powerful the analysis. | |
| Deontological | A deontological approach to distributive justice holds that the clinician's only responsibility should be to best meet the needs of the individual under her care. An alternative to the consequentialist or utilitarian view. | |
| Dependent Variable | In a regression analysis we identify predictor or independent variables and the target or dependent variable. | |

| Term | Definition | See Also |
|---|---|---|
| Detection Bias | See *Bias* | |
| Determinants of Outcome | The causal factors that determine whether or not a target event will occur. | |
| Dichotomous Outcomes | "Yes" or "no" outcomes that either happen or do not happen, such as cancer recurrence, myocardial infarction, and death. | |
| Dichotomous Variable | A variable that can take one of two values, such as pregnant or not pregnant, dead or alive, having suffered a stroke or not having suffered a stroke. | |
| Differential Diagnosis | The set of diagnoses that can plausibly explain a patient's presentation. | |
| Disability-Adjusted Life-Years (DALY) | The number of years of life after downward adjustment for disabilities that patients experience. | Quality-Adjusted Life-Year (QALY) |
| Discriminant Analysis | A statistical technique, similar to logisitic regression analysis, that identifies variables that are associated with the presence or absence of a particular outcome. | |
| Dose-Dependence | Risk of an outcome increases as the quantity or the duration of exposure to the putative harmful agent increases. Used for *Dose-Response Gradient* | |
| Dose-Response Gradient | See *Dose-Dependence* | |
| Downstream Costs | Costs due to resources consumed in the future and associated with clinical events that are attributable to the therapy. | |
| Drug Class Effects (or Class Effects) | Similar effects produced by most or all members of a class of drugs (such as beta blockers, calcium antagonists, or angiotensin converting enzyme inhibitors) | |
| Economic Analysis | A set of formal, quantitative methods used to compare two or more treatments, programs, or strategies with respect to their resource use and their expected outcomes. | |
| Economic Evaluation | Comparative analysis of alternative courses of action in terms of both their costs and consequences. | |
| Effect Size | The effect size is the difference in outcomes between the intervention and control groups divided by some measure of variability, typically the standard deviation. | |

| Term | Definition | See Also |
|------|-----------|----------|
| Efficiency | Technical efficiency is the relationship between inputs (costs) and outputs (in health, quality-adjusted life-years [QALYs]). Treatments that provide more QALYs for the same or fewer resources are more efficient. Technical efficiency is assessed using cost minimization, cost-effectiveness, and cost-utility analysis. Allocative efficiency recognizes that health is not the only goal that society wishes to pursue, so competing goals must be weighted and then related to costs. This is typically done through cost-benefit analysis. | |
| Endpoint | Endpoints refer to health events or outcomes that lead to completion or termination of follow-up of an individual in a trial or cohort study, for example, death or major morbidity. | Outcomes; Treatment Targets |
| Equivalence Studies (or Equivalence Trials) | Studies designed to determine if an intervention that has a cost (cheaper), toxicity (less toxic), or administrative (simpler to administer) advantage is equivalent in terms of its benefit to the current standard. | |
| Event Rate | Proportion of patients in a group in whom an event is observed. Control event rate (CER) and experimental event rate (EER) are used to refer to this in control and experimental groups of patients, respectively.<br><br>Used for *Experimental Event Rate (EER)* | Treatment Effects; Baseline Risk |
| Evidence-Based Medicine (EBM) | The conscientious, explicit, and judicious use of current best evidence in making decisions about the care of individual patients. The practice of evidence-based medicine requires integration of individual clinical expertise and patient preferences with the best available external clinical evidence from systematic research. | |
| Evidence-Based Practice (EBP) | See *Evidence Based Medicine* | |
| Evidence-Based Health Care (EBHC) | See *Evidence-Based Medicine* | |
| Exclusion Criteria | Criteria that render potential subjects ineligible to participate in a particular study. | |
| Experimental Event Rate (EER) | See *Event Rate* | |

| Term | Definition | See Also |
|---|---|---|
| Experimental Therapy | A therapeutic alternative, often new or innovative, to standard or control therapy. | |
| Explode | When searching Medline, the "explode" command identifies all articles that have been indexed using a given Medical Subjects Heading (MeSH) term as well as articles indexed using more specific terms. | |
| Exposure | A condition to which patients are exposed (either a potentially harmful agent or a potentially beneficial one) that may impact on their health. | |
| Face Validity | A measurement instrument has face validity if it appears to be measuring what it is intended to measure. | |
| False-Negative | In a treatment study, treatment is considered ineffective when it actually is effective. In a diagnosis study, the patient suffers from the target condition, but the test suggests the patient does not. | |
| False-Positive | In a treatment study, the treatment is deemed effective when it actually is ineffective. In a diagnosis study, the patient does not suffer from the target condition, but the test suggests the patient does. | |
| Feedback Effect | The impact of performance evaluations on clinicians' behavior. | |
| Focus Groups | Investigators use focus groups, typically gatherings of 4 to 8 people with similar background or experience, to understand their attitudes or their response to a particular situation or experience. | |
| Follow-up | The investigators are aware of the outcome in every patient who participated in a study. | |
| Generalizibility | The ability to generalize the findings of a study to a larger group of similar people. | |
| Gold Standard | See *Criterion Standard* | |
| Harm | Adverse consequences of exposure to a stimulus. | |
| Hawthorne Effect | Human performance that is improved when participants are aware that their behavior is being observed. | |

| Term | Definition | See Also |
|---|---|---|
| Hazard Ratio | Investigators may compute the relative risk over a period of time, as in a survival analysis, and call it a hazard ratio, the weighted relative risk over the entire study. | |
| Health | A state of optimal physical, mental, and social well-being; not merely the absence of disease and infirmity (World Health Organization definition). | |
| Health Care Personnel | Such persons include physicians, internists and medical doctors, nurses, nurse practitioners, physician assistants, and other allied health personnel. | Health Care Professionals |
| Health Condition | A broad term for a health state that may include diseases, disorders, syndromes, and symptoms. | Health State |
| Health Costs | These concern the use of health care resources (direct and indirect) and the inability to use the same resources for other worthwhile purposes (opportunity costs). Used for *Health Care Costs* | |
| Health Outcome | All possible changes in health status that may occur for a defined population or that may be associated with exposure to an intervention. These include changes in the length and quality of life as a result of detecting or treating disease when it is present, the false security associated with failing to detect disease when it is present, and the mislabeling associated with detecting disease when it is really absent. | |
| Health Professionals | All persons with health-based certification: physicians, nurses, medical doctors, physiotherapists, pharmacists, occupational therapists, respiratory technicians, and counselors. | Health Care Personnel |
| Health Profile | Health profiles are instruments, intended for use in the entire population (including the health, the very sick, and patients with any sort of health problem), that attempt to measure all-important aspects of Health-Related Quality of Life (HRQL). | Health-Related Quality of Life |
| Health State | The health condition of an individual or group over a specified interval of time (commonly assessed at a particular point in time). | |

| Term | Definition | See Also |
|------|-----------|----------|
| Health-Related Quality of Life | Measurements of how people are feeling or the value they place on their health state. | Health Profile |
| Heterogeneity | Differences between patients or differences in the results of different studies. | |
| Inception Cohort | A designated group of persons assembled at a common time early in the development of a specific clinical disorder (eg, at the time of first exposure to the putative cause or the time of initial diagnosis) and who are followed thereafter. | Cohort; Cohort Study |
| Incidence | Number of new cases of disease occurring during a specified period of time; expressed as a percentage of the number of people at risk. | Prevalence |
| Inclusion criteria | Investigators specify the inclusion criteria to define the population who will be eligible for a study. | |
| Incorporation Bias | See *Bias* | |
| Independent Association | When a variable is associated with an outcome after adjusting for multiple other potential prognostic factors, the association is an independent association. | |
| Independent Variables | Explanatory or predictor variables that may be associated with a particular outcome. The term is usually used in the context of a regression analysis. | |
| Index Date | The date of an important event that marks the beginning of monitoring patients for the occurrence of the outcome of interest. | |
| Indirect Costs and Benefits | The impact of alternative patient management strategies on the productivity of the patient and others involved in the patient's care. | |
| Informed Consent | A potential participant's expression of willingness, after full disclosure of the implications, to participate in a study. | |
| Intention-to-Treat (ITT) Principle (or Intention-to-Treat Analysis) | Analyzing patient outcomes based on which group into which they were randomized regardless of whether they actually received the planned intervention. This analysis preserves the power of randomization, thus maintaining that important unknown factors that influence outcome are likely equally distributed in each comparison group. | |

| Term | Definition | See Also |
|------|-----------|----------|
| Interviewer Bias | See *Bias* | |
| Inverse Rule of 3s | A rough rule of thumb, called the inverse rule of 3s, tells us the following: If an event occurs, on average, once every "x" days, we need to observe 3x days to be 95% confident of observing at least one event. | |
| Investigator Triangulation | Investigator triangulation requires more than one investigator to collect and analyze the raw data, such that the findings emerge through consensus between or among investigators. | |
| Kaplan-Meier Curve | See *Survival Curve* | |
| Kappa Statistic (or Weighted Kappa) | A measure of the extent to which observers achieve the possible agreement beyond any agreement expected to occur by chance alone. Kappa can take values from −1.0 to 1.0. | |
| Law of Multiplicative Probabilities | The law of multiplicative probabilities for independent events (where one event in no way influences the other) tells us that the probability of 10 consecutive heads can be found by multiplying the probability of a single head (1/2) 10 times over; that is, 1/2 x 1/2 x 1/2, and so on. | |
| Leading Hypothesis (or Working Diagnosis) | The clinician's single best explanation for the patient's clinical problem(s). | |
| Likelihood | See *Likelihood Ratio* | |
| Likelihood Functions | Functions constructed from a statistical model and a set of observed data that give the probability of that data for various values of the unknown model parameters. Those parameter values that maximize the probability are the maximum likelihood estimates of the parameters. | |
| Likelihood Ratio | For a screening or diagnostic test (including clinical signs or symptoms), expresses the relative likelihood that a given test would be expected in a patient with (as opposed to one without) a disorder of interest. Used for *Likelihood* | |

| Term | Definition | See Also |
|---|---|---|
| Likert-Type Scales | Scales, typically with from 3 to 9 possible values, that include extremes of attitudes or feelings (such as from totally disagree to totally agree) and that investigators present to respondents to obtain their ratings of their responses. | Visual Analogue Scale |
| Linear Regression | The term used for a regression analysis when the dependent or target variable is a continuous variable and the relationship between the dependent and independent variables is thought to be linear. | |
| Logical Operator (or Boolean Operators) | Words used by a search engine to perform specific tasks such as combining terms (AND/OR) or excluding terms (NOT) from the search strategy. | |
| Logistic Regression | A term used for a regression analysis in which the dependent or target variable is dichotomous and which uses a model that relies on logarithms. | |
| Longitudinal Study | See *Cohort Study* | |
| Lost to Follow-up | Patients whose status on the outcome or endpoint of interest is unknown. | |
| Marginal Utility | The change in a person's utility (preference or relative value) for an outcome as the outcome increases in magnitude. | |
| Masked | See *Blind* | |
| Matching | A deliberate process to make the study group and comparison group comparable with respect to factors (or confounders) that are extraneous to the purpose of the investigation but that might interfere with the interpretation of the studies' findings. For example, in case control studies, individual cases may be matched with specific controls on the basis of comparable age, gender, and/or other clinical features. | |
| Median Survival | Length of time that one half of the study population survives. | |
| Member Checking | Member checking involves sharing draft study findings with the participants to inquire whether their viewpoints were faithfully interpreted, to determine whether there are gross errors of fact, and to ascertain whether the account makes sense to participants with different perspectives. | |

| Term | Definition | See Also |
|------|-----------|----------|
| Meta-Analysis | An overview that incorporates a quantitative strategy for combining the results of several studies into a single pooled or summary estimate. | |
| Mortality | Measure of rate of death. | |
| Multivariable Regression Equation | A type of regression that provides a mathematical model that explains or predicts the dependent or target variable by simultaneously considering all of the independent or predictor variables. | Multivariate Analysis |
| Multivariate Analysis | An analysis that simultaneously considers a number of predictor variables. | Multivariable Regression Equation |
| Negative Studies | Studies in which the authors have concluded that the experimental treatment is no better than control therapy. | |
| No Test Threshold (or Test Threshold) | The probability below which the clinician decides a diagnosis warrants no further consideration. | |
| N of 1 RCT | An experiment in which there is only a single participant, designed to determine the effect of an intervention or exposure on that individual. | |
| Nomogram | Graphical scale facilitating calculation of a probability. | |
| Non randomized Trial | Experiment in which assignment of patients to the intervention groups is at the convenience of the investigator or according to a preset plan that does not conform to the definition of random. | Randomized Control Trial (RCT) |
| Null Hypothesis | In the hypothesis-testing framework, the starting hypothesis the statistical test is designed to consider and, possibly, reject. | |
| Number Needed to Harm (NNH) | The number of patients who would need to be treated over a specific period of time before one adverse side effect of the treatment will occur. It is the inverse of the absolute risk increase. | Absolute Risk Increase (ARI) |
| Number Needed to Treat (NNT) | The number of patients who need to be treated over a specific period of time to prevent one bad outcome. When discussing NNT, it is important to specify the treatment, its duration, and the bad outcome being prevented. It is the inverse of the absolute risk reduction (ARR). | Absolute Risk Reduction (AAR) |

| Term | Definition | See Also |
|------|-----------|----------|
| Observational Studies (or Observational Study Design) | Studies in which patient or physician preference determines whether a patient receives treatment or control. | |
| Odds | A ratio of probability of occurrence to nonoccurrence of an event. | |
| Odds Ratio (OR) | A ratio of the odds of an event in an exposed group to the odds of the same event in a group that is not exposed.<br><br>Used for *Cross-Product Ratio*<br><br>Used for *Relative Odds* | |
| Open-ended, Semi-structured, and Contrast Questions | Open-ended questions offer no specific structure for the respondent's answer. Semi-structured questions offer a limited structure for the respondent's answer. | |
| Opportunity Costs | The value of (health or other) benefits forgone in alternative uses when a resource is used. | |
| Outcomes | Changes in health status that may occur in following subjects or that may stem from exposure to a causal factor or to a therapeutic intervention. | Treatment targets; Endpoints |
| Overview | A type of review in which primary research relevant to a question is examined and summarized, and an effort is made to identify all available literature (published or unpublished) that pertains to that question. | Systematic Review |
| Palliate | Palliative care or treatment is a set of actions taken for patients in whom cure is unlikely. *Stedman's Medical Dictionary*, 27th edition, defines palliative as mitigating or reducing the severity of symptoms without reducing the underlying disease. These actions are often multiple and can include family members and significant others. | |
| Patient Expected Event Rate | The probability of the occurrence of the endpoint or outcome of interest. | |
| Patient Preferences | The relative value that patients place on varying health states. | |
| Performance Criteria | Concerns how interventions are performed without regard to whether they should be performed. An example would be the acceptable range of results reported for reference cholesterol samples sent to clinical laboratories. | |
| Phase I Studies | See *Studies* | |
| Phase II Studies | See *Studies* | |

| Term | Definition | See Also |
|---|---|---|
| Phase III Studies | See *Studies* | |
| Phase IV Studies | See *Studies* | |
| Phi (or Phi Statistic) | A measure of chance-independent agreement calculated by the following formula (where OR indicates odds ratio): $$\frac{\sqrt{OR} - 1}{\sqrt{OR} + 1}$$ | |
| Placebo Effect | The impact of a treatment independent of its biological effect. | |
| Placebos | Interventions (typically a pill or capsule) without biologically active ingredients. | |
| Point Estimate | The results of a study which represent the best estimates of the treatment. | |
| Positive Study or Positive Trial | A study in which the effect of experimental intervention differs from that of the control. | |
| Postmarketing Surveillance Studies | See *Studies* | |
| Posttest Odds | The odds of the target condition being present after the results of a diagnostic test are available. | |
| Posttest Probability | The probability of the target condition being present after the results of a diagnostic test are available. | |
| Power | In a comparison of two interventions, the ability to detect a difference between the two experimental if one in fact exists. | |
| Practice Guidelines | Guidelines are systematically developed statements to assist practitioner and patient decisions about appropriate health care for specific clinical circumstances. They are a set of statements, directions, or principles presenting current or future clinical rules or policy concerning the proper indications for performing a procedure or treatment or the proper management for specific clinical problems. Guidelines may be developed by government agencies, institutions, organizations such as professional societies or governing boards, or by the convening of expert panels. | |
| Predictive Value (PPV or NPV) | Two categories: Positive Predictive Value—the proportion of people with a positive test who have the disease; Negative Predictive Value—proportion of people with a negative test and who are free of disease. | |

| Term | Definition | See Also |
|---|---|---|
| Prefiltered | By prefiltered, we mean that someone has reviewed the literature and chosen only the methodologically strongest studies. | |
| Pretest Odds | The odds of the target condition being present before the results of a diagnostic test are available. | |
| Pretest Probability | The probability of the target condition being present before the results of a diagnostic test are available. | |
| Prevalence | Proportion of persons affected with a particular disease at a specified time. Prevalence rates obtained from high-quality studies can inform clinicians' efforts to set anchoring pretest probabilities for their patients. | Incidence |
| Prevent | A preventative maneuver is an action that arrests the threatened onset of disease. Primary prevention is done to stop a condition from starting. Secondary prevention stops progression of a disease or disorder when patients have a disease and are at risk for developing something related to their current disease. Very often secondary prevention is indistinguishable from treatment. An example of primary prevention is vaccination for pertussis; an example of secondary prevention is administration of an antiosteoporosis intervention to women with low bone density and evidence of a vertebral fracture to prevent subsequent fractures. | |
| Primary Care | Medical care provided by the clinician of first contact for the patient. Typically, the primary care physician is a general practitioner, family practitioner, primary care internist, or primary care pediatrician. Primary care may also be administered by health professionals other than physicians, notably specially trained nurses (nurse practitioners) and paramedics. Usually, a general practitioner, family practitioner, nurse practitioner, or paramedic provides only primary care services, but an individual with specialty qualifications may provide primary care, alone or in combination with referral services. Thus, it is the nature of the contact (first vs referred) that determines the care designation rather than the qualifications of the practitioner. | Referred Care |

| Term | Definition | See Also |
|------|-----------|----------|
| Primary Care Setting | Medical care facility that offers first contact health care only. Patients requiring specialized medical care are referred elsewhere. Some primary care centers provide a mixture of primary and referred care. Thus, it is the nature of the service provided (first contact) rather than the setting per se that distinguishes primary from more advanced levels of care. | Primary Care; Referred Care; Tertiary Care Center |
| Primary studies | Studies that collect original data. Primary studies are differentiated from systematic reviews that summarize the results of primary studies. | |
| Probability | Quantitative estimate of the likelihood of a condition existing (as in diagnosis) or of subsequent events (such as in a treatment study). | P-value |
| Prognosis | The possible outcomes of a disease and the frequency with which they can be expected to occur. | |
| Prognostic Factors | Patient or study participant characteristics that confer increased or decreased risk of a positive or adverse outcome. | |
| Prognostic Study | A study that enrolls patients at a point in time and follows them forward to determine the frequency and timing of subsequent events. | |
| Prospective Study | See *Cohort Study* | |
| Provider Adherence or Compliance | Provider adherence or compliance refers to the extent that health care providers (physicians, nurses, etc) carry out the host of diagnostic tests, monitoring equipment, interventional requirements, and other technical specifications that define optimal patient management. | |
| Publication Bias | See *Bias* | |
| Purposive Sampling | In qualitative research, the consecutive or random selection of participants, common in quantitative research, is replaced by a conscious selection of a small number of individuals meeting particular criteria—a process called purposive sampling. | |
| P-value | The probability that results as or more extreme than those observed would occur if the null hypothesis were true and the experiment were repeated over and over. | Probability |

| Term | Definition | See Also |
|------|-----------|----------|
| Qualitative Research | Qualitative research offers insight into social, emotional, and experiential phenomena in health care. | Quantitative Research |
| Quality Assurance | Any procedure, method, or philosophy for collecting, processing, or analyzing data that is aimed at maintaining or improving the appropriateness of health care services. | |
| Quality of Care | The extent to which health care meets technical and humanistic standards of optimal care. | |
| Quality-Adjusted Life-Expectancy | The number of years of expected life corrected for the quality of life that patients are expected to experience in those years. | |
| Quality-Adjusted Life-Year (QALY) | A unit of measure for survival that accounts for the effects of suboptimal health status and the resulting limitations in quality of life. For example, if a patient lives for 10 years and her quality of life is decreased by 50% because of chronic lung disease, her survival would be equivalent to 5 quality-adjusted life years. | Cost-Utility Analysis |
| Quantitative Research | Aims to test well-specified hypotheses concerning predetermined variables that yield numbers suitable for statistical analysis. | Qualitative Research |
| Random | Governed by a formal chance process in which the occurrence of previous events is of no value in predicting future events. The probability of assignment of, for example, a given participant to a specified treatment group is fixed and constant (typically 0.5), but the participant's actual assignment cannot be known until it occurs. | Randomization; Random Error |
| Random Error | We can never know with certainty the true value of a treatment effect because of random error. It is inherent in all measurement. The observations that are made in a study are only a sample of all possible observations that could be made from the population of relevant patients. Thus, the average value of any sample observations is subject to some variation from the true value for that entire population. When the level of random error associated with a measurement is high, the measurement is less precise and we are less certain about the value of that measurement. | Random; Random Sample |

| Term | Definition | See Also |
|------|-----------|----------|
| Random Sample | A sample derived by selecting sampling units (eg, individual patients) such that each unit has an independent and fixed (generally equal) chance of selection. Whether or not a given unit is selected is determined by chance, for example, by a table of randomly ordered numbers. | Random; Random Error |
| Randomization or Random Allocation | Allocation of individuals to groups by chance, usually done with the aid of table of random numbers. Not to be confused with systematic allocation (eg, on even and odd days of the month) or allocation at the convenience or discretion of the investigator. | Random; Random Sample; Random Error |
| Randomized Controlled Trial | See *Randomized Trial* | |
| Randomized Trial | Experiment in which individuals are randomly allocated to receive or not receive an experimental preventative, therapeutic, or diagnostic procedure and then followed to determine the effect of the intervention.<br><br>Used for *Controlled Trial*<br><br>Used for *Randomized Controlled Trial* | Non randomized Trial |
| Recall Bias | See *Bias* | |
| Receiver Operating Characteristic (ROC) Curve | A figure depicting the power of a diagnostic test. The ROC curve presents the test's true positive rate (ie, sensitivity) on the horizontal axis and the false positive rate (ie, 1-specificity) on the vertical axis for different cut-points dividing a positive from a negative test. An ROC curve for a perfect test has an area under the curve equal to 1.0 while a test that performs no better than by chance has an area under the curve of only .5. | |
| Recursive Partitioning Analysis | A technique for determining the optimal way of using a set of predictor variables to estimate the likelihood of an individual experiencing a particular outcome. The technique repeatedly divides the population (eg, old vs young; among young and old, the men and the women) according to their status on variables that discriminate between those who will have the outcome of interest and those who will not. | |
| Reference Standard | See *Criterion Standard* | |

| Term | Definition | See Also |
|------|-----------|----------|
| **Referred Care** | Medical care provided to a patient when referred by one health professional to another with more specialized qualifications or interests. There are two levels of referred care: secondary and tertiary. Secondary care is usually provided by a broadly skilled specialist such as a general surgeon, general internist, or obstetrician. Used for *Secondary Care* | Primary Care |
| **Regression** | A technique that uses predictor or independent variables to build a statistical model that predicts an individual patient's status with respect to a dependent or target variable. | |
| **Rehabilitation** | A set of actions designed to restore, following disease or injury, the ability to function in a normal or near-normal manner. | |
| **Relative Odds** | A synonym for odds ratio: a ratio of the odds of an event in an exposed group to the odds of the same event in a group that is not exposed. | |
| **Relative Risk (RR)** | Ratio of the risk of an event among an exposed population to the risk among the unexposed. | Relative Risk Reduction (RRR); Risk; Risk Ratio |
| **Relative Risk Reduction (RRR)** | An estimate of the proportion of baseline risk that is removed by the therapy, it is calculated by dividing the absolute risk reduction by the absolute risk in the control group. | Relative Risk (RR); Risk; Treatment Effect |
| **Reliability** | Refers to consistency or reproducibility of data. | Reproducibility |
| **Reminder Systems** | Reminder systems notify clinicians of important tasks that need to be done before an event occurs. | Alerting Systems |
| **Reproducibility** | Ability of a measure to yield the same result when reapplied to stable patients. | Reliability |
| **Review** | A general term for all attempts to obtain and synthesize the results and conclusions of two or more publications on a given topic. | |
| **Risk** | Measure of the association between exposure and outcome (including incidence, side effects, toxicity). | Absolute Risk (AR); Absolute Risk Reduction (ARR); Relative Risk (RR); Relative Risk Reduction (RRR) |

| Term | Definition | See Also |
|------|-----------|----------|
| Risk Aversion | People are said to be risk averse if they would accept a fixed outcome with certainty rather than a lottery with a higher expected value. For example, they would choose $10 for sure rather than a 50/50 chance of $0 or $30. | |
| Risk Factors | Authors often distinguish between prognostic factors and risk factors, which are those patient characteristics associated with the development of the disease in the first place. | |
| Risk Ratio | A synonym for relative risk: ratio of the risk of an event among an exposed population to the risk among the unexposed. | |
| Screening | Services, designed to detect people at high risk of suffering from a condition associated with a modifiable adverse outcome, to be offered to persons who have neither symptoms of, nor risk factors (other than age or gender) for a target condition. | Selective Screening |
| Secondary Care | See *Referred Care* | |
| Secular Trends | Changes in the probability of events with time, independent of known predictors of outcome. | |
| Selective Screening | Services to be offered to asymptomatic persons with one or more risk factors for a target condition, such as family history of the disease, certain personal behaviors, or membership in a population with increased prevalence of the disease. | Screening |
| Sensitivity | The proportion of people who truly have a designated disorder who are so identified by the test. The test may consist of, or include, clinical observations. | Sensitivity Analysis; Specificity; SnNout |
| Sensitivity Analysis | Any test of the stability of the conclusions of a health care evaluation over a range of probability estimates, value judgments, and assumptions about the structure of the decisions to be made. This may involve the repeated evaluation of a decision model in which one or more of the parameters of interest are varied. | |
| Sentinal Effect | Human performance may improve when participants are aware that their behavior is being evaluated. | |
| Sequential Sample | See *Consecutive Sample* | |

| Term | Definition | See Also |
|---|---|---|
| Sequential Tests | Tests conducted in sequence, rather than simultaneously. | |
| Sign | Any abnormality indicative of disease, discoverable by the clinician at an examination of the patient. It is an objective aspect of a disease. | |
| Sign Test | A statistical hypothesis test used when an outcome is dichotomous and in which the null hypothesis is that there is an equal likelihood of either outcome occurring. | |
| Silo Effect | One of the main reasons for considering narrower viewpoints in conducting an economic analysis is to assess the impact of change on the main budget holders, as budgets may need to be adjusted before a new therapy can be adopted (often termed the silo effect). | |
| SnNout | When a test with a high sensitivity is negative, it effectively rules out the diagnosis of disease. | Sensitivity |
| Snowball Sampling | Purposive sampling might aim to represent any of the following: typical cases, unusual cases, critical cases, cases that reflect important political issues, or cases with connections to other cases (ie, snowball sampling). | |
| Specificity | The proportion of people who are truly free of a designated disorder who are so identified by the test. The test may consist of, or include, clinical observations. | Sensitivity; SpPin |
| SpPin | When a test is highly specific, a positive result can rule in the diagnosis. | Specificity |
| Standard Error | The standard deviation of an estimate of a population parameter (thus, the standard error of the mean is the standard deviation of the estimate of the population mean value). | |
| Standard Gamble | A direct preference or utility measure that effectively asks the respondent to rate their quality of life on a scale from 0 to 1.0, where 0 is death and 1.0 is full health. The respondent chooses between a specified time x in their current health state and a gamble in which they have probability p (anywhere from 0 to .99) of full health for time x, and a probability $1 - P$ of immediate death. | |

| Term | Definition | See Also |
|------|-----------|----------|
| Standards | Authoritative statements of minimal levels of acceptable performance or results, excellent levels of performance or results, or the range of acceptable performance or results. | |
| Statistical Inference | Statistical methodologies to make deductions about underlying truth. There are two principle functions: (1) to predict or estimate a population parameter from a sample statistic, and (2) to test statistically based hypotheses. | |
| Statistical Significance | A result is statistically significant if the null hypothesis is rejected. That is, the probability of the observed results, given the null hypothesis, falls below an arbitrary threshold (most often .05). | |
| Studies or Study Design | The way a drug study is organized or constructed.<br><br>a) Phase I Studies: Studies that investigate a drug's physiological effect or ensure that it does not manifest unacceptable early toxicity, often conducted in normal volunteers.<br><br>b) Phase II Studies: Initial studies on patients, which provide preliminary evidence of possible drug effectiveness.<br><br>c) Phase III Studies: Randomized control trials designed to definitively establish the magnitude of drug benefit.<br><br>d) Phase IV Studies or Postmarketing Surveillance Studies: Studies conducted after the effectiveness of a drug has been established and the drug marketed, typically to establish the frequency of unusual toxic effects. | |
| Surrogate Outcomes (or Substitute Endpoints or Surrogate Endpoints) | Outcomes that are not in themselves important to patients, but are associated with outcomes that are important to patients (eg, bone density for fracture, cholesterol for myocardial infarction, and blood pressure for stroke). | |
| Surveillance Bias | See *Bias* | |
| Survey | Observational or descriptive non-experimental study in which individuals are systematically examined for the absence or presence (or degree of presence) of characteristics of interest. | |

| Term | Definition | See Also |
|---|---|---|
| Survival Analysis | An analysis that considers not only the proportion of patients who experience an outcome or endpoint, but also the time pattern of the occurrence of outcomes or endpoints. | |
| Survival Curve | A curve that starts at 100% of the study population and shows the percentage of the population still surviving (or free of disease or some other outcome) at successive times for as long as information is available.<br><br>Used for *Kaplan Meier Curve* | |
| Symptom | Any morbid phenomenon or departure from the normal in function, appearance, or sensation reported by the patient and indicative of disease. Symptoms are considered subjective. | |
| Syndrome | A collection of signs and/or symptoms and/or physiological abnormalities. | |
| Syndrome Diagnosis | When no reference standards exist, investigators' degree of diagnostic certainty is much lower. In these situations, known sometimes as syndrome diagnosis, diagnostic criteria usually rely on a list of clinical features required for the diagnosis. | Syndrome |
| Systematic Review | A critical assessment and evaluation of research (not simply a summary) that attempts to address a focused clinical question using methods designed to reduce the likelihood of bias. | Overview |
| Target Condition | In diagnostic test studies, the condition the investigators or clinicians are particularly interested in identifying (eg, tuberculosis, lung cancer, or iron-deficiency anemia). | |
| Target Outcomes (or Target Events or Target Endpoints) | In treatment studies, the condition the investigators or clinicians are particularly interested in identifying and which it is anticipated the intervention will decrease (eg, myocardial infarction, stroke, or death) or increase (eg, ulcer healing). | Cohort Study |
| Target-Negative | In diagnostic test studies, patients who do not have the target condition. | |
| Target-Positive | In diagnostic test studies, patients who do have the target condition. | |
| Tertiary Care | See *Referred Care* | |

| Term | Definition | See Also |
|---|---|---|
| Tertiary Care Center | A medical facility that receives referrals from both primary and secondary care levels and usually offers tests, treatments, and procedures that are not available elsewhere. Most tertiary care centers offer a mixture of primary, secondary, and tertiary care services so that it is the specific level of service rendered rather than the facility that determines the designation of care in a given study. | Referred Care; Primary Care |
| Test Threshold | Probability below which a clinician dismisses a diagnosis and orders no further tests. | Treatment Threshold |
| Theoretical Saturation (or Informational Redundancy) | The point at which iterations among data collection, analysis, and theory development yield a well-developed conceptual framework and further observations yield minimal or no new information to further challenge or elaborate the framework. | |
| Theory | Theory consists of concepts and their relationships. | |
| Theory Triangulation | Theory triangulation is a process whereby emergent findings are corroborated with existing social science theories. | |
| Time Series | Typically used in observational studies, time series design monitors the occurrence of outcomes or endpoints over a number of cycles and determines if the pattern changes coincident with an intervention or event. | |
| Treatment Effect | The results of comparative clinical studies can be expressed using various treatment effect measures. Examples are absolute risk reduction (ARR), relative risk reduction (RRR), odds ratio (OR), number needed to treat (NNT), and effect size. The appropriateness of using these to express a treatment effect and whether probabilities, means, or medians are used to calculate them depends upon the type of outcome variable used to measure health outcomes. For example, ARR, RRR, and NNT are used for dichotomous variables, and effect sizes are normally used for continuous variables. | Absolute Risk Reduction (ARR); Relative Risk Reduction (RRR); Odds Ratio (OR); Number Needed to Treat (NNT) |
| Treatment Target | The manifestation of illness (a symptom, sign, or physiological abnormality) toward which a treatment is directed. | Endpoints; Outcomes |

| Term | Definition | See Also |
|------|-----------|----------|
| Treatment Threshold | Probability above which a clinician would consider a diagnosis confirmed and would stop testing and initiate treatment. | Test Threshold |
| Trial of Therapy | In a trial of therapy, the physician offers the patient an intervention, reviews the impact of the intervention on that patient at some subsequent time, and, depending on the impact, recommends either continuation or discontinuation of the intervention. | |
| Triangulation | In the course of qualitative analysis, key findings are also corroborated using multiple sources of information, a process called triangulation. | |
| Trigger orders | Orders in response to which the computer decision support system (CDSS) would initiate action. | Corollary Orders |
| Univariable Regression (or Simple Regression) | Regression where there is only one independent variable. | Regression |
| Up-Front Costs | Costs incurred to "produce" the treatment, such as the physician's time, nurse's time, materials, and so on. | |
| Utility | Patient preferences that are measured with techniques consistent with modern utility theory. Patient preferences refer to the degrees of subjective satisfaction, distress, or desirability that patients or potential patients associate with a particular health outcome. Utility theory is based on specific axioms that describe how a rational decision-maker ought to make a decision when the outcomes of that decision are uncertain. Commonly used measures of utility include the "standard gamble" or "time trade-off" techniques. | |
| Utility Measures | Measures that provide a single number that summarizes all of Health-Related Quality of Life (HRQL) are preference- or value-weighted; these have the preferences or values anchored to death and full health and are called utility measures. | Health-Related Quality of Life (HRQL) |
| Utilization Review | An organized procedure carried out through committees to review admissions, duration of stay, and professional services furnished, and to evaluate the medical necessity of those services and promote their most efficient use. | |

| Term | Definition | See Also |
|------|-----------|----------|
| Validity | In relation to studies of diagnosis or therapy, a study is valid insofar as the results represent an unbiased estimate of the underlying truth. In relation to health-related quality of life measures, validity represents the extent to which an instrument is measuring what is intended to measure. | |
| Values | The basis for individual personal preferences. | |
| Variance | The technical term for the statistical estimate of the variability in results. | |
| Verification Bias | See *Bias* | |
| Washout Period | In a trial, the period required for the treatment to cease to act once it has been discontinued. | |
| Work-up Bias | See *Bias* | |

# CD-ROM
# INSTALLATION
# INSTRUCTIONS

## INSTALLATION INSTRUCTIONS FOR MICROSOFT WINDOWS

To run the hypertext *Users' Guides* on a PC, you must have a PC-compatible computer running Windows 95, 98, ME, NT, or 2000; a CD-ROM drive; and Microsoft Internet Explorer 4 or later installed. To run the program, follow these steps:

1. Insert the CD-ROM into your CD-ROM drive. The setup program will run automatically. If it does not, continue to Step 2.

2. Click START, select RUN, select BROWSE, and select your CD-ROM drive.

3. Select the setup.exe file form the CD-ROM and click OK or RUN.

4. Follow the instructions provided by the *Users' Guides* setup program.

A hypertext version of the *Users' Guides*, with links to an Adobe Acrobat navigable version, will appear on your computer hard drive, and a shortcut to the *Users' Guides* will be placed on your Windows desktop.

## INSTALLATION INSTRUCTIONS FOR MACINTOSH COMPUTERS

To run the read-only, PDF navigable version of the *Users' Guides* on a Macintosh, you must have a CD-ROM drive and Adobe Acrobat Reader software, version 4 or more recent, installed. If you do not have Adobe Acrobat Reader, a current version can be obtained from the Adobe Web site at www.adobe.com. Once you have Adobe Acrobat Reader installed, follow these steps:

1. Insert the CD-ROM into your CD-ROM drive.

2. Click the CD icon that appears on your desktop to open the CD-ROM.

3. Open the Mac folder.

4. Click start.pdf to open the read-only, PDF navigable version of the *Users' Guides*.

# INDEX

## A

**Absolute risk reduction (ARR)**
Definition of, 66, 355,376, 588–589, 610
Risk group and, 355, 555
vs number needed to treat (NNT),
358–360
vs relative risk reduction, 366

**Adjusted analysis**, 335

**Administrative databases**
(See Databases: Administrative)

**Alerting system**
(See also Computer decision support
systems), 295, 303

**Applicability**
Clinical manifestations of disease,
457–458
Comorbidity conditions and, 375–376
Considerations of, 371
Diagnostic tests, 134–138
Differential diagnosis, 116
Disease frequency and, 117
Economic Analysis, 636–640
Harm, 95–97
Pathophysiologic differences and,
372–373
Patient vs treatment population and, 373
Prognosis, 152
Provider standards of care and, 374–375
Qualitative research, 443–445
Summarizing the evidence, 169–170
Surrogate outcomes, 404–405
Therapy, 71–75

**ARR**
(See Absolute risk reduction)

**Assisting decision support programs**
(See also Computer decision support
systems), 295
Critiquing computer decision support
systems vs, 295

**Asymmetry**
(See also Publication bias), 534

**Autocorrelation**
(See also N of 1 randomized controlled
trial), 285

## B

**Baseline risk**, 355

**Best evidence**
Definition of, 28
Searching, 28–32

**Bias**
Channeling, 90
Definition of, 225
Detection of, 90
Incorporation, 453
Interviewer, 90
Literature selection and, 162
Lost to Follow-up and, 91, 227, 230
Outcome criteria and, 225–226
Placebo effect and, 226
Postpublication, 533
Prognostic difference and, 225–226
Publication, 163, 530
Recall, 90
Surveillance, 91
Types of, 90, 91, 126, 163, 225–227 530,
533
Unrepresentative sample, 145
Work-up, 126

**Blinding**
Clinical treatment and, 62–63
Computer decision support systems
(CDSS) and, 306
Diagnostic test vs criterion standard, 125
Harm and, 230
Lack of, 301
Patient allocation and, 62
Placebo effect and, 300
Statistical analysis and, 63

## C

**Case report**, 89

**Case series study**, 89

**Case-control study**
Definition of, 88, 365
Disadvantages of, 89
Odds ratio and, 93, 365–366

# D

# U

**Unsystematic review**
(See Nonsystematic review)

**Up-to-date**
Definition of, 36
Strategies for use of, 36–38

**Utilization review**
(See Clinical utilization review)

# V

**Validity,** 313–320
Definition of, 225
Diagnostic tests and, 124–126
Differential diagnosis and, 111–115
Economic analysis and, 630–634
Face, 316
Harm and, 83–91
Medical care outcomes, 235–241
Prognosis and, 145–149
Qualitative research and, 435–441
Quality of life and, 316
Therapy and, 58–66
Summarizing the evidence and, 159–164
Surrogate outcomes and, 396–402
Treatment recommendations and, 185

**Verification bias**
(See Work-up bias)

**Visual analogue scale,** 575

# W

**Weighted kappa,** 462, 467
(See also Chance-corrected agreement;
Kappa statistic)

**Work-up bias,** 126
(See also Bias)

**World Wide Web,** 44–45

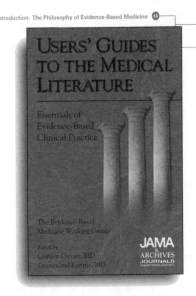

ISBN 1-57947-174-9